AF333656

Management of
Urologic Disorders

Management of
Urologic Disorders

EDITED BY

Robert R. Bahnson, MD

Associate Professor of Urologic Surgery

University of Pittsburgh School of Medicine

Pittsburgh, Pennsylvania

M WOLFE

London St. Louis Baltimore Boston Chicago Philadelphia Sydney Toronto

COPYRIGHT © 1994 Mosby–Year Book Europe, Ltd.
Published in 1994 by Wolfe Publishing, an imprint of
Mosby–Year Book Europe, Ltd.

The right of Robert Bahnson to be identified as author of
this work has been asserted by him in accordance with
the Copyright, Design and Patents Act 1988.

All rights reserved. No part of this publication may be
reproduced, stored in a retrieval system, copied or transmitted, in any form or by any means, electronic, mechanical, photocopying, recording or otherwise without written
permission from the Publisher or in accordance with the
provisions of the Copyright Act 1988, or under the terms
of any license permitting limited copying issued by the
Copyright Licensing Agency, 33–34 Alfred Place, London,
WC1E 7DP.

Any person who does any unauthorized act in relation to
this publication may be liable to criminal prosecution and
civil claims for damages.

Permission to photocopy or reproduce solely for internal
or personal use is permitted for libraries or other users
registered with the Copyright Clearance Center, provided
that the base fee of $4.00 per chapter plus $.10 per page is
paid directly to the Copyright Clearance Center, 21
Congress Street, Salem, MA 01970. This consent does not
extend to other kinds of copying, such as copying for
general distribution, for advertising or promotional purposes, for creating new collected works, or for resales.

For full details of all Mosby–Year Book Europe, Ltd. titles,
please write to Mosby–Year Book Europe, Ltd., Lynton
House, 7–12 Tavistock Square, London, WC1H 9LB,
England.

LIBRARY OF CONGRESS
CATALOGING-IN-PUBLICATION DATA
   Management of urologic disorders / edited by Robert R.
   Bahnson.
       p. cm.
     ISBN 1-56375-089-9
     1. Genitourinary organs—Diseases. I. Bahnson,
   Robert R.
     [DNLM: 1. Urologic Diseases—therapy. WJ 100
     M2666 1993]
   RC900.M25 1993
   616.6—dc 20
   93-19709

A catalogue record for this book is available from the
British Library

10 9 8 7 6 5 4 3 2 1

EDITORS: Elizabeth Greenspan, David Yoon
ART DIRECTOR/DESIGN: Kathryn Greenslade
LAYOUT/PRODUCTION: Carol Drozdyk, Irina Kogan,
   Stephanie Pinerio, John Andrews
ILLUSTRATION DIRECTOR: Carol Kalafatic
ILLUSTRATORS: Gary Welch, Nicholas Guarracino, Iris
   Nichols, Ruth Soffer (inking)
TYPESETTING: Erick Rizzotto, Madeline Carroll

Originated in Singapore by Colourscan Overseas Co.
Produced by Grafos
Printed and bound in Spain

To two inspirational physicians:

*J*anet *M*c*G*arr and *J*ohn *T.* *G*rayhack

Preface

Management of Urologic Disorders is designed to inform clinical urologists about current therapy with an emphasis on colorful, graphic presentation. Authors were selected because of their established interest and expertise in subspecialty areas. Particular gratitude is owed Reg Bruskewitz, Peter Carroll, Jon Jarow, Robert Moldwin, Glenn Preminger, and Bill Steers who agreed to author or edit major sections of text. We are pleased with the substance and style of the book, and we hope it fulfills its purpose for our urologic colleagues.

Robert R. Bahnson

Contents

Contributors

NOEL A. ARMENAKAS, MD
Clinical Instructor of Urology
Cornell University Medical College
Assistant Attending Surgeon
The New York Hospital
Adjunct Physician
Lenox Hill Hospital
New York, New York

GREGORY A. BRODERICK, MD
Assistant Professor of Urology
Director, Center for Male Sexual
    Dysfunction
University of Pennsylvania School
    of Medicine
Philadelphia, Pennsylvania

REGINALD BRUSKEWITZ, MD
Professor of Surgery
Division of Urology
University of Wisconsin
Madison, Wisconsin

JEFFREY P. BUCH, MD
Assistant Professor of Urology
Head, Section on Male Fertility
    and Sexual Function
University of Connecticut Health
    Center
Farmington, Connecticut

PETER R. CARROLL, MD
Associate Professor of Urology
School of Medicine
University of California, San
    Francisco
San Francisco, California

MICHAEL COBURN, MD
Assistant Professor of Urology
Baylor College of Medicine
Houston, Texas

MICHAEL B. COHEN, MD
Assistant Professor of Pathology
    and Urology
University of Iowa
Iowa City, Iowa

JOHN P. DONOHUE, MD
Distinguished Professor and
    Chairman
Department of Urology
Indiana University Medical Center
Indianapolis, Indiana

ROBERT DREICER, MD
Assistant Professor of Medicine
    and Urology
University of Iowa
Iowa City, Iowa

HUGH A. G. FISHER, MD
Associate Professor of Surgery
Head, Urologic Oncology
Albany Medical Center
Albany, New York

RICHARD S. FOSTER, MD
Associate Professor of Urology
School of Medicine
Indiana University
Indianapolis, Indiana

LEONARD G. GOMELLA, MD
Assistant Professor of Urology
Jefferson Medical College
Thomas Jefferson University
Philadelphia, Pennsylvania

JONATHAN P. JAROW, MD
Associate Professor of Surgical
    Sciences (Urology)
Bowman Gray School of Medicine
Wake Forest University
Winston-Salem, North Carolina

STEVEN A. KAPLAN, MD
Assistant Professor of Urology
College of Physicians and Surgeons
Columbia University
New York, New York

JACK W. McANINCH, MD
Professor and Vice-Chairman
Department of Urology
School of Medicine
University of California,
    San Francisco
San Francisco, California

DAVID E. McGINNIS, MD
Attending Physician
Department of Urology
Cooper Hospital
Camden, New Jersey

ROBERT MOLDWIN, MD
Assistant Professor of Urology
Head, Interstitial Cystitis Center
Long Island Jewish Medical Center
New Hyde Park, New York

CRAIG A. PETERS, MD
Assistant Professor of Surgery
Harvard Medical School
Assistant in Surgery (Urology)
Children's Hospital
Boston, Massachusetts

GLENN M. PREMINGER, MD
Associate Professor of Urology
    and Radiology
University of Texas Southwestern
    Medical Center
Dallas, Texas

MORTEN RIEHMANN, MD
Research Fellow
Division of Urology
University of Wisconsin
Madison, Wisconsin

CARY N. ROBERTSON, MD
Assistant Professor of Surgery
Division of Urology
Duke University Medical Center
Durham, North Carolina

PETER N. SCHLEGEL, MD
Assistant Professor of Urology
The New York Hospital–Cornell
    Medical Center
Staff Scientist
The Population Council
Associate Physician
Rockefeller University Hospital
New York, New York

WILLIAM A. SEE, MD
Assistant Professor
Department of Urology
University of Iowa
Iowa City, Iowa

MARK SIGMAN, MD
Assistant Professor of Urology
Brown University
Rhode Island Hospital
Providence, Rhode Island

WILLIAM D. STEERS, MD
Assistant Professor of Urology
University of Virginia
Charlottesville, Virginia

M. SUSAN TUCKER, MD
Division of Urology
Department of Surgery
University of North Carolina
Chapel Hill, North Carolina

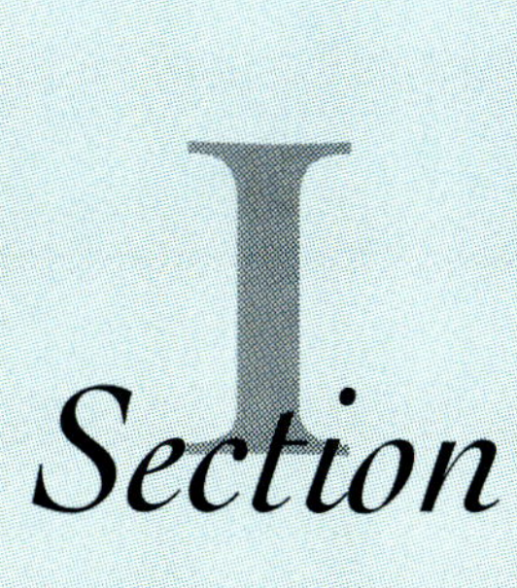

Benign Prostatic Hyperplasia

Reginald Bruskewitz, editor

CHAPTER 1

Evaluation of Benign Prostatic Hyperplasia

Morten Riehmann
Reginald Bruskewitz

Anatomy

The prostate is the largest male sexual accessory gland and the only organ that demonstrates benign neoplasia with increasing age. The gland can be divided into glandular and nonglandular portions. Within the glandular portion there are three major zones, which differ histologically and biochemically. These zones—central, transition, and peripheral—constitute approximately 25%, 5%, and 70% of the volume of the normal gland, respectively (Fig. 1.1). The nonglandular part of the prostate comprises the preprostatic and striated sphincters, anterior fibromuscular stroma, and the prostatic capsule. The preprostatic sphincter is a cylinder of smooth muscle fibers surrounding the proximal segment of the prostatic urethra. The periurethral region is located within this sphincter, which by volume comprises very little of the gland.

Histologically, the prostate is composed primarily of epithelium, glandular lumina, and stroma. Only the transition zone and the periurethral region are sites of hyperplasia. Both stromal and epithelial neoplasia exist, and the ratio demonstrates a substantial pleomorphism in resected tissue specimens. Generally, tissue from smaller glands contains a preponderance of fibromuscular stroma, whereas larger glands are dominated by epithelial nodules. This supports the hypothesis that benign prostatic hyperplasia (BPH) starts with stromal neoplasia, which in some way stimulates epithelial growth. BPH is a complex pathologic process whose incidence increases with age and histologically reveals a mixture of glandular, cystic, and stromal hyperplasia.

Pathogenesis

While it is widely accepted that testicular androgens and aging are essential for the development of BPH, it is not clear which hormone or hormones lead to the disease. Elderly men generally have a decreased serum testosterone level but maintain prostate dihydrotestosterone (DHT) level because of increased formation and reduced conversion to androstanediol. DHT is the main intraprostatic androgen and its affinity for androgen receptors is many times higher than testosterone's affinity for these receptors. The role of estrogens in the development of BPH is controversial. It has been hypothesized that an estrogen, probably estradiol, synergizes with DHT in the induction of BPH, possibly through an estradiol-induced increase in the level of androgen receptors in the prostate, but probably also through an inhibition in the rate of cell death of the prostate. A variety of growth factors have been characterized in the neoplastic prostate. These include β-fibroblastic growth factor (β-FGF), α-fibroblastic growth factor (α-FGF), transforming growth factor (TGF-β), and epidermal growth factor (EGF).

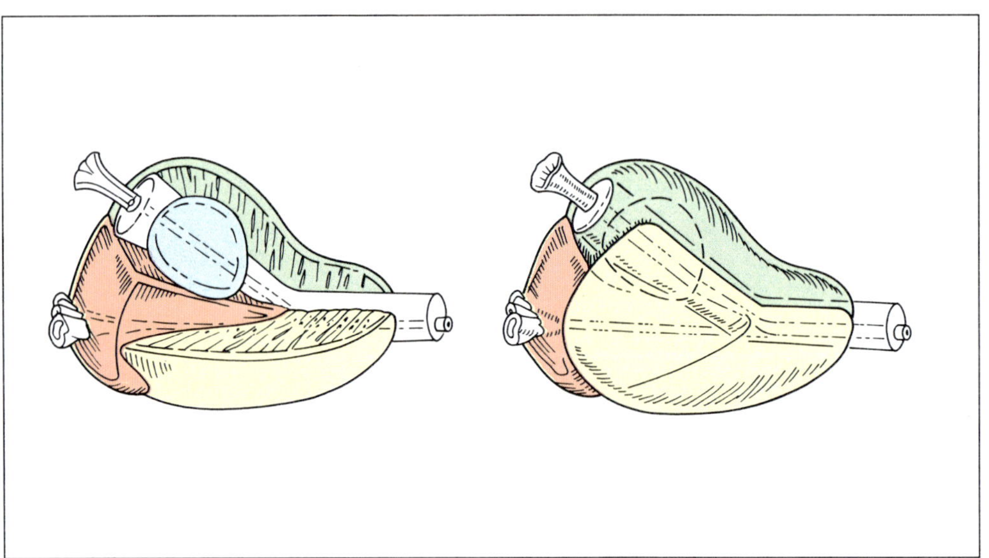

Figure 1.1 Zonal anatomy of the prostate gland. Blue = transition zone, orange = central zone, yellow = peripheral zone, green = anterior fibromuscular stroma. (Modified with permission from *Radiology.* 1989;170:609–615, courtesy of Dr. Fred Lee)

Natural History and Epidemiology

The definition of BPH is a central issue in an epidemiologic characterization of the disease. The incidence of BPH varies, depending on its classification (histologic, macroscopic, physiologic, and/or symptomatic). For example, while the clinical phase is always preceded by histologic changes of the prostate, histologic changes do not invariably lead to clinical manifestations.

The prostate undergoes the greatest growth and reaches a fully functional state during the teenage years. BPH is associated with the continued, slow increase in prostate weight after age 30, but the disease is probably initiated before this age. The prevalence of BPH increases with age; thus 50% of men between 51 and 60 years and over 85% of men older than 80 years have histologic evidence of BPH. The probability that a BPH-free 40-year-old man will develop clinical or histologic BPH if he lives until age 80 is approximately 75%.

About one half of older men with gross enlargement of the prostate will develop clinical symptoms requiring surgery. A 50-year-old man has approximately a 25% chance of having a prostatectomy during his lifetime, and almost one third of all males are destined to undergo prostatectomy.

Diagnosis

Symptoms of infravesical obstruction due to BPH are often referred to as prostatism. These symptoms are arbitrarily divided into obstructive and irritative. The obstructive symptoms are weak stream, abdominal straining, hesitancy, intermittency, incomplete bladder emptying, and terminal dribbling, whereas the irritative symptoms are frequency, nocturia, urgency, urge incontinence, and possibly dysuria. Other conditions associated with BPH are urinary tract infection, hematuria, urinary retention, and renal failure.

Some urologists feel that BPH-related symptoms of infravesical obstruction indicate surgical intervention as one of several options, while others regard these symptoms as a definitive indication for surgery. However, only hesitancy and slow stream are significantly associated with urodynamic measurements of obstruction. Correlating symptomatology to more objective criteria for bladder outlet obstruction would be desirable.

The evaluation of patients who have symptomatic BPH is often compromised by the failure to objectify subjective symptoms. Symptom scoring schemes minimize some of the uncertainty when classifying subjective urinary symptoms. A great limitation of these scoring schemes has been that questions dealing with quality of life were not included.

EXCRETORY UROGRAPHY

Though the majority of urologists in the United States perform excretory urography prior to prostatic surgery in BPH patients, this radiologic examination does not have a significant impact on the management of these patients. Urography or other urinary tract imaging in the evaluation of BPH patients should be restricted to those with symptoms or signs of upper urinary tract disease, hematuria, history of urinary tract calculi, urinary tract infections, or evidence of renal insufficiency.

CYSTOSCOPY

This endoscopic modality is not routinely indicated in the evaluation of BPH, though it is able to give information about the site of urinary obstruction (Fig. 1.2). Cystoscopy by itself cannot point out which patients require surgery, nor their postoperative outcome, mainly because some obstructed men have a normal endoscopic appearance and vice versa.

PROSTATE SIZE

There is poor correlation between prostate size and symptoms. Digital rectal examination is an unreliable method for estimation of prostate size. Weight estimated by simultaneous rectal examination and cystoscopy correlates well with resected tissue weight and preoperative obstructive symptoms. Resected weight correlates with obstructive symptoms but not urodynamic measurements of obstruction, i.e., small prostates may obstruct the urinary stream while larger prostates may not. Estimating the prostate size in BPH patients with significant urinary obstruction may help indicate the best surgical approach.

URODYNAMIC TESTING

Conventional urodynamic testing for BPH includes uroflowmetry, pressure-flow study, and cystometry.

Uroflowmetry

This test is noninvasive and it is the most often used modality in the documentation of infravesical obstruction. During uroflowmetry the urinary flow rate, volume per time unit, is recorded as a function of micturition time. The flow curve reflects the interaction between the contracting bladder and the outlet resistance. The peak flow rate is usually the most informative and valuable measurement.

Flow is dependent on intravesical or voided volume. When evaluating peak flows in male patients, voided volume should at least be 150 mL. The peak flow/voided volume relationship for volumes greater than 150 mL represents a hyperbolic curve. In order to improve the use of maximum flow rate as an index of urinary obstruction, peak flow can be corrected by using so-called flow rate nomograms.

Peak flow rates above 15 mL/sec usually exclude urinary obstruction, but it has been stated that approximately 5% of patients suffering from BPH-related infravesical obstruction are found to have "high-flow, high-pressure" bladder outlet obstruction, i.e., flow rates above 15 mL/sec combined with elevated intravesical pressure during voiding. Patients with maximum flow rate between 10 and 15 mL/sec may or may not be obstructed, and further urodynamic testing should be undertaken. Generally, flow rates less than 10 mL/sec are interpreted as a sign of infravesical obstruction, provided detrusor insufficiency is absent.

Uroflowmetry is a good screening modality in patients with symptoms of bladder outlet obstruction; however, it cannot be used to diagnose the site of a potential urinary obstruction nor to predict postoperative outcome, though there is good evidence that patients with preoperative peak flow rates above 15 mL/sec have lower postoperative success rates than those with preoperative maximum flow rates below 15 mL/sec.

Pressure Flow Studies

Synchronous recording of flow and intravesical pressure gives a rough estimate of bladder outlet resistance by the relationship maximum intravesical pressure divided by maximum flow rate squared (p/Q^2). Elevated detrusor pressure during flow and peak flow, often in combination with reduced flow, is related to infravesical obstruction. Pressure flow studies are used in the documentation of "high-flow, high-pressure" urinary obstructed men and to identify patients with primary bladder dysfunction without obstruction. Though urethral resistance is related to flow (by definition) and symptoms of infravesical obstruction, this modality is not a good index in predicting which patients will benefit from surgery. Pressure flow studies cannot be recommended as a screening modality for prostatism as voiding pressure has been found to be of limited predictive value.

Cystometry

Cystometry records intravesical pressure during filling of the bladder, and it provides information about capacity and compliance, as well as the presence of bladder contractions.

Reservoir function as well as pressure and flow are altered with BPH. Uninhibited bladder contractions or detrusor instability exist when a patient is unable to suppress increases in intravesical pressure (>15 cm of water) secondary to detrusor contractions between voidings. Detrusor instability occurs in association with infravesical obstruction as well as some neurologic diseases, and the incidence increases with age. The prevalence of uninhibited bladder contractions is about five times higher among elderly males than elderly women. This suggests that BPH and not just aging accounts for the majority of uninhibited bladder contractions found in males.

The presence of uninhibited bladder contractions is not related to the degree of urinary obstruction, and the contractions may arise when there is no obstruction,

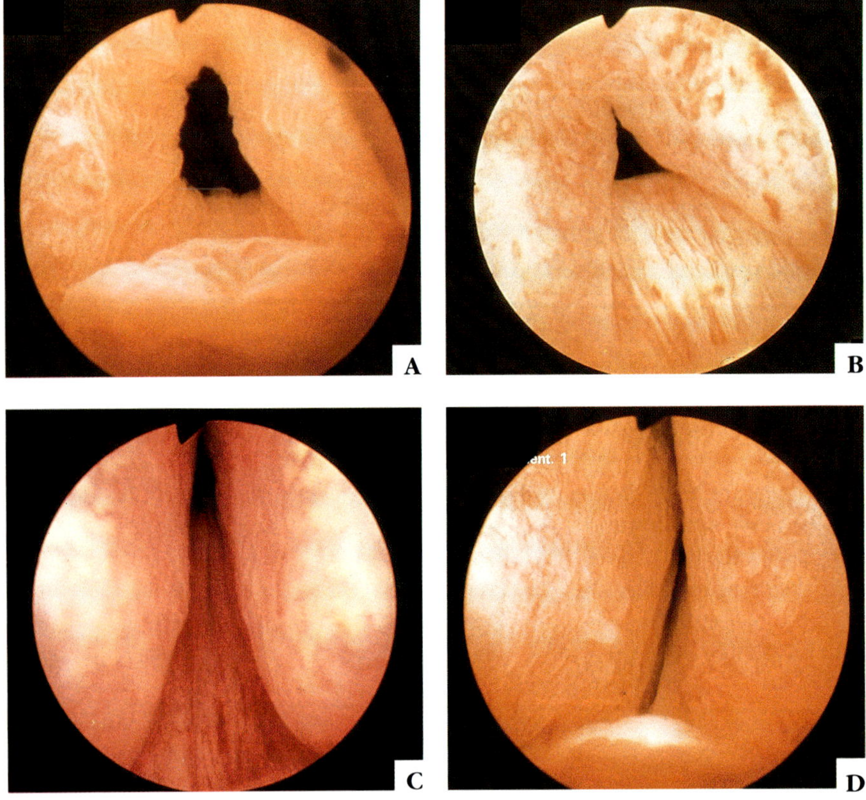

Figure 1.2 Prostatic urethra with normal appearance **A**, mild enlargement **B**, and moderate enlargement **C** of the prostate gland, and moderate to severe lateral lobe enlargement **D** of the prostate gland. (**A,B,D:** Reproduced courtesy of Maruzen Co. Ltd. and Dr. Makoto Miki)

There is controversy about the predictive value of the postoperative outcome in a patient with preoperative detrusor instability.

Conclusion

Urodynamic studies are performed to confirm the clinical impression but also to evaluate parameters that might alter diagnosis or treatment. The ultimate goal in the urodynamic investigation of patients with BPH-related infravesical obstruction is to identify those with urinary obstruction and among those the fraction who would benefit from surgery.

Symptoms of infravesical obstruction are not pathognomonic for BPH. BPH-related infravesical obstruction correlates poorly with symptoms, clinical, endoscopic, and urodynamic findings. Hesitancy and slow stream are the only symptoms that correlate to urodynamic findings of obstruction. This implies either the need for a variety of forms of objective data to confirm bladder outlet obstruction or that there is more to BPH than obstruction.

Patients often present with several of the manifestations of BPH. Several choices of treatment exist and the patient should be informed of their advantages, disadvantages, and risks and encouraged to participate in selecting the treatment. The urologist must consider comorbid disease when presenting the possibilities for treatment. Also, treatment preference varies from patient to patient. The only unequivocal contraindications to surgery are severe mental disturbance and decreased life expectancy because of comorbid disease. The indications for intervention in patients with BPH are listed in Figure 1.3.

FIGURE 1.3 *Indications for Intervention in Patients with BPH*

STRONG
Urinary retention
Azotemia with hydronephrosis
Severe gross hematuria
Urinary tract infection
Overflow incontinence

MODERATE
Symptoms
Obstruction documented urodynamically

WEAK
Cystoscopic findings
Prostate size

CHAPTER 2

Treatment of Benign Prostatic Hyperplasia

Morten Riehmann

Reginald Bruskewitz

Surgical Therapy

The current invasive options in the treatment of BPH are listed in Figure 2.1.

OPEN PROSTATECTOMY

Historically BPH has been treated with open prostatectomy, which can be performed in a simple perineal, suprapubic, or retropubic fashion. During an open prostatectomy the adenoma is enucleated and the prostatic capsule is left intact. This is to be distinguished from radical prostatectomy for cancer of the prostate, where the prostatic capsule is removed as well; this is associated with a substantially higher incidence of impotence and urinary incontinence. Of all prostatic surgery for BPH, the perineal prostatectomy carries the highest risk of impotence—it occurs in about two thirds of cases. This technique should be avoided if the patient is potent and sexually active.

Open prostatectomy ameliorates symptoms of infravesical obstruction in BPH and is applicable and indicated in 5% to 10% of the patients with BPH. This surgery may reduce morbidity in those with very large adenomatous glands (prostate size limit varies widely among urologists). The major disadvantages of this procedure are that it has a higher rate of morbidity than other procedures and requires a lengthier hospital stay than after endoscopic resection.

TRANSURETHRAL RESECTION OF THE PROSTATE (TURP)

Over the last 50 years, TURP has become the primary choice of treatment for symptomatic BPH, with approximately 400,000 procedures done each year in the United States. It is a safe procedure with high efficacy; over 80% of the patients experience regression in voiding symptoms, and postoperative improvement in urinary flow is significant.

Fifteen percent of the patients experience no benefit 1 year after TURP. Only patients with severe symptoms or acute urinary retention show significant regression in voiding symptoms and improvement in quality of life following prostatectomy. Reoperations after TURP are significantly higher than following open prostatectomy. Recent outcome studies indicate that the long-term age-specific mortality rate associated with TURP is considerably high-

---

FIGURE 2.1 *Invasive Options in the Treatment of BPH*

Prostatectomy
    Open
    TURP
    Transurethral ultrasound-guided
        laser-induced prostatectomy (TULIP)
    Ultrasonic tissue ablation
Transurethral incision of the prostate (TUIP)
    Knives
        Cold
        Electrocautery
    Resectoscope
    Laser
        Free-beam
        Contact
    Cutting balloons
Balloon dilation
Prostatic stents and coils
    Temporary
    Permanent
Hyperthermia of the prostate
    Transrectal
    Transurethral
        +/− urethral cooling

---

er than that of open surgery. There is wide variation in the rate at which TURP is performed in the United States. These differences are significantly higher than might be expected due to differences in access to medical care throughout the country or in the prevalence of BPH, which indicates substantial uncertainty about the indications for this operation.

The equivocal safety of TURP as well as uncertainty about which patients are likely to benefit from this technique have been factors in the increasing interest in different approaches to the management of BPH.

LASER ABLATION

The neodymium:yttrium-aluminum-garnet (Nd:YAG) laser is a potent energy source that was introduced into experimental medical use about 30 years ago. It has been used in the treatment of prostate and bladder cancer, as well as urethral strictures.

The TULIP® (TULIP is a trademark of Intra-Sonix) system consists of a side-firing Nd:YAG laser positioned within an ultrasound transducer that is designed to improve the directional control of the laser beam, which is always in the center of the ultrasound image (Figs. 2.2, 2.3). The distal end of the probe is enclosed within a small transparent balloon (Fig. 2.4). No irrigating fluid is used, but during ablation of the prostate the bladder is filled with fluid (Fig. 2.5). Since November 1990 the TULIP procedure has been the subject of a prospective, multicenter clinical trial.

The potential advantages of the TULIP procedure compared to TURP are shorter hospitalization, no fluid absorption, short operative time, little bleeding, and a decreased incidence postoperatively of retrograde ejaculation and bladder neck contracture. However, the laser-induced prostatectomy is not optimal in the treatment of large median lobes, and large prostate glands may require several passes. Postoperative urinary retention is often seen due to the edema from the coagulation necrosis. Other concerns are that no tissue is available for histology and the risk of using a free-beam laser. The results are preliminary, and the procedure's ultimate utility in the treatment of BPH is unknown until data from large prospective, *randomized*, multicenter clinical trials are available.

TRANSURETHRAL INCISION OF THE PROSTATE (TUIP)

An alternative to TURP that comes closest to matching its results in terms of relief of symptoms and improvement in uroflow is TUIP. The incision can be performed unilaterally or bilaterally at a variety of locations around the bladder neck. Different instruments have been and are used in the incision of the bladder neck and prostate. Recently a cutting balloon as well as a laser-induced incision (free-beam and contact laser) have been introduced (Figs. 2.6, 2.7).

Indications for resection and incision of the prostate are nearly equal. Because of the increased incidence of retrograde ejaculation after TURP, TUIP is preferred in

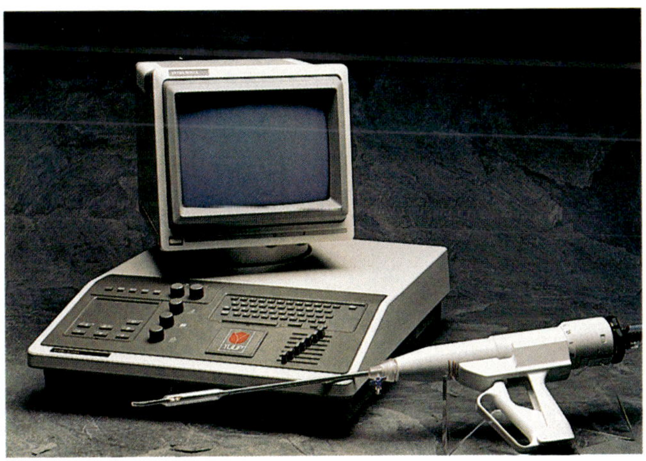

Figure 2.2 The TULIP® System for transurethral ultrasound-guided laser-induced prostatectomy consists of a 20 Fr transurethral probe, a control handle, and an ultrasound console. (TULIP® is a trademark of Intra-Sonix. Reproduced with permission of Intra-Sonix)

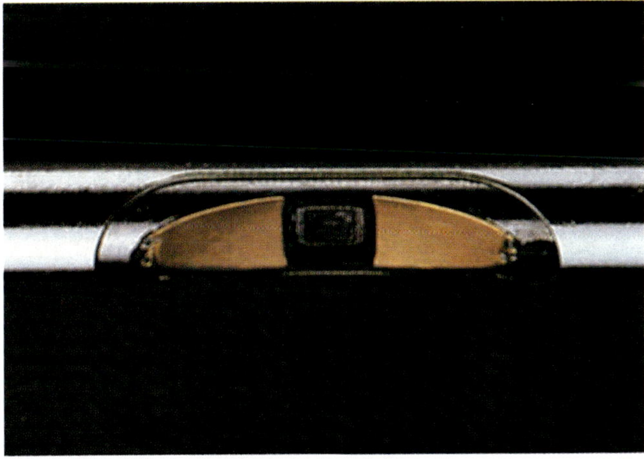

Figure 2.3 The transurethral probe incorporates at its distal tip a side-firing Nd:YAG laser positioned within an ultrasound transducer. (Reproduced with permission of Intra-Sonix)

younger and/or sexually active BPH patients. TUIP should be reserved for smaller glands (estimated resected weight <20 g) because of the increased incidence of complications and difficulties as well as decreased incidence of symptom regression when larger glands are incised. TURP is preferable to the incision procedure in BPH patients with 1) symptoms of urinary obstruction and large prostate glands, 2) severe recurrent gross hematuria, and 3) prostatitis when the aim is to remove the infected prostatic tissue and calculi.

BALLOON DILATION

Balloon dilation has been employed as an alternative to prostatectomy for the last several years (Fig. 2.8). The procedure is simple and safe, and its advantages over TURP are lower initial costs, minimal or no hospitalization, and that it does not preclude later alternate or standard treatment. Neither incontinence nor impotence has been reported following balloon dilation, but the efficacy varies considerably from study to study and does not reach the level of TURP.

Patients with severe symptoms, urinary retention, large residual urine volumes, median lobe hyperplasia, bladder neck contractures, or urethral strictures are less likely to experience relief of symptoms after dilation, and some or all of these conditions are regarded as relative contraindications to this procedure. Candidates who are most likely to benefit from balloon dilation of the

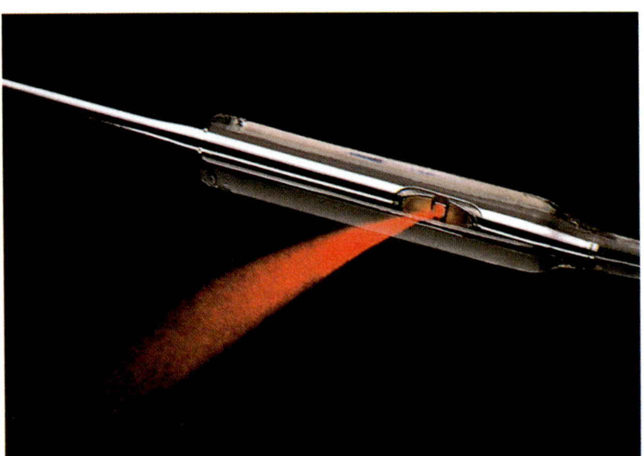

Figure 2.4 The distal end of the transurethral probe of the TULIP device is enclosed within a small transparent balloon. (Reproduced with permission of Intra-Sonix)

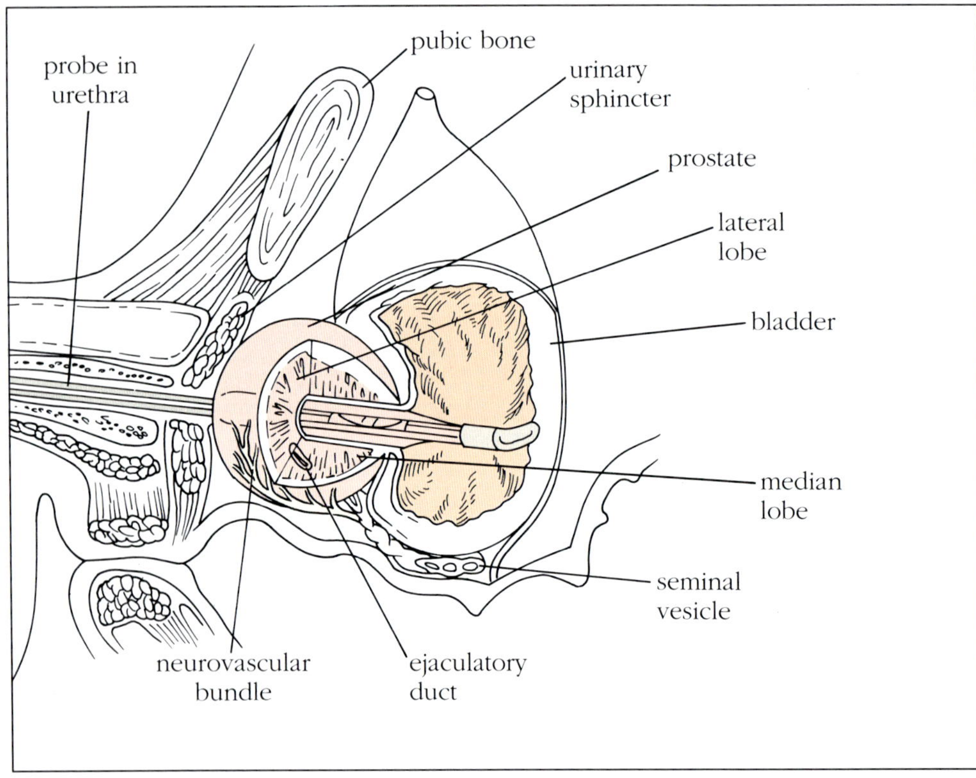

Figure 2.5 The distal end of the surgical probe in position during the TULIP procedure. (Modified with permission of Intra-Sonix)

prostate are BPH patients with moderate obstructive symptoms, small to moderate-sized glands, and lateral lobe enlargement.

PROSTATIC STENTS AND COILS

Stents used in coronary and peripheral arteries to maintain patency after transluminal angioplasty inspired attempts to treat urethral strictures, dyssynergic external urinary sphincters, and prostate and bladder neck obstructions with indwelling stents and coils. These stents are of two types: temporary and permanent (Figs. 2.9–2.11).

BPH candidates for these devices generally have an excessively high operative risk or refuse surgery. The advantages of this modality in the treatment of BPH are a short operative time (30 minutes or less) and the potential for insertion as an outpatient procedure. It is difficult,

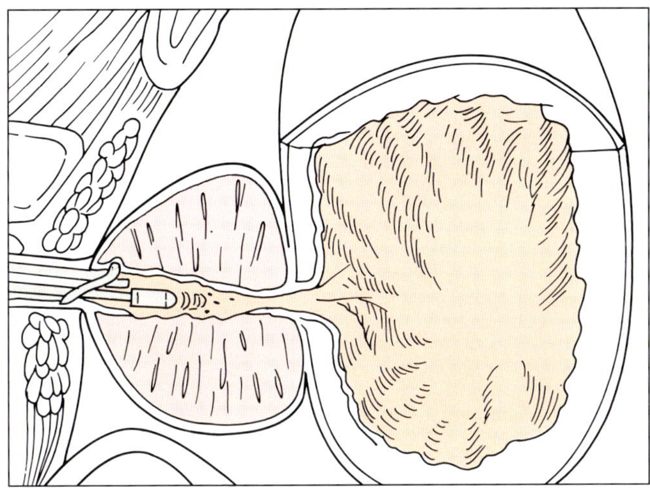

Figure 2.6 Incision of the prostate performed with a SLT contact laser. (Modified with permission of Surgical Laser Technologies)

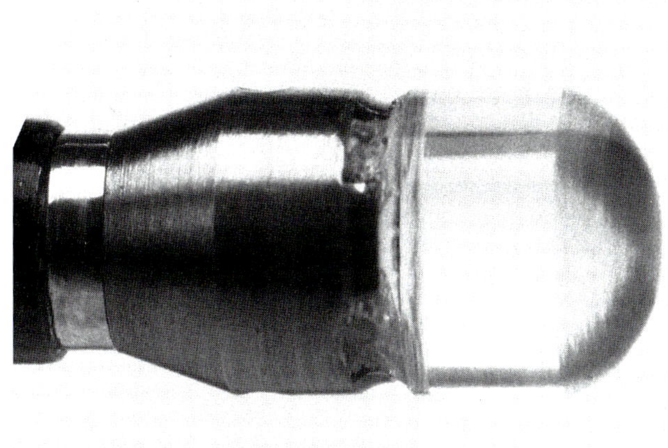

Figure 2.7 The SLT contact laser probe. (Reproduced with permission of Surgical Laser Technologies)

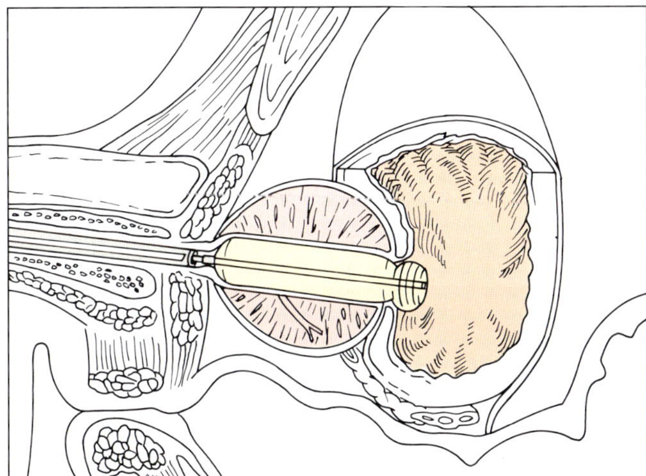

Figure 2.8 Inflated dilation balloon in prostatic urethra. The proximal balloon marker is positioned at the external sphincter and the sheath just beyond the sphincter. Before performing balloon dilation of the prostate, the anatomic length of the prostatic urethra is determined with markings on a calibration catheter in order to apply the right balloon size. (Reproduced with permission of Advanced Surgical Intervention)

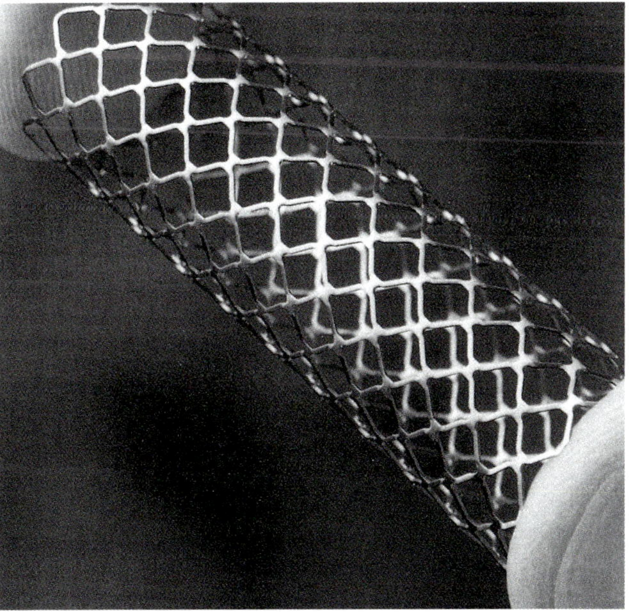

Figure 2.9 This prostatic stent (Advanced Surgical Intervention) is made from pure titanium and designed for permanent epithelialization, which usually occurs within 3 months after placement. If removal should be necessary, this can be performed transurethrally using a specially designed removal system.

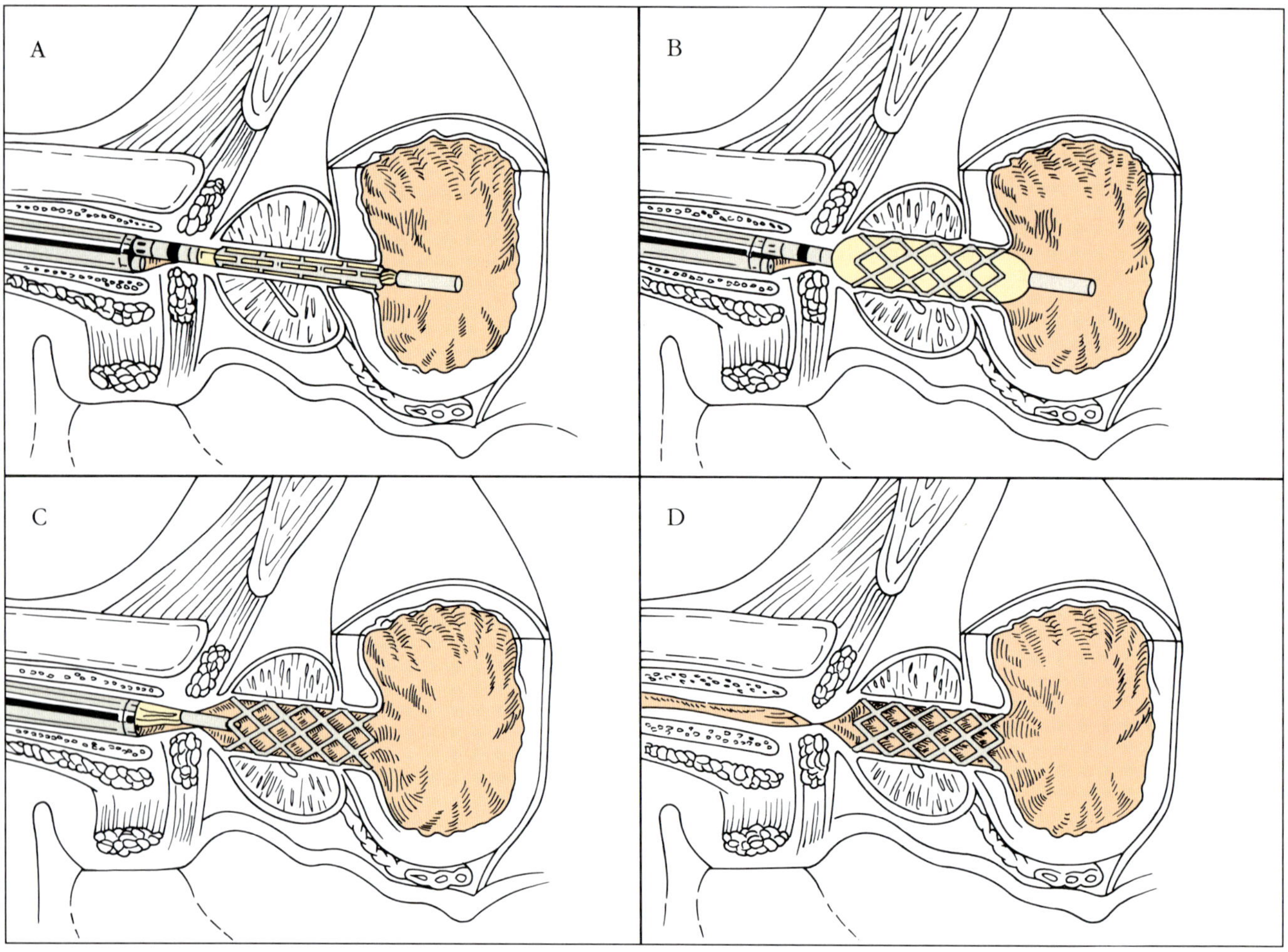

Figure 2.10 **A** The length of the prostatic urethra is meaured with a Foley calibration catheter before placement of the titanium stent. Picture shows delivery catheter placed in the prostatic urethra under endoscopic vision. The marker band is distal to the external sphincter. **B** Inflation of the delivery balloon and full expansion of the stent to a diameter of 12 mm. **C** After expanding the stent the inflation balloon subsequently is deflated and withdrawn through the sheath. **D** The stent in place in the prostatic urethra. (Modified with permission of Advanced Surgical Intervention)

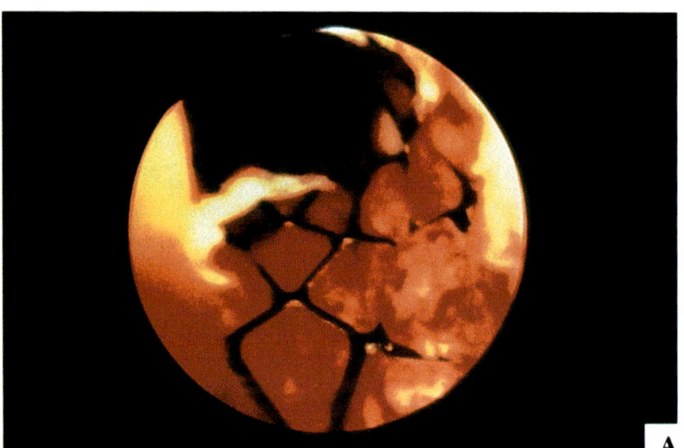
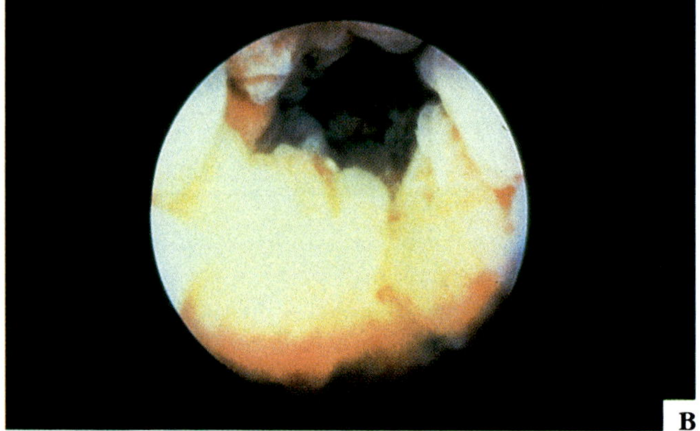

Figure 2.11 **A** Cystoscopic view of the prostatic urethra immediately after stent placement. Minor adjustments of the position of the stent can be performed using grasping forceps through the cystoscope. **B** Cystoscopic view of the same patient showing epithelialization of the stent seven months after placement. (Reproduced with permission of Advanced Surgical Intervention)

however, to define precise indications for this procedure in BPH patients who do not have urinary retention and do not have a potential operative risk. The role of this modality in the management of BPH can only be determined after the results of long-term follow-up, ongoing, prospective, randomized studies are available.

HYPERTHERMIA OF THE PROSTATE

Hyperthermia of the prostate was introduced to treat cancer of the prostate because it was recognized that due to changes in vascularity cancer tissue is more sensitive to heating than normal tissue when using temperatures in the range of 42° to 44°C.

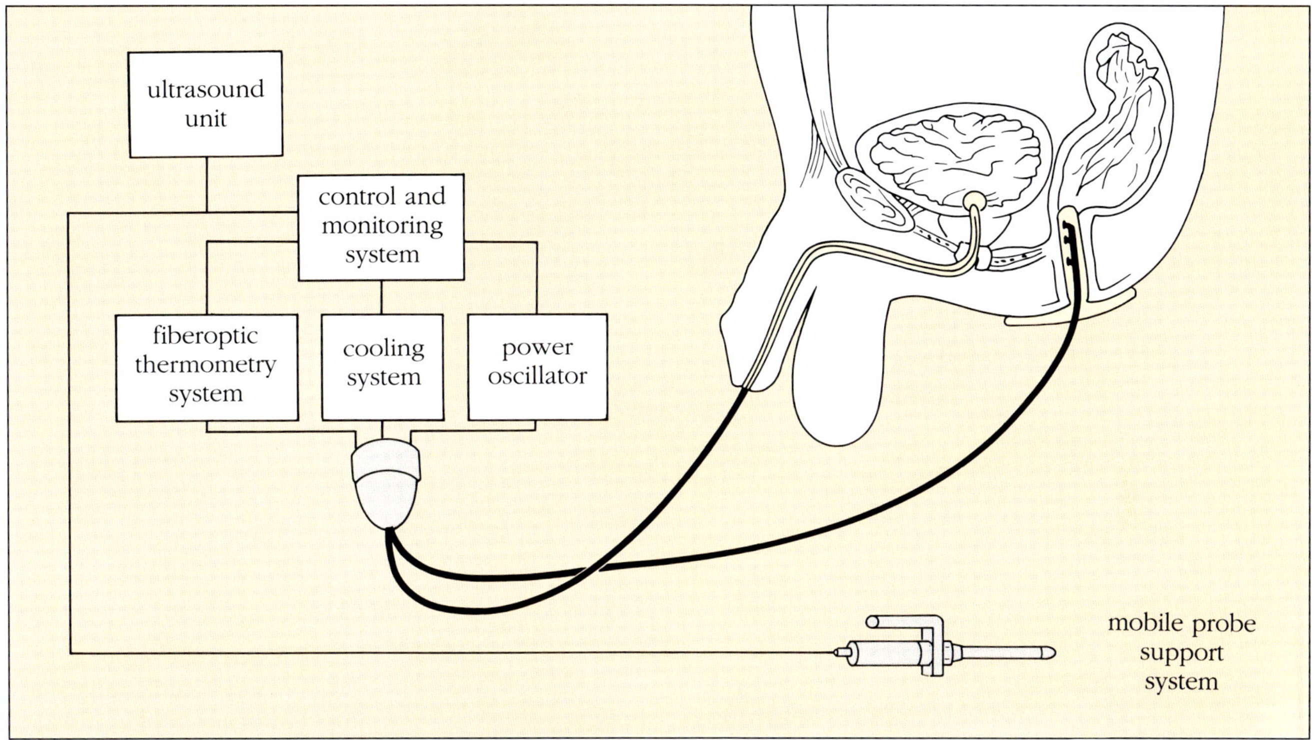

Figure 2.12 Diagram of the integrated system used in transurethral microwave thermotherapy of the prostate (TUMT). The treatment is performed in a single setting without regional or general anesthesia. Temperatures of 45°C or more are achieved for at least 45 minutes in the targeted tissue. The cooling system is designed to achieve therapeutic temperatures deep within the prostate gland and adenoma while preserving the prostatic urothelium, and without damaging bladder, rectum, or external sphincter. (Modified with permission of Technomed International)

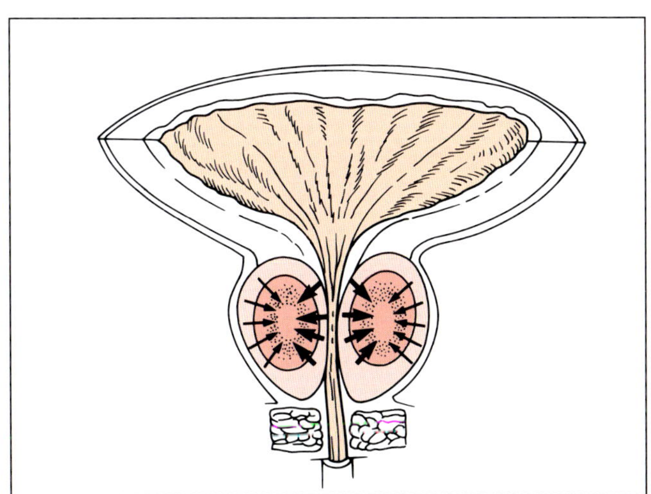

Figure 2.13 The microware heat causes the targeted hyperplastic tissue to shrink because of cell death. This ultimately leads to improvements in urinary flow rate and regression in severity of symptoms.

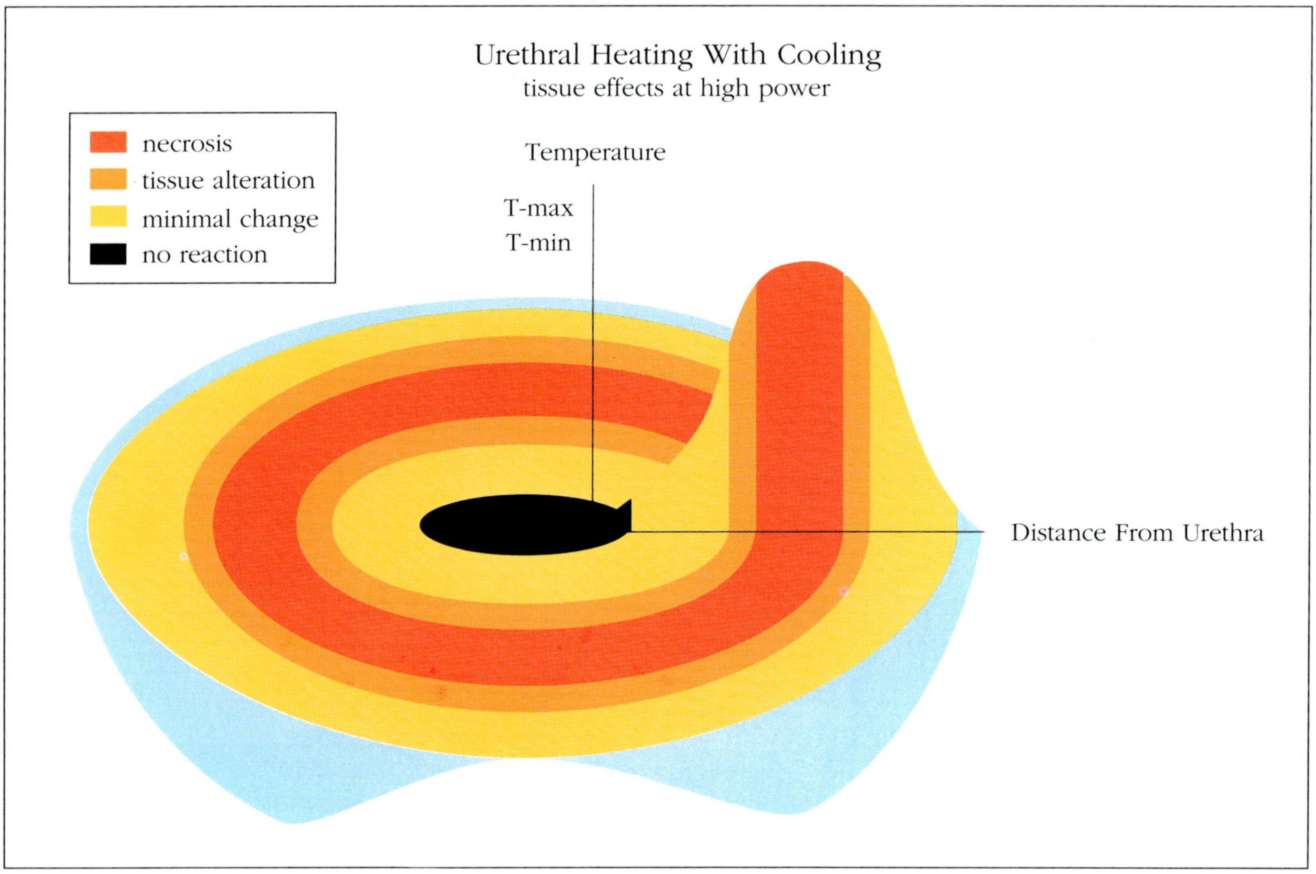

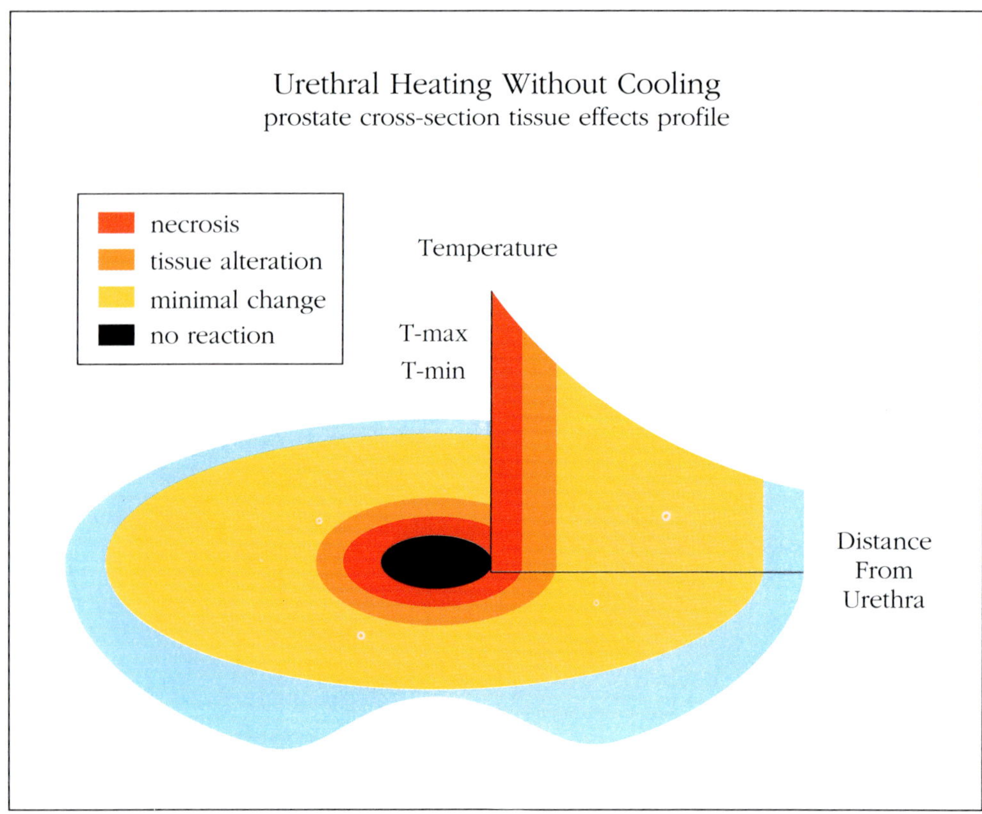

Figure 2.14 Zonal temperature ranges in the prostatic urethra and prostate gland during microwave thermotherapy with **A** and without **B** urethral cooling.

Thermotherapy is used in the treatment of BPH and the procedure is performed either transrectally or transurethrally. In thermotherapy, target temperatures higher than 45°C are used, which lead to cell death in normal, benign hyperplastic, and malignant tissue. Recently, transurethral microwave thermotherapy (TUMT) combined with conductive cooling of the prostatic urethra has been introduced in the treatment of BPH. Cooling of the urethra allows higher temperatures to be employed so that therapeutic temperatures can be achieved deeper within the prostate (Figs. 2.12–2.16). Consequently, the procedure has the potential for definitive treatment in one session.

Thermotherapy is at the experimental stage in the United States and the data for treatment of BPH are preliminary. Randomized studies are not yet available, but the method seems safe, with urinary retention being the only adverse effect. Retrograde ejaculation has not been reported after treatment. The procedure causes an improvement in objective and symptomatic criteria for urinary obstruction.

Medical Therapy

Relaxation of the prostate smooth muscle fibers through α-adrenergic receptor inhibition and regression of the neoplastic tissue volume by hormonal manipulation are the main goals of medical intervention for symptomatic BPH. The prostatic smooth muscle tone and physical presence of the hyperplastic tissue account for the dynamic and mechanical components of obstruction, respectively.

The medical options in the treatment of BPH are listed in Figure 2.17.

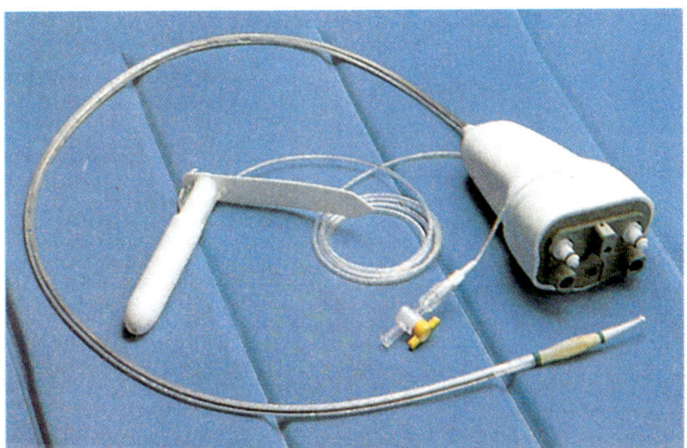

Figure 2.15 Foley catheter integrating microwave antenna, cooling system, and fiberoptic thermosensor, which continuously provides measurements of urethral temperatures. Rectal probe with fiberoptic thermosensors provides continuous monitoring of rectal temperatures. (Reproduced with permission of Technomed International)

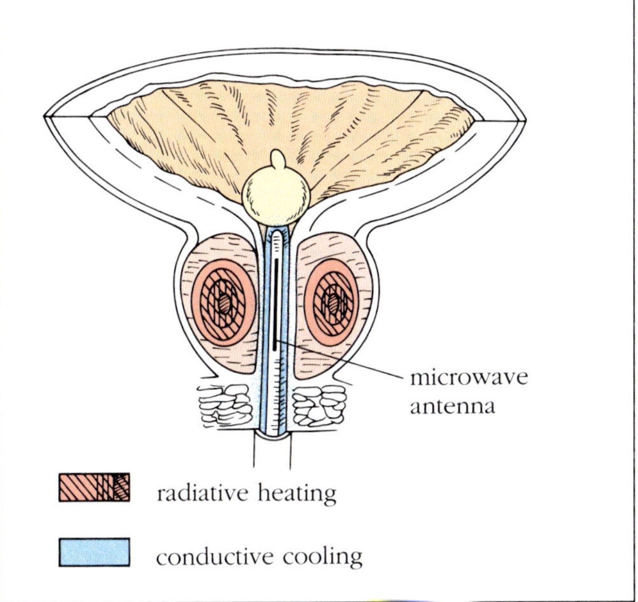

Figure 2.16 The Foley catheter in place. (Modified with permission of Technomed International, courtesy of Dr. Michael L. Blute)

FIGURE 2.17 *Medical Options in the Treatment of BPH*

	PRIMARY SITE OF ACTION	SIDE EFFECTS/ADVERSE REACTIONS
ANDROGEN SUPPRESION		
DES	Inhibition of LH secretion → T↓ + DHT↓	Hot flashes Impotence/loss of libido Vascular disease Gynecomastia

LHRH Agonists
  Nafarelin
  Buserelin
  Goserelin
  Leuprolide
	Desensitization of LHRH receptors in the pituitary → inhibition of LH secretion → T↓ + DHT↓	Hot flashes
		Impotence/loss of libido
		Gynecomastia

Cyproterone acetate	Androgen receptor inhibition Inhibition of LH secretion → T↓ + DHT↓	Impotence/loss of libido
Flutamide	Androgen receptor inhibition through competitive blockade of T + DHT binding to androgen receptors	Gynecomastia (Impotence) Gastrointestinal symptoms

Progestins
  Megestrol acetate
  Hydroxyprogesterone caproate
  Medrogestone
	Inhibition of LH secretion → T↓ + DHT↓
	Androgen receptor inhibition
		Impotence/loss of libido
		Heat intolerance

Finasteride	5α-reductase inhibitor → T↛DHT	Impotence/loss of libido
Ketoconazole	Potent inhibitor of gonadal and adrenal steroid biosynthesis through inhibition of 17α-hydroxylase and 17,20-desmolase activity Aromatase inhibition	Gynecomastia Impotence Oligospermia Drowsiness Gastrointestinal symptoms Hypersensitvity reaction (Hepatotoxicity)
Spironolactone	Diuretic and antihypertensive Aldosterone antagonist with anti-androgenic action through competitive inhibition of androgen receptors, and inhibition of androgen biosynthesis by inhibiting 17α-hydroxylase and 17,20-desmolase activity	Gynecomastia

FIGURE 2.17 *(Continued) Medical Options in the Treatment of BPH*

H$_2$-RECEPTOR ANTAGONIST Cimetidine	H$_2$-receptor antagonist with antiandrogenic action	Drowsiness Gastrointestinal symptoms
AROMATASE INHIBITORS	Δ4-Androstenedione ↛ estrone Testosterone ↛ estradiol	Loss of libido Headache Nausea Gastrointestinal symptoms
Nonsteroidal Ketoconazole Miconazole Clotrimazole		
Steroidal 1-Methyl-1,4-androstadi- ene-3,17-dione 1,4,6-Androstatriene- 3,17-dione Testolactone		
α-ADRENERGIC RECEPTOR ANTAGONISTS		
Nonselective	Antihypertensive smooth muscle relaxant through α_1- and α_2-adrenoreceptor blockade	Postural hypotension Tachycardia Inhibition of ejaculation
Phenoxybenzamine		Gastrointestinal symptoms Drowsiness
Thymoxamine		Dizziness
Selective	Antihypertensive smooth muscle relaxant through α_1-adrenorecep-tor blockade	Postural hypotension Tachycardia Inhibition of ejaculation
Prazosin Alfuzosin Terazosin Doxazosin YM 617 Nicergoline		Gastrointestinal symptoms Drowsiness Dizziness

ANDROGEN SUPPRESSION

The current approach in suppression of androgens is directed toward drugs that block the synthesis or action of testosterone and especially dihydrotestosterone (DHT) (Fig. 2.18). This therapy can be directed toward any of the regulatory steps in the synthesis or action of androgens (Fig. 2.19). Though older men generally have decreased serum testosterone levels, aging causes maintenance of intraprostatic DHT levels due to increased formation and reduced conversion to androstanediol. DHT is the main active intraprostatic androgen, and its affinity for androgen receptors is many times higher than that of testosterone.

A 20% to 30% reduction of prostate volume as well as regression in severity of sympyoms and improvement in objective criteria for urinary obstruction are seen after antiandrogen therapy. However, the efficacy of this modality cannot match that of the surgical approach. The optimal time to initiate hormonal therapy is another concern. Should treatment be administered prophylactically before the BPH process begins? If so, which patients would be eligible, and when?

AROMATASE INHIBITION

The enzyme aromatase is found predominantly in gonads, adipose tissue, and the hypothalamus. Aromatase catalyzes the final step in estrone and estradiol synthesis. These estrogens are thought to stimulate growth of the fibromuscular stroma in the prostate. Aromatase inhibitors can be steroidal or nonsteroidal (see Fig. 2.17).

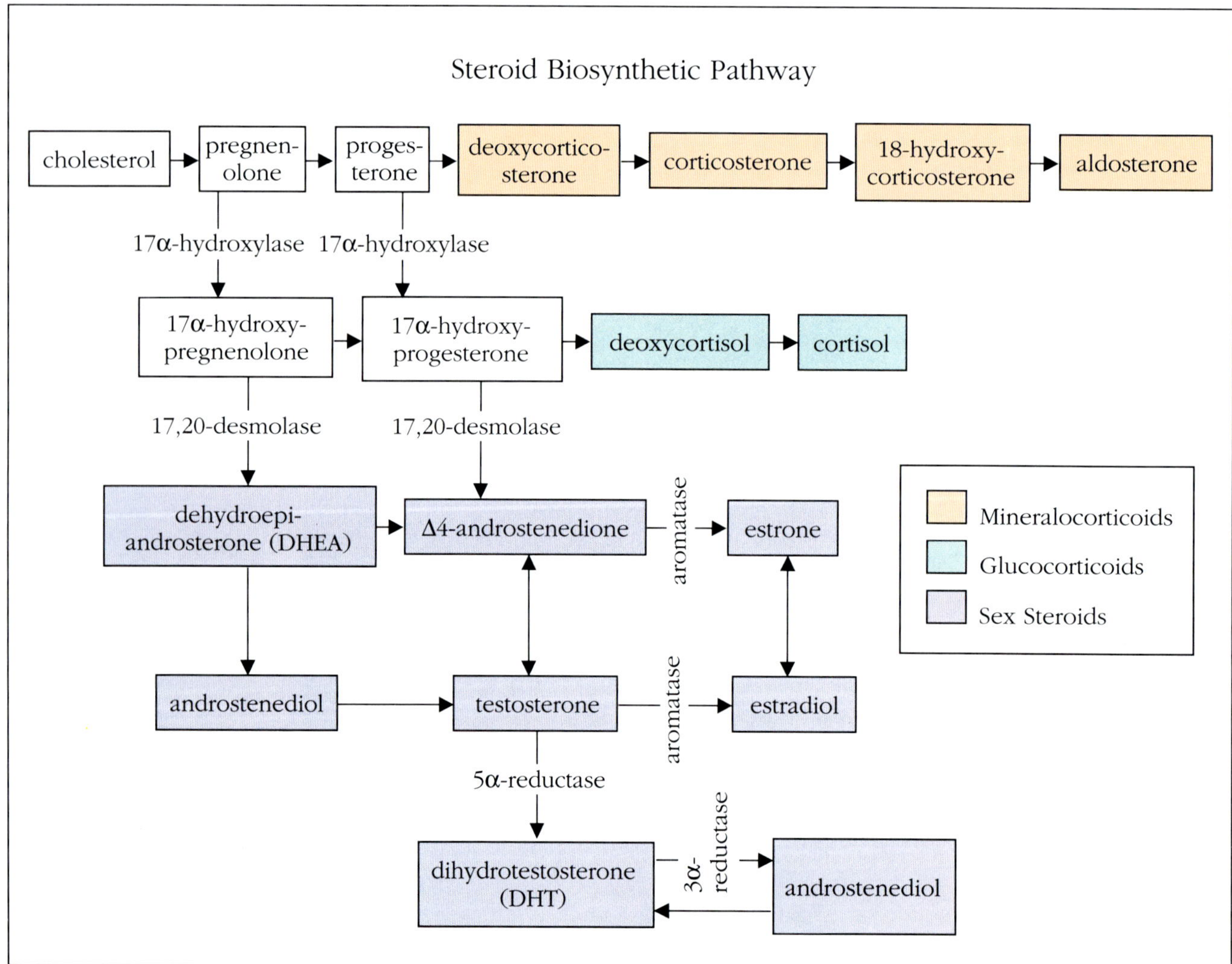

Figure 2.18 Diagrammatic representation of steroid biosynthetic pathways. Testosterone, whether from direct secretion or peripheral formation, is processed further by sexual tissue to DHT, which is the nuclear androgen in the prostate. Much of the DHT is further metabolized locally to androstanediol before entering circulation.

Treatment of symptomatic BPH patients with aromatase inhibitors is currently at the experimental stage in the United States. From animal models it is known that an aromatase inhibitor in combination with an antiandrogen will synergically inhibit the glandular and stromal components of the prostate.

α-ADRENERGIC RECEPTOR INHIBITION

α-Adrenergic receptors are found in high concentration in the smooth muscle fibers in the adenoma and capsule of the hyperplastic prostate. Inhibition of these receptors by selective and nonselective adrenergic blockers (Fig. 2.20) causes smooth muscle relaxation, which ultimately results in improved urinary flow and regression in urinary symptoms. These improvements are significant during therapy with adrenergic receptor blockers. It is reasonable to offer this therapy to men with moderate symptoms of urinary obstruction who have no strong indications for surgery.

As indicated earlier, the stroma to epithelium ratio is changed with BPH. The stroma consists of smooth muscle fibers and intermuscular components such as collagen. The ease of contraction and relaxation of smooth muscle fibers is to some extent affected by collagen. This implies that the efficacy of α-blockers is partly dependent on the magnitude of these nonmuscular components, which probably varies with age. Currently, very little is known about these age-related changes in collagen.

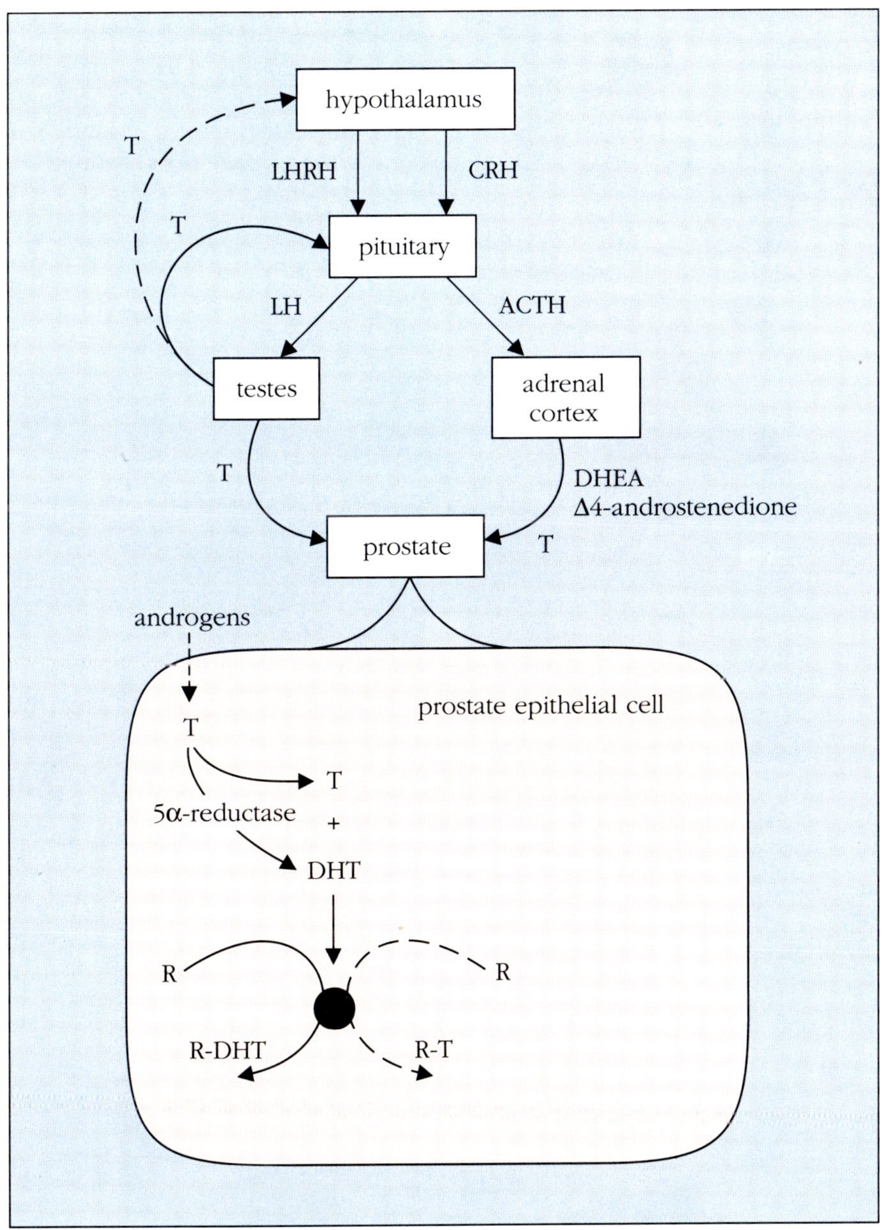

Figure 2.19 Regulation and secretion of androgens. Within the prostate epithelial cell, testosterone—and especially DHT—binds to androgen receptor proteins. Within the prostate gland DHT has a much higher affinity for androgen receptors than does testosterone. The formed steroid-receptor complex ultimately leads to protein synthesis, causing tissue growth. (Modified from Riehmann M, Bruskewitz R. *Mediguide to Urology,* 1992) T = testosterone; DHT = dihydrotestosterone; R = androgen receptor protein; LH-RH = luteinizing hormone-releasing hormone; CRH = corticotropin-releasing hormone; LH = luteinizing hormone; ACTH = adrenocortico-tropic hormone; DHEA = dehydroepiandrosterone.

Conclusion

In the evaluation of therapies for BPH, it is worthwhile to remember the natural history of prostatic hyperplasia. Approximately 30% of men with untreated symptomatic BPH will experience regression in subjective symptoms and more than 20% will show improvement of objective criteria for infravesical obstruction when followed over approximately 2.5 to 5 years.

The efficacies of TUIP and TURP are nearly equal and are not likely to be matched by the newer surgical and medical options. The alternative invasive and medical options in the management of benign prostatic hyperplasia are hampered by the presence of few randomized, published studies that contain valuable information about the ultimate usefulness of these procedures.

Urologists should carefully study all new BPH treatment options and be prepared to implement them, while resisting pressure from industry, the press, and patients to rush toward these newer modalities before their efficacy and safety are proven.

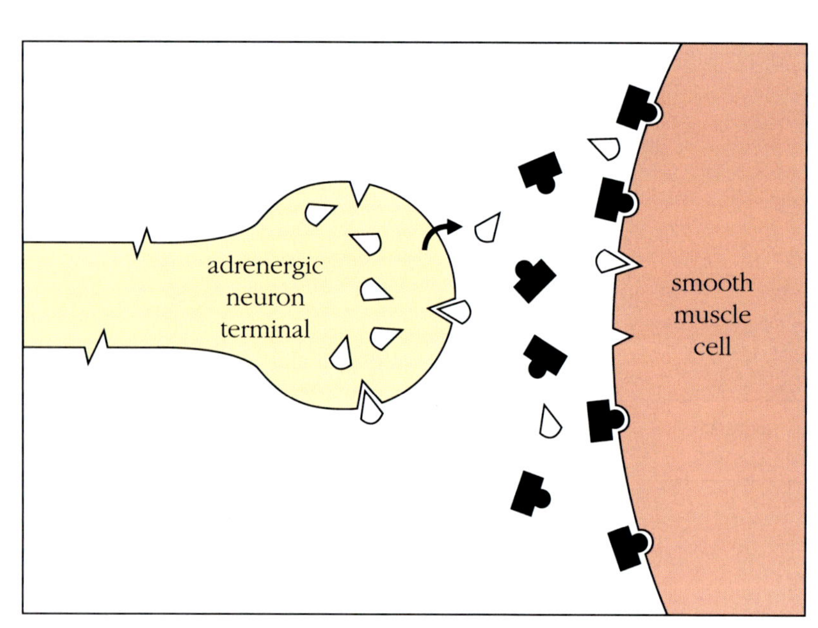

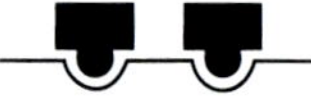

Figure 2.20 Selective α-blockers prevent norepinephrine from occupying the α_1-receptor sites, which triggers contraction of the smooth muscle fibers in the prostatic adenoma and capsule. The α_1-receptor antagonist causes smooth muscle cell relaxation, thereby ultimately facilitating urinary flow through the prostatic urethra.

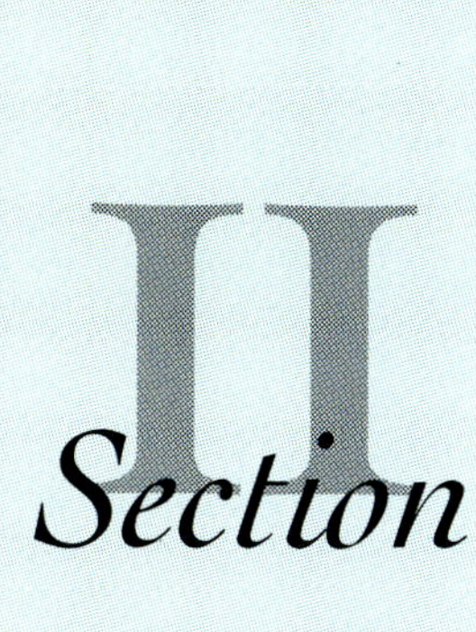

Section

II

Adult Tumors

Robert R. Bahnson, editor

CHAPTER 3

Renal Tumors

Cary N. Robertson

Renal neoplasms arise from the renal cortex, tubular epithelium, juxtaglomerular apparatus, renal capsule, residual embryonal tissue, and renal collecting system (Fig. 3.1). Local extirpation is the treatment of choice for all malignant renal tumors. Although benign tumors can be followed expectantly, radiographic characteristics are rarely uniquely distinguishing, and diagnosis of benign lesions is usually made by pathologic examination of a surgical specimen.

This chapter focuses on the evaluation and surgical management of renal tumors, benign and malignant. Approaches for small, well-confined tumors are contrasted to those for large, locally extensive neoplasms. Management of renal cell carcinoma is discussed extensively. Renal adenoma is subclassified in relation to renal cell carcinoma as an early manifestation of this most interesting neoplasm.

Malignant Tumors

RENAL CELL CARCINOMA

Renal cell carcinoma is the most common renal neoplasm, accounting for 85% of renal tumors (Fig. 3.2).[1] Described as resembling yellowish adrenal tissue, this tumor was initially believed to arise from adrenal rests within the kidney. Subsequent studies have proven that the cell of origin is within the proximal convoluted tubule of the nephron, hence the term *renal cell carcinoma.*[2] Small tumors of less than 2 cm are termed *cortical adenomas* and are histologi-cally indistinguishable from larger renal cell carcinomas. It is unclear whether these adenomas can develop into renal cell carcinomas or, conversely, represent a benign form of neoplasm with a distinct natural history.

Incidence

The annual incidence of renal cell carcinoma in the United States approaches 27,000 cases, with 11,000 deaths each year.[1] The male to female ratio is 2:1, with a median age at occurrence of 55 years. This malignancy is uncommon in younger age groups but is not rare, occasionally occurring in children and young adults. There are four histologic subtypes of renal cell carcinoma: clear cell, granular cell, papillary adenocarcinoma, and sarcomatoid variant. They may be present in various combinations in the same tumor.

Etiology

No specific etiologic agent has been identified for renal cell carcinoma, although a genetic basis is strongly supported by studies of familial clusters and patients with von Hippel-Lindau (VHL) disease. Patients with VHL disease exhibit associated retinal angiomas, hemangioblastomas of the central nervous system, pancreatic cysts, and epididymal cysts. Renal cell carcinoma frequently develops in these patients at an incidence of almost 60% and is commonly bilateral.

Patients undergoing chronic hemodialysis develop renal cysts at a rate that is correlated with the length of

---

FIGURE 3.1
Renal Neoplasms

NOMENCLATURE	SITE OF ORIGIN
Renal cell carcinoma	Proximal tubular epithelium
Renal adenoma	Proximal tubular epithelium
Reninoma	Juxtaglomerular apparatus
Renal pelvic tumor	Collecting system transitional epithelium
Duct of Bellini tumor	Collecting ducts
Angiomyolipoma	Embryonal rests
Wilms' tumor	Embryonal rests
Sarcoma	Renal capsule

FIGURE 3.2
Malignant Tumors of the Kidney

TYPE	PERCENTAGE OF CASES
Adenocarcinoma	83%
Tumors of the renal pelvis	8%
Wilms' tumor	6%
Sarcoma	3%

Courtesy of Greg Fontana, MD

dialysis dependence. Acquired renal cystic disease occurs in up to 50% of dialysis patients. Renal cell carcinoma subsequently develops in approximately 6% of such patients, usually involving cysts directly.

Sporadic cases of renal cell carcinoma reveal a consistent deletion in the short arm of chromosome 3.[3] This is similar to the translocation deletions observed in a family cohort with an autosomal dominant inheritance pattern. It is hoped that genetic markers and environmental hazards will eventually be identified, allowing screening of populations at risk.

Clinical Presentation

Fifty percent of renal cell carcinomas are detected incidentally during imaging studies for other conditions. These tumors are usually small. The remainder of cases may present with a combination of symptoms and signs thought to be distinctly characteristic (Fig. 3.3). Signs of hematuria, abdominal/flank pain, and a palpable mass represent the "classic" triad, yet this occurs in only 10% of patients and usually portends a dire prognosis. Hematuria is the most common presenting sign, occurring in 50% of cases. Other more obscure manifestations of disease are secondary to systemic factors associated with the tumor, not always in proportion to tumor size. These include anemia, cachexia, fever, and hypertension (Fig. 3.4). Polycythemia, believed to be secondary to erythropoietin production, is seen in 5% of cases. Hypercalcemia occurs in 15% of patients and is secondary to secretion of a prim-

itive parathyroid-like protein. The hepatic dysfunction observed in 15% of cases may reverse after nephrectomy. Additional phenomena include hyperreninemia, secondary amyloidosis, polyneuropathy, elevated serum human chorionic gonadotropin, and gynecomastia.[4]

Diagnostic Imaging

The predominant feature of renal cell carcinoma is that of a mass effect on renal parenchyma. This is detected by a variety of imaging techniques. A distinction between benign and malignant renal masses is frequently impossible, requiring surgical removal for final diagnosis. However, certain characteristics of renal cell carcinoma are highly predictive, with a confidence level of 95%. In short, contrast-enhancing solid renal masses are presumed to be renal cell carcinomas until proven otherwise. Algorithms for evaluations of all renal masses are often clinically helpful (Fig. 3.5). Because hematuria is the most common presenting complaint, intravenous pyelography may be the first study to identify an abnormality in renal tissues. Small tumors of less than 1 cm may be missed, however, and if clinical concern for a mass is high (e.g., pain, hypercalcemia) ultrasonography can be employed as a simple, inexpensive technique to evaluate the renal parenchyma further. Computed tomography of the abdomen provides the greatest anatomic detail, allowing evaluation of renal vasculature, adjacent organs (liver, colon, spleen), and lymphadenopathy (Fig. 3.6).

FIGURE 3.3 *Symptoms and Signs Associated With Renal Cell Carcinoma*

SYMPTOM	PERCENT OCCURRENCE
Pain	41
Hematuria	38
Weight loss	36
Mass	24
Hypertension	22
Fever	18
Classic triad	10
Hypercalcemia	6

FIGURE 3.4 *Paraneoplastic Syndromes Noted in RenalCell Carcinoma*

EFFECT	RATIO	PERCENT
Raised erythrocyte sedimentation rate	362/651	55.6
Hypertension	89/237	37.5
Anemia	473/1300	36.3
Cachexia, weight loss	338/979	34.5
Pyrexia	164/954	17.2
Abnormal liver function	65/450	14.4
Raised alkaline phosphatase	64/434	10.1
Hypercalcemia	44/886	4.9
Polycythemia	43/1212	3.5
Neuromyopathy	13/400	3.2
Amyloidosis	12/573	2.0

Adapted from Chisholm GD, 1974

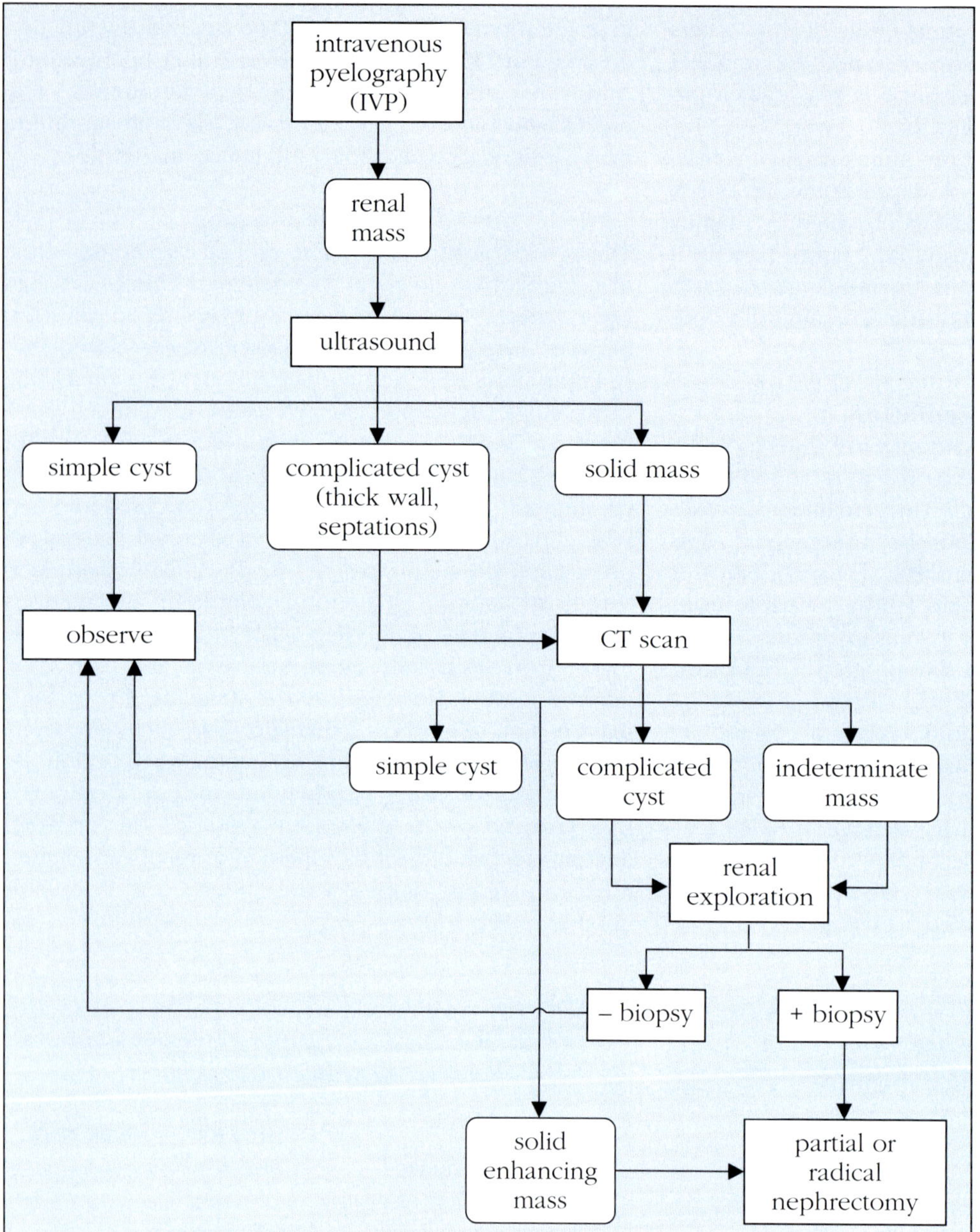

Figure 3.5 Algorithm for evaluation of renal mass noted on IVP.

FIGURE 3.6 *Keys to Renal Tumor Imaging*

MODALITY	UNIQUE FEATURES
IVP	Urothelial involvement (renal pelvis/calyces)
Ultrasound	Hepatic–renal interface distinguished by simultaneous movement of renal mass ± movement of liver
CT	Renal cell carcinoma distinguished from avascular mass by contrast enhancement
	Fatty tumor characteristic of angiomyolipoma
	Thickness of cystic wall
	Septations of complicated cyst
	Dynamic CT sensitive for renal vein thrombus
MRI	Extrarenal extent of tumor distinguished on coronal views
	Extent of renal vein and vena cava thrombus determined on coronal plane
Venacavogram	Occlusion by renal vein or vena cava thrombus noted

Staging and Prognosis

The staging system most commonly employed in the past has been Robson's classification (Fig. 3.7).[5] This is a modification of a previous classification of Flocks and Kadesky. Grouping of renal vein, vena cava, and lymph node involvement into a single stage with this system has resulted in a mixture of results, depending on the extent of involvement of the renal vein and vena cava. Specifically, vena cava invasion has a dire prognosis, whereas vena cava thrombus without attachment is associated with no worse a prognosis than organ-confined tumors.

The TNM system, as proposed by the International Union Against Cancer (UICC), offers a more subselected classification of tumor involvement. This classification has most recently been updated by the American Joint Committee on Cancer, as outlined in Figure 3.8.[6] Tumors of less than 2.5 cm are considered T1 tumors. Tumors greater than 2.5 cm are T2 tumors and are likely to distort the renal parenchyma. Tumor involvement of major veins of the adrenal gland or perinephric tissues is classified as T3, with a subclassification of T3c for tumors involving the vena cava with thrombus above the diaphragm (Fig. 3.9). Organ-confined renal tumors are associated with a 5-year survival rate near 90% and a very high likelihood of cure.

Lymph node involvement is a predictor of poor outcome, associated with a negligible 5-year survival. The regional distribution of lymph nodes draining either kidney is diffuse and may involve multiple channels both anterior and posterior to the vena cava and aorta.

The 5-year survival rate for patients with metastatic renal cell carcinoma ranges between 0% and 20%. After undergoing nephrectomy, patients with primarily pul-

FIGURE 3.7 *Robson and 1986 TNM Staging Systems for Renal Cell Carcinoma*

TUMOR STAGE	ROBSON*	TNM†
No primary tumor	—	T0
Small primary tumor, minimal distortion	A	T1
Large tumor, renal distortion	A	T2
Perinephric tissues involved	B	T3a
Renal vein involved	C	T3b
Renal vein and infradiaphragmatic vena cava involved	C	T3c
Invasion of adjacent structures	D	T4
Superior vena cava involved	C	—
No nodes involved	A,B	N0
Single ipsilateral node involved	C	N1
Multiple regional nodes involved	C	N2
Fixed regional nodes	C	N3
Juxtaregional nodes involved	C	—
Distant metastases	D	M1

*After Robson CJ, et al, 1968
†After Beahrs OH, et al, 1992

FIGURE 3.8 *1992 TNM Staging of Renal Cell Carcinoma*

TX	Primary tumor cannot be assessed.
T0	No evidence of primary tumor.
T1	Tumor 2.5 cm or less in greatest dimension limited to the kidney.
T2	Tumor more than 2.5 cm in greatest dimension limited to the kidney.
T3	Tumor extends into major veins or invades the adrenal gland or perinephric tissues but not beyond Gerota's fascia.
T3a	Tumor invades the adrenal gland or perinephric tissues but not beyond Gerota's fascia.
T3b	Tumor grossly extends into the renal vein(s) or vena cava below the diaphragm.
T3c	Tumor grossly extends into the vena cava above the diaphragm.
T4	Tumor invades beyond Gerota's fascia.

Adapted from Beahrs OH, et al, 1992

monary metastases may experience spontaneous regression at an incidence rate of 0.4%, but this is usually temporary. There are occasional reports of patients who have prolonged periods with no apparent disease after metastectomy. It is this aspect of renal cell carcinoma that proves most fascinating.

Surgical Management

PREOPERATIVE ASSESSMENT AND PLANNING   The median age for onset of renal cell carcinoma is 55 years. Many patients are in good physical condition and have no outward signs of disease. However, weight loss and liver dysfunction may accompany tumors of significant size, and this should be anticipated. Patients with hematuria, fever, flank pain, weight loss, and anemia can be categorized as having a poor performance status. Similarly, patients with hypercalcemia may pose the challenges of confusion and cardiac arrhythmias.

It is important to consider expected blood loss based on the vascularity and size of the tumor. Preoperative arteriography and angioinfarction of renal tumors may be helpful as an adjunct to nephrectomy. Angioinfarction should preferably be carried out on the day of surgery, as pain, discomfort, and fever from acute infarction of renal tumors and renal parenchyma may be significant. Previous techniques of angioinfarction to enhance the immunologic response to disease have proven marginally beneficial and should not constitute the major reason for angioinfarction.

Preoperative intravenous hydration as well as antibiotic and mechanical bowel preparation should be employed in all patients with tumors of significant size, since the possibility of tumor invasion of bowel, pancreas, and spleen must be considered.

Tumor imaging preoperatively is critical. Figure 3.6 depicts the unique abilities of each imaging modality. Patients with right-sided tumors that may be invading the liver substance should undergo ultrasound examination, with palpation and movement of the tumor during the exam to determine if the liver interface is attached to the kidney, in which case the liver should also move. Magnetic resonance imaging is quite helpful in distinguishing the extent of renal vein and vena cava thrombus superiorly and inferiorly (Fig. 3.10). Distinction between the liver and kidney can be assisted by this technique and by abdominal ultrasound, as previously discussed. CT scanning reveals the greatest amount of detail for lymphadenopathy and extension to psoas musculature. In addition, pancreatic and colonic involvement can be predicted on the basis of CT scanning. Cases of metastatic disease with involvement of spinal structures (Fig. 3.11), as well as metastases to lung parenchyma with associated pulmonary effusion, may influence the choice of a flank or a thoracoabdominal approach as opposed to a pure transabdominal approach.

Body habitus and the location and extent of the tumor (i.e., lower pole vs. upper pole) dictate the surgical approach. Three basic approaches are useful for removal of renal tumors. The traditional approach is a *flank approach* through a tenth, eleventh, or twelfth rib interspace, proceeding in a retroperitoneal fashion only (Fig. 3.12). An extension of this approach is the *thoracoabdom-*

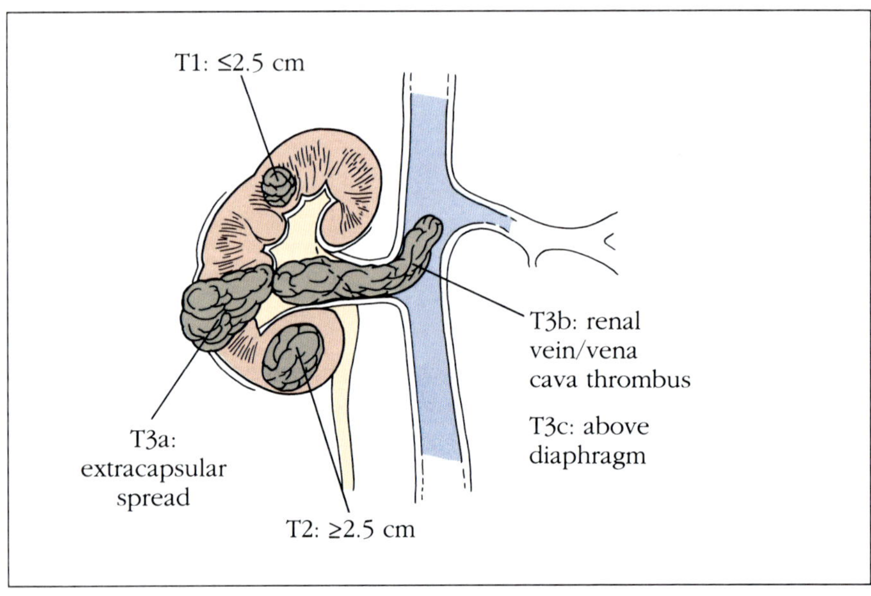

Figure 3.9 Renal cell carcinoma staging (TNM classification).

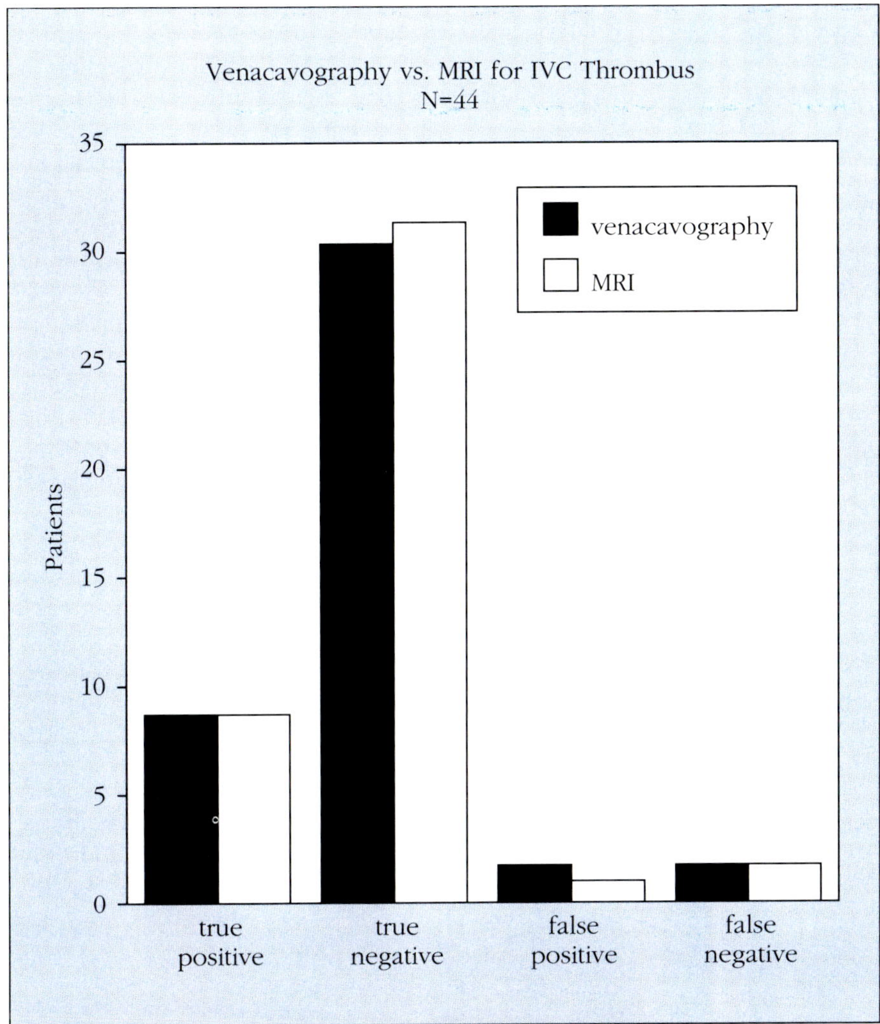

Figure 3.10 MRI is equivalent to venacavography for the detection of venous thrombosis in renal cell carcinoma. (Adapted with permission from Horan JJ, et al, 1989)

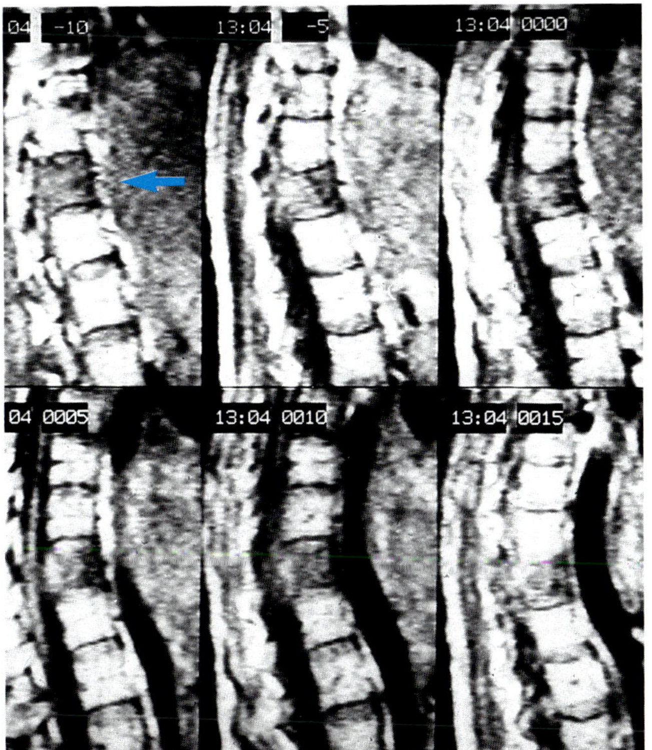

Figure 3.11 MR image showing vertebral metastasis (arrow pointing to dark image). Bone scanning may not reveal this during the early phase of involvement with renal cell carcinoma.

inal approach, with a tenth or ninth rib incision connecting to an abdominal midline incision (Fig. 3.13). This represents a transthoracic, transabdominal approach to the kidney. A third approach is the *bilateral subcostal abdominal approach,* or so-called chevron approach, which is strictly transabdominal (Fig. 3.14).

RADICAL NEPHRECTOMY   Robson abandonded simple nephrectomy in favor of radical nephrectomy after cure rates were shown to be improved with the more extensive surgical procedures.[5] Radical nephrectomy involves removal of the ipsilateral adrenal gland, associated perirenal fat, and associated lymphatic structures (Fig. 3.15). A separate regional lymphadenectomy may be combined with radical nephrectomy. There is minimal evidence to suggest that this is beneficial in terms of survival, but it does provide ample prognostic information concerning lymph node status. The area to which regional lymphadenectomy should extend is debatable, but it usually involves removal of adjacent tissue overlying the ipsilateral great vessel (aorta, vena cava). Additional removal of pararenal fat, leaving the psoas fascia bare, may make the surgical procedure simpler.

Gerota's fascia extends in a separate compartment around the adrenal gland and inferiorly surrounding the upper third of the ureter. There is an easily demarcated plane of dissection overlying the medial extent of the gonadal vein adjacent to the vena cava. Cleansing of fascia from the anterior surface of the vena cava and/or aorta on the left side renders a medial extent of dissection extending to the renal vein and inferiorly to the proximal ureter. The lateral extent of dissection is defined by pararenal fat attachments to the posterior abdominal wall and the posterior peritoneum. The plane between posterior peritoneum and Gerota's fascia can be quite delicate but is readily identified if care is taken during initial dissection. It is possible to remain completely retroperitoneal, thus providing complete exposure by an extraperitoneal and extrapleural approach. The renal vessels may be approached best anteriorly (Figs. 3.16–3.19). Survival rates for radical nephrectomy in stage T1,N0,M0 disease are quite acceptable, approaching 90% at 5 years.[7]

PARTIAL NEPHRECTOMY   For patients with renal carcinoma and a solitary kidney or abnormal renal function due to either stone disease or renal insufficiency, partial

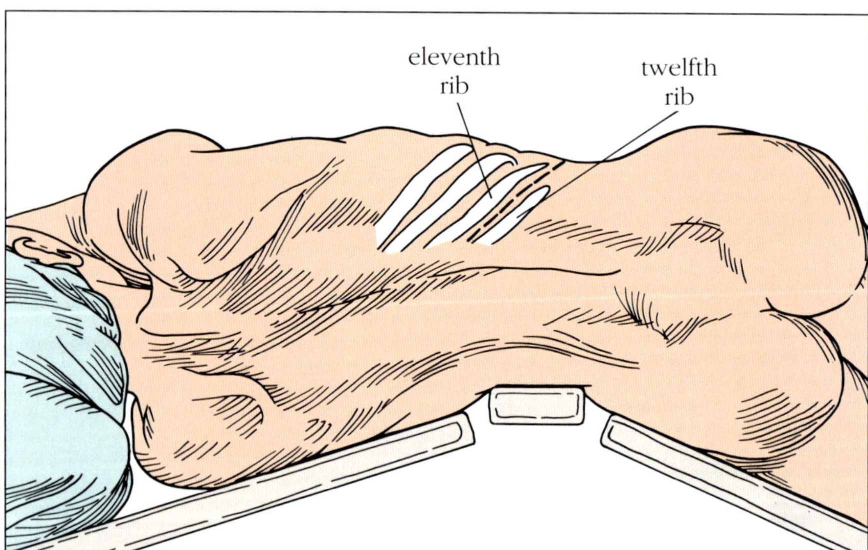

Figure 3.12 Traditional position for flank approach to the kidney.

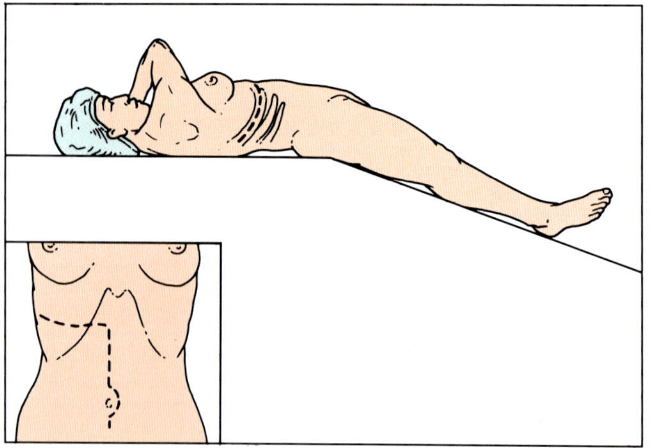

Figure 3.13 Thoracoabdominal approach for extensive or high-lying renal tumors.

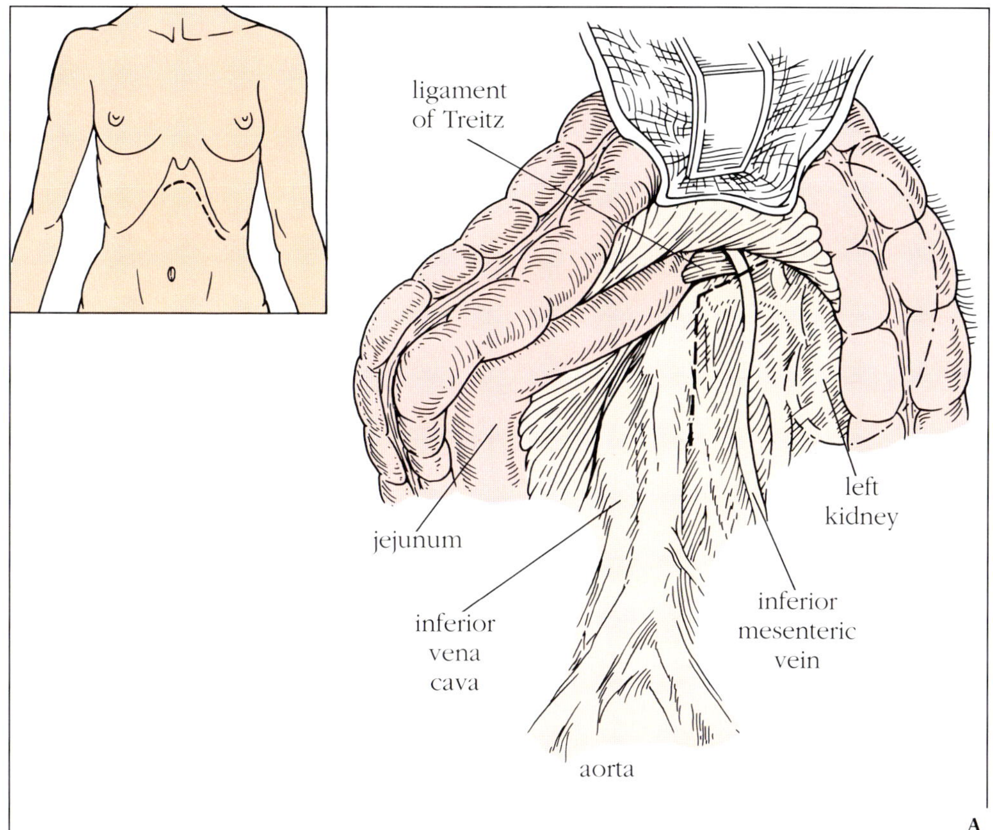

Figure 3.14 **A** Transabdominal approach to the kidney affords exposure to the great vessels, inferior vena cava, and aorta. **B** Position for bilateral subcostal (chevron) incision to be used for anterior exposure to the renal hilum and in cases of bilateral renal tumors. **C** Anterior subcostal abdominal incision, left side for resection of left renal tumor. This represents one half of a "chevron" incision.

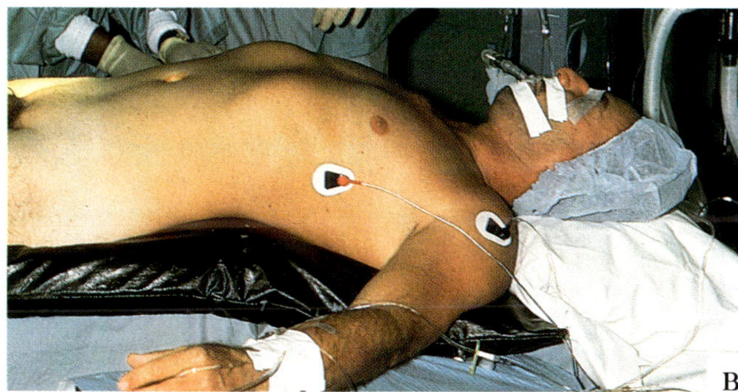

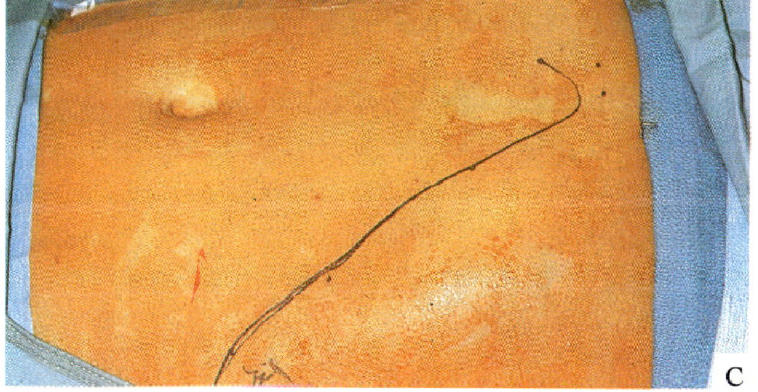

Figure 3.15 Gerota's fascia should be removed intact with the kidney and renal tumor to complete the radical nephrectomy.

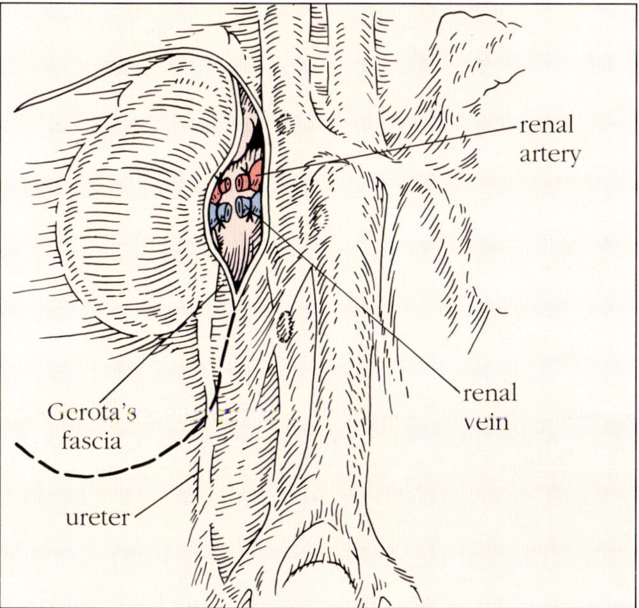

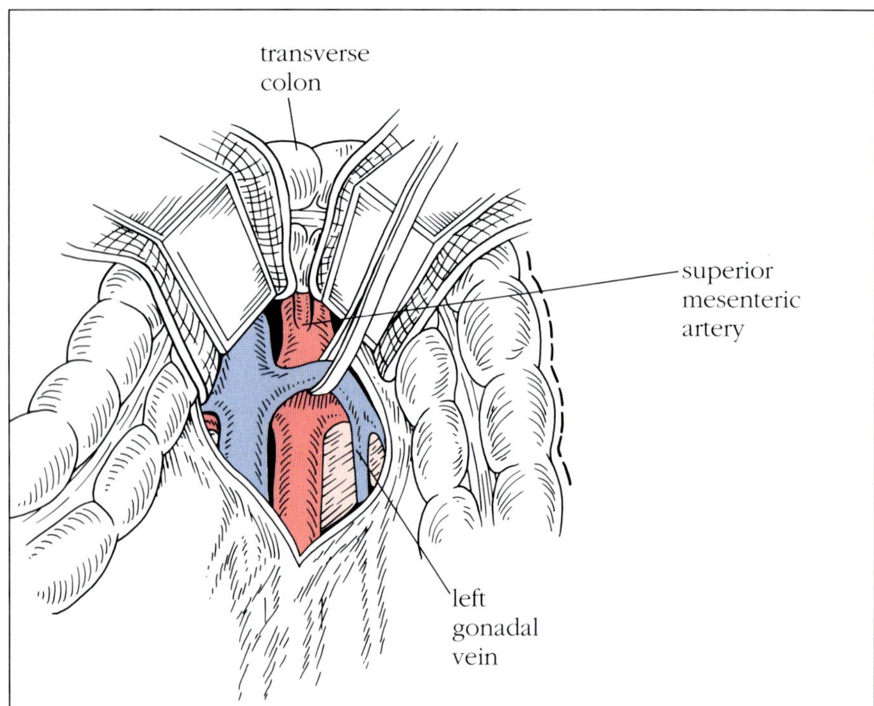

Figure 3.16 Manipulation of the renal vein permits access to the renal artery from an anterior approach.

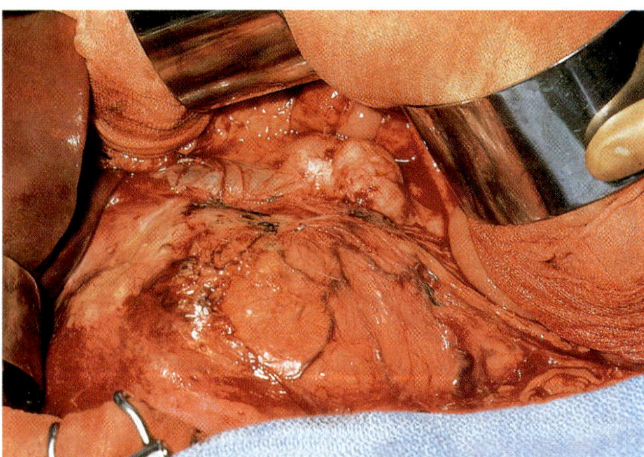

Figure 3.17 Initial exposure of right-sided renal cell carcinoma revealing inferior vena cava and liver with associated lymphadenopathy.

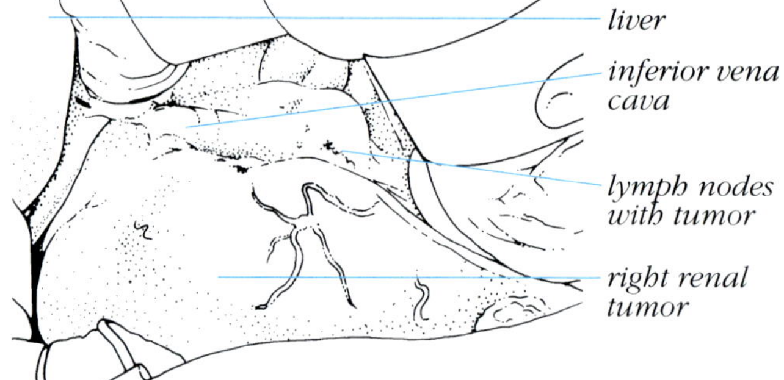

Figure 3.18 Classic radical nephrectomy specimen demonstrating intact Gerota's fascia as well as adrenal gland.

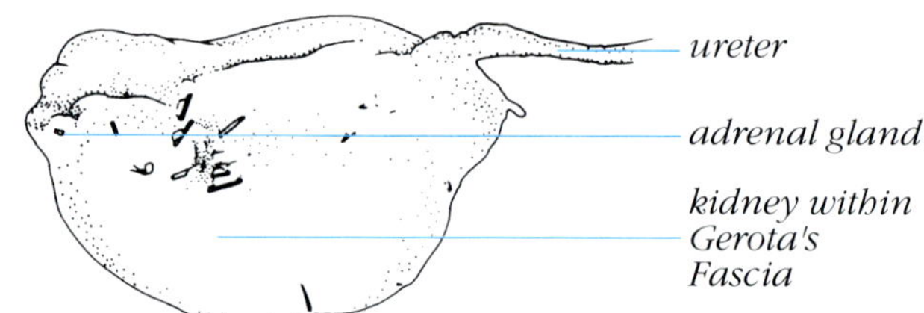

nephrectomy can be performed as a nephron-sparing procedure. Exophytic masses are most amenable to a wedge resection of renal parenchyma in addition to renal tumor (Figs. 3.20, 3.21). Deeply embedded renal tumors involving the renal collecting system may require extensive in situ dissection, necessitating prolonged clamping of the renal artery and perfusion cooling of the renal parenchyma. Warm ischemia times of 20 minutes or less are well tolerated; cold ischemia time may exceed 60 minutes with minimal renal effects. Surgical judgment must be exercised before beginning wedge resection, as the renal parenchyma is quite vascular and unexpected hemorrhage may require hurried renal artery occlusion with possible risk of intimal injury and renal spasm.

Because 50% of renal tumors are found incidentally on CT scanning of the abdomen, enthusiasm has increased in recent years for partial nephrectomy of incidentally noted small tumors that are favorably located on the periphery or on the superior or inferior pole of the kidney. Surgical techniques are not altered under these circumstances, and the decision to proceed with a partial nephrectomy is based more on the assessment for possible residual satellite tumors in the ipsilateral kidney; the incidence of such ipsilateral tumors may be as high as 12%.[8] In addition, if a choice is made for enucleation rather than wedge resection of the tumor, residual disease may be present in the enucleation bed in 20% to 40% of cases.[9] Extracorporeal (bench) surgery for extensive dis-

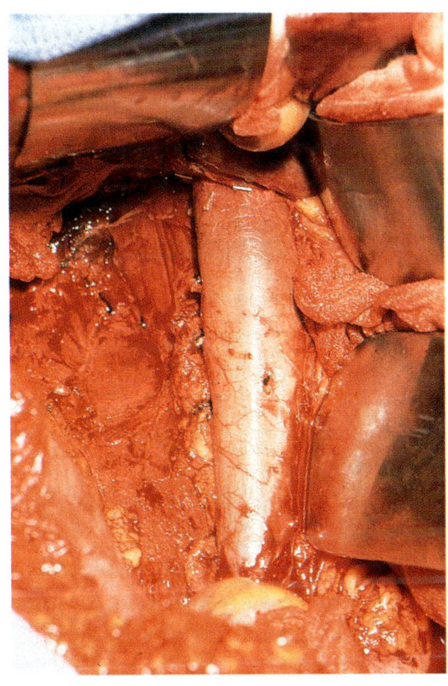

Figure 3.19 Renal bed after right radical nephrectomy leaving posterior abdominal wall musculature exposed as well as the surface of the inferior vena cava.

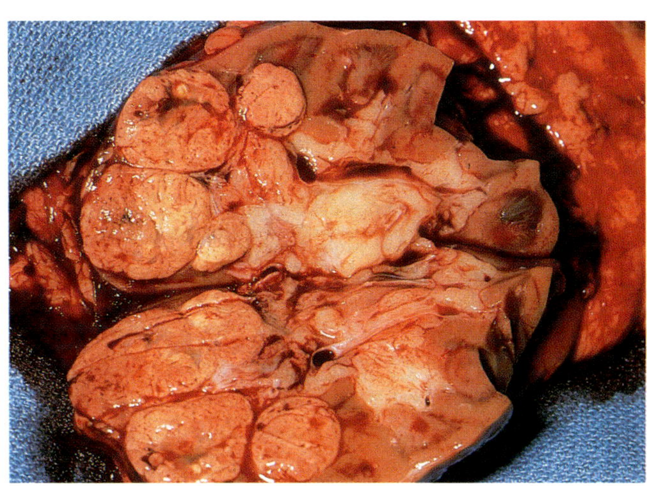

Figure 3.20 Bivalved renal tissue demonstrating multifocal renal cell carcinoma in a 67-year-old female patient with bilateral synchronous tumors.

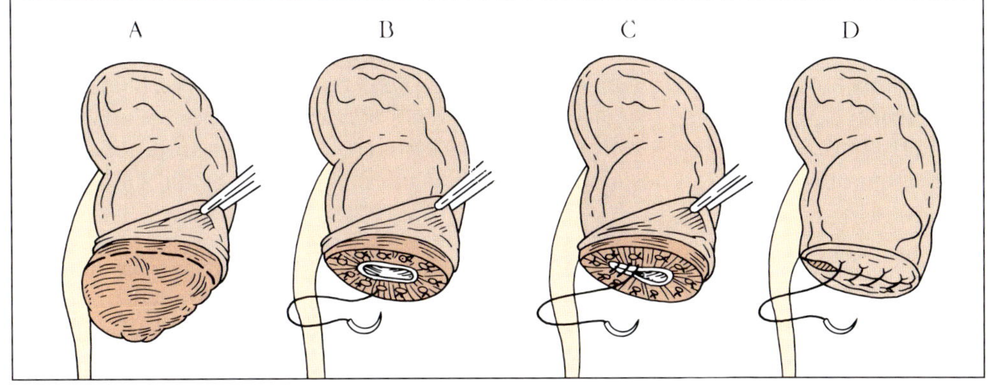

Figure 3.21 Partial nephrectomy may be performed in exophytic tumors. Suture ligation of blood vessels and closure of renal capsule must be accompanied by repair of the collecting system to prevent urinary fistula formation. **A** Line of intended excision. **B** Ligation attained by suture ligation. **C** Collecting system being closed. **D** Capsule closed over the severed parenchyma.

section of tumors in solitary kidneys has been reported, but if in situ dissection can be accomplished with regional cooling perfusion, that is the preferred technique.

SURGICAL TECHNIQUE   Before arterial occlusion with vascular bulldogs or clamps, mannitol (12.5 g) should be given intravenously to promote osmotic diuresis and preserve nephron function during ischemia. The perfusate solution can be prepared by adding 50 g of albumin to 1000 mL of lactated Ringer's solution. The solution should be chilled to 4°C and infused through an 18-gauge butterfly needle proximal to the vascular clamping. A clamp on the renal vein should precede venting of the renal vein with a small incision. Perfusate will flush through the renal parenchyma rapidly if elevated 100 cm above table height. In addition to perfusate, ice slush of normal saline should be available to pack around the renal parenchyma to augment cooling. A plastic or foam jacket can be placed around the kidney to prevent associated organ cooling or loss of irrigant into the abdomen or flank (Fig. 3.22).

Entry points of catheters and the venting incision in the renal vein can be repaired by standard vascular technique with fine, monofilament, nonabsorbable sutures. Frozen section analysis of renal parenchymal margins should be performed at the time of the in situ or ex vivo dissection to ensure that complete tumor excision has been accomplished. Collecting system violations can be detected by intravenous indigo carmine testing. Urinary staining should be promptly noted. The renal collecting system can be repaired with interrupted and running small-caliber chromic sutures. Renal vessels are visualized easily on end and can be occluded with figure-of-eight chromic sutures. Renal repair is effected before release of clamps on the renal vessels to allow renal capsule suturing with large, horizontal mattress, chromic sutures. Renal parenchyma turgidity will increase with reperfusion, allowing compression of small vessel bleeders.

Special Circumstances

REGIONAL LYMPH NODE DISSECTION   As discussed earlier, the utility of extensive regional lymph node dissection in renal cell carcinoma is dubious because of the diffuse lymphatic communications to the renal parenchyma. Nevertheless, extensive dissection of the paraaortic and interaortocaval and paracaval tissues may be a useful adjunct to nephrectomy when extensive lymph node involvement is present. The template for this dissection is very similar to that for retroperitoneal dissection for testicular tumors. Care should be taken to avoid extensive suprahilar dissection above the left renal artery, as injury to the lymphatic trunk and cisterna chyli may predispose to lymphocele formation. Caution should be exercised in dissecting the anterior surface at the aorta superior to the left renal artery, since the superior mesenteric artery may be confused with a renal vessel in cases of distorted anatomy associated with large renal tumors.

BILATERAL TUMOR   In cases of bilateral renal cell carcinoma, it is recommended that bilateral partial nephrectomies be performed when possible. In cases of extensive unilateral disease, a contralateral partial nephrectomy should be performed first to verify viability of that renal unit before proceeding to radical nephrectomy. Bilateral enucleation of renal cell carcinoma in cases of VHL disease seems reasonable, as the biologic potential of these tumors appears to be less aggressive than synchronous sporadic renal cell carcinoma.

VENOUS THROMBUS   The propensity for renal cell carcinoma to invade vascular spaces is well recognized. In small venules, renal cell tumor emboli and thrombi may be noted microscopically in 70% of tumors. Involvement of renal vein by renal cell carcinoma is very common, occurring in 20% of patients (Fig. 3.23). Vena cava involvement may be present in 5% to 10% of patients (Figs. 3.24–3.26).

There is a greater likelihood of vena cava involvement with right-sided tumors. Preoperative MRI should be performed for all moderate-sized tumors involving the right kidney and for most large left-sided tumors (see Fig. 3.10). Venous involvement of the adrenal vein may also be noted, by direct extension to the adrenal parenchyma and the adrenal vein. It is imperative that the superior and inferior extent of the vena cava thrombus be noted preoperatively: the choice of surgical incision is influenced significantly by the distinction between infrahepatic and suprahepatic tumor thrombus. If tumor thrombus is pre-

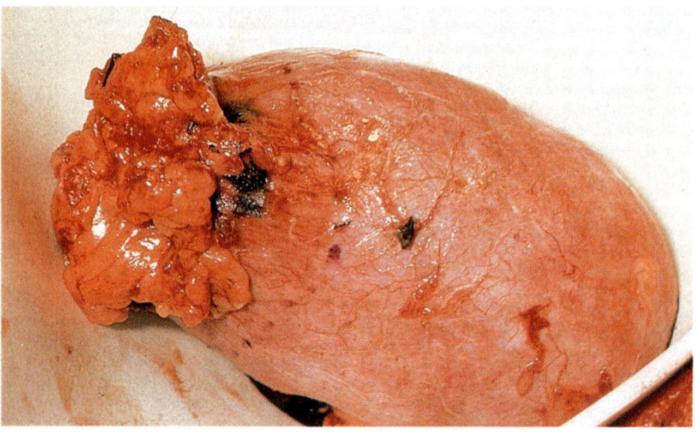

Figure 3.22 Upper pole renal cell carcinoma immediately before partial nephrectomy. Note surrounding fat preserved on tumor surface, also the surrounding dam (white) preventing slushed ice contacting other tissues.

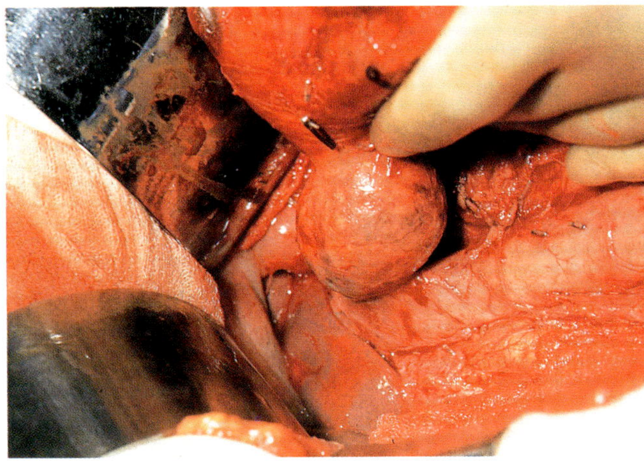

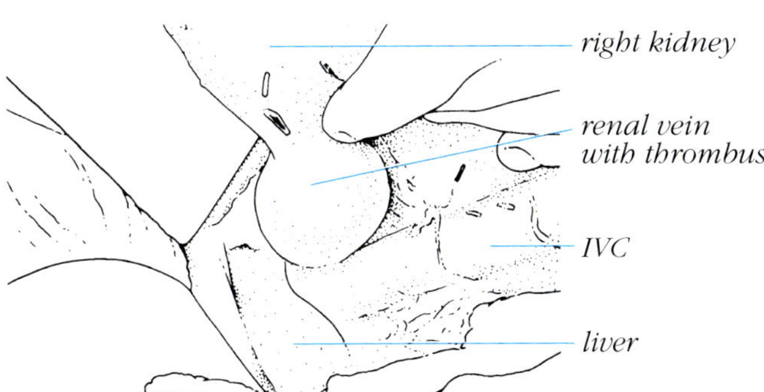

Figure 3.23 Renal cell carcinoma tumor thrombus in the renal vein immediately adjacent to the inferior vena cava (IVC).

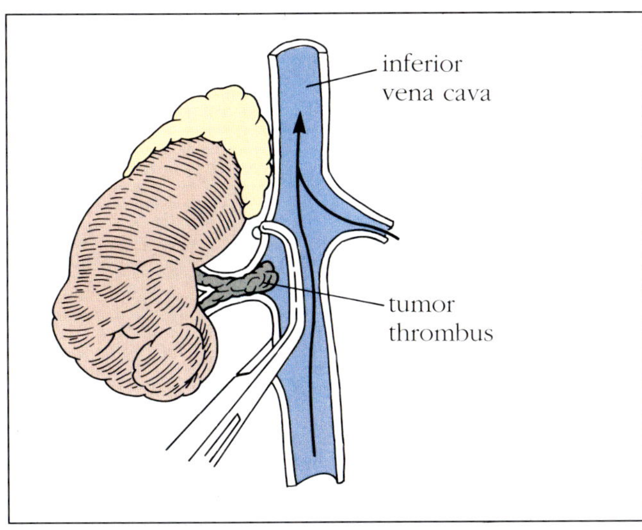

Figure 3.24 Placement of a partial occlusion clamp on the inferior vena cava permits opening of the renal vein and extraction of any free-floating tumor thrombus at the time of kidney removal.

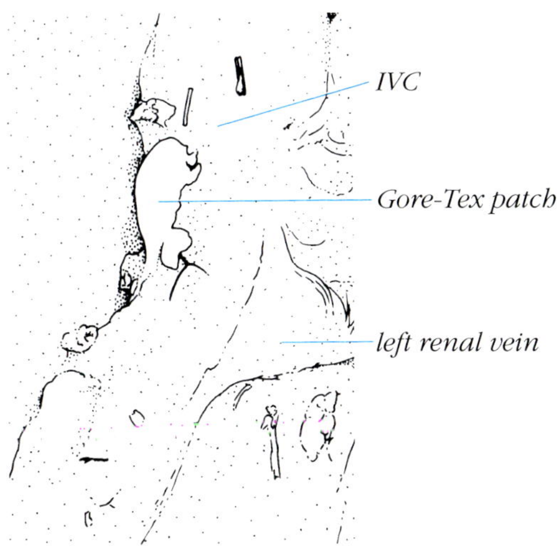

Figure 3.25 Satinsky vascular clamp partially occluding the inferior vena cava (IVC) for resection of tumor thrombus within renal vein and IVC.

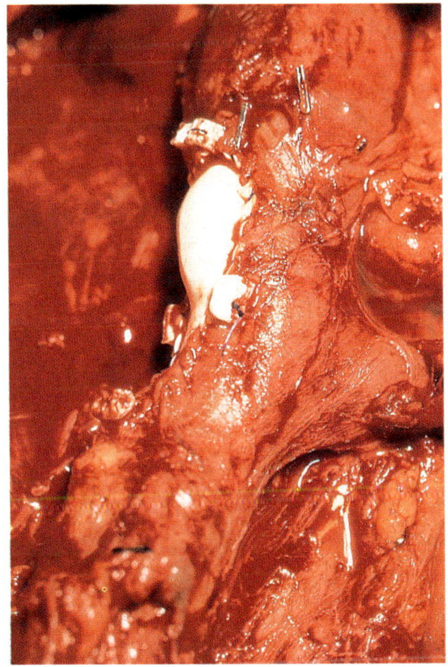

Figure 3.26 Gore-Tex patch repair of the inferior vena cava (IVC) after venous resection for tumor thrombus. (Courtesy of H.I. Pass, MD)

sent above the liver, there is significant risk for right atrial involvement (Fig. 3.27). Transesophageal echocardiography may be helpful in identifying thrombus in the right atrium, as may MRI and superior venacavography. The distribution of tumor thrombi in a group of patients with T (any),M+ disease is shown in Figure 3.28.[10]

Incomplete excision of direct invasion of the vena cava wall results in a median survival rate similar to that of other poor prognostic groups, including lymph-node-positive patients and patients with local extension to adjacent organs. The 5-year survival rate of all patients who undergo nephrectomy, regional lymphadenopathy, and vena cava tumor thrombectomy for renal cell car-cinoma is between 20% and 60%. The previously reported poor survival rate of patients with vena cava wall invasion may reflect inadequate resection with positive margins. For T3c,N0,M0 patients with negative vena cava surgical margins, the 5-year survival rate is 55%.[10] These data suggest that the ability to distinguish ad-herence of tumor thrombus is a strong predictor of outcome and may be important intraoperatively.

Intraoperative ultrasonography of vena cava thrombus allows such a determination and may obviate extensive heroic surgery in selected patients (Figs. 3.29–3.31). The ability to characterize the vena cava intraoperatively may also clarify contradictory results of MRI and venacavography, suggesting the presence or absence of vena cava thrombus.[11]

METASTECTOMY   Solitary metastases are is present in 2% to 4% of renal cell carcinoma patients at initial diagnosis. Resection of a solitary metastasis of renal cell carcinoma may be indicated in selected cases, as a survival time of 4 or 5 years can be seen in 15% to 50% of patients. Metastectomy is justified when technically feasible. In most cases the metastasis takes the form of a pulmonary nodule, frequently on the ipsilateral side. This favors a thoracoabdominal approach with simultaneous nephrectomy and pulmonary wedge resection.[12]

Medical Management

Metastatic renal cell carcinoma is for all practical purposes a uniformly fatal condition. A unique pattern of metastasis

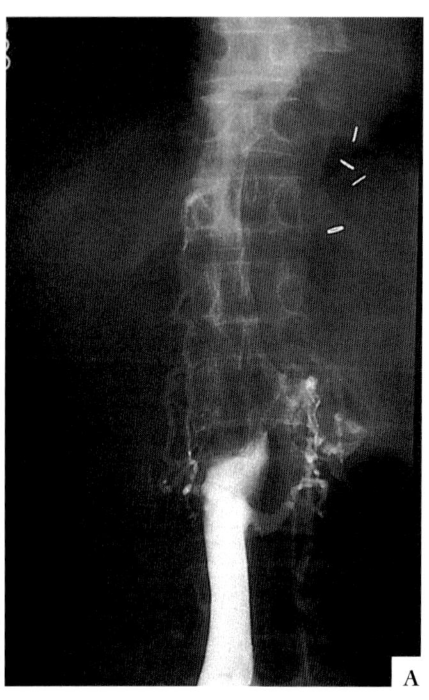

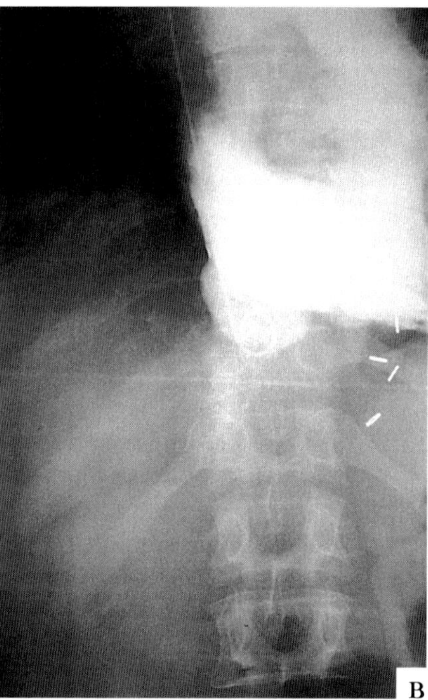

Figure 3.27 Complete occlusion of inferior vena cava in a 72-year-old female with right renal cell carcinoma. Inferior **A** and superior **B** venacavograms show involvement of the right atrium. Cardiopulmonary bypass was required for extraction of thrombus. Attachment of thrombus to hepatic veins was encountered intraoperatively and was not predicted by preoperative studies.

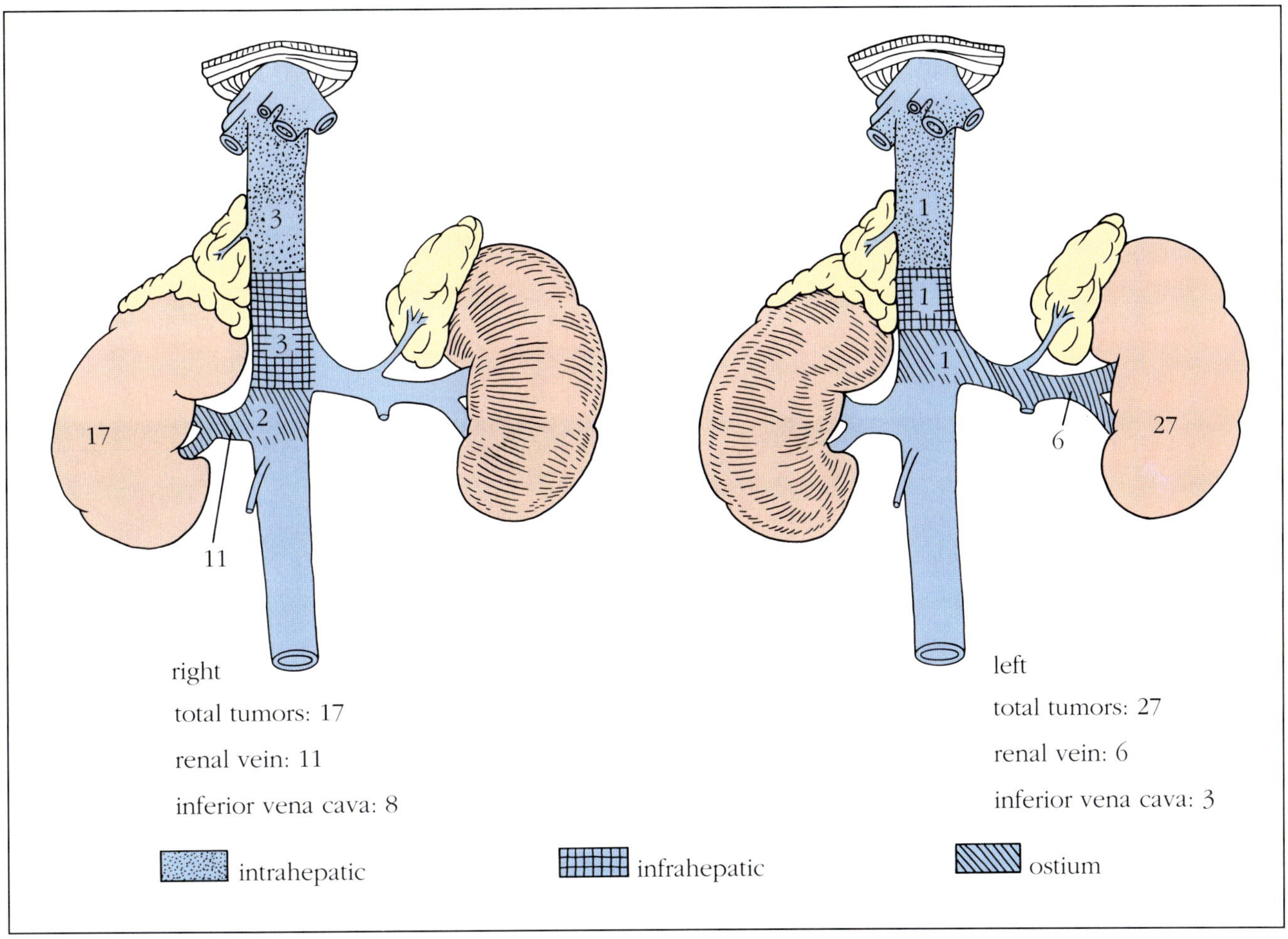

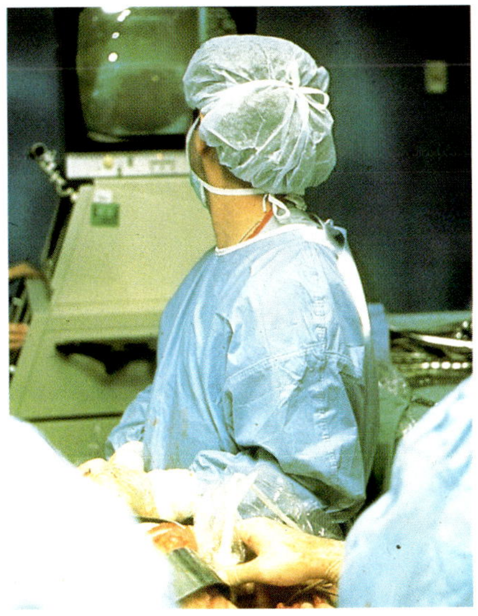

Figure 3.28 Venous thrombosis of renal tumors may be variable in extent. This diagram depicts the distribution in M+ disease in 44 patients. (Adapted from Horan JJ, et al, 1989)

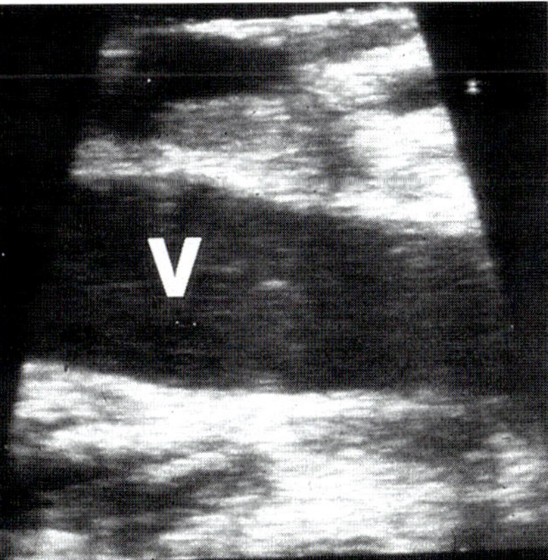

Figure 3.30 Intraoperative ultrasound may be used to assess the vena cava in cases of conflicting preoperative imaging studies. Here the vena cava (V) is free of thrombus.

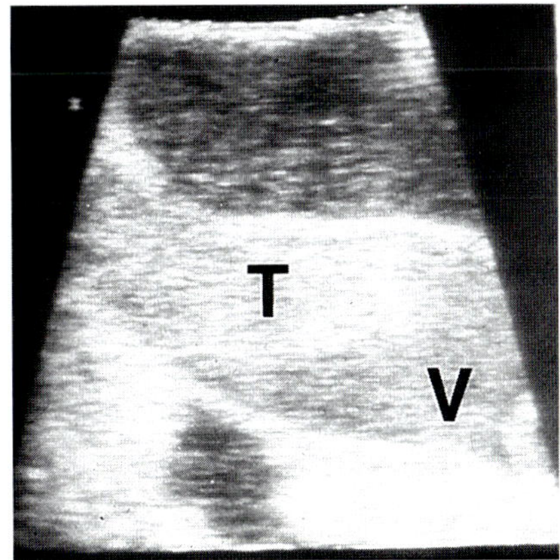

Figure 3.31 Tumor thrombus (T) within the vena cava (V) as shown by intraoperative ultrasound.

Figure 3.29 Intraoperative ultrasound of the vena cava may differentiate between attached and nonattached thrombi of renal tumors (renal cell carcinoma or Wilms'). Note the use of a hand-held probe and video monitor.

may be confounding at presentation (Figs. 3.32–3.35). Renal cell carcinoma is disturbingly refractory to traditional chemotherapy. For unclear reasons, no single chemotherapeutic agent seems to have any significant activity in this disease.[13] Vinblastine, a vinca alkaloid, appears to be the most effective form of single-agent therapy, with an objective response rate of up to 20% (Fig. 3.36). Renal cell carcinoma exhibits a phenomenon of multidrug resistance. Efforts to reduce *p*-glycoprotein activity have not been associated with significant therapeutic responses. Biologic therapy is more promising in the short term. Interferon-

alpha and interferon-gamma have been tested in many trials, yielding minimal activity for interferon-gamma and a 10% response rate for interferon-alpha (Fig. 3.37).[14] Adoptive immunotherapy with transferred lymphokine-activated lymphocytes and high-dose intravenous interleukin-2 is associated with complete resolution of metastatic disease in 10% of patients and partial resolution of metastatic disease in an additional 15% to 20%.[15] An alternative strategy has been the development of cultures of tumor-infiltrating lymphocytes and sensitization with interleukin-2 and interferon-alpha; it is hoped that this will yield tumor-specific

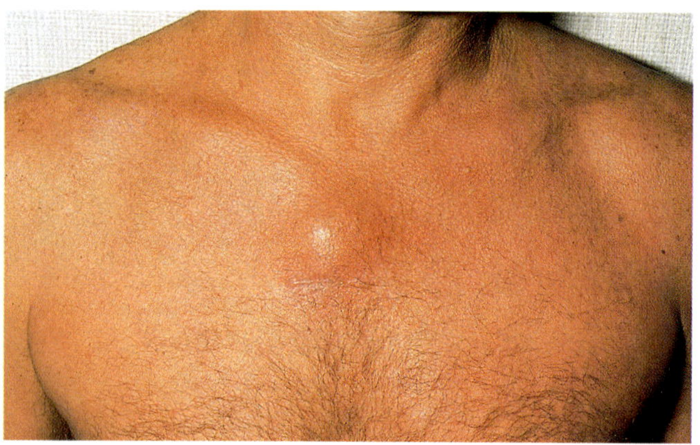

Figure 3.32 Metastatic renal cell carcinoma to the sternum as a presenting sign. The most common metastatic tumor to the sternum is renal cell carcinoma.

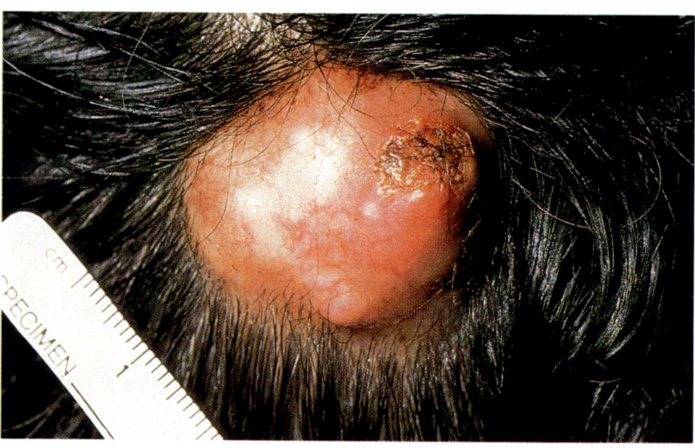

Figure 3.33 Metastatic renal cell carcinoma to the scalp as a presenting sign in a 55-year-old male. This is an example of the variable metastatic potential of renal cell carcinoma.

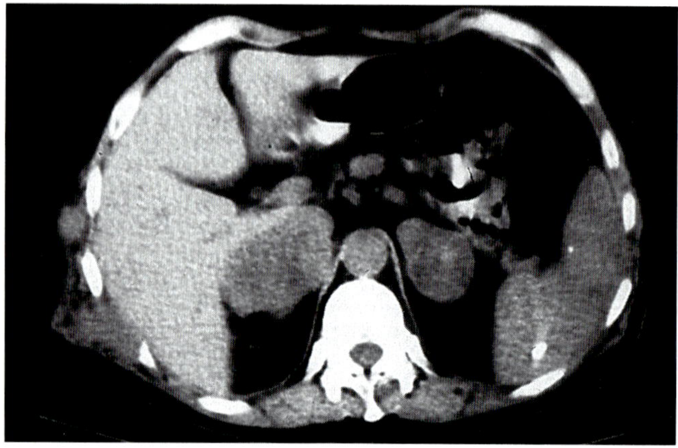

Figure 3.34 Metastasis to right chest wall associated with right renal tumor.

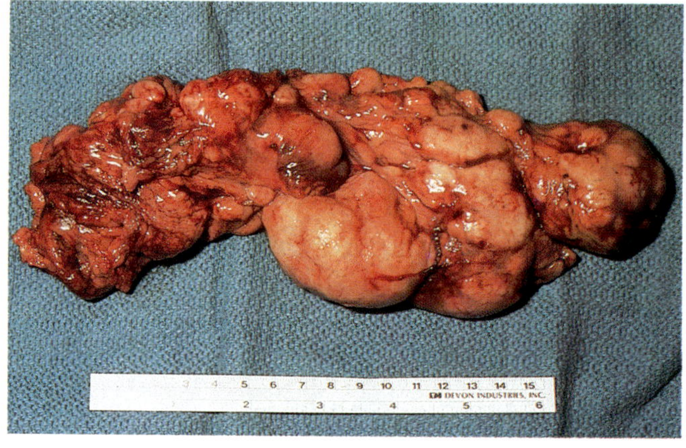

Figure 3.35 Omental metastases in a 54-year-old male patient with right-side renal cell carcinoma.

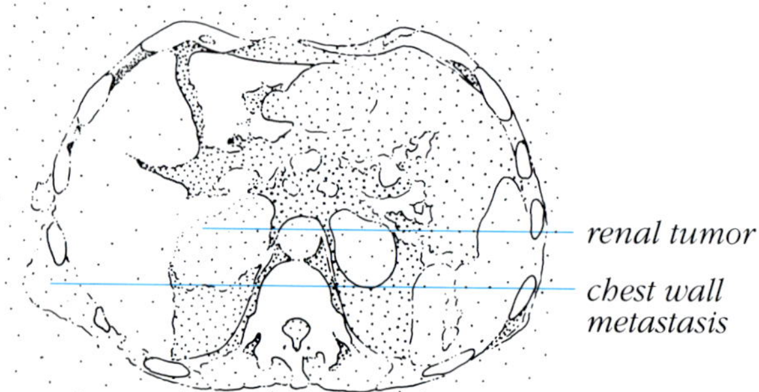

FIGURE 3.36 *Response of Metastatic Renal Cell Carcinoma to Traditional Chemotherapy*

SINGLE-AGENT CHEMOTHERAPY

DRUG	RESPONSE		
Single-Agent Chemotherapy	**Patients**	**Complete**	**Partial**
4′(9-acridinylamine) methanesulfon-*m*-aniside	37	0	1
Baker's antifol	17	1	0
Methotrexate	20	0	2
Ifosfamide	15	0	1
Cyclophosphamide (high-dose)	12	0	0
Methyl-GAG	76	1	6
Chloroethyl-cyclohexy-nitrosourea	23	0	4
5-Fluorouracil	12	0	0
Hydroxyurea	24	0	1
Vinblastine	15	0	2
Actinomycin D	65	0	1
Triazimate	59	1	2
Cis-platinum	32	0	0
Multiple-Agent Chemotherapy			
Vinblastine, chloroethyl-cyclohexy-nitrosourea	93	3	9
Vinblastine, methyl-chloroethyl-cyclohexy-nitrosourea	15	0	1
Vinblastine, methotrexate, bleomycin	14	0	5
Vinblastine, methotrexate, bleomycin, tamoxifen	14	0	5
Vinblastine, cyclophosphamide, 5-fluorouracil	10	0	0
Vinblastine, cyclophosphamide, hydroxyurea, medroxyprogesterone acetate, prednisone	45	1	6
Cyclophosphamide, 5-fluorouracil, vincristine, methotrexate	18	0	0
Vinblastine, cyclophosphamide, doxorubicin, bleomycin, bacillus Calmette-Guérin	14	0	3

FIGURE 3.37 *Minimal Effectiveness of Interferon Gamma in Renal Cell Carcinoma*

AUTHOR	DATE	THERAPY	PATIENTS	PARTIAL RESPONSE	COMPLETE RESPONSE	DURATION/ SURVIVAL
Garnick	2/88	IFN-gamma 30–3000 μg/m² 7/28 d IV	42	3/41	1/41	6, 2, 9, 13 months' duration
Rec. IFN gamma Research Group in RCC	9/87	IFN-gamma 8–12 × 10⁶ U/m² qd × 4 wk IV	32	9.4%	1/30	
		IFN-gamma 40 × 10⁶ U/m² intermittent admin × 8 wk	30	5/30		

lymphocytes that can be reinfused for an augmented effect (Fig. 3.38).[16] Biologic response modification, such as interferon and interleukin-2 therapy, may mediate regression of metastatic disease in 10% to 30% of patients, and these responses may be lasting. Expected survivals have been doubled in selected cases. Further experimental studies will be needed to establish a sufficient impact on metastatic renal cell carcinoma before these therapies can be widely adopted. Cytoreductive surgery may be useful for such immunotherapies (Figs. 3.39, 3.40).

RENAL PELVIC TUMOR

Primary tumors of the renal pelvis are relatively unusual and account for less than 5% of all renal tumors. These tumors are predominantly of transitional cell origin but may occasionally be derived from squamous cells. For purposes of discussion, transitional cell carcinoma is the tumor of concern. Like bladder carcinoma, transitional cell carcinoma of the renal pelvis may be linked to chronic exposure to aniline dyes. Cigarette smoking is also a strongly associated etiologic factor. In addition, phenacetin abuse is specifically associated with upper tract transitional cell carcinomas. *Balkan nephropathy* is an inflammatory process of the renal interstitium of unknown etiology, which has been described in patients of Balkan or Greek origin. It is associated with development of tumors of the renal pelvis. These tumors are usually superficial and of limited biologic potential.

Renal pelvic tumors present predominantly with a history of hematuria and may be associated with pain. Bladder irritation and/or bladder tumor by history may also be present. Histologic grading of transitional cell tumors permits distinction between well-differentiated grade I, moderately well-differentiated grade II, and poorly differentiated grade III and grade IV tumors. Urinary cytology may be unremarkable in grade I and grade II tumors. Grade III to grade IV tumors typically shed obviously malignant cells and may prompt specific diagnostic

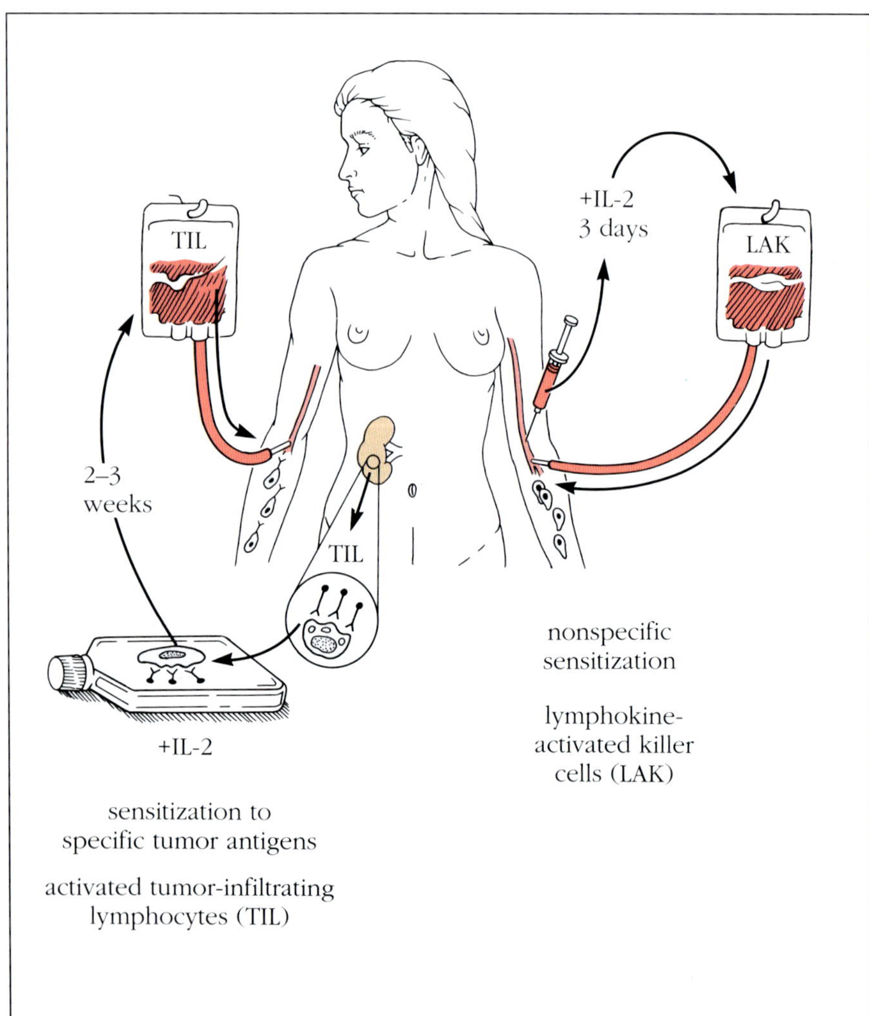

Figure 3.38 Adoptive immunotherapy in renal cell carcinoma may employ tumor-infiltrating lymphocytes (TIL) or lymphokine-activated lymphocytes (LAK cells). (Modified from deKernion JB, Belldegrun A, 1992)

procedures when detected in a voided urine specimen. Patients who present with a history of hematuria should undergo urinary cytology evaluation. If positive, intravenous pyelography and possibly retrograde pyelograms should be performed to delineate further the upper urinary tract. A filling defect noted on intravenous pyelography is a classic sign of renal pelvic tumor; however, it must be distinguished from blood clot, nonopaque urinary calculus, or sloughed renal papillary tissue (Fig. 3.41). To accomplish this discrimination, a noncontrasted CT scan should be performed and compared to a contrasted CT scan. Urinary calculi are readily distinguished in this manner. Retrograde pyelography with associated selected cytologic specimens, comparing the normal side to the abnormal side, should be performed, in addition to brush biopsies of any suspicious lesions noted on intravenous pyelography. Avoidance of retrograde injection of contrast

before collection of selective cytologic specimens and/or brushings may prevent false-positive readings generated by contrast hyperosmolarity. Ureteroscopy can be especially helpful in direct visualization of indeterminate filling defects in the renal pelvis, particularly in cases of negative urinary cytology.

Treatment of renal pelvic tumors is very similar to that for renal cell carcinoma. Radical nephrectomy should be accompanied by ureterectomy and excision of the distal ureter with a bladder cuff. The incidence of distal ureteral carcinoma during the lifetime of the patient is sufficiently high to warrant this additional resection of tissue: tumor recurrence in the ureteral stump may develop in more than 30% of patients treated by nephrectomy and partial ureterectomy alone.[17] Well-differentiated noninvasive lesions are associated with a good prognosis and prolonged survival; however, invasion beyond the muscularis

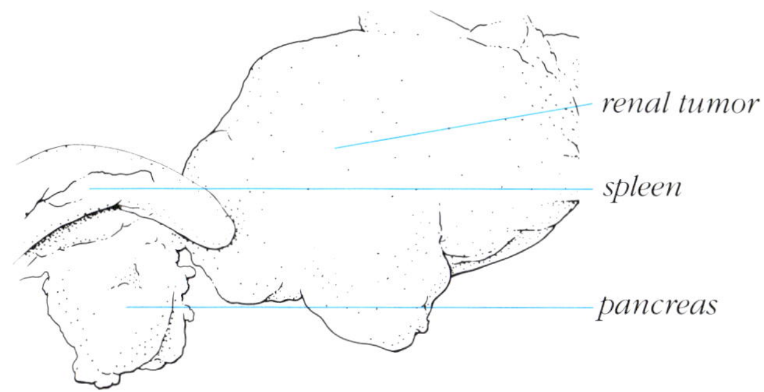

Figure 3.39 Spleen and tail of pancreas resected in continuity with a left-side renal cell carcinoma.

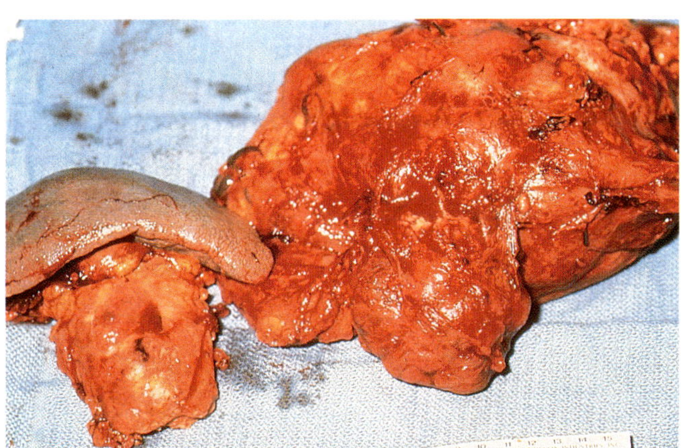

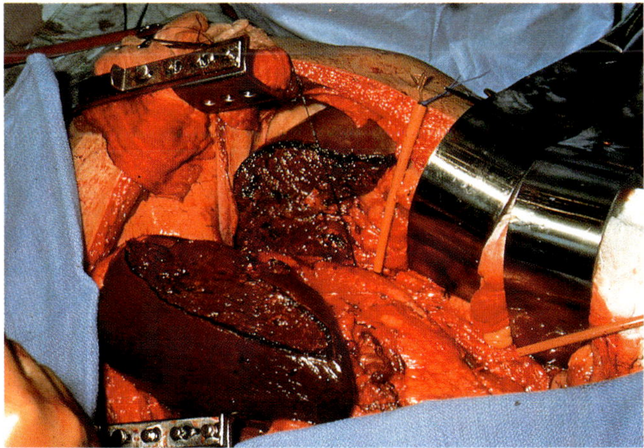

Figure 3.40 Partial hepatectomy in progress for locally invasive right-sided renal cell carcinoma. Note vascular tapes on inferior vena cava.

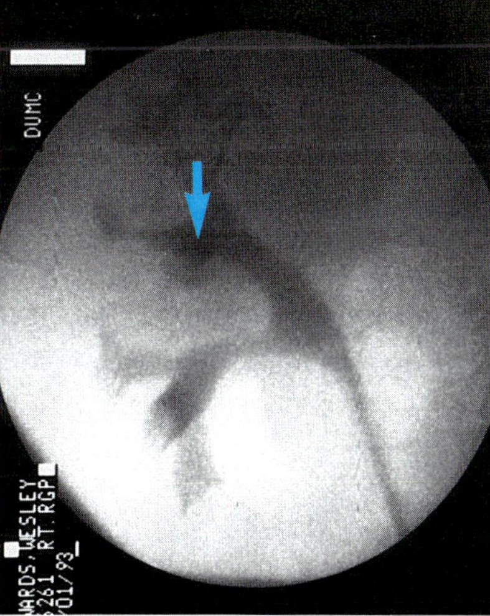

Figure 3.41 Renal pelvic tumor noted on retrograde pyelogram in the right upper pole calyx (arrow) of the right kidney in a 63-year-old male with a history of hematuria. Final pathology revealed noninvasive grade II/III transitional cell carcinoma.

into peripelvic fat may be associated with a remarkably poor course and a 5-year survival rate of 25% (see Figure 3.42 for staging of neoplasms of the renal pelvis and ureter). In solitary kidneys with isolated polypoid tumors, ureteroscopy and partial resection with adjunctive laser therapy may be considered, as well as nephroscopy and excision and laser therapy.

WILMS' TUMOR

Wilms' tumor is the most common malignant neoplasm of the genitourinary tract in children. Each year, 7.8 cases per one million children are reported in a relatively constant rate of incidence. This constitutes approximately 500 new cases annually in the United States.[18] Wilms' tumor occurs most commonly during the first 7 years of life, peaking between ages 3 and 4 years, with an equal distribution between boys and girls. There is a genetic component to this tumor, approximately 1% of patients having a familial variety with an autosomal dominant inheritance pattern. Microscopically, this tumor shows evidence of origin from metanephrogenic blastema, with blastemal stromal and epithelial cell components. This gives rise to a unique mixture of very primitive cells and highly differentiated tubular cells resembling embryonic glomeruli and tubules.[19] Grossly, the tumor appears to be quite fleshy but may have areas of necrosis that lead to cavity formation (Fig. 3.43). Clinically, most cases of Wilms' tumor involve a palpable abdominal mass. Vague abdominal symptoms may occur in 30% of patients. In addition, hypertension may be present in almost 50% of diagnosed children. Bilateral Wilms' tumors are not uncommon and are a hallmark of the familial type.

The management of Wilms' tumor is dependent on stage at diagnosis. Initial therapy for stages I through IV, as well as for high-risk types, includes surgery. Enucleation of bilateral tumors is routinely practiced in an effort to preserve nephron mass before chemotherapy. Vena cava thrombosis is noted in Wilms' tumor, as in renal cell carcinoma, and this should be considered in preoperative therapy. An abdominal approach is preferred for bilateral exploration and confirmation of the extent of disease. Flank approaches are not recommended, as adequate staging cannot be performed and increased tumor spillage is likely. Lymph node involvement strongly

FIGURE 3.42 *TNM Staging for Renal Pelvis and Ureteral Carcinoma*

PRIMARY TUMOR (T)

TX	Primary tumor cannot be assessed.
T0	No evidence of primary tumor.
TA	Papillary noninvasive carcinoma.
Tis	Carcinoma in situ.
T1	Tumor invades subepithelial connective tissue.
T2	Tumor invades the muscularis.
T3	(for renal pelvis only) Tumor invades beyond the muscularis into peripelvic fat or the renal parenchyma.
T3	(for ureter only) Tumor invades beyond the muscularis into periureteric fat.
T4	Tumor invades adjacent organs, or through the kidney into the perinephric fat.

REGIONAL LYMPH NODES (N)*

NX	Regional lymph nodes cannot be assessed.
N0	No regional lymph node metastasis.
N1	Metastasis in a single lymph node, 2 cm or less in greatest dimension.
N2	Metastasis in a single lymph node, more than 2 cm but not more than 5 cm in greatest dimension; or multiple lymph nodes, none more than 5 cm in greatest dimension.
N3	Metastasis in a lymph node more than 5 cm in greatest dimension.

DISTANT METASTASIS (M)

MX	Presence of distant metastasis cannot be assessed.
M0	No distant metastasis.
M1	Distant metastasis.

Adapted from Beahrs OH, et al, 1992
*Laterality does not affect N classification.

affects the prognosis for disease-free survival, and regional lymphadenectomy with selective sampling of abnormal nodes is therefore recommended. Second-look operations are also useful and may dictate the choice of chemotherapy for patients felt to be initially unresectable. Second-look operations may be useful for accurate staging in patients initially treated by a flank approach to nephrectomy. At present, radiation therapy is reserved for stage III and stage IV patients and for all

stages of high-risk patients with clear cell sarcoma (see Figure 3.44 for the National Wilms' Tumor Study 4 protocols). With multidisciplinary therapy including surgery, chemotherapy, and selective radiation therapy, node-negative patients can expect a 2-year survival rate close to 80%, and a 55% survival rate can be expected for node-positive patients. Wilms' tumor may recur at distant time points, which have been described at 9, 10, and 11 years.[20]

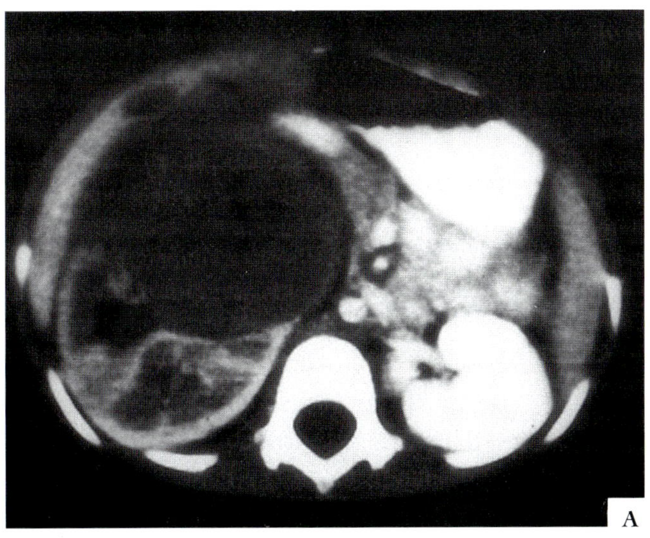
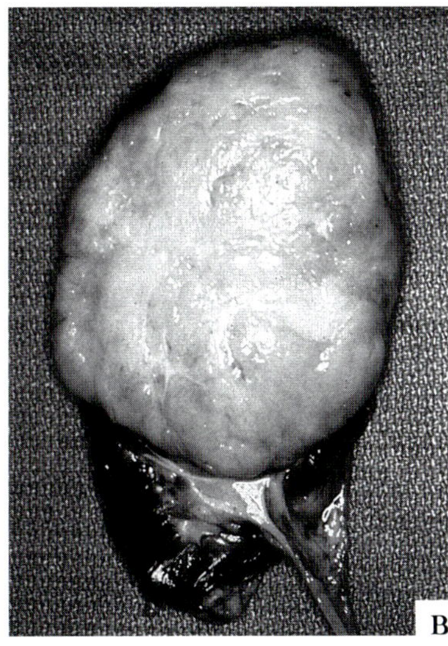

Figure 3.43
A Wilms' tumor with areas of necrosis on right renal mass. **B** Fleshy gross appearance of the same Wilms' tumor.

FIGURE 3.44 *National Wilms' Tumor Study 4 Protocol*

DISEASE	INITIAL THERAPY	RADIOTHERAPY	CHEMOTHERAPY REGIMEN
Stage I/favorable histology, I/anaplastic	Surgery	None	EE—actinomycin D plus vincristine (24 wk) EE—4-pulsed, intensive actinomycin D plus vincristine (15 wk)[†]
Stage II/favorable histology	Surgery	None	K—actinomycin D plus vincristine (22 and 65 wk) K—4-pulsed, intensive actinomycin D plus vincristine (24 and 60 wk)[†]
Stage III/favorable histology	Surgery	1080 cGy	DD—actinomycin D, vincristine, and doxorubicin (26 and 65 wk) DD—4-pulsed, intensive actinomycin D, vincristine, and doxorubicin (24 and 52 wk)[†]
High risk (clear cell sarcoma, all stages) and stage IV/favorable histology	Surgery	Yes*	DD—actinomycin D, vincristine, and doxorubicin (26 and 65 wk) DD—4-pulsed, intensive actinomycin D, vincristine, and doxorubicin (24 and 52 wk)[†]

Data from Mesrobian HG. Wilms' tumor: past, present, future. *J Urol.* 1988;140:231–238.
*Clear cell sarcoma patients receive 1080 cGy and stage IV/favorable histology cancer patients are given 1080 cGy if the primary tumor would qualify as stage III were there no metastases.
[†]Refer to latest National Wilms' Tumor Study protocol for dosage and length of treatment.

COLLECTING DUCT TUMOR

Collecting duct carcinoma is a rare tumor of the collecting ducts of the renal parenchyma. To date, 26 cases have been described in the literature. These tumors typically present as medullary masses, often invading the parenchymal collecting system and giving rise to hematuria. CT scanning reveals a parenchymal mass with necrosis and relative hypovascularity. A histologic papillary pattern is frequently confused with papillary adenocarcinoma of the kidney, a subtype of renal cell carcinoma. Papillary ovarian adenocarcinoma may also be the initial incorrect diagnosis; futile searches for primary ovarian lesions should direct the astute clinician to the renal parenchyma as a primary source for malignancy. These tumors typically present in a younger age group than is usual for renal cell carcinoma, are often associated with metastatic disease, and have an aggressive clinical course and a poor prognosis. Surgical therapy is identical to that for renal cell carcinoma. Embryologically, the collecting ducts represent the terminal differentiation point from the ureteral bud, which may influence the choice of chemotherapy. Some transitional cell carcinomas are responsive to multiagent chemotherapy, and this may offer direction for future cases.[21]

SARCOMA

Sarcomas represent 1% to 3% of malignant renal tumors, and are of mesenchymal origin. Sarcomatoid variants of renal cell carcinoma and the rhabdoid type of Wilms' tumor are not true sarcomas. In addition, retroperitoneal sarcomas may extend into renal parenchyma and be mistakenly identified as primary renal sarcomas.

The clear cell sarcoma of childhood, otherwise known as the bone-metastasizing renal tumor of childhood, is an extremely aggressive primary renal sarcoma. It is more accurately classified with Wilms' tumor, however, and will not be considered in this discussion. Similarly, sarcomatoid renal cell carcinoma is a subtype that demonstrates spindle cells and other features consistent with sarcomas. These tumors have a relatively aggressive clinical course. Rhabdoid tumor of the kidney is a relatively rare pediatric tumor. Mesenchymal elements are present on immunohistochemical evaluation. Treatment strategies are similar to that for clear cell carcinoma and Wilms' tumor.

Among the primary adult renal sarcomas, the most common clinical presentation is that of an enlarging retroperitoneal mass associated with pain and cachexia. Hematuria is not a prominent feature of these tumors. On arteriographic studies, these tumors are avascular or hypovascular. Such a finding should suggest an alternate diagnosis to renal cell carcinoma when large renal masses are evaluated.

The most common type of renal sarcoma is leiomyosarcoma, accounting for between 20% and 60% of cases.[22] Grossly, these tumors are firm and multinodular. Microscopically, bundles and whorls of spindle-shaped cells are present. Fibrosarcomas comprise the remaining bulk of commonly found renal sarcomas, and may represent between 10% and 20% of primary renal sarcomas. This tumor is characterized by a propensity towards renal vein invasion, which occurs in 40% of patients. It grows rapidly and may be confused with undifferentiated adenocarcinoma. Sheets of bland, benign-appearing spindle cells may be seen in association with very anaplastic cells. Rhabdomyosarcoma and liposarcoma occur with equal frequency and have a typical histologic pattern and biologic behavior as for other sites in the retroperitoneum. Local occurrence of liposarcoma is very common. Renal hemangiopericytoma has been reported only occasionally. It is believed that this tumor arises from the renal capsule and has little potential to invade the parenchyma. Hypoglycemia may be associated with this disease.

Treatment of renal sarcomas is predicated on strategies designed to prevent local recurrence. A large, expansive incision should be chosen to allow en bloc resection of contiguous structures, including adjacent organs and possibly great vessels. Adjuvant radiotherapy may be of some benefit in reducing local recurrence rates. Chemotherapy appears to be partially effective, particularly the combination of vincristine, cyclophosphamide, actinomycin D, and doxorubicin.[23]

Benign Tumors

ONCOCYTOMA

Renal oncocytoma is a benign neoplasm composed of oncocytic cells similar to granular cells frequently seen in renal cell carcinoma. Oncocytoma accounts for 3% to 6% of all renal tumors. The median age for this tumor is 60 years. More than two thirds of oncocytomas are discovered incidentally, one third presenting with symptoms of hematuria, flank pain, or palpable mass. Hypertension may be prominent in 25% of cases.

On gross pathologic examination, these tumors appear as solitary, well-circumscribed neoplasms, usually tannish brown to mahogany in color, with a central scar. This is in contrast to the yellowish orange color of a typical renal cell carcinoma. Bilateral and multifocal tumors may occur and the central scar, which is not specific for oncocytoma, may be absent. Microscopically, there is an almost uniform composition of epithelial cells with abundant granular cytoplasm. These cells are typically larger than the granular cells of renal cell carcinoma.

Prognostically, CT scanning of renal oncocytoma usually reveals a distinctly smooth-contoured, marginated, hypodense solid mass (Fig. 3.45).[24] There are no pathonomonic features of oncocytoma on CT scanning. Homogeneous enhancement on contrast imaging is not clearly distinguishable from renal cell carcinoma. Angiography may be more useful, as a distinctive spoked-wheel arterial pattern has been seen in approximately 20% to 30% of patients. Central scarring may be noted on CT scanning. Ultrasonography may be helpful but, again, not clearly diagnostic of a benign tumor. MRI may detect central scarring and demonstrate a homogeneous medium signal intensity. Fine-needle aspiration biopsy may reveal grade I tumor characteristics distinguishable from renal cell carcinoma. These cells may appear similar to normal hepatocytes.

Renal-sparing strategies may be justified in cases where preoperative fine-needle aspiration of a suspected oncocytoma reveals compatible cells. Further experience with preoperative needle aspiration and nephron-sparing surgery must be obtained before this can be uniformly recommended as a treatment strategy. At present, enhancing solid renal tumors are probably best considered primary renal cell carcinomas until proven otherwise.[25]

RENAL ADENOMA

Small tumors histologically indistinguishable from renal cell carcinoma but less than 3 cm in diameter have been termed *renal adenomas.* However, a review of 180 cases of such tumors from the Armed Forces Institute of Pathology did allow a histologic distinction to be made between renal adenoma and renal carcinoma.[26] True renal adenomas may represent premalignant tumors destined to become renal cell carcinomas. Because renal CT scanning carries a limit of resolution well below 1 cm, renal masses between 1 and 3 cm can easily be detected and found to be enhancing, suggesting renal cell carcinoma.

The decision to perform total nephrectomy for such lesions must hinge on the relative risks for incomplete resection. It is probable that alternate foci of "renal adenomas" will be left undisturbed with nephron-sparing surgery, but metastasis arising from a small adenoma is unlikely.

At present, small enhancing renal masses are thought to be renal tumors until proven otherwise, and extirpative strategies are recommended. In cases of planned surveillance of lesions that later proved to be renal cell carcinomas, the growth rate of the tumors has been approximately 0.5 cm annually. No clear mandate for expectant management of these tumors exists at the present time.

ANGIOMYOLIPOMA

Angiomyolipoma is a benign lesion of the renal parenchyma, which may also be termed a *renal hamartoma.* These lesions have a propensity towards spontaneous hemorrhage, partially because of their composition of blood vessels, fat cells, and smooth muscle cells. They may be associated with tuberous sclerosis, and 45% to 80% of such patients develop angiomyolipomas and/or renal cysts by the third or fourth decade of life. For angiomyolipomas associated with tuberous sclerosis, a distinct clinical pattern is recognized (Fig. 3.46). The most common distinguishing features are that bilat-

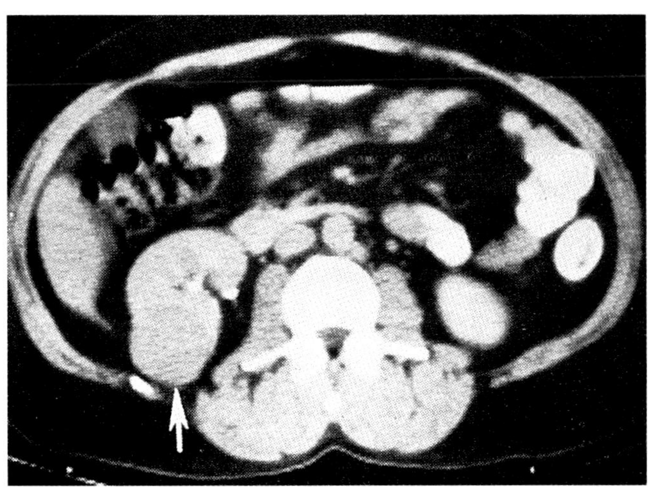

Figure 3.45 Oncocytoma as seen on CT. The initial impression was renal cell carcinoma.

erality is much more frequent in association with tuberous sclerosis and that these tumors are usually small and multifocal. Conversely, solitary large lesions, more commonly noted in women and more commonly unilateral, are associated with angiomyolipoma in patients without tuberous sclerosis.

Symptomatically, these tumors are characterized by sudden hemorrhage of the renal parenchyma with acute pain. Local pressure and invasion of adjacent structures may cause chronic pain, and renal infection may be associated with these lesions. Large tumors may manifest initially by abdominal or flank pain (Fig. 3.47). Small tumors may manifest by sudden spontaneous hemorrhage.

Diagnostic imaging with abdominal CT scanning may reveal pathognomonic features of low-attenuation areas consistent with fat. No other renal neoplasm exhibits such a distinctive appearance. Comparison of imaging modalities for angiomyolipoma detection is useful, but for most practical purposes CT scanning is the primary procedure (Fig. 3.48).

Management of renal angiomyolipoma is dependent on tumor size. Asymptomatic small lesions can be followed annually with ultrasonography. Symptomatic patients can undergo embolization or can be treated by enucleation or partial nephrectomy. Asymptomatic lesions greater than 4 cm are usually observed, whereas larger symptomatic lesions may require complete nephrectomy, subselective embolization or enucleation, or partial nephrectomy (Fig. 3.49).[27]

RENINOMA

Reninoma, or juxtaglomerular cell tumor, may a treatable form of hypertension in young patients. To date, 35 cases have been described in the literature.[28] Ages range from 7

FIGURE 3.46
Clinical Features of Renal Angiomyolipoma With and Without Tuberous Sclerosis

	WITH TUBEROUS SCLEROSIS	WITHOUT TUBEROUS SCLEROSIS
Age (average)	31	48
Sex predilection	Women 2:1	Women 4:1
Renal involvement	Bilateral (80%)	Unilateral (90%)
Number	Multifocal	Solitary
Size	Small	Large

Adapted from Anderson, 1990 (Courtesy of E. Everett Anderson, MD)

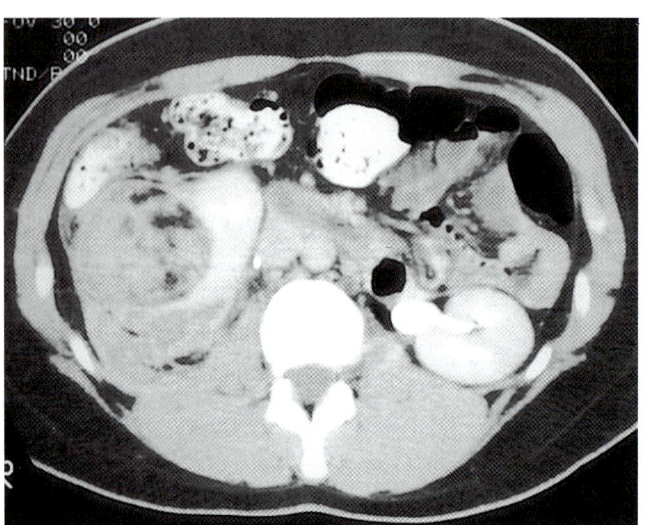

Figure 3.47 Angiomyolipoma in a 26-year-old female with sudden onset of flank pain and hematuria. Note low-density fat in right renal mass.

to 58 years, with a mean age of 24 years. Severe hypertension in young patients may be the only hallmark of this unusual and rare tumor.

Pathologically, these tumors are whitish gray and are well demarcated and encapsulated. They are typically solid but may be cystic. Scattered hemorrhage may be present. Renin-secreting granules may be noted on special stains of involved cells. Electron microscopy reveals the characteristics of human juxtaglomerular cells.

Severe hypertension and elevated peripheral renin activity with associated secondary hyperaldosteronism may prompt initial investigations. In most patients the intravenous pyelogram is normal; however, renal ultrasonography may reveal a solid mass. CT reveals a renal mass but a normal CT scan does not always exclude the diagnosis, as witnessed by description of postmortem cases.

Renal angiography performed in patients undergoing evaluation for renal artery stenosis will reveal normal renal arteries and a hypovascular solid renal mass. This is the scenario in approximately 50% of reninoma patients. The average reported size for this tumor is approximately 3 cm, with a range from 0.2 to 6 cm. Lateralization of elevated renin levels in the setting of normal renal arteries and no renal mass suggests the diagnosis of a small juxtaglomerular cell tumor.

Partial nephrectomy may be possible in selected patients. A majority of previously reported patients have undergone total nephrectomy for therapy.

FIGURE 3.48
Diagnostic Imaging Distinctions Between Renal Carcinoma and Renal Angiomyolipoma

MASS	ULTRASOUND	CT	ARTERIOGRAPHY
Renal cell carcinoma	Echogenic	No fat	80% Vascular
			20% Hypovascular
			Neovascularization
			Arteriovenous fistulas
			Pseudoaneurysms
			Vascular "whorls"
			Invasion of renal vein
Angiomyolipoma	Very echogenic	Fat present	Findings identical to renal cell carcinoma

Adapted from Anderson EE, 1990 (Courtesy of E. Everett Anderson, MD)

FIGURE 3.49 Strategies for Angiomyolipoma Management

Asymptomatic lesion less than 4.0 cm	Annual ultrasonogram
Symptomatic lesion less than 4.0 cm	Observation; renal angiography, subselective arterial embolization; enucleation or partial nephrectomy
Asymptomatic lesion greater than 4.0 cm	Ultrasonogram every 6 months
Symptomatic lesion greater than 4.0 cm	Entire renal unit involvement, do nephrectomy; segmental renal unit involvement, do angiography, subselective renal arterial embolization; enucleation or partial nephrectomy

Adapted from Anderson EE, 1990 (Courtesy of E. Everett Anderson, MD)

References

1. Silverberg E, Boving CC, Squires TS. Cancer statistics 1990. *Cancer.* 1990;40:9.
2. Tannenbaum M. Ultrastructural pathology of human renal cell tumors. *Pathol Annu.* 1971;6:259.
3. Zbar B, Brauch H, Talmadge C, Linehan WM. Loss of alleles of loci on the short arm of chromosome 3 in renal cell carcinoma. *Nature.* 1987;327:721.
4. Chisholm GD. Nephrogenic ridge tumors and their syndromes. *Ann NY Acad Sci.* 1974;230:403.
5. Robson CJ, Churchill BM, Anderson W. The results of radical nephrectomy for renal cell carcinoma. *Trans Am Assoc Genitourin Surg.* 1968;60:122.
6. Beahrs OH, Henson DE, Hutler RVP, Kennedy BJ. *Manual for Staging Cancer.* 4th ed. Philadelphia: JB Lippincott; 1992:201.
7. Selli C, Hinshaw WM, Woodard BH, Paulson DF. Stratification of risk factors in renal cell carcinoma. *Cancer.* 1983;52:899.
8. Blackley SK, Ladaga L, Woolfett RA, Schellhammer PF. Ex situ study of the effectiveness of enucleation in patients with renal cell carcinoma. *J Urol.* 1988;140:6.
9. Marshall FF, Taxey JB, Fishman EK, Chang R. The feasibility of surgical enucleation for renal cell carcinoma. *J Urol.* 1986;135:231.
10. Horan JJ, Robertson CN, Choyke PL, et al. The detection of renal cell carcinoma extension into the renal vein and inferior vena cava. *J Urol.* 1989;142:943.
11. Hatcher PA, Anderson EE. The management of renal cell carcinoma with renal vein and vena cava tumor thrombus. *Probl Urol.* 1990;4:273.
12. Long JP, Choyke PL, Shawker TA, Robertson CN, Pass HI, Walther MM, Linehan WM. Intraoperative ultrasound in evaluation of tumor involvement of inferior vena cava. *J Urol.* 1993;150:13.
13. Pouillson DR, deVere White R. Surgery of renal cell carcinoma. *Urol Clin North Am.* 1993;20:263.
14. Vugrin D. Systemic therapy of metastatic renal cell carcinoma. *Semin Nephrol.* 1987;7:156.
15. Muss HB. Interferon therapy for renal cell carcinoma. *Semin Oncol.* 1987;14:36.
16. Rosenberg SA. The development of new immuno-therapies for the treatment of cancer using interleukin 2. *Ann Surg.* 1988;203:121.
17. deKernion JB, Belldegrun A. Renal tumors. In: Walsh PC, et al, eds. *Campbell's Urology.* 6th ed. Philadelphia, Pa: WB Saunders Co; 1992:1053.
18. Robertson CN, Linehan WM, Pass HI, et al: Preparative cytoreductive surgery in patients with metastatic renal cell carcinoma treated with adoptive immunotherapy with IL2 or IC2 plus LAK cells. *J Urol.* 1990;144:614.
19. Strong DW, Pearse HD. Recurrent urothelial tumors following surgery for transitional cell carcinoma of the upper urinary tract. *Cancer.* 1976;38:2173.
20. Young JL, Miller RW. Incidence of malignant tumors in US children. *J Pediatr.* 1975;86:254.
21. Kramer SA. Wilms' tumor. *Probl Urol.* 1990;4:237.
22. Clausen N. Late recurrence of Wilms' tumor. *Med Pediatr Oncol.* 1982;10:557.
23. Kennedy SM, Marino MJ, Linehan WM, Roberts JR, Robertson CN, Newmann RD. Collecting duct carcinoma of the kidney. *Hum Pathol.* 1990;21:449.
24. Srinivas V, Sogani PC, Hayden SI, Whitmore WF. Sarcomas of the kidney. *J Urol.* 1984;132:13.
25. Beccia DJ, Elkort RJ, Krane RJ. Adjuvant chemotherapy in renal leiomyosarcoma. *Urology.* 1979;13:652.
26. Cohan RH, Dunnick NR, Tegesys GE, Korobkin M. Computed tomography of renal oncocytoma. *J Comput Assist Tomogr.* 1984;8:284.
27. Moul JW. Renal oncocytoma. *Probl Urol.* 1990;4:207.
28. Murphy GP, Mostofi FK. Histologic assessment and clinical prognosis of renal adenoma. *J Urol.* 1970;103:31.
29. Lingeman JE, Donohue JP, Radwin JA, Selke F. Angiomyolipoma: emerging concepts in management. *Urology.* 1982;20:566.
30. Perinelli R, Graziadei Z. A renin-secreting tumor. *Nephron.* 1987;46:380.
31. Anderson EE. Renal angiomyolipoma. *Probl Urol.* 1990;4(2):230.

CHAPTER 4

Adult Tumors
of the
Ureter and Bladder

William A. See

Robert Dreicer

Michael B. Cohen

Epidemiology

In 1991 approximately 50,000 new patients presented with tumors of the urinary collecting system.[1] These tumors represent the most common neoplasm involving the urinary tract in women, and the second most frequent genitourinary tumor in men. Urothelial neoplasms have a male to female preponderance of 4:1. These lesions typically manifest in the sixth and seventh decades of life; however, there is a broad range from the pediatric to the geriatric population. Although they may occur at any site along the urinary collecting system, the vast majority of urothelial neoplasms occur in the bladder. Figure 4.1 shows the relative distribution of urothelial tumors within the urinary tract.

Etiology

As with any organ, tumors involving the urinary collecting system may arise from any tissue element: epithelial, mesenchymal, or hematopoietic. Figure 4.2 lists the spectrum of histologic neoplasms that have been reported to arise in the urinary bladder. Despite this apparent diversity, most tumors involving the urinary bladder and upper tract collecting system arise from epithelial elements. The majority of these are transitional in histology (90%), followed distantly by squamous cell carcinoma (5%) and adenocarcinoma (2%). The ensuing discussion will be limited to these three most common histologic types.

TRANSITIONAL CELL CARCINOMA

Neoplasms of the transitional epithelium were one of the earliest types of tumor to be associated with environmental risk factors. In 1895 Rehn noted a markedly increased incidence of bladder tumors in German workers employed in the aniline dye industry.[2] Since this original report, an increased risk of bladder tumor formation has been identified in a number of other industries, including leather, rubber, and paint manufacturing.[3,4] Other risk factors identified as a result of epidemiologic studies include smoking (thought to be related to nicotinic acid), residing in an urban environment, age (80% of transitional cell carcinomas are found in those patients over 50 years), sex (about 4:1 male to female ratio), and race (a higher incidence among whites).[3,5] Chronic use of cyclophosphamide or analgesics containing phenacetin is known to predispose to bladder neoplasms, although the contribution of these etiologies to the total number of bladder cancers is small.[6,7] Lastly, there are a number of other chemicals that have been implicated, most notably artificial sweeteners, but the evidence remains controversial.[3,4]

The general mechanism by which environmental carcinogens predispose to transitional cell tumors has been established. Systemic absorption followed by urinary excretion of the primary carcinogenic compound and its metabolites exposes the urinary epithelium to "concentrated" drug levels for prolonged periods of time. Interaction of the urine-solubilized carcinogen with the

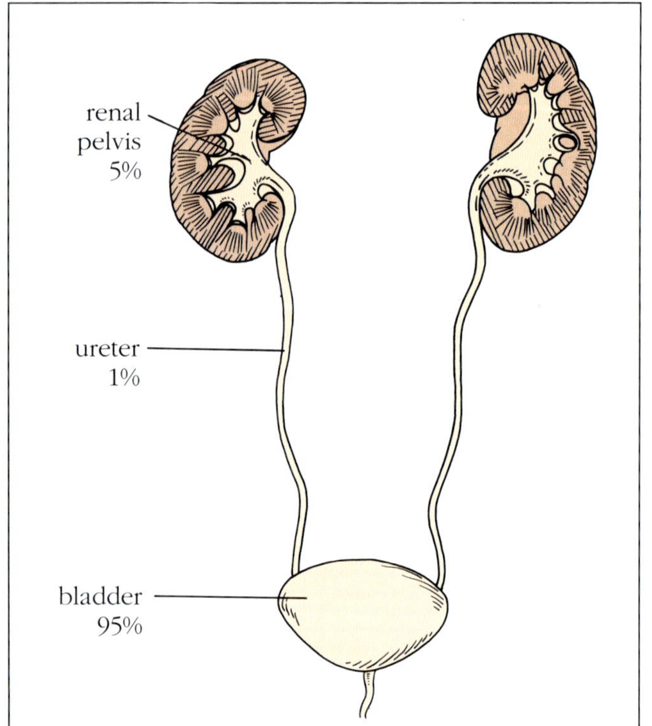

Figure 4.1 The distribution of urothelial malignancies within the urinary tract.

urinary epithelium at the bladder–lumen interface results in what has become known as contact chemical carcinogenesis.[8] In 1954 McDonald and Lund performed the classic experiment that excluded a "blood-borne" etiology, when they showed that bladder pouches isolated from the urinary stream of carcinogen-fed animals failed to develop the tumors observed in urothelium that remained exposed to the urine.[9]

While it is clear that carcinogens excreted in the urine predispose to neoplastic transformation of the transitional epithelium, the precise molecular mechanism by which they do so remains undefined. Although the initiation and promotion phases of general chemical carcinogenesis may be said to apply to urothelial transformation as well, in reality these terms only serve to mask a misunderstanding of molecular events that ultimately result in the malignant phenotype.

SQUAMOUS CELL CARCINOMA

Squamous cell carcinoma is relatively rare in this country, accounting for less than 5% of cancers in the bladder and ureter. The prevalence of this histologic phenotype in other nations has been attributed to the presence of the blood-borne parasite *Schistosoma haematobium*. In areas where schistosomiasis is endemic, up to 75% of all bladder cancers have a squamous histology.[10] However, the incidence of upper tract tumors remains low. Chronic inflammation resulting from the host response to the parasite and its egg in the bladder wall is felt to be etiologic in the tumor development. Like transitional cell carcinoma in these sites, there is a male predominance of about 60%.

In this country, chronic bladder irritation has been implicated as an etiologic factor for the development of squamous cell carcinoma. Risk factors that have been associated with this tumor include prolonged placement of urinary catheters, particularly in paraplegic individuals, recurrent urinary tract infections, and bladder stones.[3,4] Between 10% and 25% of bladder and ureteral squamous cell carcinomas are associated with stones at some time in the patient's history.[4] It is assumed that the prolonged inflammatory response leads to squamous metaplasia, which ultimately undergoes neoplastic transformation.

ADENOCARCINOMA

Adenocarcinomas of the bladder and ureter are extremely rare, accounting for less than 2% of all bladder and ureteral cancers. The sex distribution is very similar to transitional cell carcinoma, with 70% having been reported in men.[4] Bladder extrophy is a well-recognized risk factor for the development of adenocarcinoma, although this association accounts for only a small percentage of all adenocarcinomas seen in this location. Similarly, adenocarcinomas have been associated with urachal remnants but, again, are relatively uncommon. Interestingly, 40% of patients with adenocarcinomas of the bladder have a concurrent or previous history of stones.[4]

FIGURE 4.2 *Classification of Primary Bladder Neoplasms*

	BENIGN	**MALIGNANT**
Epithelial	Transitional cell papilloma	Transitional cell carcinoma
	Squamous cell papilloma	Squamous cell carcinoma
	Villous adenoma	Adenocarcinoma
		Mixed carcinoma
	Carcinoid	Small cell undifferentiated carcinoma
	Pheochromocytoma	
		Malignant melanoma
		Germ cell neoplasm
Mesenchymal	Leiomyoma	Leiomyosarcoma
		Rhabdomyosarcoma
	Hemangioma	
	Neurofibroma	
	Granular cell tumor	
		Osteosarcoma
Hematophetic		Plasmacytoma
		Malignant lymphoma
Miscellaneous		Carcinosarcoma

Gross Morphology

On the basis of gross morphology, transitional cell carcinomas of the bladder and ureter can be divided into papillary (exophytic) and sessile types. Papillary tumors account for about 70% of all bladder cancers and are most commonly located on the lateral walls and trigone (Figs. 4.3, 4.4). Sessile neoplasms, which have a similar distribution in the bladder, may or may not be associated with a minor papillary component and usually have a large ulcerating crater in the midportion (Figs. 4.5, 4.6). Hemorrhage and necrosis may be found in these sessile tumors. Similar gross morphologic findings have been observed in transitional cell neoplasms involving the ureter, but there is a marked disparity in location, with most tumors arising in the distal third. Transitional cell carcinoma in situ typically has no identifiable gross findings, although endoscopically it has classically been associated with a "patchy, velvety red" appearance. Because transitional cell carcinomas are very often multifocal, a careful examination is necessary to record the number of tumors in addition to their location and size.

The gross morphologic findings of squamous cell carcinoma are most similar to the sessile transitional cell tumors, typically presenting as a single nodular, ulcerating mass in the region of the trigone. Squamous cell carcinoma in situ, particularly if it is keratinizing, may appear as leukoplakia. Adenocarcinomas are also usually single and often involve the trigone and dome. In the latter instance, consideration must be given to an adenocarcinoma arising from a urachal remnant.

Pathology

HISTOLOGIC MORPHOLOGY

The pathologist provides important information to the urologist relevant to the subsequent management of individuals with urothelial neoplasms. In examining histologic sections of these lesions the pathologist must discuss a number of important features. The three most important are the histologic type, the grade, and the stage of the tumor.

The histologic type is readily recognized in most tumors. Focal squamous and/or glandular differentiation may be seen in poorly differentiated transitional cell carcinomas, but the tumor should still be classified as such. Only if the tumor is "purely" squamous or glandular should it be classified as a squamous cell carcinoma or

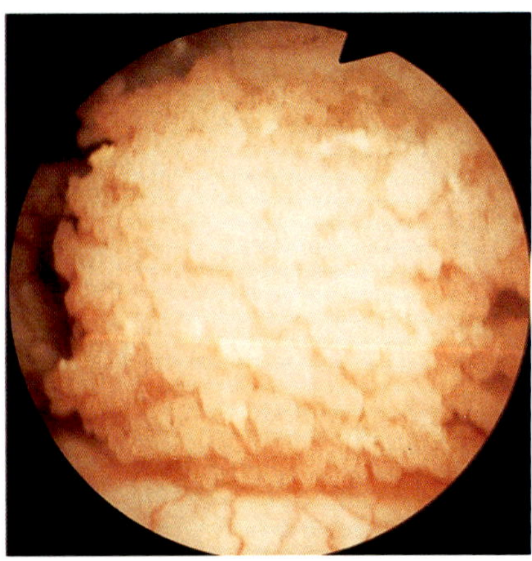

Figure 4.3 An endoscopic photograph of a typical, papillary, low-grade, transitional cell bladder neoplasm.

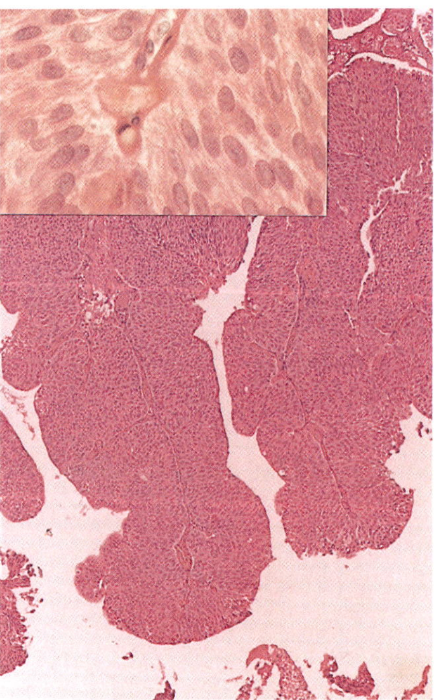

Figure 4.4 Low-power (×40) and high-power (×400) photomicrographs of a low-grade (I), papillary transitional cell bladder carcinoma. Note the clear frond formation in the low-power view and the lack of atypia seen at higher power.

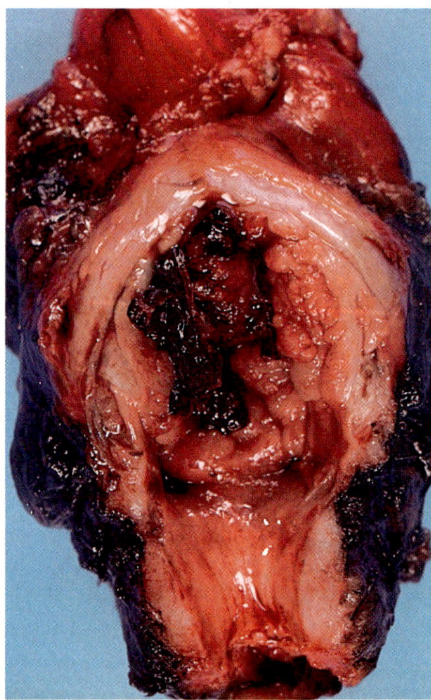

Figure 4.5 Gross specimen from a radical cystoprostatectomy done for muscle-invasive transitional cell bladder cancer. The sessile neoplasm can be seen protruding into the bladder lumen on the left side of the photograph.

adenocarcinoma. Particularly in the case of adenocarcinomas, another primary site must be excluded, i.e., prostate, colon, or a metastasis from a distant site. Although there are other histologic types of bladder tumors (see Fig. 4.2), they account for less than 2% of all bladder tumors.

Grading of tumors has been shown to be relatively subjective.[11] Over time there has been a trend towards collapsing the number of grades that are used to describe transitional cell tumors (Fig. 4.7). Broders originally introduced a four-grade scheme that was modified by the World Health Organization (WHO) to three.[12,13] More recently Murphy has introduced a two-grade scheme that needs further evaluation before it becomes accepted.

The grading of squamous cell and adenocarcinomas has been more difficult to apply reproducibly. Although three grades—well, moderately, and poorly differentiated—have been applied, it is Murphy's contention that all these types of tumors are high-grade since they do not at all resemble normal transitional epithelium.

Histologic grading is a useful prognostic indicator. For example, Gilbert et al., in a retrospective study of 365 patients with papillary transitional cell carcinoma, were able to correlate recurrence and progression with the histologic grade.[14] Of 155 patients with initial grade I tumors, 146 (94%) were alive or died of intercurrent disease. Eighty-three (57%) of these 146 patients had recur-

rences, 83% of which were of the same grade. Nine (6%) patients died of bladder cancer, all of whom had recurrences, and in 78% of the cases these were of higher grade. In contrast, of 23 patients with grade III superficial bladder cancer, 15 (65%) were alive or died of intercurrent disease. Seven (47%) of these 15 patients had recurrences, 5 of which were muscle-invasive. Of the 8 (35%) patients who died of bladder cancer, 5 (63%) died of the initial tumor. There were 70 patients with grade III muscle-invasive disease at presentation. Fifty-eight (83%) died of bladder cancer, and in 71% of the patients it was from the initial tumor.

As is the case for tumor grading, the staging system is in a process of evolution. Jewett's original 1946 classification for the bladder has been modified to the current TNM system, introduced about 15 years ago (Fig. 4.8).[15–17] By and large, all of these staging schemes are based on the depth of invasion into the wall of the bladder. In assessing histologic material, it is important to pay particular attention to the involvement of muscle. It has only recently been recognized that the bladder has a muscularis mucosae, and thus the subepithelial tissue can be divided into lamina propria and submucosa.[18] The muscularis mucosae is often interrupted and therefore may be difficult to identify, particularly in small transurethral biopsies. The distinction between muscularis

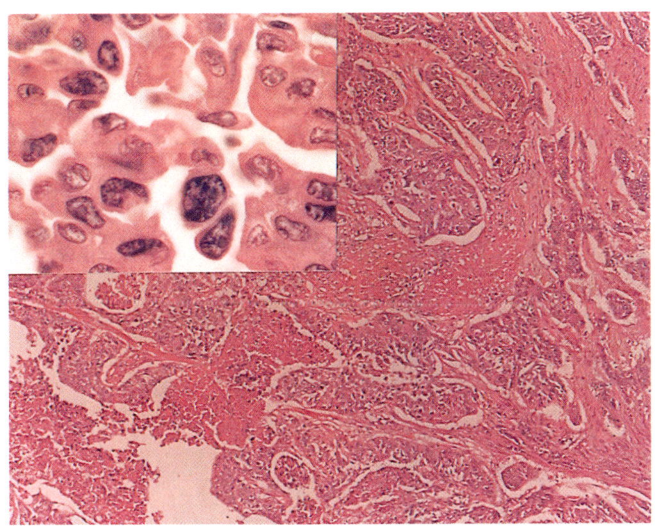

Figure 4.6 Low-power (×40) and high-power (×400) photomicrographs of a high-grade (III), muscle-invasive, transitional cell bladder carcinoma. Nests of cells are seen infiltrating between smooth muscle bundles of the bladder wall. Marked nuclear pleomorphism is present in the high-power view.

FIGURE 4.7 *Grading Schemes for Transitional Cell Neoplasms*

	BRODERS	**WHO**	**MURPHY**
Papilloma	No	Yes	Yes
Carcinoma	4 Grades	3 Grades	2 Grades

mucosae and muscularis propria is crucial, since invasion of the muscularis mucosa has different implications than invasion of the muscularis propria. The distinction between lamina propria invasion and submucosal invasion has recently been suggested to be an important prognostic factor and in the future may therefore be important therapeutically as well.[19] Careful distinction between these two muscle bundles is critical to proper staging and, consequently, patient management.

The staging system for the ureter was adapted from that of the bladder (Fig. 4.9).[17] One important difference, however, is the absence of a muscularis mucosae in the ureter. Further, the distinction between superficial and deep muscle bundles of the muscularis propria has not been applied. Nonetheless, there is striking similarity in both staging systems.

There is correlation between the stage and the grade of the tumor. Typically, noninvasive papillary tumors are grade 1/3, whereas sessile tumors are grade 3/3; the correlation is far from perfect, but both provide important prognostic information.

The staging systems for both these sites recognize local and distant tumor spread as high-stage disease. Local spread involves extension to adjacent structures, which obviously varies with the site of the primary tumor. Distant tumor spread includes the regional and paraaortic lymph nodes and the liver, lung, and bone, in decreasing order of frequency.[4] The cause of death in patients with bladder or ureteral cancer is most often uremia, carcinomatosis, or pneumonia.[4]

Like grading, staging is a useful, independent, but imperfect predictor of biologic behavior of bladder and ureteral cancers. In a study of 850 patients by the National Bladder Cancer Group (NBCG), 67% had superficial disease (TA/T1), 20% had muscle-invasive disease, and 10% presented with metastatic disease.[20] Although more than 95% of the patients with superficial disease attained disease-free status, prolonged follow-up showed about a 45% recurrence rate at 2 years, but only a 3% progression rate to higher-stage disease. In patients with muscle-invasive disease, about 70% can be rendered disease-free, although the 5-year survival varies between 38% for T2 tumors and 16% for T3b tumors.

In addition to tumor type, grade, and stage, additional histologic features should be addressed. Besides confirming the gross morphologic findings of the location, size, and number of tumors, lymphatic and vascular invasion should also be diligently sought, as well as the extent of disease and the adequacy of the margins of resection. Finally, careful assessment of the adjacent urothelium is important. The finding of carcinoma in situ in the neighboring urothelium should be specifically mentioned in the pathology report. Lesser degrees of intraepithelial atypia and dysplasia should probably also be mentioned, although the therapeutic implications remain controversial.

Dysplasia is a concept that is not well accepted in the bladder, unlike other anatomic sites such as the cervix or colon. It is reasonable to assume that there is a spectrum of intraepithelial atypia that should be recognizable mor-

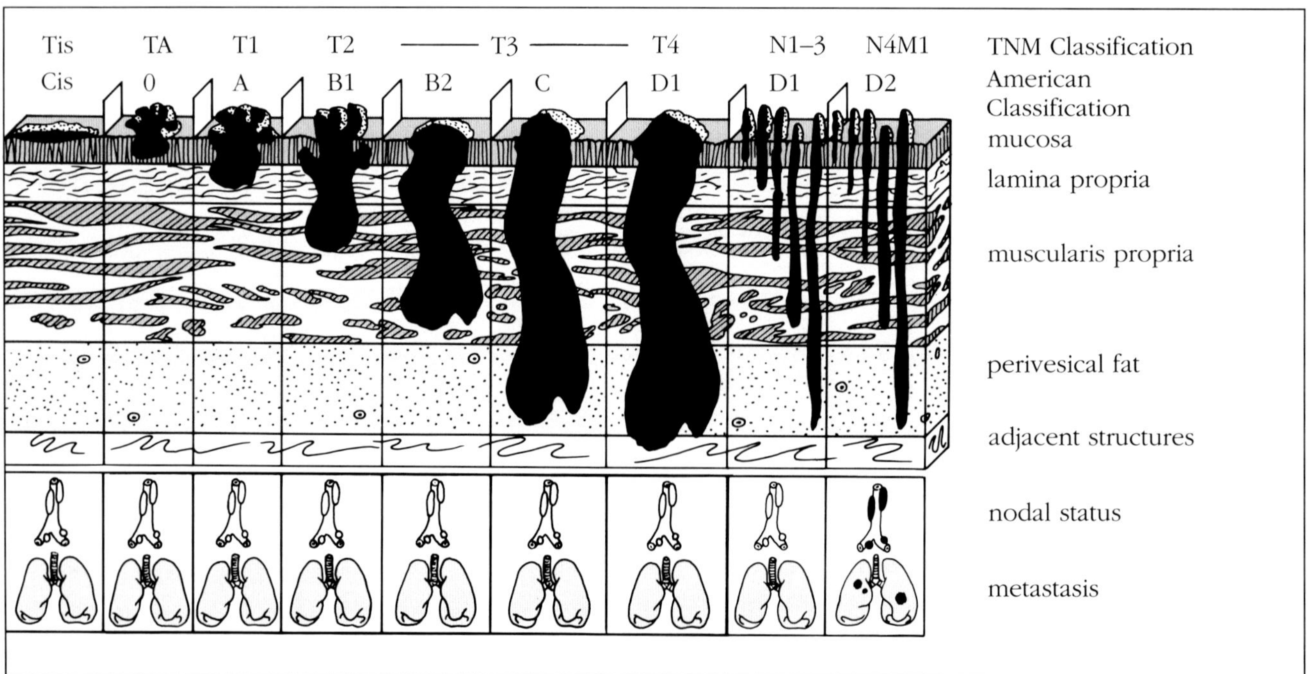

Figure 4.8 The TNM and Jewett (American) staging systems for bladder neoplasms.

phologically prior to the development of carcinoma in situ. The major advocate of this term is Murphy, but his comments are based on a rodent model of chemically induced bladder cancer, which may not apply to human bladder cancer.[3] However, most pathologists recognize *atypia* in flat lesions that do not fulfill their criteria of malignancy and will report them. The biggest problem in this area is that the natural history of dysplasia is unknown, and thus it may not be a precursor/preneoplastic lesion as is generally accepted in the cervix. Clearly, additional studies need to be done.

There are some other difficulties that face the histopathologist. The identification of the muscularis mucosae in the bladder has already been discussed. Another is the diagnosis of papilloma. The more recent grading schemes recognize this entity, although in reality the diagnosis is very unusual. The morphologic criterion is basically one of exclusion—a papillary tumor with a covering epithelium that lacks atypia. Grade 1/3 papillary carcinomas may demonstrate a mild degree of atypia. The distinction is often very subjective. Further, the biology of both of these types of tumors is indolent. Low-grade pap-

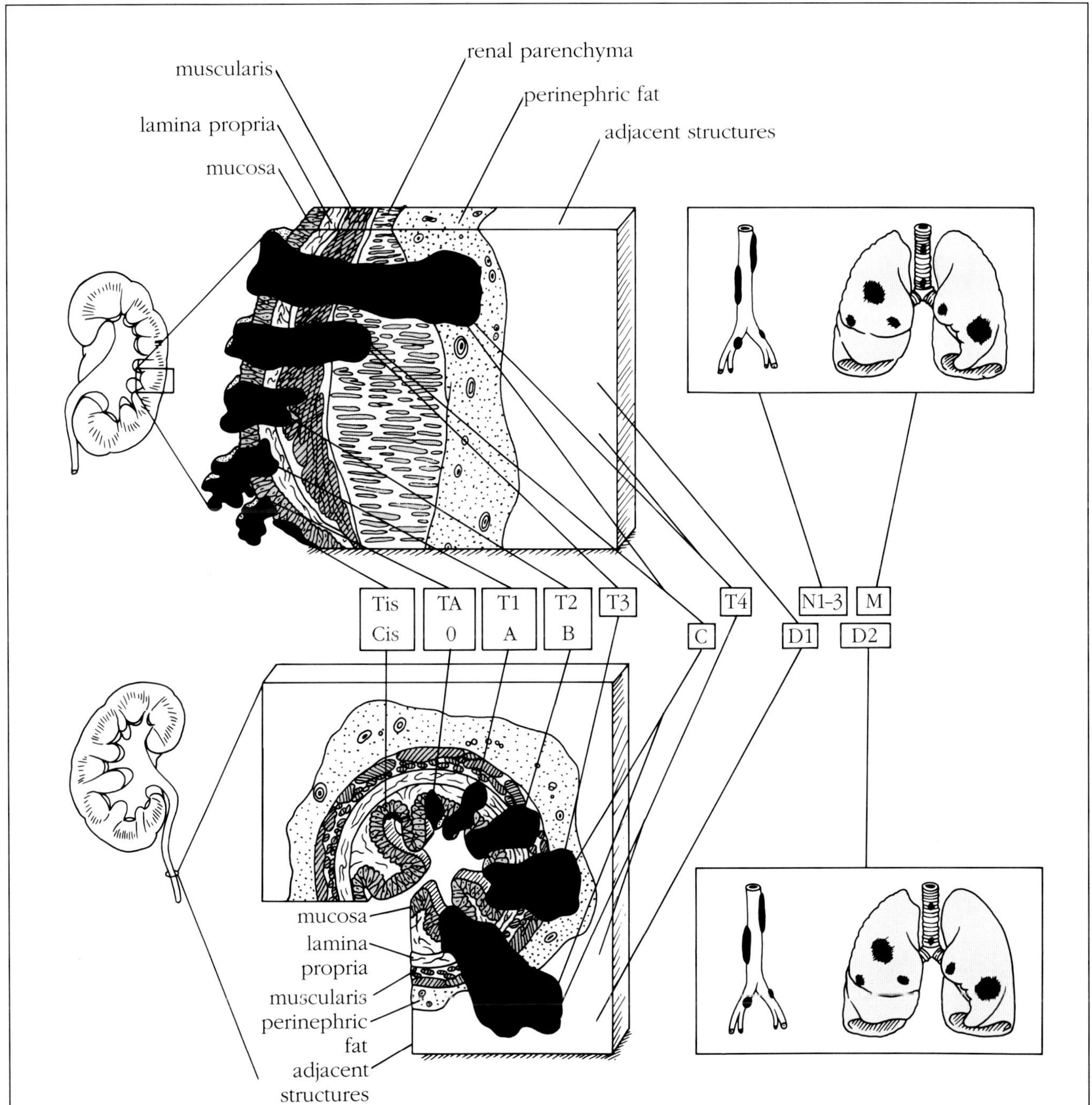

Figure 4.9 The TNM staging system for neoplasms involving the upper tract collecting system.

illary transitional cell carcinomas "recur" but do not often progress to higher grade or stage tumors. Therefore, the distinction between papilloma and low-grade papillary carcinoma may not be therapeutically important.

CYTOLOGY

As an organ readily accessible for the collection of exfoliated cells, the bladder is ideally suited to cytologic assessment. Indeed the role of cytology in the diagnosis and follow-up of patients with bladder cancer is generally accepted. Its role for upper tract disease, i.e., the ureter, is more limited.[21] This technique has been particularly useful for monitoring patients with histories of bladder cancer and, to a lesser extent, certain high-risk groups.[22] With patients falling into the former category, urinary cytology is a relatively noninvasive means of following patients. In the latter instance, this approach has been of use in detecting primary tumors, particularly carcinoma in situ.

The literature suggests that the accuracy of cytology in detecting bladder malignancies is quite variable. In El-Bolkainy's 1980 review, urinary cytology had a mean diagnostic sensitivity of 74% (range 44% to 97%).[23] To a large extent this is related to the grade of the tumor. In early studies by Esposti and coworkers and Farrow and coworkers, the accuracy of cytologically diagnosing histologic grade I tumors was under 25%.[24,25] More recently Murphy and coworkers and Shenoy and coworkers have reported accuracies in the 60% to 70% range.[26,27] Thus, even in the best of hands, about one third of low-grade transitional cell carcinomas, usually papillary tumors, will not be recognizable to the cytologist. Higher-grade tumors (WHO grades II and III) are diagnosed with much greater degrees of accuracy. For example, in the four studies cited above, the mean sensitivity for grade III tumors was about 87%.[24–27] Carcinoma in situ, which is morphologically a high-grade tumor, is also readily recognized.

The cytologic morphology of bladder cancer, i.e., transitional cell carcinoma, has been described by numerous authors (Figs. 4.10, 4.11).[22,27,28] As noted earlier, the major difficulty is in diagnosing low-grade, predominantly papillary tumors. This difficulty is illustrated in Figure 4.12; there is not often concordance of the cystoscopic, histologic, and cytologic findings. This is in part related to the limitations of cytology. However, the three aspects of patient evaluation, cystoscopy, histology, and cytology, must be correlated (Fig. 4.13). There are a number of

FIGURE 4.10 *Key Cytologic Textures of Transitional Cell Carcinoma*

	BENIGN	LOW-GRADE	HIGH-GRADE
Cell size	Uniform	Uniform	Variable
Cytoplasm	Finely vacuolated	Homogeneous	Variable
Nuclear location	Central	Eccentric	Eccentric
N/C*	Low	Increased	Increased
Nuclear size	Small	Enlarged	Variable
Nuclear pleomorphism	Absent	Minimal	Prominent
Chromatin	Finely granular	Finely granular	Coarsely granular
Nucleoli	Variable	Absent	Variable

* Nuclear-cytoplasmic ratio
Modified from Murphy WE, 1989

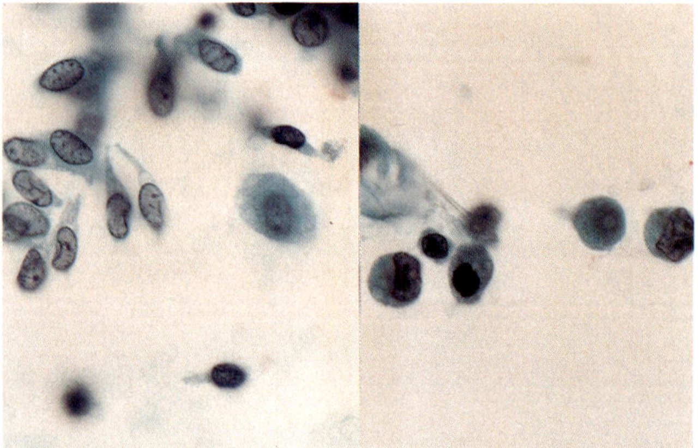

Figure 4.11 Cytologic specimens from low-grade (left) and high-grade (right) transitional cell carcinomas (both ×400).

other morphologic pitfalls, including polyoma virus infection, radiation effects, chemotherapy-induced alterations, and stones. In such cases patient history is important in order to report clinically useful results. To some extent a variety of nonmorphologic features influence the accuracy of urinary cytology. These have been summarized by Farrow and include the number of tumors, tumor size, and tumor configuration (papillary versus sessile).[25]

From the pathologist's and urologist's standpoints, both false-negative and false-positive diagnoses are of particular concern. A brief discussion of the issue of false-negative diagnoses was mentioned above. In large part this is related to the grade of the tumor, although there may be other contributing factors. Farrow et al. have nicely shown that actual false-positive diagnoses are relatively rare.[25] In a careful follow-up of such patients, more than 85% subsequently had cystoscopic and/or histologic evidence of tumor. Therefore, apparent false-positive diagnoses, especially if they are high-grade, should not be ignored.

ANCILLARY STUDIES

There are a variety of special studies available to the pathologist to obtain additional information regarding the tumors. By and large, these remain within the realm of the research laboratory and have not been routinely used clinically.

Electron microscopy provides little additional information, particularly as it applies to the management of individual patients. Its main use has been in the classification of poorly differentiated tumors. Immunohistochemistry has been extensively studied, particularly with the use of cytokeratins and blood group antigens. Cytokeratin expression has been studied in an attempt to delineate neoplastic transformation and to predict the biologic behavior.[29] By and large, no consistent phenotypic alteration has been identified. A correlation between tumor progression and specific blood group antigen loss has been noted.[30,31] However, the separation is far from perfect and is not routinely applied. A variety of other bladder-cell-related antigens have been studied, and some of these seem to correlate with the biologic potential of the tumors.[32,33] Further studies in the area of biomarkers are needed.

Most studies of bladder tumors have focused on the use of ploidy analysis, that is, measuring DNA content. As a rule, diploid tumors have a better prognosis than aneuploid tumors, but again the separation is not perfect.[34] Ploidy analysis has been applied to histologic and cytologic samples, but in some laboratories it is not routinely used for the diagnosis or management of patients with bladder or ureteral tumors.

In a related series of studies, attempts are being made to correlate the biologic behavior of tumors with their proliferative activity. Using a variety of techniques to

FIGURE 4.12 *Typical Case of "Recurrent" Low-Grade Bladder Cancer*

DATE	CYTOSCOPY	HISTOLOGY	CYTOLOGY
6/80	−	nd	−
7/81	+	nd	−
7/81	+	PTCC	Dysplasia
10/81	−	nd	Suspicious
3/82	−	nd	Suspicious
6/82	+	PTCC	Suspicious
8/82	−	nd	−
12/82	−	nd	−
3/83	−	nd	−
6/83	−	nd	−
9/83	−	PTCC	−
3/84	−	nd	+
6/84	+	nd	−
7/84	+	PTCC	−
10/84	−	Dysplasia	+

nd = not done
PTCC = papillary transitional cell carcinoma

assess proliferation, most of which are immunohisto-chemical, the percent of cells in S-phase can be correlated with the grade and stage of the tumor.[35,36]

In attempting to understand the etiology and patho-genesis of bladder cancer, recent work has focused on the role of oncogenes. Although deletion, overexpression, and the expression of a mutant form of the oncogene product have been identified, the role of oncogenes remains unknown. To date, most of the study has focused on the *ras* gene family.[37] At this time, the altered expression of oncogenes, or tumor suppressor genes, has been shown to be useful in predicting tumor progression or response to treatment.

Presentation

MICROSCOPIC HEMATURIA

Hematuria is by far the most common presenting symptom for both upper and lower urinary tract tumors. Over 85% percent of patients with urothelial neoplasia will have this associated finding.[38,39] For this reason, a clear understanding of the evaluation of the patient presenting with hematuria is germane to the discussion of tumors of these organs.

Up to 13% of asymptomatic adult patients may present with microscopic hematuria.[40] Figure 4.14 lists an abbreviated differential diagnosis for this common finding. It is the clinician's responsibility to distinguish those patients with benign conditions from those with malignant urinary tract diseases. Since tumors of the urinary tract primarily affect the adult population, the following discussion will focus on this group of patients.

As with any disease, a thorough history and physical examination constitute the framework for further evaluation. Clearly, the differential diagnosis in an elderly male with flank pain and a palpable flank mass will be different from that of a sexually active female who presents with urinary frequency and urgency, despite the fact that both may have microscopic hematuria. Historical evaluation must include any record of urologic diseases or urologic manipulation, as well as any background of urinary tract infections, calculus disease, or prior neoplasms. A history of local or constitutional symptoms as well as prior traumatic injury must be sought. A complete physical examination with special attention to the abdomen, flank, and external genitalia in men and a pelvic exam in women is essential.

Repeat urinalysis should be performed in all patients seen for microscopic hematuria. In the microscopic evaluation of the centrifuged urinary sediment, observation of more than one to three erythrocytes per high-power field is considered abnormal.[41,42] The presence or absence of associated pyuria, bacteriuria, or proteinuria may be important in establishing the etiology of hematuria. Red cell morphology may aid in distinguishing glomerular hematuria from that of more distant sites.[43,44] All patients with microscopic hematuria require a urine culture.

Failure to establish a clear diagnosis at this point in the evaluation indicates the need for further study. The subsequent work-up should include excretory urography or renal ultrasonography in combination with cystoscopy. Crowin and Silverstein have suggested that renal ultrasonography in combination with cystoscopy is the most cost-effective strategy for the evaluation of asymptomatic

FIGURE 4.13 *Correlation Between Cytoscopic, Histologic, and Cytologic Findings*

CYTOSCOPY	CYTOLOGY	HISTOLOGY	COMMENT
+ (papillary)	−	+	low-grade PTCC
+ (papillary)	+ (low-grade)	+	low-grade PTCC
+ (papillary)	+ (high-grade)	+	PTCC; ? Cis
+ (sessile)	+	+	TCC
−	+ (low-grade)	−	PTCC; false +
−	+ (high-grade)	−	Cis, upper tract
−	+	+	Cis

+ = present
− = absent
PTCC = papillary transitional cell carcinoma
Cis = carcinoma in situ

microscopic hematuria.[45] The sensitivity and specificity of this approach were identical to strategies that included excretory urography. We prefer to perform our upper tract imaging study prior to cystoscopy as findings in the upper tract may influence the nature and extent of our endoscopic evaluation. Upper tract filling defects may warrant retrograde pyelography, upper tract cytology, and/or ureteropyeloscopy as part of the diagnostic evaluation.

GROSS HEMATURIA

The above discussion has been limited to patients who are asymptomatic and present with microscopic hematuria. In addition to history, physical examination, urinalysis, and urine culture, all patients presenting with gross hematuria or symptoms attributable to the urinary tract in association with microhematuria warrant excretory urography and cystoscopy. Only rarely will the above diagnostic studies fail to establish a clear diagnosis in individuals with gross hematuria. Historically, such unusual patients required interval evaluation with excretory urography and cystoscopy to preclude an occult malignancy. However, recent advances in fiberoptic instrumentation now enable urologists routinely to access the upper tract for direct visualization. Recent reports have established flexible ureteropyeloscopy as an important diagnostic study in patients with otherwise unexplained gross hematuria.[46,47]

VOIDING DYSFUNCTION

Irritative voiding symptoms, including frequency and dysuria, are additional common findings in patients with bladder malignancies, particularly those with carcinoma in situ. Bladder irritability, with detrusor instability, represents a "final common path" response of the bladder to a spectrum of pathologic processes. While commonly associated with bladder outflow obstruction due to prostatism, the clinician must be careful not to ascribe isolated symptoms of bladder irritability prematurely to prostatism in male patients in the age group at risk for both prostatism and urothelial malignancies.

Tumors of the Upper Urinary Tract

Transitional cell neoplasms involving the upper urinary tract account for less than 10% of urothelial tumors.[48] These lesions may occur anywhere along the course of the upper tract collecting system. Most, however, are identified in the distal ureter.[49] Hematuria remains the most common presenting symptom, occurring in up to 80% of cases.[50] Although 40% to 50% of patients will develop ureteral obstruction with superimposed hydroureteronephrosis, the insidious onset of this phenomenon results in renal colic in a minority of individuals.

Excretory urography followed by cystoscopy constitutes the initial diagnostic evaluation. In cases where renal nonfunction secondary to long-standing obstruction precludes unilateral contrast excretion, or when excretory urography is nondiagnostic, retrograde pyelography is the

FIGURE 4.14 *Causes of Hematuria*

HEMATOLOGIC
Coagulopathy
Anticoagulation
Sickle cell anemia and trait

RENAL (GLOMERULAR)
Acute proliferative glomerulonephritis (GN) (e.g., poststreptococcal GN)
Primary mesangiopathic GN (e.g., Berger's disease and other nonsystemic focal proliferative GN)
Focal proliferative GN associated with systemic disease (e.g., Henoch-Schönlein purpura, vasculitis, etc.)
Lupus nephritis
Membranoproliferative GN
Alport syndrome
Benign familial hematuria

RENAL (NONGLOMERULAR)
Nephrosclerosis secondary to hypertension
Renal infarct
Renal vein thrombosis (infants)
Tuberculosis
Pyelonephritis
Polycystic disease
Medullary sponge kidney
Interstitial nephritis (drug allergy, infection, etc.)
Tumors
Vascular malformations
Trauma
Papillary necrosis
Cortical necrosis
Perirenal hematoma (infants)

POSTRENAL
Stones
Tumors of lower urinary tract
Cystitis (schistosomal, bacterial, viral, drug-induced, radiation-induced, idiopathic)
Prostatitis
Epididymitis
Meatal ulceration (circumcised boys)
Urethral stenosis
Foreign bodies of bladder or urethra (including Foley catheter)
Strenuous exercise
Urethritis
Phimosis
Benign prostatic hypertrophy
Obstruction
Vascular malformations
Endometriosis
Vesicoureteral reflux

Adapted from Abuelo JG. Evaluation of hematuria. *Urology.* 1983;21:215.

study of choice. Further evaluation may include upper tract cytology and/or direct visualization and biopsy with rigid or flexible ureteropyeloscopy. Care should be taken to exclude other radiolucent ureteral filling defects, which include sloughed papillae, radiolucent stones, and fungus balls. Figure 4.15 shows the classic goblet sign that is characteristic of ureteral transitional cell neoplasms.

Treatment is determined by the tumor location, stage, grade, and status of the contralateral kidney. A chest x-ray, abdominal CT, and bone scan are necessary to determine the local and systemic extent of disease. Due to difficulty in excluding local invasion, most patients with these lesions are treated with extirpative surgery. As a result of their unique propensity for downstream metachronous recurrence, tumors involving the renal pelvis and/or calyces have been classically treated with nephroureterectomy. Depending on stage and grade, distal ureteral tumors may be amenable to local excision with subsequent ureteral implantation.[51] Recently, highly selected groups of patients with unifocal, low-grade, low-stage neoplasms, or a contraindication to nephrectomy, have been successfully managed with endoscopic tumor ablation.[52]

Prognosis for these patients is stage- and grade-dependent. Figure 4.9 outlines the TNM and Jewett staging systems used for ureteral and upper tract transitional cell neoplasms. Fortunately, most cases are low-stage and low-grade and therefore have an excellent prognosis. Muscle invasion and/or direct local extension are poor prognostic signs.

The high rate of downstream metachronous tumor recurrence in these patients necessitates careful follow-up. While less than 5% of patients will develop a contralateral upper tract lesion, 50% to 60% of patients will eventually present with a bladder neoplasm.[53,54] For this reason, repeat cystoscopy at 3-month intervals is recommended until the patient remains tumor-free for a period of one year. Semiannual or annual surveillance is then warranted.

The prognosis for patients presenting with or subsequently developing metastatic disease is poor. However, recent improvements in the treatment of transitional cell bladder carcinoma using multidrug chemotherapy are promising and argue for the use of these regimens in the treatment of disseminated upper tract transitional cell carcinoma.[55]

SPECIAL ISSUES IN THE MANAGEMENT OF UPPER TRACT TUMORS

Patients with synchronous bilateral upper tract neoplasms or those with tumors involving a solitary kidney represent a difficult management problem. While surgery rendering the patient anephric is an option, it should only be embarked upon following extensive patient counseling regarding the sequelae of such an intervention. Depending on the location and stage of the lesion or lesions, alternative treatments would include open local excision, transurethral or percutaneous ablation, or intraluminal chemotherapy. A single small series has reported success with BCG instilled into the upper tract.[56,57]

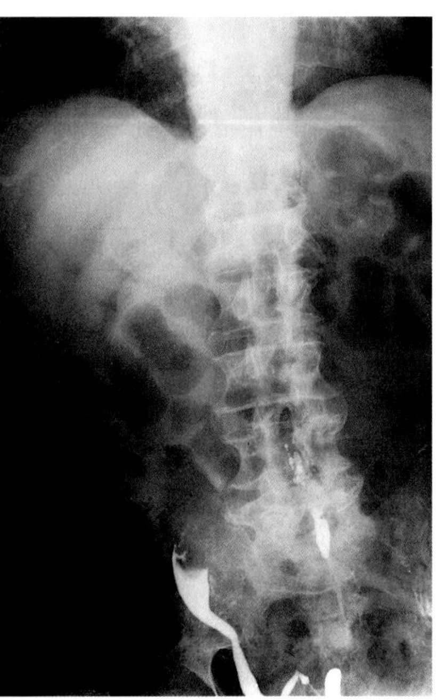

Figure 4.15 Retrograde pyelogram demonstrating the classic "goblet" sign of a ureteral filling defect caused by a ureteral transitional cell carcinoma.

Tumors of the Urinary Bladder

The diagnostic work-up for bladder neoplasms is identical to that described for upper tract lesions. Careful cystoscopy with urinary cytology is sufficient to exclude the presence of lower tract disease. When identified, bladder abnormalities should be treated with transuretheral excisional biopsy and examination under anesthesia. Selected mucosal biopsies of adjacent areas of urothelial abnormality may be necessary to define the presence of associated carcinoma in situ. For lesions that appear to be of high grade and those that involve the bladder neck, transurethral prostate biopsies are recommended to exclude prostatic duct or stromal involvement.

In assessing prostatic fossa involvement, the clinician must be careful to distinguish epithelial confined disease from that invading the prostatic parenchyma. Epithelial confined disease falls into the category of superficial tumors and may be managed with therapies appropriate for this category. In contrast, prostatic stromal invasion is a harbinger of poor outcome and warrants immediate aggressive therapy. If intravesical chemo/immunotherapy is chosen for the treatment of superficial prostatic involvement, one must be certain that an intact bladder neck does not prevent drug access to the target site.

Electrosurgical resection remains the time-honored and most widely used technique for bladder tumor removal. Recently, the Nd:YAG laser has been used with success for this same purpose. Which of these two techniques, if either, confers distinct advantages is unclear. Figure 4.16 lists some of the advantages and disadvantages of the laser relative to conventional electrocautery. For the most part they are of relatively minor consequence. The most pertinent issue—whether laser tumor ablation results in a lower incidence of tumor recurrence—remains unanswered. While existing laboratory data suggest that laser surgery may reduce implantation-mediated tumor recurrence, clinical studies have led to conflicting results.[58] A single prospective, randomized study found a lower incidence of recurrence in laser-treated patients. Unfortunately a large percentage of patients in the laser group received primary treatment with electrocautery followed by a second intervention with the laser.[59] The validity of comparing a "two treatment" arm involving laser to a single treatment arm managed with electrocautery is questionable.

Select sites within the bladder may be more easily treated with the laser. The ability of the laser fiber to pass through flexible instrumentation makes it a useful tool for treating sites such as the bladder dome, which can be difficult to reach with rigid instrumentation. Additionally, the preservation of tissue collagen ultrastructure subsequent to the absorption of laser energy makes the laser ideal for managing tumors involving the the ureteral orifice. The use of electrocautery at this site may predispose to ureteral stricture formation. Tumors involving the lateral wall, in areas at risk for obturator muscle spasm, represent a final site at which the laser has select advantages. However, obturator nerve blockade is an easily performed technique that all but obviates the risk of muscle spasm associated with electrocautery-induced nerve stimulation.

The stage and grade of the tumor defined by excisional biopsy will dictate further evaluation and/or therapy. Tumors are broadly divided into superficial and invasive categories. Figure 4.8 demonstrates the TNM classification for neoplasms of the bladder. Tumors of stage T1 or less are defined as superficial, with stage T2 or greater defined as invasive. All decisions regarding the management of patients with "superficial bladder carcinoma" must be based on adequate bladder biopsies. An absence of muscularis propria in the biopsy specimen suggests inadequacy of the sample and the need for additional tissue.

SUPERFICIAL BLADDER CARCINOMA

Seventy percent of patients have superficial lesions at presentation.[60] The major disease-related issues for this group of patients can be divided into the risks of tumor recurrence and tumor progression.

The biologic behavior of superficial bladder carcinoma is characterized by polychronotropism, that is, multiple occurrences in space and time. One-year and overall recurrence rates of 56% and 70% respectively have been reported in the literature.[61,62] The etiology of this exceptionally high rate of recurrence is an issue of debate. Urothelial field change disease resulting from diffuse

---

FIGURE 4.16 *Laser Tumor Ablation Versus Electrosurgical Resection*

ADVANTAGES

Painless (no current conduction)
Bloodless "no touch" technique
No catheter required
No obturator nerve spasm
Minimal risk of bladder perforation
Maintenance of collagen structure
    (ideal for lesions involving ureteral orifice)
Outpatient procedure
?Lower recurrence rate

DISADVANTAGES

No pathology or pathology difficult to interpret
Instrument cost
Usage risk to OR personnel
Requires special training
Unique complications (bowel injury)
Large lesions require combined approach
    (electrosurgery)

urothelial contact carcinogenesis clearly plays some role.[63] However, when one compares metachronous recurrence rates of different organ sites at risk for diffuse contact carcinogenesis (nasopharynx, lung, stomach, colon), the bladder is unique in terms of both its frequency and pattern of recurrence.[64–68] This finding is particularly striking considering the low grade and otherwise low malignant potential of the majority of superficial bladder neoplasms.

Tumor implantation represents a unique mechanism that may account for the idiosyncratic behavior of superficial bladder carcinoma.[69–73] Transurethral bladder tumor removal is novel in that it releases large numbers of viable tumor cells into a fluid medium in direct contact with areas of bladder injury. In vivo studies have shown that areas of urothelial injury represent preferential sites for tumor cell adherence and growth.[58,74] A number of iatrogenic and tumor-associated variables, including concentration of tumor cells, surface area of urothelial injury, duration of urothelial exposure, and intravesical pressure at the time of exposure, demonstrate a positive correlation with the size of the adherent inoculum.[75] The size of the adherent inoculum in turn determines risk of tumor growth.

An additional iatrogenically mediated factor that may influence implantation-associated recurrence is the local milieu at the site of tumor cell adherence. Traumatic urothelial injury initiates the process of epithelial repair involving cell division, migration, and neovascularization. The same factors that regulate normal reparative processes may influence the growth of tumor cells adhering to the injury site.

Incomplete resection of the primary tumor is an additional factor that may contribute to local tumor recurrence. A recent article noted a 40% incidence of residual tumor at the time of a "second look" tumor resection in patients with T1 disease.[76] The authors suggested this residual tumor could account in part for the high incidence of tumor recurrence.

To date, of myriad variables investigated only tumor size and the number of tumors at presentation correlate with risk of recurrence.[77,78] While bladder tumor recurrence is a cause of significant patient morbidity, it rarely represents a life-threatening process. Patients who are at high risk for recurrence may be treated in an effort to prevent recurrence of their first tumor, but due to the morbidity associated with treatment, most clinicians withhold therapy until the first recurrence.

Tumor Progression

Risk of tumor progression, defined as recurrence at a higher tumor stage or grade, is dependent upon initial tumor stage and grade. While less than 2% of grade I TA lesions ultimately progress, 69% to 83% of cases with grade III lamina propria invasion (T1) and associated carcinoma in situ will recur as muscle-invasive disease (>T2).[79] As disease progression has a potentially lethal outcome, careful attention must be paid to individual patient risks for this phenomenon. Patients at high risk must be followed closely with cystoscopy, biopsy, and urinary cytology and the most effective agent chosen for first-line therapy.

Clinical Management

Depending upon tumor stage and grade, excisional biopsy may serve as definitive therapy for a subset of patients with superficial bladder malignancies. Observation alone can be easily justified in patients with single, small to moderate volume, grade I tumors confined to the epithelium. However, in treating any patient with a superficial bladder neoplasm, the physician should always decide if the patient would benefit from adjuvant intravesical therapy. To effectively address this question one must assess the patient's risk for both tumor recurrence and progression. Factors associated with increased risk of recurrence include number of tumors, tumor size, completeness of resection, and prior recurrence history. Variables that influence the risk of progression include tumor stage, grade, and associated Cis. The risk/benefit ratio of therapy versus no therapy in a given individual will determine the need for, and appropriateness of, adjuvant measures.

Therapy to prevent recurrence is founded upon the intravesical administration of chemo- or immunotherapeutic agents. Thiotepa, doxorubicin, mitomycin C, and bacillus Calmette-Guérin (BCG) have been administered in an effort to decrease recurrence rates.[80] There is little evidence to support a clear advantage of one of these agents over the others. Figure 4.17 lists frequently used intravesical chemotherapeutic regimens.

FIGURE 4.17 *Frequently Used Intravesical Chemotherapeutic Regimens*

AGENT	Thiotepa	Doxorubicin	Mitomycin	BCG
CONCENTRATION	30 mg/30 mL	50 mg/30 mL	20-40 mg/40 mL	120 mg/50 mL
FREQUENCY/ INTERVAL	Weekly × 6	Weekly × 6	Weekly × 8	Weekly × 6

In selecting an agent for intravesical therapy, the clinician must weigh not only risk of recurrence but also potential for disease progression as well as the toxicity associated with the chosen therapeutic agent. Figure 4.18 lists some of the complications observed with intravesical agents. For patients with low-stage, low-grade lesions at low risk for progression, thiotepa, a low-cost, low-morbidity agent, represents a reasonable initial choice.

Of the immunotherapeutic agents studied to date, BCG appears to be the most effective intravesical agent for preventing recurrence. Forty percent to 60% of treated patients will benefit from BCG.[80] Unfortunately, intravesical BCG treatment is associated with moderate toxicity in a significant percentage of patients.[81,82] Life-threatening complications have been reported in a few individuals.[83,84] The toxicity of BCG argues against its routine use as first-line therapy in patients for whom the sole treatment objective is prevention of recurrence.

Alpha interferon is another agent with proven efficacy, particularly in the treatment of tumors refractory to other drugs.[85] Although relatively well tolerated, the financial cost of therapy precludes its routine use in uncomplicated patients.

All patients at high risk for disease progression should be treated at the time of presentation. This would include patients with grade III tumors and/or grade II or III lesions demonstrating invasion of the lamina propria. Intravesical BCG administered in 6 weekly courses of 120 mg is the therapeutic agent of choice. Patients failing a 6-week induction course of BCG may benefit from an additional 6-week course.[86] Patients who fail a second induction course are at high risk for tumor progression and disease-related death and should be considered for exenterative surgery. Current data suggest that maintenance BCG is of little benefit.[87]

Although it is categorized with the superficial bladder carcinomas, carcinoma in situ (Cis) is an aggressive form of urothelial neoplasia. Either alone or in conjunction with papillary neoplasia, Cis frequently progresses to muscle invasion and may represent the precursor lesion to invasive disease. Patients with isolated or mixed lesions containing CiS should be treated aggressively with intravesical BCG at the time of presentation. The intravesical administration of BCG was recently approved by the FDA specifically for this purpose. Persistent positive bladder cytology following therapy in the face of negative bladder mucosal biopsy may indicate disease persistence in the upper tract or prostatic fossa.[88,89]

Timing and Duration of Intravesical Chemotherapy

There is little evidence on the optimal timing of administration of intravesical chemotherapy. The use of intravesical therapy in a "neoadjuvant" setting remains largely unstudied. A small trial at the University of Iowa comparing recurrence rates in patients randomized to receive thiotepa either 1 hour preoperatively or on the first day postoperatively failed to demonstrate any difference in tumor recurrence.

The administration of chemotherapeutic agents in the immediate postoperative period has potential theoretical advantages in terms of preventing implantation-mediated tumor recurrence. However, to date, no study has demonstrated a significant difference in efficacy between immediate and delayed drug administration. Given that the risk of systemic drug absorption and therefore systemic toxicity appears to be increased in patients given intravesical therapy immediately following TURBT, perioperative administration of chemotherapy should be used with caution.

The use of BCG in the immediate postoperative setting is associated with an inordinate risk of toxicity. The majority of fatal complications associated with the use of this agent have resulted from systemic dissemination of the bacterium through traumatized urothelium. Active lower tract bleeding and/or areas of significant bladder injury represent an absolute contraindication to the intravesical administration of this agent. For this reason, BCG should not be administered in the immediate perioperative period.

The postoperative period is the most widely accepted time for the initiation of both chemo- and immunotherapy. Not only is the risk of systemic toxicity decreased, but the

FIGURE 4.18 *Complications With Intravesical Agents*

	THIOTEPA	DOXORUBICIN	MITOMYCIN	BCG
Hematuria	Yes	Yes	Yes	Yes
Myelosuppression	Yes	Rare	No	No
Vesical irritability	Yes	Yes	Yes	Frequent
Bladder contraction	Yes	Yes	Yes	Yes
Cutaneous rash	No	No	Yes	Rare
Fever	No	No	No	Yes
Tuberculosis sepsis	No	No	No	Yes

availability of pathologic tumor stage and grade allows a more accurate assessment of recurrence and progression so that one may optimize the choice of therapeutic agents.

Therapy is typically administered at weekly intervals for a total of six treatments. Patients are instructed to hold the drug for 1 to 2 hours prior to voiding. Having patients change their position at intervals during drug administration to "expose the entire bladder surface" makes no sense in the case of soluble agents, which, in the absence of intravesical air, uniformly and continuously bathe the bladder surface. The exception to this is BCG, which, being particulate in nature, could settle out in the dependent portion of the bladder. Given that studies suggest that BCG must adhere to the urothelial surface in order to exert its antitumor effect, it is not unreasonable to have patients reposition themselves to place various portions of the bladder sequentially in a dependent state.

Patients should undergo reevaluation 4 to 6 weeks after the completion of therapy. Failure of intravesical therapy to effect the treatment objective necessitates consideration of alternate modalities. Possible decision paths after the failure of an initial therapeutic agent include additional cycles of the same agent, institution of alternative nonsurgical therapy, and surgical intervention alone or in combination with one of the above. As was the case for the decision regarding the initial choice of therapy, recommendations regarding subsequent therapies must be founded upon a clear assessment of the patient's risks of recurrence and progression. Given that the choice of therapy has the potential to affect the outcome profoundly, the patient must be allowed to participate in the decision-making process. For some patients the fear of developing invasive cancer overrides any concern for bladder preservation. Others may choose to subject themselves to an increased risk of disease progression in an effort to avoid surgery.

Follow-up

Patients are followed with cystoscopy and cytology every 3 months until they have been tumor-free for 1 year. Surveillance then proceeds on a semiannual and, ultimately, annual basis. The predictive value of other "bladder monitors," including DNA ploidy and a spectrum of immunohistochemical markers, remains unclear. Although existing preliminary data suggest that some of these studies may prove useful, at the time of this writing they remain largely investigational tools. Figure 4.19 illustrates an algorithm for management and follow-up of patients with bladder neoplasms.

MUSCLE-INVASIVE BLADDER CARCINOMA

Tumor stages greater than or equal to T2 constitute invasive disease. Treatment options are determined by the local extent of disease and the presence of systemic spread. The staging evaluation should include a chest x-ray, abdominal and pelvic CT, and bone scan. If cystecto-

my is a consideration, the decision regarding a concomitant urethrectomy and urinary diversion options depends on the degree to which the disease has extended in the prostatic fossa and proximal urethra. For this reason, staging should include biopsies of these sites.

Accepted single-modality treatment options for the patient with organ-confined disease include radical radiotherapy or cystectomy. Studies suggest that radical cystectomy confers the greatest likelihood of cure.[90] Advances in modern urologic oncology in the past decade have markedly reduced the morbidity and mortality associated with radical cystectomy. Selected individuals may be candidates for potency-sparing dissections.[91] New methods of continent urinary diversion afford improved body image and quality of life for both male and female patients.[92,93]

Despite advances in surgical techniques and postoperative management, the 5-year survival of patients with advanced organ-confined disease ($\geq$T2) remains only 50%.[94] Local recurrence after radical surgery is relatively rare, with most patients succumbing to metastatic disease. This observation highlights the failure of current therapy to treat effectively the population of patients who have occult metastases at the time of radical surgery. Radiotherapy and chemotherapy alone or in combination and administered in both the neoadjuvant and adjuvant settings have been used in an attempt to improve long-term survival.

Preoperative Radiotherapy

Historically, preoperative external beam radiotherapy followed by radical cystectomy represents the earliest use of combination therapy in an attempt to improve outcome. The rationale for administering preoperative radiotherapy includes: 1) attempting to sterilize small tumor aggregates either in the bladder or regional lymph nodes that might be left behind during surgery; 2) preventing tumor seeding into the operative field during cystectomy; and 3) attempting to downstage an unresectable tumor mass into a resectable lesion.[95] For patients with muscle-invasive disease the two most relevant clinical end points for evaluating the efficacy of any new strategy, including preoperative radiotherapy, are its effects on local recurrence rates and overall survival.

Unfortunately, attempting to glean the incidence of pelvic recurrences after preoperative radiotherapy followed by surgery or after cystectomy alone is problematic. The vast majority of studies reported are retrospective in nature, and the majority date from the pre-CT era. Variability in staging (clinical versus pathologic), surgical procedures (with or without lymph node dissection), radiotherapy dose and schedule, and use of adjuvant chemotherapy all complicate interpretation of the available data. Batata et al. reported a decrease in the risk of pelvic recurrence from 37% following surgery alone to 14% following preoperative radiotherapy and cystectomy.[96] Skinner et al. noted a 7% local failure rate following surgery alone versus a 9% rate in patients receiving

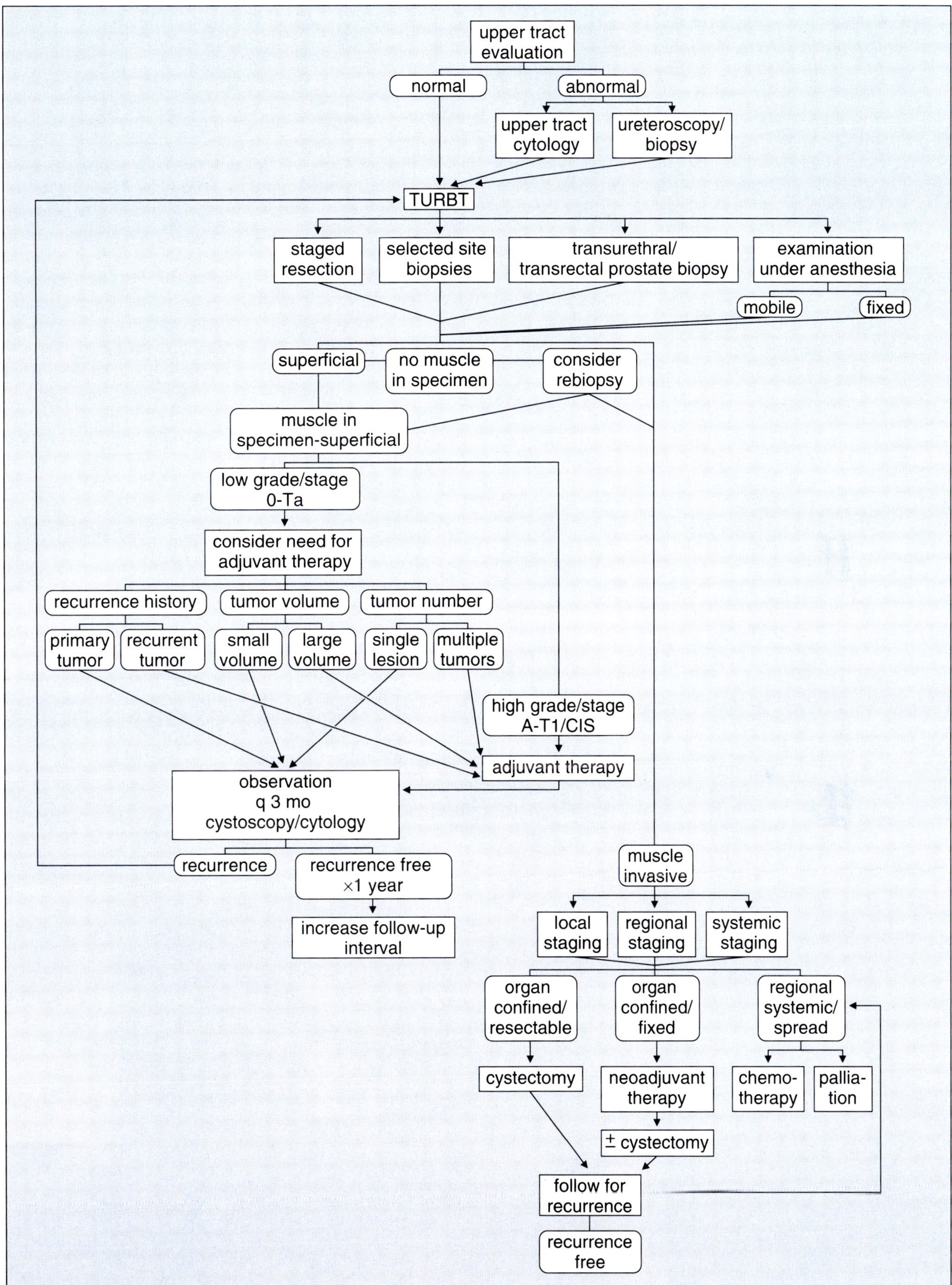

Figure 4.19 Algorithm for the initial evaluation, treatment, and follow-up of patients with newly diagnosed bladder tumors.

both modalities.[97] At best these data are contradictory, at worst uninterpretable.

Most available data for the impact of preoperative radiation followed by cystectomy on survival come from retrospective analyses using both historic and contemporary controls. Parsons and Million have argued that there is compelling evidence that preoperative irradiation followed by cystectomy improves 5-year survival by almost 50% in patients with clinical stage B2–C (T3) when compared with patients undergoing cystectomy alone.[95] They support their contention with data from a selected group of contemporary (1960 to 1980), retrospective, single-institution experiences (cystectomy alone and preoperative radiotherapy followed by surgery), encompassing 1185 patients. The only prospective, randomized clinical trial using patients with muscle invasive (T2–T4), primarily transitional cell histology was conducted by the National Surgical Adjuvant Bladder Project (NSABP).[98] Notable findings from this study included a significant percentage of patients randomized to radiotherapy whose bladder tumors were downstaged to P0, compared to patients undergoing surgery alone (34% versus 9%). Most important, however, was the lack of a statistically significant difference in survival of patients receiving preoperative radiotherapy versus patients undergoing surgery alone. While the controversy regarding the benefits of preoperative radiotherapy persists, the consensus of opinion in the urologic oncology community is that there is no compelling evidence to support the routine use of preoperative radiotherapy.

Neoadjuvant Chemotherapy

In the early 1980s several investigators recognizing the activity of cisplatin-based chemotherapy in the treatment of metastatic bladder cancer began to evaluate the utility of multiagent chemotherapy in the neoadjuvant setting.[99–101] In contrast to preoperative radiotherapy, chemotherapy offered the potential for improving both regional and systemic control. By addressing micrometastases as well as local tumor burden, this strategy held significant theoretical advantage for dealing with the issue of distant recurrence.[96,97]

In 1987 Scher et al. reported their experience with neoadjuvant M-VAC (methotrexate, vinblastine, doxorubicin, and cisplatin) (Fig. 4.20) in 50 patients.[101] Patients with muscle-invasive bladder cancer (T2–T4,N0,M0) received from one to five cycles of M-VAC. Thirty-nine of the 50 patients also underwent an aggressive transurethral resection of the bladder (TURBT) after cycle one or two. Forty-one of the 50 patients had pure transitional cell histology and 42 had clinical (c) T3 or T4 disease. In 44 patients deemed evaluable there was a 63% clinical response rate (24% complete clinical response [cCR] + 39% partial clinical response [pCR]) and a 50% pathologic (p) response rate (33% cPR + 17% pPR).

Zincke et al. treated 16 patients with locally advanced transitional cell carcinoma of the bladder with two to four cycles of neoadjuvant M-VAC.[102] Ten patients underwent postchemotherapy pelvic lymphadenectomy and radical cystectomy. The overall response rate was 69%, with a complete remission rate (pathologic and clinical) of 50%.

FIGURE 4.20 *Cisplatin-Based Adjuvant Regimens*

M-VAC	Cycle every 28 days
Methotrexate	30 mg/m^2 days 1, 14, 21
Vinblastine	3 mg/m^2 days 1, 14, 21
Doxorubicin	30 mg/m^2 day 2
Cisplatin	70 mg/m^2 day 2
CMV	Cycle every 21 days
Cisplatin	100 mg/m^2 day 2
Methotrexate	30 mg/m^2 days 1 and 8
Vinblastine	4 mg/m^2 days 1 and 8
CISCA	Cycle every 28 days
Cisplatin	70 mg/m^2 day 2
Cyclophosphamide	500 mg/m^2 day 1
Doxorubicin	50 mg/m^2 day 1

One of the well-recognized difficulties in interpreting the impact of neoadjuvant chemotherapy on local tumor burden is the error associated with clinical versus pathologic staging. The Memorial Sloan-Kettering Group reported a 63% overall (clinical-T and/or pathologic-P) response rate in 41 patients with pure transitional cell carcinoma.[101] While this group reported a relatively modest 38% staging error, 45% of all responders in this study underwent clinical and endoscopic staging only. In contrast, Skinner et al. reported a staging error rate of 64% (41% understaged, 23% overstaged) in 131 patients who were treated with preoperative radiation therapy followed by radical cystectomy and pelvic node dissection.[103] The Eastern Cooperative Oncology Group recently reported a pilot study of perioperative M-VAC in a small series of well-studied patients with locally advanced bladder cancer.[104] Eighteen patients with T2–T3 disease received two preoperative cycles of M-VAC followed by cystectomy, then two adjuvant cycles of M-VAC. Radical cystectomy was performed in 17 of 18 patients. There were three (17%) pathologic partial responses and two (11%) pathologic complete responses, for an overall response rate of 28% (95% confidence limits, 10% and 53%). The lower response rate in this study compared to other, larger experiences may merely reflect its small sample size. Alternatively, it may represent a more accurate representation of response rates, since all patients were pathologically staged.

The role of surgery following neoadjuvant chemotherapy has not yet been firmly established. Several preliminary observations from the emerging experience can be made. Radical surgery following neoadjuvant chemotherapy can be done without an increase in morbidity and mortality.[104,105] Endoscopic procedures, when done with therapeutic intent as part of the neoadjuvant therapy, can increase the difficulty in interpreting the clinical response to therapy, especially in patients with T2–T3a disease. Patients who are clinically downstaged to Tis or T0–T1 disease would appear to benefit most from cystectomy.[105] The benefit of surgery in patients with residual T3–T4 disease after chemotherapy is uncertain; however, it remains the most likely intervention to allow long-term survival. Patients downstaged to T0 remain at risk for persistent, invasive tumor not appreciated at endoscopy and development of recurrent or invasive disease. The role of partial cystectomy and other bladder-sparing therapies in this group remains unproven. Available data consist primarily of single-institution phase II studies, which provide only limited preliminary information.[106] Until convincing data from ongoing phase III studies demonstrate that patient survival is not affected by bladder preservation, patients should undergo definitive surgery unless they are enrolled in a clinical trial.

While many questions remain unanswered, certain facts have come to light from the available phase II studies. Patients with nontransitional cell histology have poorer response rates than those with transitional cell histol-ogy.[101,107] Morbidity from M-VAC is moderate, with several groups reporting an unusually high incidence of thromboembolic events.[104,108] Neoadjuvant chemotherapy is capable of downstaging bladder cancer in selected individuals to P0. Whether this approach increases survival or merely selects patients with a good prognosis is unclear. Hopefully, results from the ongoing Intergroup study comparing three cycles of preoperative M-VAC followed by cystectomy versus cystectomy alone will provide badly needed guidance.

Another experimental approach using a variation of neoadjuvant therapy is combination chemotherapy and radiation therapy in an attempt to preserve the bladder and decrease distant metastases. Kaufman and Shipley et al. recently reported their pilot study of bladder-sparing therapy in 40 evaluable patients with T2–T4 bladder cancer.[109] Patients underwent transurethral surgery and two cycles of methotrexate, cisplatin, and vinblastine (MCV), followed by 4000 cGy pelvic x-ray therapy plus two cycles of cisplatin. Patients demonstrating a clinical complete response (cCR) at the time of repeat TURBT continued radiotherapy to a dose of 6480 cGy. With 30 months median follow-up, 27 (68%) patients are alive and disease-free and 25 (63%) are alive without evidence of distant metastases. Additional confirmation of this experience awaits the results of the ongoing RTOG phase III study of neoadjuvant MCV/radiotherapy.

Adjuvant Chemotherapy

Another approach to attempt to decrease the high recurrence rate in patients with high-risk (deep muscle invasion, high-grade tumors) bladder cancers involves the use of adjuvant chemotherapy. In contrast to neoadjuvant trials, adjuvant therapy trials allow pathologically staged patients to be stratified appropriately for known risk factors (depth of muscle invasion, node status etc).

In 1985 the National Bladder Cancer Group presented preliminary data from their prospective, randomized trial of adjuvant cisplatin following preoperative radiotherapy and cystectomy.[110] Of 220 patients, 180 completed the primary therapy. There were 83 patients with residual disease in the resected specimens eligible for randomization to either observation or eight cycles of cisplatin at 70 mg/m^2 every 3 weeks. While there was no significant difference in disease-free survival between the two treatment arms, it must be kept in mind that only nine of 43 patients randomized to receive cisplatin actually completed the intended eight cycles of therapy (median cycles: four), thus significantly compromising the dose intensity delivered.

Two recent studies using cisplatin-based regimens provide most of the available data regarding the efficacy of adjuvant chemotherapy for bladder neoplasms. In 1988, Logothetis et al. reported their institutional experience utilizing CISCA (cisplatin, cytoxan, doxorubicin) (see Fig. 4.20) in a retrospective analysis using a contemporary control group.[111] Over a 5-year period, 71 patients with pathologic features thought to indicate high risk for recurrence received up to five cycles of CISCA initiated approximately 6 weeks after cystectomy. These features included the presence of resected nodal metastases, extravesical involvement of tumor, or pelvic visceral invasion. A group of 62 patients with these high-risk features were not treated with chemotherapy for reasons including patient refusal, medical contraindications, and physician preference. A third group of 206 patients were considered to be at low risk and were not treated with adjuvant therapy. A significant disease-free survival advantage was demonstrated for patients who received adjuvant therapy when compared to high-risk patients who did not receive therapy (p = 0.00012). When compared to low-risk patients, there was no significant difference in disease-free survival of the high-risk patients receiving adjuvant therapy.

In a recently reported, randomized, prospective trial, Skinner et al. compared adjuvant chemotherapy to observation in 91 patients with P3, P4, or node-positive disease.[112] Patients randomized to receive chemotherapy during the early phase of this trial were given therapy tailored to the individual patient based on results from tumor clonal assays; the remaining patients were treated with cisplatin, cytoxan, and doxorubicin for four cycles. Of the 44 patients randomized to receive chemotherapy, 12 did not receive protocol therapy, but other, primarily cisplatin-based therapy, and 11 patients ultimately refused chemotherapy. Significant increases in both time to progression and survival were demonstrated in patients with pure transitional cell or mixed histology. While all patients benefited from adjuvant therapy, the most significant improvement in survival was seen in patients with 0 or 1 positive nodes. Toxicity was a significant problem affecting compliance, and only 21 of 44 patients completed the planned 4-month course.

The appropriate role of adjuvant therapy in patients with high-risk bladder cancer remains to be established. The most effective drug(s) and optimal number of cycles have not been determined. Both of the large reported adjuvant experiences used CISCA as primary therapy; however, Logothetis et al. recently reported the superior activity of M-VAC versus CISCA in patients with advanced bladder cancer.[113] Given the significant morbidity associated with this therapy, a clear benefit will have to be demonstrated before it should be considered the standard of care. A large prospective study will be required ultimately to answer this question; however, as has been amply demonstrated with the current neoadjuvant intergroup study, such a study will be a difficult undertaking.

SPECIAL ISSUES IN LOWER TRACT TUMORS

While bladder preservation is a laudable goal in the management of bladder neoplasms, it must not take precedence over the primary objective of cancer cure. The "field change" nature of urothelial neoplasms precludes the use of partial cystectomy in the majority of patients.

However, in carefully selected individuals this technique may prove appropriate. Neoplasms limited to bladder diverticula may represent a singular indication. The absence of a diverticular muscle layer precludes any assessment of tumor invasion and makes transurethral excision hazardous. Diverticulectomy, including a cuff of normal bladder, may prove curative in patients whose remaining bladder has mapped negative at earlier biopsy.

NONTRANSITIONAL CELL BLADDER NEOPLASMS

Nontransitional cell bladder neoplasms account for less than 10% of all bladder tumors, with the most common histologic types being squamous cell carcinoma and adenocarcinoma. Squamous cell carcinoma and adenocarcinoma are commonly seen in the adult population and are usually invasive at presentation. These are aggressive, radioresistant neoplasms, which do not respond to drug regimens proven efficacious against transitional cell lesions. Surgical extirpation of organ-confined disease at the time of presentation affords the greatest chance of cure.

Management of Disseminated and Locally Advanced Bladder Cancer

Despite the progress that has been made in both surgical and medical therapy, the management of local or distant recurrences subsequent to definitive therapy remains a significant clinical problem. Single-agent chemotherapy has a long track record; however, response rates are modest (10% to 30%) and are typically partial and nondurable.[114] In the mid 1980s, several groups reported response rates in patients with advanced disease ranging from 50% to 80% using the CMV (cisplatin, methotrexate, vinblastine) (see Fig. 4.20), M-VAC, and CISCA regimens.[115–117] In an attempt to clarify the role of single-agent versus multiagent therapy, four prospective studies have been performed comparing multiagent therapy versus cisplatin alone. Three studies comparing cisplatin alone to cisplatin and cyclophosphamide, cisplatin with cyclophosphamide and doxorubicin, and cisplatin plus methotrexate have failed to demonstrate a significant improvement in survival.[118–120] However, Loehrer et al. recently reported preliminary results of a large intergroup study of 266 patients with advanced bladder cancer randomized to receive cisplatin alone or M-VAC.[121] Patients treated with cisplatin alone had a response rate of 9% and a median survival of 8.7 months, which was significantly different from the 33% and 12.6 months for the M-VAC group.

Despite the relatively short period during which "effective" systemic therapy for advanced bladder cancer has been used, certain observations have been made that may help guide the clinician in determining appropriate therapy. While there are no prospective studies demonstrating a survival benefit from combination chemotherapy, an update of the Memorial experience in 133 patients with metastatic urothelial cancer noted that 36% of patients obtained a complete response.[122] This response has proven durable in approximately one third of patients, with the median survival exceeding 38 months. An additional observation suggesting that systemic therapy has affected the natural history of disseminated disease is the 16% incidence of brain metastases observed in recent trials. The emergence of these heretofore uncommon lesions suggests that therapy may be affecting non-sanctuary sites and in doing so selecting for metastases in protected environments. As has been described by various investigators, primary adenocarcinomas, squamous cell carcinomas, and mixed histologies (TCC and adeno/squamous) have response rates inferior to pure transitional cell lesions.[116] Patient selection is clearly important in predicting outcome. The Memorial group noted that a higher percentage of patients with nodal metastases achieved a complete response than did patients with nonnodal distant metastases, and that while all metastatic sites showed evidence of tumor regression, hepatic metastases appeared the least responsive to M-VAC.[122] An additional noteworthy observation is that age per se is not a contraindication to therapy. Several groups have noted that performance status irrespective of age is a much more relevant prognostic factor.[123,124]

Chemotherapy-induced toxicity has historically represented a major impediment to both patient acceptance of treatment and the ability of the clinician to deliver optimal dose intensity. Two new classes of drugs, representatives of which have recently been approved by the FDA, are having significant impact on these management issues.

Nausea and vomiting associated with chemotherapy administration have been a major cause of treatment-related morbidity. Serotonin antagonists represent a new class of antiemetic agent that appears more effective and less sedating than other conventional antiemetics. Multiple clinical trials have demonstrated the efficacy of serotonin antagonists in lessening the morbidity of systemically administered therapy and support the conclusion that a significant improvement in the care of these patients has been achieved.[125,126]

Myelosuppression is frequently the dose-limiting toxicity associated with chemotherapy. Granulocyte-colony-stimulating factor (G-CSF) is a glycoprotein produced by monocytes, macrophages, fibroblasts, and endothelial cells, which stimulates committed granulocytic precursors, increasing the number and function of neutrophils.[127] Gabrilove et al. evaluated the ability of human recombinant G-CSF to prevent chemotherapy-induced neutropenia or increase neutrophil recovery time in 27 patients receiving M-VAC chemotherapy for urothelial cancer.[128] Patients receiving G-CSF after chemotherapy had significantly fewer days on which antibiotics were used to treat febrile neutropenia and had a significant increase in their ability to receive chemotherapy on day 14 of the treatment cycle. Interestingly, there was also an unanticipated statistically significant decrease in the incidence of mucositis. Whether the use of colony-stimulating factors to increase the dose intensity of chemotherapy is of clinical benefit is uncertain. However, Logothetis et al., reporting a phase I trial of granulocyte-macrophage colony-stimulating factor (GM-CSF) with escalated doses of M-VAC in 32 patients with metastatic urothelial tumors refractory to "standard" dose M-VAC, noted a 40% response rate with 23% of patients obtaining a complete response.[129]

Summary

We have summarized the current "state of the art" for the diagnosis and treatment of the spectrum of urothelial neoplasms. Hopefully this discussion has illustrated to the reader not only where we are with respect to this disease, but what issues remain to be addressed in the management of the second most common urologic malignancy. Despite a solid foundation of clinical understanding, urologists are limited in their ability to predict the behavior of a given tumor and to intervene effectively. Issues ranging from the pathogenesis of development to correlates of biologic potential must be addressed for the gamut of these tumors. For superficial lesions, the mechanisms involved in tumor recurrence and progression argue for further study. In the case of invasive disease, inroads into bladder-sparing approaches for organ-confined disease and improved systemic therapy for disseminated disease are badly needed. Despite being a chemosensitive neoplasm, metastatic bladder cancer, like metastatic breast cancer, appears ultimately to develop drug resistance and appears incurable with the therapies currently available. While the primary management of this disease is, and should remain, the responsibility of the urologic oncologist, it is only through a multidisciplinary effort performed in conjunction with our colleagues in pathology and medical and radiation oncology that this complex problem will be dealt with effectively.

Acknowledgement
The authors wish to thank Kristina Gaunt for her editorial assistance.

This work was supported in part by American Cancer Society Career Development Award #91-269.

References

1. Silverberg E, Lubera JA. Cancer statistics. *CA*. 1989;39:3.

2. Rehn L. Über Basentumoren bei Fuchsinarbeitern. *Arch Klin Chir*. 1895;50:588.

3. Murphy WM. Diseases of the urinary bladder, urethra, ureters, and renal pelves. In: Murphy WM, ed. *Urological Pathology*. Philadelphia, Pa: WB Saunders Co; 1989.

4. Petersen RO. Urinary bladder. In: Petersen RO, ed. *Urologic Pathology*. Philadelphia, Pa: JB Lippincott; 1986.

5. Ross RK, Paganini-Hill A, Henderson BE. Epidemiology of bladder cancer. In: Skinner DG, Lieskovsky G, eds. *Genitourinary Cancer*. Philadelphia, Pa: WB Saunders; 1988.

6. Wall RL, Clausen KP. Carcinoma of the urinary bladder in patients receiving cyclophosphamide. *N Engl J Med*. 1975;293:271.

7. Bengtssan U, et al. Transitional cell tumors of the renal pelvis in analgesic abusers. *Scand J Urol Nephrol*. 1968;2:145.

8. Lower GM Jr. Concepts in causality chemically induced human urinary bladder cancer. *Cancer*. 1982;49:1056.

9. McDonald DF, Lund RR. The role of the urine in vesical neoplasm, 1: experimental confirmation of the urogenous theory of pathogenesis. *J Urol*. 1954;71:560.

10. El-Bolkainy MN, Mokhtar NM, Ghoneim MA, Hussein MH. The impact of schistosomiasis on the pathology of bladder carcinoma. *Cancer*. 1981;48:2643.

11. Ooms ECM, Anderson WAM, Alons CL, Boon ME, Veldhuizen RW. Analysis of the performance of pathologists in the grading of bladder tumors. *Hum Pathol*. 1983;14:140.

12. Broders AC. Epithelium of the genito-urinary organs. *Ann Surg*. 1922;75:574.

13. Mostofi FK, Sobin LH, Torloni H. *Histological Typing of Urinary Bladder Tumours*. Geneva: WHO; 1973. International Classification of Tumors 19.

14. Gilbert HA, Logan JL, Kagan AR, et al. The natural history of papillary transitional cell carcinoma of the bladder and its treatment in an unselected population on the basis of histologic grading. *J Urol*. 1978;119:488.

15. Jewett HJ, Strong GH. Infiltrating carcinoma of the bladder: relation of depth of penetration of the bladder wall to incidence of local extension and metastases. *J Urol*. 1946;55:366.

16. Marshall VF. The relation of the preoperative estimate to the pathologic demonstration of the extent of vesical neoplasms. *J Urol*. 1952;68:714.

17. American Joint Committee on Cancer. *Manual for Staging of Cancer*. Philadelphia, Pa: JB Lippincott; 1988.

18. Dixon JS, Gosling JA. Histology and fine structure of the muscularis mucosae of the human urinary bladder. *J Anat*. 1983;136:265.

19. Younes M, Sussman J, True LD. The usefulness of the level of the muscularis mucosae in the staging of invasive transitional cell carcinoma of the urinary bladder. *Cancer*. 1990;66:543.

20. Cutler SJ, Heney NM, Friedell GH. Longitudinal study of patients with bladder cancer: factors associated with disease recurrence and progression. In: Bonney WW, Prout GR, eds. *Bladder Cancer*. Baltimore, Md: AVA Monographs, Williams & Wilkins; 1982.

21. Kannan V. Papillary transitional-cell carcinoma of the upper urinary tract: a cytological review. *Diagn Cytopathol*. 1990;6:204.

22. Koss LG. *Diagnostic Cytology and Its Histopathologic Bases*. 3rd ed. Philadelphia, Pa: JB Lippincott; 1961.

23. El-Bolkainy MN. Cytology of bladder carcinoma. *J Urol*. 1980;124:20.

24. Esposti PL, Zajicek. Grading of transitional cell neoplasms of the urinary bladder from smears of bladder washings. *Acta Cytol*. 1972;16:529.

25. Rife CC, Farrow GM, Utz DC. Urine cytology of transitional cell neoplasms. *Urol Clin North Am*. 1979;6:599.

26. Murphy WM, Soloway MS, Jukkola AF, et al. Urinary cytology and bladder cancer: the cellular features of transitional cell neoplasms. *Cancer*. 1984;53:1555.

27. Shenoy UA, Colby TV, Schumann GB. Reliability of urinary cytodiagnosis in urothelial neoplasms. *Cancer*. 1985;56:2041.

28. Kern WH. The cytology of transitional cell carcinoma of the urinary bladder. *Acta Cytologica*. 1975;19:420

29. Schaafsma HE, Ramaekers FCS, van Muijen GNP, et al. Distribution of cytokeratin polypeptides in human transitional cell carcinomas, with special emphasis on changing expression patterns during tumor progression. *Am J Pathol*. 1990;136:329.

30. Coon JS, Weinstein RS. Blood group-related antigens as markers of malignant potential and heterogeneity in human carcinomas. *Hum Pathol*. 1986;17:1089.

31. Sheinfeld J, Reuter VE, Melamed MR, et al. Enhanced bladder cancer detection with the Lewis X antigen as a marker of neoplastic transformation. *J Urol*. 1990;143:285.

32. Fradet Y, Cordon-Cardo C, Thomson T, et al. Cell surface antigens of human bladder cancer defined by mouse monoclonal antibodies. *Proc Natl Acad Sci USA*. 1984;81:224.

33. Fradet Y, Tardif M, Bourget L, Robert J. Clinical cancer progression in urinary bladder tumors evaluated by multiparameter flow cytometry with monoclonal antibodies. *Cancer Res*. 1990;50:432.

34. Murphy WM. DNA flow cytometry in diagnostic pathology of the urinary tract. *Hum Pathol*. 1987;18:317.

35. Tsujihashi H, Matsuda H, Uejima S, Akiyama T, Kurita T. Cell proliferation of human bladder tumors. *J Urol*. 1989;142:113.

36. Okamura K, Miyake K, Koshikawa T, Asai J. Growth fractions of transitional cell carcinomas of the bladder defined by the monoclonal antibody Ki-67. *J Urol*. 1990;144:875.

37. Hayward NK, Keegan R, Nancarrow DJ, et al. c-Ha-*ras*-1 alleles in bladder cancer, Wilms' tumour and malignant melanoma. *Hum Genet*. 1988;78:115.

38. Varkarakis MJ, Gaeta J, Moore RN, Murphy GP. Superficial bladder tumor: aspects of clinical progression. *Urology*. 1974;4:414.

39. Skinner DG, Calvin RB, Vermillian CD, et al. Diagnosis and management of RCC: a clinical and pathologic study of 309 cases. *Cancer*. 1971;28:1165.

40. Mohr DN, Offord KP, Woen RA, Melton LJ III. Asymptomatic microhematuria and urologic disease: a population-based

study. *JAMA*. 1986;256:224.

41. Larcom RC Jr, Carter GH. Erythrocytes in urinary sediment: identification and normal limits with note on nature of granular casts. *J Lab Clin Med*. 1948;33:875.

42. Wright WT. Cell counts in urine. *Arch Intern Med*. 1959;103:76.

43. Birch DF, Fairley KF, Whitworth JA, et al. Urinary erythrocyte morphology in the diagnosis of glomerular hematuria. *Clin Nephrol*. 1983;20:78.

44. Sayer J, McCarthy MP, Schmidt JD. Identification and significance of dysmorphic versus isomorphic hematuria. *J Urol*. 1990;143:545.

45. Corwin HL, Silverstein MD. The diagnosis of neoplasia in patients with asymptomatic microscopic hematuria: a decision analysis. *J Urol*. 1988;139:1002.

46. Kumon H, Tsugawa M, Matsumura Y, Ohmori H. Endoscopic diagnosis and treatment of chronic unilateral hematuria of uncertain etiology. *J Urol*. 1990;143:554.

47. Bagley DH, Allen J. Flexible uretheroplyeloscopy in the diagnosis of benign essential hematuria. *J Urol*. 1990;143:549.

48. Bennington JL, Beckwith JB. Tumors of the kidney, renal pelvis, and ureter. In: Firminger HI, ed. *Atlas of Tumor Pathology, Second Series*. Washington, DC: AFIP; 1975.

49. Anderstrom C, Johansson SL, Pettersson S, Wahlqvist L. Carcinoma of the ureter: a clinicopathologic study of 49 cases. *J Urol*. 1989;143:280.

50. McCarron JP, Mills C, Vaughn ED Jr. Tumors of the renal pelvis and ureter: current concepts and management. *Semin Urol*. 1983;1:75.

51. Babaian RJ, Johnson DE. Primary carcinoma of the ureter. *J Urol*. 1980;123:357.

52. Huffman JL, Bagley DH, Lyon ES, et al. Endoscopic diagnosis and treatment of upper-tract urothelial tumors. *Cancer*. 1985;55:1422.

53. Grabstald, Whitmore WF, Melamed MR. Renal pelvic tumors. *JAMA*. 1971;218:845.

54. Kakizoe T, Fujita J, Murase T, et al. Transitional cell carcinoma of the bladder in patients with renal pelvic and ureteral cancer. *J Urol*. 1980;124:17.

55. Sternberg CN, Yagoda A, Scher HI, et al. M-Vac (methotrexate, vinblastine, doxorubicin and cisplatin) for advanced transitional cell carcinoma of the urothelium. *J Urol*. 1988;139:461.

56. Herr HW. Durable response of a carcinoma in situ of the renal pelvis to topical bacillus Calmette-Guerin. *J Urol*. 1985;134:531.

57. Schoenberg MP, Van Arsdalen KN, Wein AJ. The management of transitional cell carcinoma in solitary renal units. *J Urol*. 1991;146:700.

58. See WA, Chapman WH. Tumor cell implantation following neodymium-YAG bladder injury: a comparison to electrocautery injury. *J Urol*. 1987;137:1266.

59. Beisland HO, Seland P. A prospective, randomized study on neodymium-YAG laser irradiation for treatment of urinary bladder tumors. *Scand J Urol Nephrol*. 1986;20:209.

60. American Cancer Society. *Cancer Facts and Figures, 1981*. New York, NY: American Cancer Society; 1982.

61. Loening S, Narayana A, Yoder L. Factors influencing the recurrence rate of bladder cancer. *J Urol*. 1980;123:29.

62. Pyrah LN, Raper FP, Thomas GJ. Report of follow-up of papillary tumors of the bladder. *Br J Urol*. 1964;36:14.

63. Caplan JH, McDonald JR, Thompson GJ. Multicentric origin of papillary tumors of the urinary tract. *J Urol*. 1951;66:792.

64. Massberg A, Samit AM. Early detection, diagnosis and management of oral and oropharyngeal cancers. *CA*. 1989;39:67.

65. Wu S, Lin ZQ, Xu CW, et al. Multiple primary lung cancers. *Chest*. 1987;92:892.

66. Marrano D, Biti G, Gringioni W, Marr A. Synchronous and metachronous cancer of the stomach. *Eur J Surg Oncol*. 1987;13:493.

67. Kellokumpu I, Husa A. Colorectal adenomas: morphologic features and the risk of developing metachronous adenomas and carcinomas in the colorectum. *Scand J Gastroenterol*. 1987;22:833.

68. Cumliffe WJ, Hasleton PS, Tweedle DEF, Schofield PF. Incidence of synchronous and metachronous colorectal carcinoma. *Br J Surg*. 1984;71:941.

69. Albarran J, Imbert L. *Les tumeurs du rein*. Paris: Masson et Cie; 1903:452.

70. Weyrauch HM, Crossfield JH. Dissemination of bladder neoplasms by endoscopic electroresection. *J Urol*. 1972;97:391.

71. Soloway MS, Masters S. Urothelial susceptibility to tumor cell implantation: influence of cauterization. *Cancer*. 1980;46:1158.

72. McDonald DF, Thornson T. Clinical implications of transplantability of induced bladder tumors to intact transitional epithelium in dogs. *J Urol*. 1956;75:960.

73. Hinman F. Recurrence of bladder tumor by surgical implantation. *J Urol*. 1956;75:695.

74. See WA, Miller JS, Williams RD. Pathophysiology of transitional tumor cell adherence to sites of urothelial injury in rats: mechanisms mediating intravesical recurrence due to implantation. *Cancer Res*. 1989;49:5414.

75. See WA, Chapman PH, Williams RD. Kinetics of tumor cell line 4909 adherence in injured urothelial surfaces in (F-344) rats. *Cancer Res*. 1990;50:2499.

76. Klan R, Loy V, Huland H. Residual tumor discovered in routine second transurethral resection in patients with stage T1 transitional cell carcinoma of the bladder. *J Urol*. 1991;146:316.

77. Parmar MKB, Freedman LS, Hargreave TB, Tolley DA. Prognostic factors for recurrence and followup policies in the treatment of superficial bladder cancer: report from the British Medical Research Council subgroup on superficial bladder cancer. *J Urol*. 1989;142:284.

78. National Bladder Cancer Collaborative Group A. Superficial bladder cancer: progression and recurrence. *J Urol*. 1983;130:1083.

79. Herr HW. Carcinoma in situ of the bladder. *Semin Urol*. 1983;1:15.

80. Herr HW, Laudone VP, Whitmore WF Jr. An overview of intravesical therapy for superficial bladder tumors. *J Urol*. 1987;138:1363.

81. Lamm DL, Stogdill VD, Stogdill BJ, Crispen RG. Complications of bacillus Calmette-Guérin immunotherapy in 1278

patients with bladder cancer. *J Urol.* 1986;135:272.

82. Orihuela E, Herr HW, Pinsky CM, Whitmor WF. Toxicity of intravesical BCG and its management in patients with superficial bladder tumors. *Cancer.* 1987;60:326.

83. Marans HY, Bekirov HM. Granulomatous hepatitis following intravesical bacillus Calmette-Guérin therapy for bladder carcinoma. *J Urol.* 1987;137:111.

84. Deresiewicz RL, Stone RM, Aster JC. Fatal disseminated mycobacterial infection following intravesical bacillus Calmette-Guérin administration for bladder cancer. *J Urol.* 1990;144:1331.

85. Torti F, Shortliffe LD, Williams RD, et al. Alpha-2 interferon in superficial bladder cancer: an NCOG study. *J Clin Onc.* 1988;6:476.

86. Kavoussi LR, Torrence RJ, Gillen DP, et al. Results of 6 weekly intravesical bacillus Calmette-Guérin instillations of the treatment of superficial bladder tumors. *J Urol.* 1988;139:935.

87. Hudson MA, Ratliff TL, Gillen DP, et al. Single course versus maintenance bacillus Calmette-Guérin therapy for superficial bladder tumors: a prospective randomized trial. *J Urol.* 1987;138:295.

88. Herr HW, Whitmore WF Jr. Ureteral carcinoma in situ after successful intravesical therapy for superficial bladder tumors: incidence, possible pathogenesis and management. *J Urol.* 1987;138:292.

89. Hardeman SW, Perry A, Soloway MS. Transitional cell carcinoma of the prostate following intravesical therapy for transitional cell carcinoma of the bladder. *J Urol.* 1988;140:289.

90. Skinner DG, Lieskovsky G. Management of invasive and high grade bladder cancer. In: Skinner DG, Lieskovsky G, eds. *Diagnosis and Management of Genitourinary Cancer.* Philadelphia, Pa: WB Saunders Co; 1988.

91. Walsh PC, Mostwin JL. Radical prostatectomy and cysto-prostatectomy with preservation of potency: results utilizing a new nerve-sparing technique. *Br J Urol.* 1984;56:694.

92. Skinner DG, Lieskovsky G, Boyd SD. Continuing experience with the continent ileal reservoir (Kock pouch) as an alternative to cutaneous urinary diversion: an update after 250 cases. *J Urol.* 1987;137:1140.

93. Rowland RG, Mitchell ME, Bihrle R, Kahnoski RJ, Piser JE. Indiana continent urinary reservoir. *J Urol.* 1987;137:1136.

94. Caldwell WC. Carcinoma of the urinary bladder. *JAMA.* 1974;229:1643.

95. Parsons JT, Million RP. Planned preoperative irradiation in management of clinical stage B2–C (T3) bladder carcinoma. *Int J Radiat Oncol Biol Phys.* 1988;4:797.

96. Batata MA, et al. Preoperative whole pelvis versus true pelvis irradiation and/or cystectomy for bladder cancer. *Int J Radiat Oncol Biol Phys.* 1981;7:1349.

97. Skinner DG, Lieskovsky G. Contemporary cystectomy with pelvic node dissection compared to preoperative radiation therapy plus cystectomy in management of invasive bladder cancer. *J Urol.* 1984;131:1069.

98. Slack NH, Bross ID, Prout GR Jr. Five-year follow-up results of a collaborative study of therapies for carcinoma of the bladder. *J Surg Oncol.* 1977;9:393.

99. Fagg SL, Dawson-Edwards P, Hughes MA, Latief TN, Rolfe EB, Fielding JW. Cis-diamminedichloroplatinum (DDP) as initial treatment of invasive bladder cancer. *Br J Urol.* 1984;56:296.

100. Pearson BS, Raghaven D. First-line intravenous cisplatin for deeply invasive bladder cancer: update on 70 cases. *Br J Urol.* 1985;57:690.

101. Scher HI, et al. Neoadjuvant M-VAC (methotrexate, vinblastine, doxorubicin, and cisplatin) effect on the primary bladder lesion. *J Urol.* 1988;139:470.

102. Zincke H, Sen SE, Hahn RG, Keating JP. Neoadjuvant chemotherapy for locally advanced transitional cell carcinoma of the bladder: do local findings suggest a potential for salvage of the bladder? *Mayo Clin Proc.* 1988;63:16.

103. Skinner DG, Tift JP, Kaufman JJ. High dose, short course preoperative radiation therapy and immediate single stage radial cystectomy with pelvic node dissection in the management of bladder cancer. *J Urol.* 1982;127:671.

104. Dreicer R, Messing EM, Loehrer PJ, Trump DL. Perioperative methotrexate, vinblastine, doxorubicin and cisplatin (M-VAC) for poor risk transitional cell carcinoma of the bladder: an Eastern Cooperative Oncology Group pilot study. *J Urol.* 1990;144:1123.

105. Herr HW, Whitmore WF Jr, Morse MJ, Sogani PC, Russo P, Fair WR. Neoadjuvant chemotherapy in invasive bladder cancer: the evolving role of surgery. *J Urol.* 1990;144:1083.

106. Kaufman DS, Shipley WU, Heney NM, et al. The integration of transurethral surgery, chemotherapy and radiation with bladder sparing in patients with invasive bladder cancer. *Proc Am Soc Clin Oncol.* 1991;10:163. Abstract 516.

107. Sternberg CN, Yagoda A, Scher HI, et al. M-VAC (methotrexate, vinblastine, doxorubicin and cisplatin) for advanced transitional cell carcinoma of the urothelium. *J Urol.* 1988;139:461.

108. Tannock I, Gospodarowicz M, Connolly J, Jewett M. M-VAC (methotrexate, vinlbastine, doxorubicin and cisplatin) chemotherapy for transitional cell carcinoma: the Princess Margaret Hospital experience. *J Urol.* 1989;142:289.

109. Fung CY, et al. Prognostic factors in invasive bladder carcinoma in a prospective trial of preoperative adjuvant chemotherapy and radiotherapy. *Clin Oncol.* 1991;9:1533.

110. Einstein AB Jr, et al. Cisplatin adjuvant therapy following preoperative radiotherapy plus radical cystectomy for invasive bladder carcinoma: a randomized trial of the national bladder group. *Am Urol Assoc.* 1985;133:222. Abstract 433.

111. Logothetis CJ, et al. Adjuvant cyclophosphamide, doxorubicin, and cisplatin chemotherapy for bladder cancer: an update. *Clin Oncol.* 1988;6:1590.

112. Skinner DG, et al. The role of adjuvant chemotherapy following cystectomy for invasive bladder cancer: a prospective comparative trial. *J Urol.* 1991;145:459.

113. Logothetis CJ, Dexeus FH, Sella A, Amato Ri, Finn LD. A prospective randomized trial of CISCA vs M-VAC chemotherapy for patients with metastatic urothelial tumors. *J Clin Oncol.* 1990;8:1050.

114. Yagoda A. Chemotherapy of metastatic bladder cancer. *Cancer.* 1980;45(suppl):1879.

115. Harker WG, Meyers FJ, Freiha FS, et al. Cisplatin, methotrexate and vinblastine (CMV): an effective chemotherapy regimen for metastatic transitional cell carcinoma of the urinary tract: a Northern California Oncology Group study. *J Clin Oncol.* 1985;3:1463.

116. Sternberg CN, Yagoda A, Scher HI, et al. M-VAC (methotrexate, vinblastine, doxorubicin and cisplatin) for advanced transitional cell carcinoma of the urothelium. *J Urol.* 1988;139:461.

117. Logothetis CJ, Samuels ML, Ogden S, et al. Cyclophosphamide, doxorubicin and cisplatin chemotherapy for patients with locally advanced urothelial tumors with or without nodal metastases. *J Urol.* 1985;134:460.

118. Soloway MS, Einstein A, Corder MP, Bonney W, Prout GR Jr, Coombs JA. Comparison of cisplatin and the combination of cisplatin and cyclophosphamide in advanced urothelial cancer: a National Bladder Cancer Collaborative Group A study. *Cancer.* 1983;52:767.

119. Khandekar JD, Elson PJ, DeWys WD, Slayton RE, Harris DT. Comparative activity and toxicity of cisdiamminedichloroplatinum (DDP) and a combination of doxorubicin, cyclophosphamide, and DDP in disseminated transitional cell carcinomas of the urinary tract. *J Clin Oncol.* 1985;3:539.

120. Hillcoat BI, Raghavan D, Matthews J, et al. A randomized trial of cisplatin versus cisplatin methotrexate in advanced cancer of the urothelial tract. *J Clin Oncol.* 1989;7:706.

121. Loehrer PJ Sr, Elson P, Kuebler JP, et al. Advanced bladder cancer: a prospective intergroup trial comparing single agent cisplatin (CDDP) versus M-VAC combination therapy (INT 0078). *Proc Am Soc Clin Oncol.* 1990;8:132. Abstract 511.

122. Sternberg CN, Yagoda A, Scher HI, et al. Methotrexate, vinblastine, doxorubicin, and cisplatin for advanced transitional cell carcinoma of the urothelium. *Cancer.* 1989;64:2448.

123. Geller NL, Sternberg CN, Penenberg D, Scher H, Yagoda A. Prognostic factors for survival of patients with methotrexate, vinblastine, doxorubicin, and cisplatin chemotherapy. *Cancer.* 1991;67:1525.

124. Raghavan D, Grundy R, Greenaway TM, et al. Preemptive (neo-adjuvant) chemotherapy prior to radical radiotherapy for fit septuagenarians with bladder cancer: age itself is not a contra-indication. *Br J Urol.* 1988;62:154.

125. Roila F, Tonato M, Cognetti F, et al. Prevention of cisplatin-induced emesis: a double-blind multicenter randomized crossover study comparing ondansetron and ondansetron plus dexamethasone. *J Clin Oncol.* 1991;9:675.

126. Hainsworth J, Harvey W, Pendergrass K, et al. A single-blind comparison of intravenous ondansetron, a selective serotonin antagonist with intravenous metoclopramide in the prevention of nausea and vomiting associated with high-dose cisplatin chemotherapy. *J Clin Oncol.* 1991;9:721.

127. Lindemann A, Herrmann F, Oster W, et al. Hematologic effects of recombinant human granulocyte colony stimulating factor in patients with malignancy. *Blood.* 1989;74:2644.

128. Gabrilove JL, Jakubowski A, Scher H, et al. Effect of granulocyte colony-stimulating factor on neutropenia and associated morbidity due to chemotherapy for transitional-cell carcinoma of the urothelium. *N Engl J Med.* 1988;318:1414.

129. Logothetis CJ, Dexeus FH, Sella A, et al. Escalated therapy for refractory urothelial tumors: methotrexate-vinblastine-doxorubicin-cisplatin plus unglycosylated recombinant human granulocyte-macrophage colony-stimulating factor. *J Natl Cancer Inst.* 1990;82:667

CHAPTER 5

Tumors of the Prostate

David E. McGinnis

Leonard G. Gomella

Epidemiology

Carcinoma of the prostate is an increasingly common problem in American men, and the management of prostate cancer continues to be controversial. Carcinoma of the prostate is the most common cancer in men in 1993, with an estimated 165,000 cases. It is the second most common cause of mortality from cancer, with an estimated 35,000 deaths.[1] Occult prostate cancer is even more prevalent than clinically evident prostate cancer. Autopsy studies indicate that 20% of men aged 50 to 59, 25% of men aged 60 to 69, 40% of men aged 70 to 79, and over 50% of men over age 80 have occult cancer of the prostate.[2] These data are derived from autopsy series of men who died of causes other than prostate cancer. The clinical dilemma in prostate cancer treatment is whether a given cancer will remain clinically silent or will be life-threatening. According to these statistics, over his lifetime a 50-year-old man has a 42% chance of having prostate cancer, a 10% chance of having clinically evident carcinoma of the prostate, and a 3% chance of dying from carcinoma of the prostate.[2] How to determine which carcinomas of the prostate are life-threatening is difficult and complicates prostate cancer screening.

Detection of Prostate Cancer

In its earliest stages, prostate cancer is often asymptomatic. It is usually found on routine screening examinations, although sometimes patients present with symptoms of advanced disease. Cancer may also be an incidental finding on pathologic examination of tissue from prostatectomy for presumed benign disease. Voiding symptoms, hematuria, hematospermia, pelvic or perineal pain, bone pain, or azotemia may be the first presentation of prostate cancer.

Prostate cancer is now often detected by routine screening. Currently, the American Cancer Society recommends that all men aged 50 to 70 undergo an annual digital rectal examination (DRE) and serum prostate-specific antigen (PSA) assay. This should start at age 40 if there is a strong family history or in African Americans.[3] Abnormalities of either DRE or PSA are indications for prostate biopsy. Findings suggestive of prostate cancer on DRE include nodularity, marked asymmetry, induration, or fixation. A PSA of 0 to 4 ng/mL (monoclonal assay) is considered "normal," but cases of prostate cancer can be diagnosed with a PSA of less than 4 ng/mL. An abnormal PSA may be due to benign prostatic hypertrophy (BPH), prostate cancer, prostatitis, prostatic infarcts, prostatic biopsy, surgery, or other causes. Significant elevations of PSA, greater than 10 to 20 ng/mL, in the absence of prostatitis or recent prostate biopsy, are strongly suggestive of cancer of the prostate.

Two new methods of interpreting PSA levels have recently been studied: PSA velocity and PSA density. Carter and colleagues studied the rate of change of serum PSA (PSA velocity) in patients with 1) no prostatic disease, 2) benign prostatic hypertrophy (BPH) requiring prostatectomy, or 3) prostate cancer. They found that PSA velocities were markedly different in each group. A velocity greater than 0.75 ng/mL per year (in the 5 years prior to the diagnosis of cancer)[4] was associated with the presence of prostate cancer. Other investigators have

---

FIGURE 5.1 *Summary of the Positive Predictive Value of DRE, TRUS, and PSA in the Detection of Prostate Cancer*

POSITIVE PREDICTIVE VALUE (IN %, LISTED IN ASCENDING ORDER)

5.4%	DRE −, TRUS +, PSA −
6.4%	DRE +, TRUS −, PSA −
15.2%	DRE +, TRUS +, PSA −
27.3%	DRE +, TRUS −, PSA +
32.8%	DRE −, TRUS +, PSA +
62.2%	DRE +, TRUS +, PSA +

DRE = digital rectal examination; TRUS = transrectal ultrasound; PSA = prostatic-specific antigen

PSA positive is defined as a value >4.0 ng/mL on Hybritech assay.

Based on data from Littrup PJ, Lee F, Mettlin C. Prostate cancer screening: current trends and future applications. *CA.* 1992;42:198.

studied the relation of prostate size to PSA in order to distinguish between PSA elevated because of a large volume of BPH and PSA elevated because of prostate cancer (in a proportionally small prostate). Early studies do seem to indicate that a higher PSA density (serum PSA divided by prostatic volume) determined by transrectal ultrasound (TRUS)[5] correlates with risk of prostate cancer. Further study with a screening population and a large number of patients will be required to determine exactly how helpful PSA velocity and PSA density will be in screening patients for prostate cancer.

There was some enthusiasm in the 1980s for using TRUS (transrectal ultrasound) as a screening modality in prostate cancer. Typically, prostate cancers appear hypoechoic on TRUS; however, at least 30% of prostate cancers are isoechoic.[6] Currently, TRUS does not appear to have a role in screening, but it is useful in directing the biopsy and increasing the accuracy of prostate biopsies and allows determination of prostate volume (for the calculation of PSA density).

PSA has recently been evaluated as a screening tool. In a study by Catalona and associates,[7] patients with a PSA level of 4 to 10 ng/mL (Hybritech) had a one-third chance of having prostate cancer, whereas patients with a PSA level greater than 10 ng/mL had a two-thirds chance of having carcinoma of the prostate. Most investigators believe that digital rectal exam and PSA should be used in combination to screen for prostate cancer.

Current data from the American Cancer Society National Prostate Cancer Detection Project summarize the positive predictive value of digital rectal examination, transrectal ultrasound, and PSA measurement (Fig. 5.1).

Pathology

More than 95% of prostatic malignancies are adenocarcinomas. The treatment of other histologic types, such as squamous, transitional, or endometrial carcinomas, will not be discussed here. Most grading systems for adenocarcinoma of the prostate are based on acinar configurations, while some other systems also consider nuclear morphology, tumor volume, and invasion.

The most common system in use today is the Gleason grading scale. Tumors are graded on a scale of 1 to 5 and then given a score based on the grade of the two most common histologic patterns seen within the tumor (Fig. 5.2). The grade correlates with the biologic potential of prostate cancer. Studies of lymph node metastases show a higher rate of metastases in higher-grade tumors.[8] According to Paulson's data, 15% of patients with Gleason score 2 to 5, 50% with score 7, and more than 75% with score 8 to 10 have lymph node metastasis.[9] DNA ploidy also broadly correlates with the biologic potential of prostate cancer. Although studies are still in progress, patients with diploid tumors are more likely to respond to hormonal therapy and less likely to experience tumor progression, and have a better overall survival than patients with aneuploid tumors.

Staging

The Whitmore-Jewett staging system has been the most commonly used system. Stage A denotes nonpalpable cancer; stage B denotes palpable cancer that is confined to the prostate gland; stage C denotes cancer that has

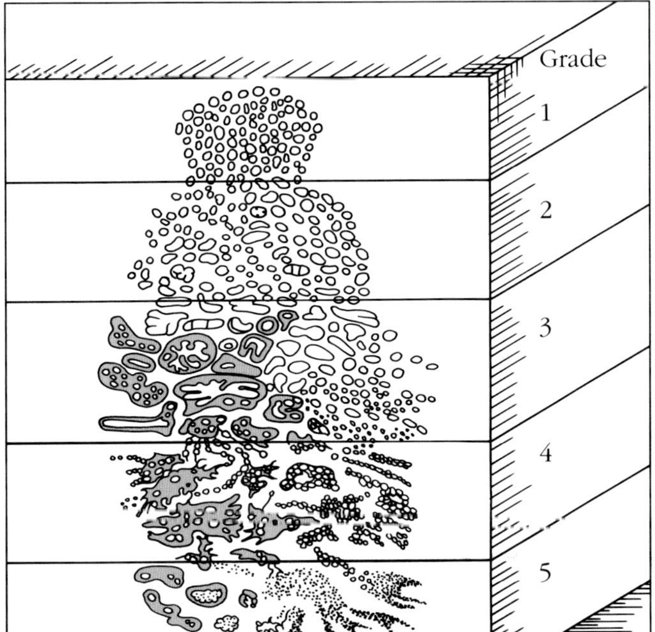

Figure 5.2 Gleason grading system for prostate cancer.

locally invaded beyond the prostate gland into either the capsule or the seminal vesicles; stage D indicates metastatic disease (Fig. 5.3). More recent investigators have been using the TNM system of staging. Prostate cancer staging systems may require further modification to accommodate tumors discovered by PSA screening or transrectal ultrasound. It is not clear whether these tumors behave the same as traditional stage A tumors discovered by transurethral resection of the prostate.

The staging evaluation of prostate cancer is a matter of controversy. Digital rectal exam (DRE) is required in all patients. However, compared to pathologic staging, digital rectal exam understages as many as 50% of patients.

Serum PSA and prostatic acid phosphatase measurements should be obtained initially in all patients with prostate cancer. A PSA level greater than 10 ng/mL has been found to be associated with a higher rate of locally advanced cancer.[7] Routine screening digital rectal exam will not spuriously elevate PSA unless the patient has acute prostatitis at the time of the exam.[10] Acid phosphatase is not sensitive enough to be used as a screening tool; however, elevation of prostatic acid phosphatase should make one suspicious of locally advanced or metastatic disease. Prostatic acid phosphatase is elevated in 10% to 80% of patients with localized carcinoma of the prostate; it is elevated in 50% to 90% of patients with metastatic disease.[11]

Radionuclide bone scan is a standard staging study in prostate cancer since bone is the next most common site of metastases after the pelvic lymph nodes. The use of

FIGURE 5.3 *Prostate Cancer Staging*

TNM CLASSIFICATION		AMERICAN UROLOGICAL ASSOCIATION CLASSIFICATION (A–D) (MODIFIED)		
T0	No evidence of primary tumor	Stage	A	No palpable lesion
T1a	Three or fewer microscopic foci of carcinoma		A1	Focal
T1b	More than 3 microscopic foci of carcinoma		A2	Diffuse
T2	Tumor present clinically or grossly, limited to the gland	Stage	B	Confined to prostate
T2a	Tumor 1.5 cm or less in greatest dimension with normal tissue on two sides		B1	Small discrete nodule
T2b	Tumor more than 1.5 cm in greatest dimension or in more than one lobe		B2	Large or multiple nodules or areas
T3	Tumor invades the prostatic apex or into or beyond the prostatic capsule, bladder neck, or seminal vesicle but is not fixed	Stage	C	Localized to periprostatic area
			C1	No involvement of seminal vesicle, <70 g
T4	Tumor is fixed or invades adjacent structures other than those listed in T3		C2	Involvement of seminal vesicles, >70 g
N1	Metastasis in a single lymph node, 2 cm or less in greatest dimension	Stage	D	Metastatic disease
			D0	Elevated markers only
N2	Metastasis in a single lymph node, more than 2 cm but not more than 5 cm in greatest dimension, or multiple lymph nodes, none more than 5 cm in greatest dimension		D1	Pelvic lymph node metastases
N3	Metastasis in a lymph node more than 5 cm in greatest dimension		D2	Bone or distant lymph node or organ or soft tissue metastases
			D3	Hormone-refractory
M1	Distant metastasis			

Adapted with permission from Gomella L. *Clinicians Pocket Reference.* 7th ed. Norwalk, Conn: Appleton and Lange; 1993:277.

bone scans in every prostate cancer patient has recently been questioned. In a study from the Mayo Clinic, the results of bone scans were compared with PSA levels. Of patients who had PSA levels less than 20 ng/mL, only 1 out of 306 had a positive bone scan.[12] However, a bone scan is still recommended for the baseline staging of all prostate cancer patients by most clinicians.

Local staging of carcinoma of the prostate is more problematic. Studies by Rifkin et al.[13] and McSherry et al.[14] have compared pathologic staging to local staging by pre-operative digital rectal exam, transrectal ultrasound (TRUS), and magnetic resonance imaging (MRI). All of these staging modalities suffer difficulties of understaging. If the studies predicted stage C disease, they were correct in 70% to 100% of cases; however, if they predicted disease confined to the prostate (i.e., stage B), this was confirmed pathologically in 30% to 40% of cases. Rifkin's study showed that transrectal ultrasound was slightly more accurate than digital rectal exam and MRI was slightly more accurate than transrectal ultrasound. Studies are now ongoing to evaluate endorectal coil MRI of the prostate. It is unclear yet whether this modality will improve our accuracy of staging localized prostate cancer.

Evaluation of the pelvic lymph nodes for metastasis is another important aspect of staging prostate cancer.[15] This is important since patients with lymph node metastases have a markedly different prognosis and merit different treatment. Imaging studies of the pelvic lymph nodes have largely been unsatisfactory. Trials of lymphangiography, CT, and MRI have shown the inability of these modalities to detect lymph node involvement until it is quite advanced (i.e., nodes larger than 1 cm). Surgical staging of the pelvic lymph nodes has been the standard method; however, open surgical dissection of the pelvic lymph nodes has the usual morbidity of an abdominal operation. A new technique, laparoscopy, has been used recently for pelvic lymph node dissection in selected patients. The chief advantages of laparoscopy are the accuracy of surgical staging and lower morbidity; the technique is discussed below.

Prostate Biopsy

Core needle and fine needle aspiration biopsies (FNAB) of the prostate, often combined with ultrasound guidance, are the modalities most widely used to diagnose prostate cancer. Whether the diagnosis should be established by FNAB or core tissue biopsy is unsettled. FNAB has been used most extensively in Europe and recently has become more popular in the United States. FNAB has the advantages of being relatively easy to perform, requiring no anesthesia, having a very low complication rate, and allowing rapid pathologic interpretation. The main disadvantage is that it requires a cytopathologist who is experienced in the interpretation of FNAB. Transurethral prostate biopsy is not currently widely used.

Abnormal DRE or PSA is the main indication for prostate biopsy to detect prostate cancer. Patients with palpable nodules and patients with normal exams but abnormal serum PSA levels should undergo prostate biopsy. Biopsy may also be used to assess the efficacy of definitive radiation therapy in a patient with previously diagnosed prostate cancer. The addition of PSA density and PSA velocity may further define the indications for biopsy of the prostate (see Detection above).

PREOPERATIVE PREPARATION

Patients should be screened to rule out a bleeding diathesis and should refrain from ingesting aspirin or non-steroidal antiinflammatory agents for 1 week prior to biopsy. If the transperineal approach is used, shaving is not necessary, but the skin should be prepared with a cleansing solution (e.g., povidone-iodine). For the transrectal biopsy, an oral antibiotic (usually a fluoroquinolone) is administered 30 to 60 minutes before the procedure and is continued for 2 to 3 days. A cleansing enema is usually given just before the procedure.

Prostatic biopsy can be performed under general, regional, local, or no anesthesia. With advances in technique, biopsies are now most often performed without anesthesia. Intermediate-sized 18-gauge core biopsy needles and rapid-fire, spring-loaded biopsy guns allow patients to tolerate biopsies by the transrectal approach easily without anesthesia. If the transperineal approach is used, 1% lidocaine anesthesia is needed. Fine needle aspiration of the prostate is most often performed transrectally without any anesthesia.

OPERATIVE TECHNIQUES
Digitally Directed Core Biopsy

The Vim-Silverman needle has been used for many years; however, the 18-gauge core biopsy needle, with or without the spring-loaded biopsy gun, is preferred by most urologists. The Vim-Silverman needle works by trapping tissue in its core needle, which is then sheared off by rotating the outer cutting sheath. Its disadvantages are that it is larger, and therefore more likely to require anesthesia as well as more cumbersome. More commonly used are the intermediate-sized 18-gauge biopsy needles (e.g., Tru-cut), and the spring-loaded, rapid-fire biopsy gun (e.g., Biopty). Figure 5.4 shows various biopsy needles and devices.

The patient is placed in the dorsal lithotomy position. A transrectal or transperineal approach can be taken. The transrectal approach permits more accurate needle placement into the lesion and does not require any anesthesia, but it is associated with a higher incidence of septic and bleeding complications (see below). The transperineal approach is associated with fewer complications, but it requires local anesthesia and directing the needle into the lesion is often more difficult than in the transrectal technique.

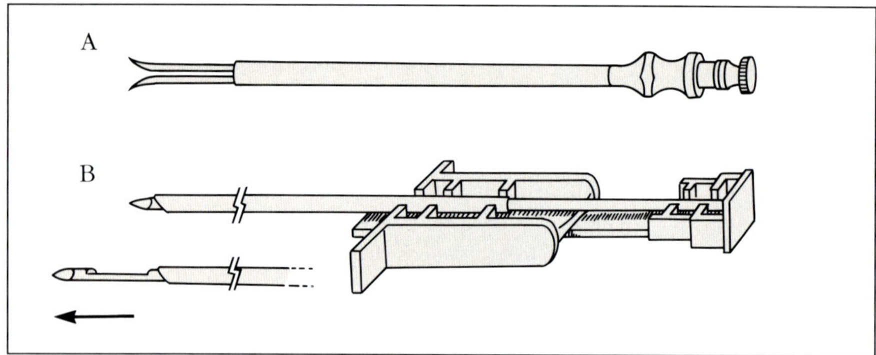

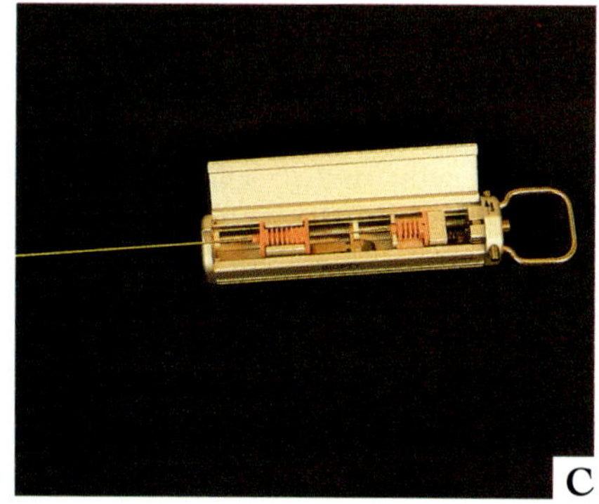

Figure 5.4 Prostate biopsy devices. **A** Vim-Silverman needle. **B** Trucut needle. **C** Biopsy gun. A biopsy needle is loaded into the device and the spring is loaded. (Courtesy of BARD Urologic, Covington, Ga)

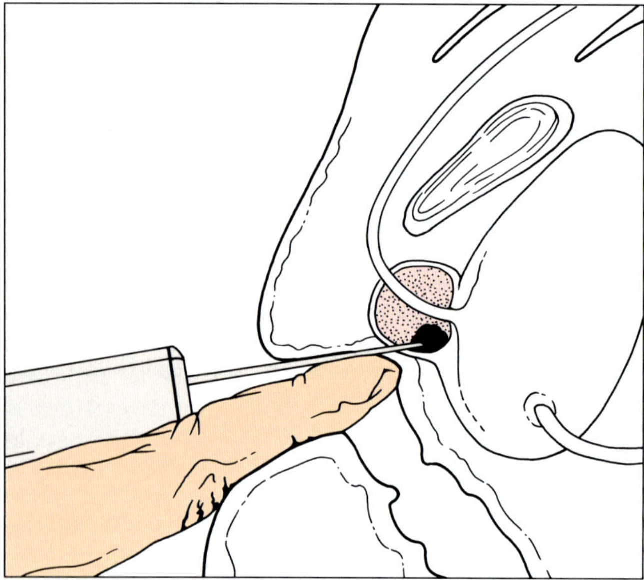

Figure 5.5 Transrectal needle biopsy of the prostate. The 18-gauge core biopsy needle is loaded in the rapid-fire biopsy gun. The trigger is activated and with digital guidance the biopsy needle passes rapidly into the prostate.

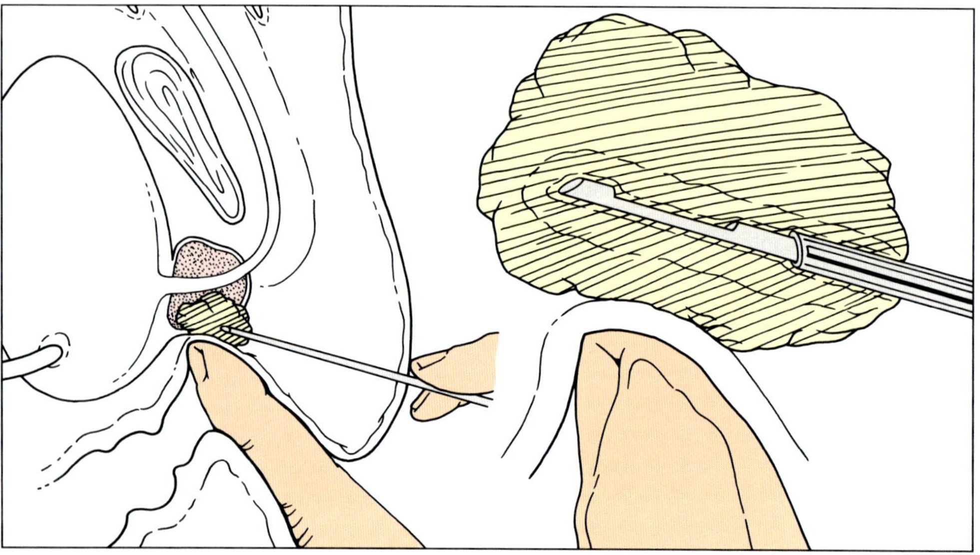

Figure 5.6 Transperineal prostate biopsy. After the perineum is anesthetized, the transperineal biopsy needle is passed into the prostate nodule using digital rectal guidance.

Digitally Directed Transrectal Core Biopsy

The biopsy needle is inserted along with the well-lubricated index finger. The lesion is palpated and the needle is advanced through the rectal wall into the lesion (Fig. 5.5). If the biopsy gun is used, the needle tip is positioned at the lesion and the gun is activated, causing rapid passage of the cutting needle and the outer sheath through the rectal wall into the lesion. The needle is removed and the core of prostatic tissue is recovered.

Transperineal Core Biopsy

The perineal skin above the rectum is anesthetized with 1% lidocaine, and the deeper tissues and periprostatic area are anesthetized with a 22-gauge spinal needle. A small stab wound with a #11 blade eases passage of the needle into the skin. The core biopsy needle is then inserted into the perineum while the examining finger is in the rectum. The needle is advanced under bimanual control to the suspicious area and the sample is taken (Fig. 5.6).

Digitally Directed Fine Needle Aspiration

FNAB of the prostate can be done with various patient positions: dorsal lithotomy position, knee-chest position, or leaning over the examining table with the feet spread apart slightly. The Franzen style (22-gauge) biopsy needle is prepared by aspirating approximately 1 mL of saline into the needle and expelling the saline (Fig. 5.7). A needle guide is placed over a gloved index finger (Fig. 5.8A). The Franzen needle is then attached to a 10 mL aspirating syringe (Fig. 5.8B). A second glove is placed over the needle guide. The needle is passed through the glove into the needle guide (Fig. 5.8C). The index finger is lubricated and passed into the rectum, and the prostatic abnormality is palpated (Fig. 5.8D). Negative pressure is applied and the needle is passed using a back and forth motion throughout the area for 20 to 30 seconds. The negative pressure is released and the needle is withdrawn. Failure to release the negative pressure prior to

removing the needle will result in fecal material contaminating the specimen.

Depending on the pathologist's requirements, the aspirate can be handled in either of two ways. The usual FNAB procedure is to use an air-filled syringe to expel the needle's contents onto a glass slide. A "smear" is made by quickly passing a second clean slide over the drop expelled from the needle. The slide is then either air dried or placed in alcohol fixative for later staining. Some laboratories now ask that the aspirate be drawn into a clean syringe using 2 mL of saline and expelled into fixative solution. This procedure should be repeated for a total of three to four collections. It is more comfortable for the patient if the examining finger is left in the rectum between collections.

Ultrasound-Directed Biopsy

Core needle and aspiration biopsy both can be performed under TRUS guidance. Core biopsy is more commonly performed using ultrasound guidance.

The role of TRUS in biopsy of the prostate is controversial. When a clearly palpable abnormality is present, the diagnostic accuracy of digitally directed biopsy appears similar to that of ultrasound-directed biopsy in some studies; other investigators show improved accuracy using ultrasound guidance. Ultrasound guidance is probably most useful when the prostate is palpably normal but the PSA is elevated, in cases where a suspicious gland has been previously biopsied without a definitive diagnosis, or if the findings on rectal exam are subtle. Although prostate cancer is classically described as hypoechoic on TRUS, it is now recognized that prostatic malignancies may also be hyperechoic, isoechoic, or of mixed echogenicity. Since up to 30% of cancers may be isoechoic and therefore not well visualized on TRUS, random biopsies of four to six ultrasonically normal areas will increase the diagnostic accuracy.[16,17] Newer color Doppler imaging shows promise in identifying cancerous

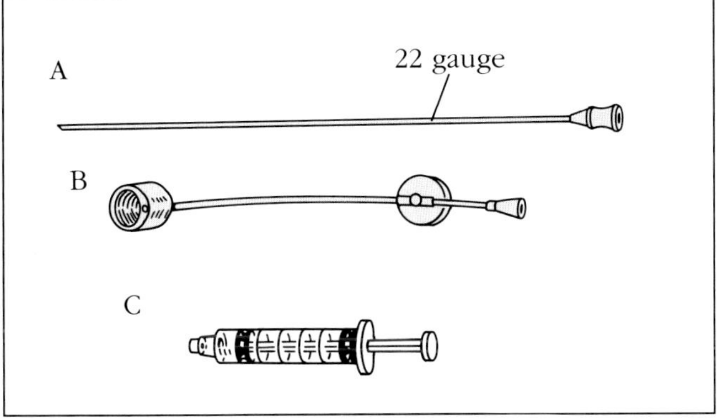

Figure 5.7 Fine needle aspiration biopsy. A 22-gauge Franzen needle **A**, needle guide with adjustable palm plate **B**, and special double-stoppered aspirating syringe **C** are the basic equipment needed for fine needle aspiration biopsy.

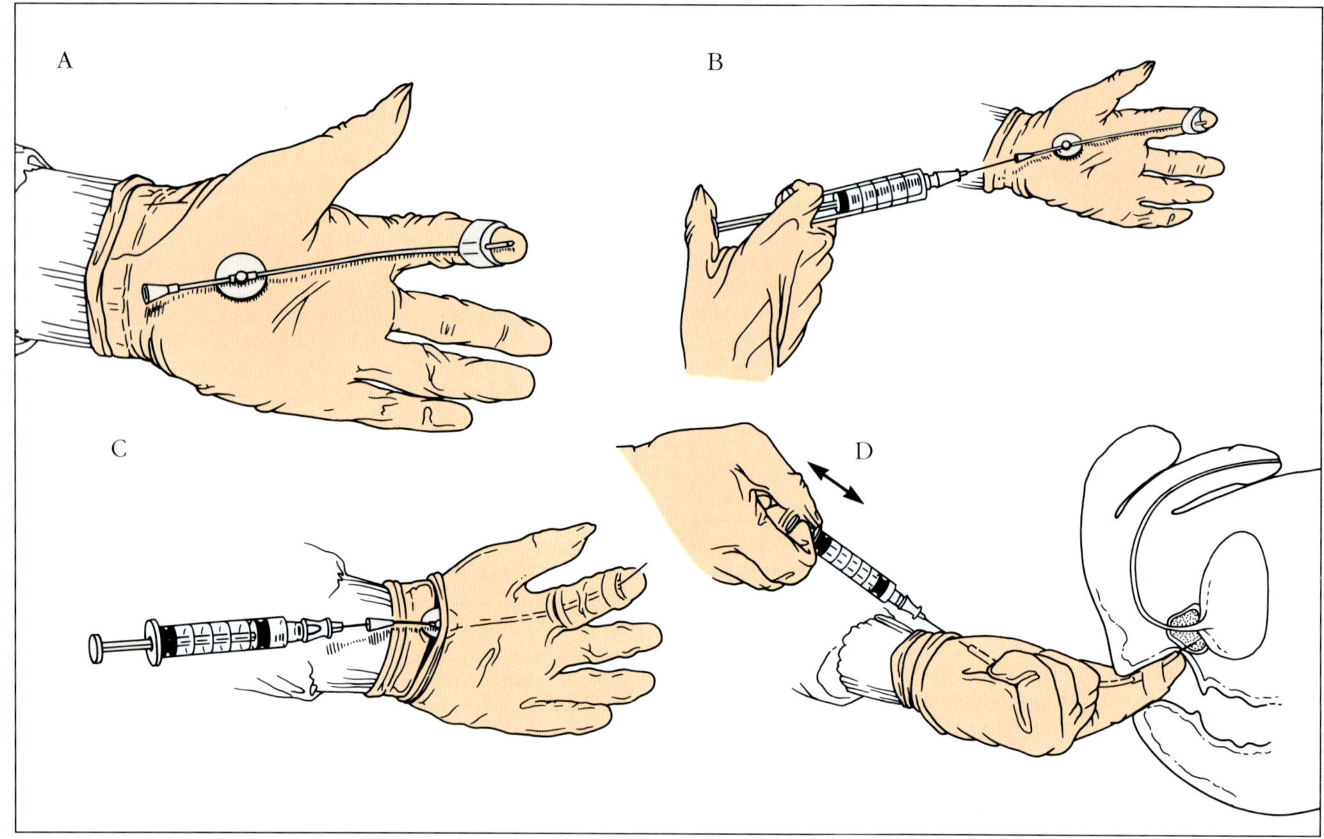

Figure 5.8 Fine needle aspiration biopsy. To perform fine needle aspiration biopsy, the needle guide is placed over the index finger of the gloved examining hand and the palm plate is adjusted **A**. The needle is connected to the syringe **B**. A second glove is applied and the needle is passed through it into the guide **C**. The finger is then lubricated and passed into the rectum, where the needle tip is passed repeatedly into the lesion while aspirating on the needle **D**.

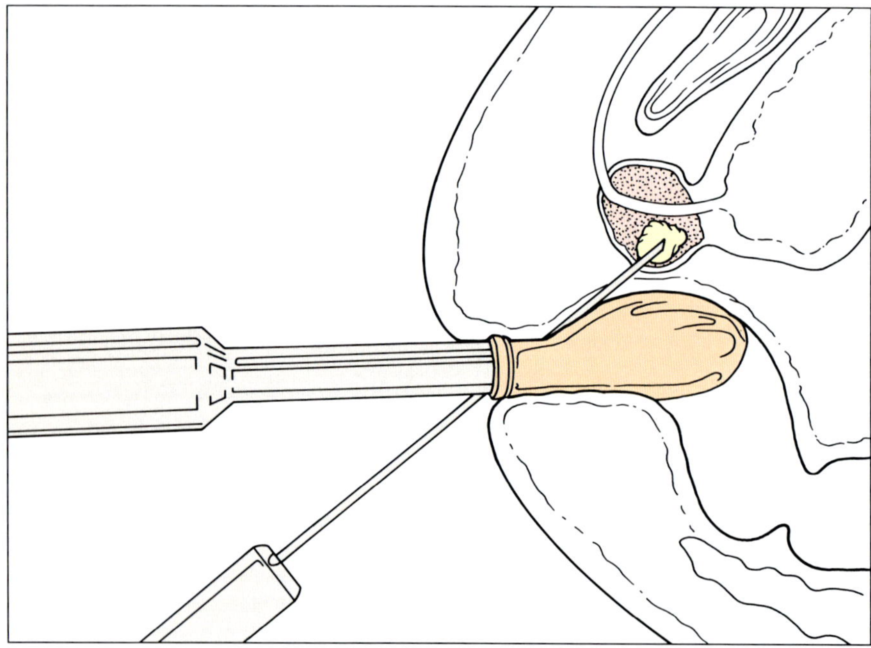

Figure 5.9 Transrectal ultrasonically directed biopsy using a state-of-the-art probe that can visualize the prostate in both transverse and longitudinal (sagittal) planes. The needle guide is intrinsic to the probe and the biopsy is done here using the spring-loaded biopsy gun.

lesions.[18] Patient preparation is identical to that for a digitally directed core biopsy. The dorsal lithotomy position is most frequently used for the transperineal biopsy. Transrectal biopsy is usually performed in the lateral decubitus position.

Ultrasound transducers are typically in the 5.0 to 7.5 MHz range and can produce real-time imaging of the gland. Newer biplanar probes allow scanning of the prostate in both longitudinal (sagittal) and transverse planes with the same instrument. Transverse scanning is best for defining the lateral margins of the prostate and longitudinal scanning is most useful for the prostate biopsy, since the entire needle can be visualized and the exact tissue being biopsied can be clearly identified.

The ultrasound probe is prepared according to manufacturer's specifications. All transducers are covered with a protective condom; some require that the condom be filled with 40 to 60 mL of water as an acoustic interface. If the transducer requires a water interface, all air bubbles should be aspirated prior to insertion of the probe. The condom is lubricated and inserted into the rectum. The entire prostate is examined for abnormalities before the biopsy is performed. Biopsy can be performed "freehand"; however, needle guides, either built into or attached onto the probe, are most commonly used (Fig. 5.9).

POSTOPERATIVE CARE

Patients are observed until they are able to void. Hematuria is common, but grossly bloody urine may occasionally require catheterization and irrigation. Oral broad-spectrum antibiotics (fluoroquinolones) are continued for 2 to 3 days. Patients are to refrain from any heavy exertion for 1 week and should be informed that hematospermia is not unusual for several weeks after prostate biopsy.

COMPLICATIONS

Transrectal core needle biopsy is associated with higher complication rates, including hematuria (37%), bloody bowel movements (9.4%), and sepsis (2%). Complications of FNAB and transperineal biopsy are infrequent.

Lymphadenectomy for Staging

The lymphatic drainage of the prostate includes three primary chains of lymph nodes: external iliac, internal iliac, and presacral. The external iliac nodes run from lateral to the external iliac artery laterally to the obturator fossa medially. The internal iliac nodes are found along the branches of the artery of the same name, and the presacral nodes are found anterior to the sacral promontory. Whitmore suggests that a modified pelvic lymph node dissection (obturator), including the internal iliac nodes and the medial aspect of the external iliac nodes, is sufficient for staging prostate cancer. There was no change in the incidence of positive nodes compared with a standard lymph node dissection, which includes the lateral external iliac nodes. The advantages of the modified pelvic lymphadenectomy are less edema of the genitals and lower extremities and a shorter operating time when compared to the standard (extended) node dissection.

LAPAROSCOPIC PELVIC LYMPHADENECTOMY

Laparoscopic pelvic lymphadenectomy for staging prostate cancer is a rapidly evolving new technique. The advantages over open surgical lymphadenectomy include shorter hospitalization (0 to 2 days rather than 5 to 7 days), less patient discomfort, lower cost, and quicker resumption of normal activities (1 week rather than 4 weeks).[19,20]

Although there have been previous laparoscopic applications in urology (such as the localization of undescended testicles), transperitoneal lymphadenectomy for staging prostate and bladder cancer is a recent application of this technology.[21,22] Carcinoma of the prostate is the leading solid tumor in males, so there is currently widespread interest in this technique.

In spite of advances in imaging techniques, pathologic staging of the pelvic lymph nodes remains the most accurate modality for staging localized prostate cancer.[23] Laparoscopic transperitoneal lymphadenectomy is a major advance in minimally invasive surgery.[24,25] Early studies indicate that the number of pelvic lymph nodes removed with the laparoscope is similar to the number removed with open lymph node dissection.[26]

Indications

Not all patients with prostate cancer need to be staged with a laparoscopic pelvic lymph node dissection.[27] At present, the procedure is most useful where there is concern that the patient may have stage D1 prostate cancer (pelvic node involvement) but this cannot be conclusively established by less invasive studies, or if definitive therapy (e.g., radiation) is being considered and accurate staging of the nodes is critical. Perineal prostatectomy is enjoying a resurgence of interest now that a minimally invasive node dissection technique is available.

Contraindications include the inability to tolerate a general anesthetic or pneumoperitoneum (due to heart or lung disease), extreme obesity, large intraabdominal masses, ileus or obstruction, extensive lower abdominal surgery, aneurysmal disease, previous vascular graft surgery, inflammatory bowel disease, history of peritonitis, and diaphragmatic hernia.

Preoperative Preparation

A mild bowel prep (milk of magnesia the afternoon before and a Fleets enema the morning of the procedure) is used. Patients are also encouraged to avoid dairy products for 2 days before the procedure to help control intestinal gas. Broad-spectrum prophylactic antibiotics (such as ceftriaxone) are given preoperatively and for several doses postoperatively.

General endotracheal anesthesia is used. Nitrous oxide is to be avoided since it can cause bowel distention.

Operative Technique

Instrumentation used in interventional gynecology or in laparoscopic cholecystectomy is easily adapted to laparoscopic lymph node dissection. It is advisable to have a laparotomy set-up available in the room in case it is needed. Two operating surgeons and a camera assistant are needed. The operation is viewed by all participants on one or two video monitors and close teamwork must be emphasized in the practice of laparoscopic surgery. Early experience is being gained in the preperitoneal laparoscopic approach. At present, most laparoscopic pelvic lymphadenectomy is being performed by the transperitoneal route.

A nasogastric tube and Foley catheter are placed to decompress the bladder and stomach, and pneumatic compression stockings are used to prevent deep venous thrombosis. The patient is positioned supine on the operating table with a roll of towels under the buttocks. The table is broken slightly to allow easier access to the pelvis. The entire abdomen is prepped from the genitalia to the subcostal area. The Trendelenberg position will displace the small intestine out of the operative field, and rolling the table to the side opposite the dissection also helps to improve visualization.

Four ports are usually used: one for the laparoscope and three working ports (Fig. 5.10). A new modification is the "fan" technique using five working ports. The five trocars are particularly useful for obese patients (Fig. 5.11).[28] Usually the umbilical port is placed first. A small skin incision is made inferior or superior to the umbilicus. The abdominal wall is lifted upward, usually with the aid of towel clips placed on either side of the umbilicus, and a Veress needle is passed through the fascia and into the abdominal cavity (Fig. 5.12). The spring-loaded tip of the Veress needle helps prevent inadvertent bowel injury. Various tests can then be performed to verify that the needle is inside the peritoneum. Five to 10 mL of saline can be injected into the needle: if the needle is in the correct position, the water cannot be aspirated. Alternatively, a drop of saline is placed on the Veress needle hub and the abdominal wall is lifted upward. If the needle is inside the peritoneum, the negative pressure will draw the drop into the abdomen. Lastly, if the initial pressure reading is less than 6 to 8 mm Hg, the needle is probably within the peritoneal cavity. False-positive results can be seen with any of these techniques.

The Veress needle is then connected to the CO_2 insufflator and approximately 4 to 5 L of CO_2 at 12 to 15 mm Hg pressure is introduced to create the pneumoperitoneum. The insufflation of the abdomen can be monitored by percussing for diffuse abdominal tympany indicating proper insufflation and symmetric distention. A high-flow CO_2 insufflator (capable of flow rates of 3 to 10 L/min) is essential to maintain an adequate pneumoperitoneum. Pressure is maintained at approximately 15 mm Hg during the procedure.

After the Veress needle is removed, a 10/11-mm trocar is passed into the abdominal cavity and directed into the hollow of the pelvis (Fig. 5.13). Trocars have a retractable safety shield that covers the sharp needle tip

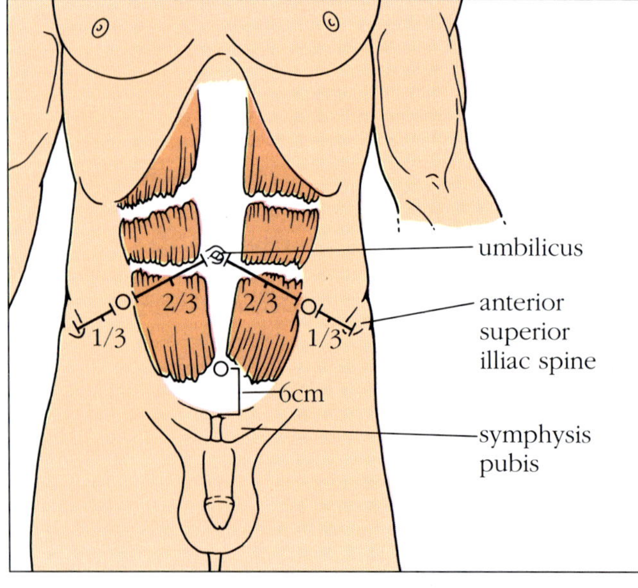

Figure 5.10 The standard trocar insertion sites ("diamond configuration") and sizes for laparoscopic pelvic lymphadenectomy. A 10 or 10/11 mm trocar is required at the umbilicus for the laparoscope. The three additional working ports should include at least one 10 or 10/11 mm trocar to pass larger instruments.

after it enters the peritoneal cavity. The laparoscope is placed in this umbilical port, the video camera is attached, and a brief visual inspection of the abdomen is performed to rule out injury. For the four-trocar technique, three of the remaining working trocars are inserted under direct vision. The choice of size of the trocars is up to the operator's preference; some prefer to use 10/11 trocars laterally and a 5-mm port medially. At least one 10- or 10/11-mm working port is needed so that larger instruments, such as clip appliers and specimen extractors, can be introduced. One trocar is placed approximately 6 cm above the pubic symphysis and two additional trocars are placed in the right and left lower quadrants just lateral to the rectus muscles at a point approximately one third of the way between the umbilicus and the anterior superior iliac spine. Additionally, secondary trocar insertion should be visualized with the laparoscope to help prevent injury to the epigastric vessels laterally.

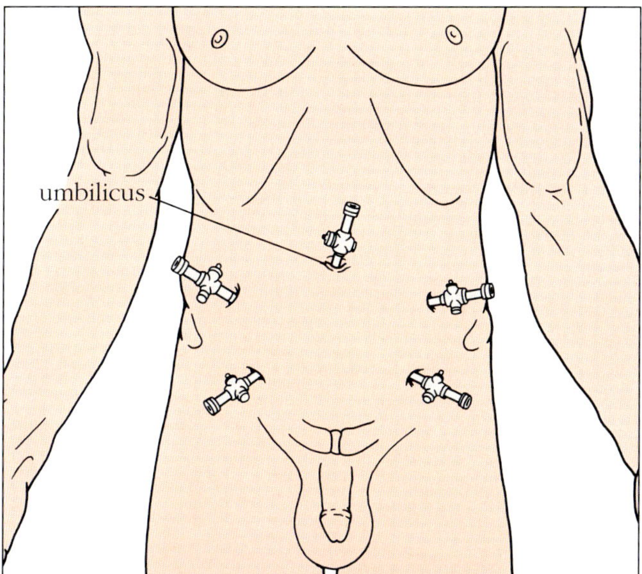

Figure 5.11 A newer five-trocar technique ("fan configuration") for laparoscopic pelvic lymphadenectomy is useful for obese patients and for training purposes. Trocars of 10/11 mm are used in the umbilical and upper positions, with 5-mm trocars in the lower positions.

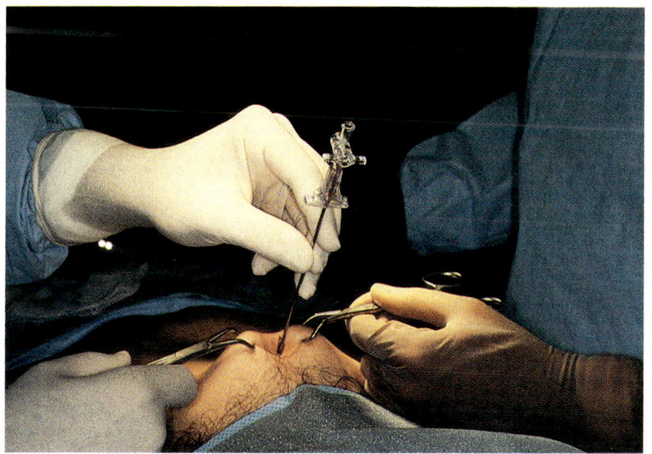

Figure 5.12 Placement of Veress needle. The abdominal wall is elevated by towel clips in order to minimize the risk of bowel injury, although this is controversial. The Veress needle has a spring-loaded inner cannula so that its sharp tip is covered once the abdominal wall and peritoneum have been penetrated. The needle is directed into the hollow of the pelvis.

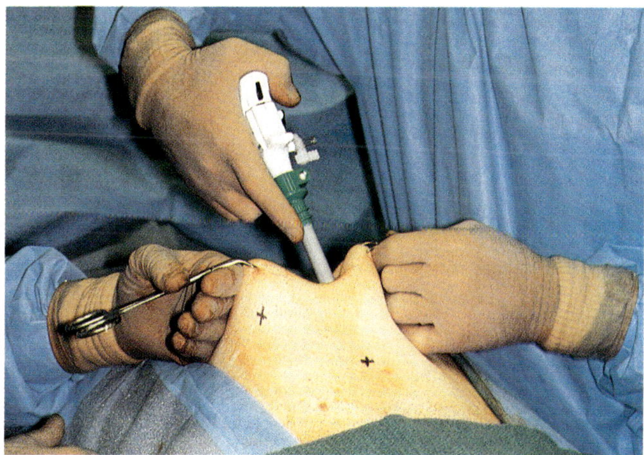

Figure 5.13 Proper technique for trocar insertion. The abdominal wall is stabilized with towel clips, a finger is placed down the shaft to prevent "uncontrolled entry," and pressure is applied with the palm.

Node dissection is usually done on the right side first, with the primary surgeon on the patient's left and the assistant on the right. For the left side, the primary surgeon stands on the patient's right side. The video monitor is placed near the patient's feet.

Figure 5.14 shows the key landmarks at the pelvic side wall visualized through the peritoneum: median umbilical ligament (obliterated umbilical artery), epigastric vessels, vas deferens, internal inguinal ring, external iliac vessels, and spermatic vessels. In some patients the ureter can be seen more proximally as it crosses the iliac vessels. The position of the ureter should be rechecked before removing the proximal external iliac lymph node tissue.

The limits of the dissection are identical to those in open pelvic lymph node dissection. For staging prostate cancer, the limited obturator lymph node dissection is used. The dissection begins using the medial umbilical ligament as the initial landmark; this defines the medial extent of the dissection. With medial traction on the ligament, a longitudinal incision is made in the peritoneal reflection just lateral to the ligament at the approximate level of the internal inguinal ring, across the vas and gently curving laterally in the direction of the bifurcation of the iliac vessels (Fig. 5.15). The Nd:YAG contact laser (10 W continuous power) or electrocautery with endoscopic scissors may be used for the peritoneal incision. The peritoneum is opened and the vas is identified as it crosses the middle of the incision (Fig. 5.16). The vas is clipped with hemoclips and transected with the laser or scissors; this permits maximal medial retraction of the umbilical ligament and exposure of the obturator fossa.

At the distal end of the incision, the pubic ramus is identified, initially by feeling for the bone and then visually after the loose fibroareolar tissue is gently stripped. Accessory obturator vessels are often found that require careful dissection or ligation with a hemoclip.

The tissue is swept medially using blunt dissection until the obturator nerve and vessels are identified medially and the external iliac vein is seen laterally. Countertraction makes the dissection easier. The nodal tissue

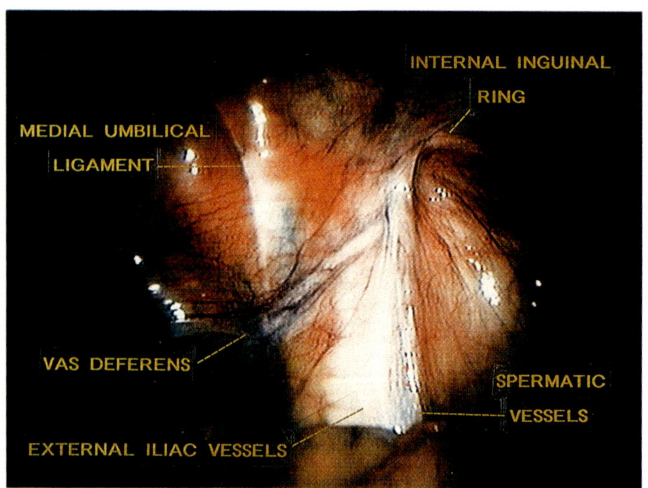

Figure 5.14 Right pelvic sidewall anatomy viewed through the laparoscope from the umbilical insertion site.

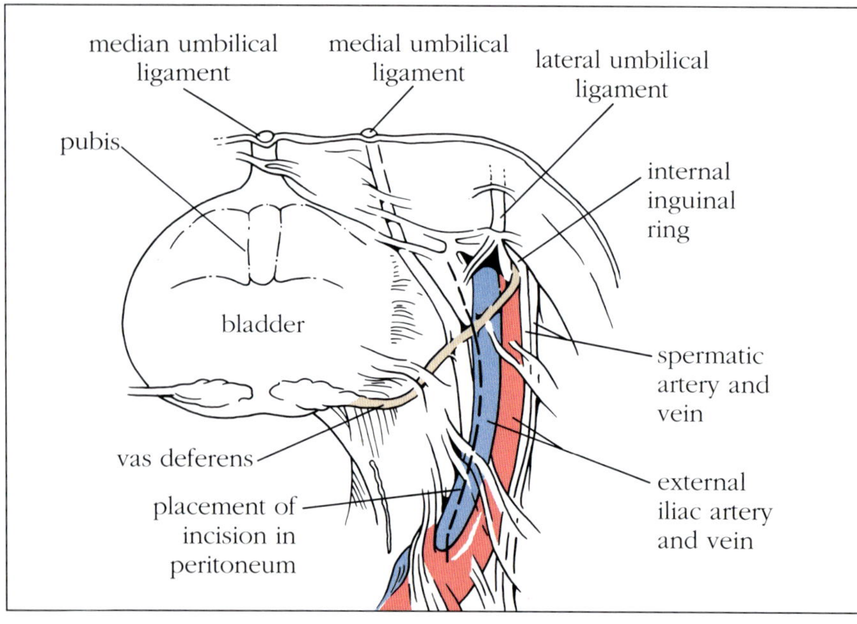

Figure 5.15 The initial incision in the peritoneum should be lateral to the medial umbilical ligament and extend across the vas to the region of the bifurcation of the internal and external iliac vessels (right side).

between the obturator nerve and external iliac vein is the primary specimen. The dissection continues medially along the umbilical ligament, proximally to the point where the obturator nerve, umbilical ligament, and external iliac vein meet, and laterally along the external iliac vein. The ureter should be noted as it crosses the vessels more proximally; the obturator node dissection is always distal to the ureter. A proximal dissection is difficult since the internal iliac vein often cannot be seen well. The lymphadenectomy packet can then be removed either en bloc or in separate segments through the 10/11 port. A completed right-side dissection is shown in Figure 5.17.

The left-side lymphadenectomy is completed in a similar fashion. Sigmoid adhesions are frequently encountered on the left side that are easily taken down with the contact Nd:YAG laser or scissors. In all other aspects, the dissection is identical.

After the procedure is completed, the right and left sides are inspected for bleeding. As the trocars are removed, inspect for bleeding with the laparoscope. The laparoscopic port is the last to be removed, and as much CO_2 as possible should be expelled from the abdomen while the flapper valve is held open on the trocar. The scrotum should also be manually compressed to expel as much CO_2 as possible if pneumoscrotum has developed. Smaller (5 mm) trocar insertion sites are closed with absorbable suture on the skin; the 10 or 10/11 trocar sites should have fascial closure with 2-0 absorbable suture and absorbable suture on the skin.

Postoperative Care

Clear liquids are begun within several hours of surgery and the patients are quickly advanced to a regular diet. The majority of patients are discharged within 24 hours of the procedure and return to full activities within 1 week.

Complications

Laparoscopic lymphadenectomy complications include bleeding, inadvertent bowel, bladder, or ureter injury, equipment failure, atelectasis, and other general anesthetic complications. Complications unique to laparoscopic surgery (related to the CO_2 pneumoperitoneum) can include subcutaneous emphysema, pneumoscrotum, hypercarbia and hypothermia, hypotension, and failure to complete the procedure due to equipment failure. Lymphocele formation is rare since the bed of the dissection is open to the peritoneum, but it has been reported.[29]

OPEN PELVIC LYMPHADENECTOMY
Indications

Staging pelvic lymphadenectomy is performed most often prior to definitive treatment of localized prostate cancer. Pelvic lymphadenectomy is routinely done at the same operation with radical retropubic prostatectomy for patients with clinically localized disease. In patients with clinical stage C disease, who have a 50% chance of nodal metastasis, pelvic lymphadenectomy is done in some cases to help determine whether local therapy (radiation) or hormonal therapy is best.[30]

The indications for laparoscopy versus laparotomy in pelvic lymph node dissections are still being developed. Laparoscopy carries a lower morbidity than open surgery but is more time-consuming and has a high equipment cost. Laparoscopic lymphadenectomy is currently indicated for patients with a high likelihood of nodal metastasis,

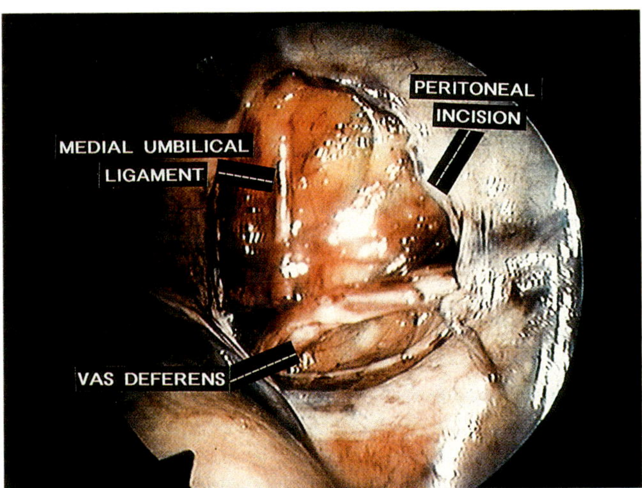

Figure 5.16 After the peritoneum is opened, the vas is exposed (right side), clipped, and transected.

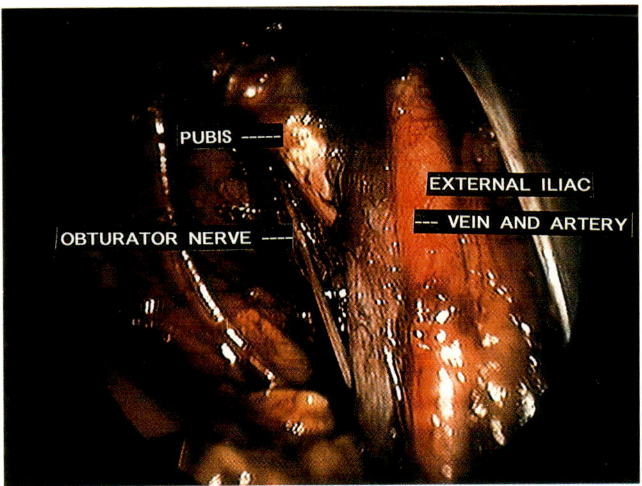

Figure 5.17 Right pelvic sidewall view after the laparoscopic lymphadenectomy is completed.

who might be saved the morbidity of an incision if their nodes are positive. Clinical stage C and stages A and B with poor prognostic factors such as high Gleason scores or markedly elevated PSAs are most likely to benefit from a laparoscopic approach, especially if radiation therapy is being considered.

Preoperative Preparation

If this procedure is performed concomitantly with radical prostatectomy, no additional preoperative preparation is necessary. If it is performed as a separate procedure, broad-spectrum prophylactic antibiotics are given perioperatively and pneumatic compression stockings are used as prophylaxis against deep venous thrombosis. Perioperative heparin should be avoided since it increases the rate of postoperative lymphoceles. General, spinal, or epidural anesthesia may be used.

Operative Technique

Most surgeons employ a lower midline incision, although a Pfannenstiel incision also provides adequate exposure (see Figure 5.18 for positioning and incision). The anterior rectus fascia is incised and the peritoneum is swept bluntly off the iliac vessels. Division or retraction of the vas deferens also may aid in exposure. A self-retaining retractor, such as a Balfour or Bookwalter, with a malleable blade to retract the bladder and peritoneum is helpful. The fibrous tissue over the external iliac vein is incised and swept medially. Lymphatic channels posterior to Cooper's ligament are ligated or clipped and divided until the obturator nerve and vessels are identified. Ligation of lymphatic channels reduces the rate of lymph leakage and symptomatic lymphocele. Care should be taken to avoid or ligate any accessory obturator veins. The obturator nerve and vessels are not disturbed, and the lymphatic tissue is swept off the obturator nerve, the pelvic sidewall, and the underside of the external iliac vein (Fig. 5.19). A vein retractor helps with exposure at this point. Dissection is followed superiorly until the package is removed where the external iliac vein crosses the internal iliac artery, and again lymphatic channels are ligated or clipped and divided. Once hemostasis is verified, closed suction drains are placed on each side and the incision is closed in a standard fashion or the radial prostatectomy can begin.

Postoperative Care

Most patients have a mild ileus lasting 1 to 3 days. Hospitalization averages around 5 days, with the pelvic drains being removed prior to discharge.

Complications

Complications include lower extremity and genital edema, wound infection, deep venous thrombosis, and pulmonary embolism. Excessive bleeding and vascular, ureteral, or obturator nerve injury are rare with good surgical technique. Symptomatic lymphocele is sometimes seen.[31,32]

Treatment Options for Localized Prostate Cancer

In the last 30 years, many treatment options for localized prostate cancer have come in and out of favor. Radical surgery and radiation therapy are the mainstays of treatment of localized prostate cancer (i.e., stages A and B). Twenty years ago, radical surgery fell out of favor due to problems with excessive blood loss and high rates of incontinence as well as impotence. With careful study of prostatic and pelvic anatomy, Walsh has made improvements in surgical technique, bringing a renaissance of radical surgery based on low complication rates. Radiation therapy also has a role in prostate cancer treat-

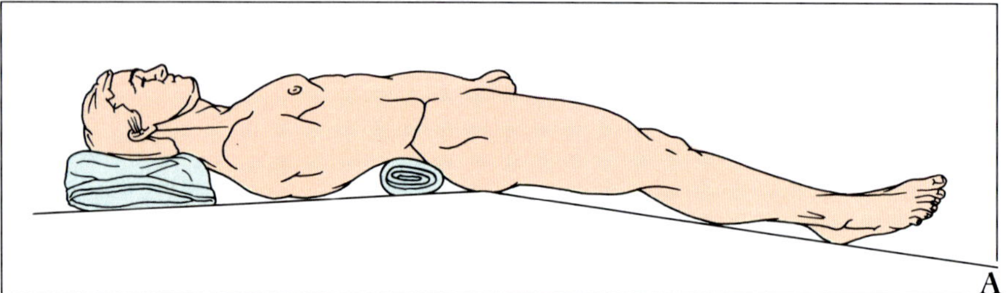

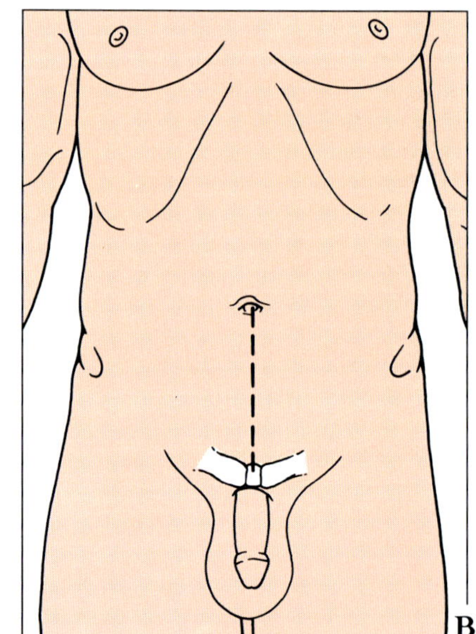

Figure 5.18 Patient positioning **A** and standard incision **B** for open pelvic lymphadenectomy.

ment. Brachytherapy by seed implantation into the prostate, using iodine-125, was pioneered at the Memorial Sloan-Kettering Cancer Center. Poor local control has led to the abandonment of seed implantation by many centers. Newer techniques are being investigated using ultrasound guidance for seed placement. External beam radiation is an option for treatment of localized prostate cancer, and its morbidity has declined over the last 30 years due to improvements in technique.[8,33]

Determining which therapy is best for localized carcinoma of the prostate is highly controversial. Studies of each mode of therapy are difficult to evaluate for several reasons. One problem is patient selection. It is difficult to control comorbid conditions in a population of patients. Also it is difficult to control the various factors that determine the biologic potential of a given tumor, such as grade, age, PSA level, and DNA ploidy. A second difficulty is the absence of objective and accurate local staging methods for prostate cancer. No method exists that can accurately determine the local extent of prostate cancer: digital rectal exam, MRI, and TRUS are all inadequate. In addition, digital rectal examination is highly subjective. There is probably a tendency for urologists to expand the group of stage B patients to include some that are actually stage C, in order to make them candidates for radical prostatectomy. The reverse tendency is probably true of radiation therapists. A third problem is the lack of pathologic staging in radiation therapy trials, which makes them difficult to compare to surgical trials, where lymph node and prostatic pathology is known. Furthermore, the variable and often lengthy course of prostate cancer means that any interpretable study must have 15 years or more of patient follow-up.

Several findings from studies indicate that radical prostatectomy may be more efficacious than radiation therapy, although some data indicate that the overall survival of patients with localized prostate cancer treated with radiation therapy is no different from age-matched controls.[34] Looking at disease-specific actuarial survival, survival is higher in patients treated with radical surgery than in those treated with radiotherapy. The disease-specific survival at 15 years was 86% with radical prostatectomy and 64% with radiation therapy.[35] The only prospective randomized trial to date is by Paulson and associates. In that study, treatment failure (local and distant) at 5 years was 10% for radical prostatectomy and 40% for radiation therapy.[36] Although local recurrence rates have been considered low with radiation therapy as evaluated by digital rectal exam, recent studies evaluating local recurrence by PSA and ultrasound-guided biopsies have indicated an alarming rate of local failure. Five years after radiation therapy, biopsy studies have shown positive biopsies in 40% to 80% of patients. Also, serial PSA levels after radiation therapy have shown that although PSA levels initially fall, the PSA levels subsequently rise in the majority of patients.[37,38] All of these factors, while not conclusive, tend to support the notion that radical prostatectomy may be the treatment of choice for localized prostate cancer, especially in the younger, healthy patient. Longer studies of survival and progression using these newer techiniques are needed to help answer these difficult questions.

RADICAL PROSTATECTOMY

Radical prostatectomy involves en bloc resection of the prostate and seminal vesicles and a portion of the bladder neck. Two approaches are used for radical prostatectomy: retropubic or perineal. The retropubic approach is currently used most often, because the staging pelvic lymphadenectomy may be performed through the same incision and because of improvements in technique developed by Walsh, as noted above. However, several

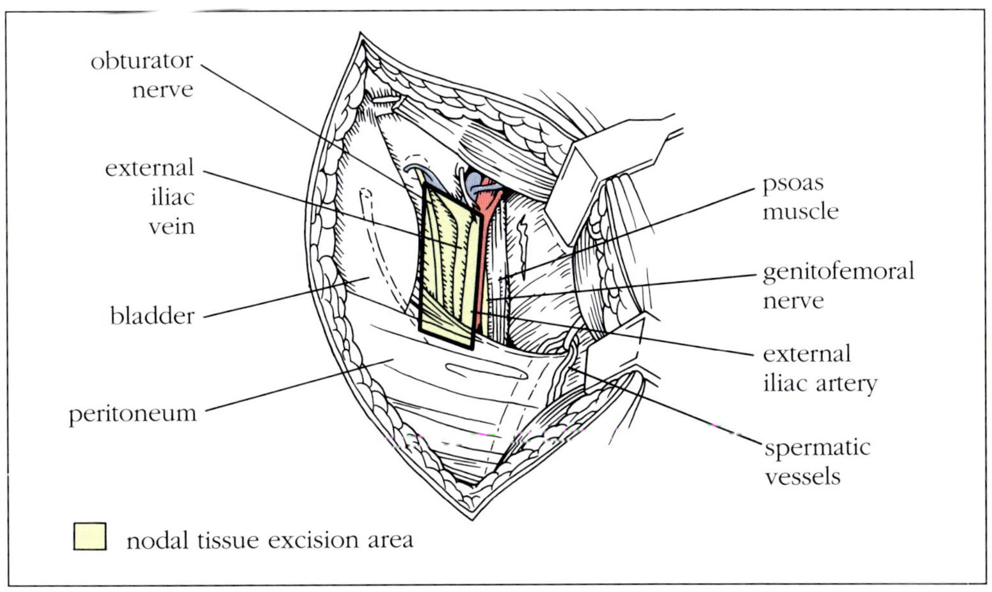

Figure 5.19
Open pelvic lymphadenectomy on the right side. The margins of dissection for the staging of prostate cancer are noted by the shaded area. A vein retractor is useful to expose the lymph node tissue below the external iliac vein.

considerations make the perineal approach attractive. First, perineal prostatectomy is performed without traversing the dorsal vein complex, thereby reducing the risk of extensive blood loss. Second, access to the urethra is more direct via a perineal approach. Third, the postoperative morbidity and hospitalization for the perineal approach are less than with an abdominal incision. The disadvantages are a more difficult surgical exposure, poor access to the seminal vesicles, and a high incidence of impotence, although potency-sparing perineal prostatectomy is being investigated.[39] Another argument against perineal prostatectomy has been the inability to evaluate the pelvic lymph nodes at the same time; however, laparoscopic lymphadenectomy is overcoming this objection.[39,40]

Indications

Patients with cancer localized to the prostate are considered for radical prostatectomy. The exact indications are controversial, but certainly patients who are good surgical risks and have stage A2, B1, or B2 prostate cancer are candidates. The treatment of older patients (e.g., older than age 75) with early stage A disease (low grade, low PSA) is not entirely clear, since the natural history of the disease may follow a more benign course. Some clinicians also suggest that radical prostatectomy is beneficial in some stage C and D1 prostate cancer, but this is not universally accepted.

Preoperative Preparation

Patients should be carefully screened for medical diseases (particularly cardiovascular ones), which would make them a higher surgical risk. High-risk patients may be better served by radiation therapy. Patients are encouraged to bank 3 or 4 units of their own blood over a 3 to 4 week period before surgery. Admission the day before surgery allows a mechanical and antibiotic bowel prep to be performed (oral laxative such as GoLYTELY, magnesium citrate, or mannitol, oral erythromycin base and neomycin in three divided doses, and cleansing enemas). Broadspectrum antibiotics (such as cefoxitin) are used perioperatively, and sequential pneumatic compression stockings are used to help prevent deep venous thrombosis.

General endotracheal or epidural anesthesia is most commonly used. Advocates of epidural anesthesia feel that operative blood loss is less, possibly due to less distention of the pelvic venous plexus. Epidural anesthesia also allows the use of postoperative epidural narcotics for pain control.[41]

Radical Retropubic Prostatectomy: Operative Technique

Before the advances in surgical technique pioneered by Walsh,[42] radical prostatectomy was feared by both patients and surgeons for its high rate of complications. Blood loss was typically greater than several liters, and incontinence and impotence were common. As reported in Walsh's series, the average blood loss is now 400 mL, incontinence occurs postoperatively in less than 1% of patients, and postoperative potency is reported in more than 70% of patients. This is a direct result of techniques to control bleeding from the dorsal vein complex, thus allowing good visualization for the remainder of the operation. Recognizing and preserving the neurovascular bundles is also critical to maintaining potency.

A lower midline abdominal incision is used; the incision and positioning are as described in Figure 5.18. After the staging lymphadenectomy, the operation is begun. Control of the dorsal vein complex is important for reducing blood loss and allowing visibility that the remainder of the operation may be performed in a careful fashion. The retropubic adipose tissue anterior to the apex of the prostate contains one or more veins (Santorini's plexus) that are the most troublesome source of bleeding. In the majority of cases a single midline vein is found, although 20% or more of patients have one or more side branches. To control these veins effectively, an incision of the endopelvic fascia laterally is required. Incising the endopelvic fascia medially can injure the plexus of veins along the prostate. The puboprostatic ligaments must be dissected out and incised close to the pubis. These ligaments are avascular and may be safely incised as long as there are no immediately adjacent veins. Cutting the puboprostatic ligaments allows the prostate to fall posteriorly, allowing better exposure for subsequent dissection. The dorsal vein complex can then be controlled by a ligature around the entire packet of tissue anterior to the urethra at the apex of the prostate. After ligating and dividing these veins, the remainder of the dissection can be done in a relatively bloodless field (Fig. 5.20).[43]

Nerves that are important to erectile function run immediately posterolateral to the prostate in a neurovascular bundle. Identification of the neurovascular bundle and avoidance of injury to this bundle is important to nerve-sparing radical prostatectomy. If there is any question of cancerous involvement close to the neurovascular bundle, nerve-sparing operation should be abandoned on that side. Sparing one neurovascular bundle does result in a significant (although lower) rate of postoperative potency. The neurovascular bundle must be avoided at three particularly important parts of the dissection. The neurovascular bundle runs very close to the urethra and the apex of the prostate, and care must be taken when transecting the urethra and incising the rectourethralis muscle. The neurovascular bundle also runs close to the midportion of the prostate posterolaterally in the groove between the prostate and the rectum. The third location where the neurovascular bundle is apt to be injured is where the lateral pedicle is ligated at the junction of the prostate and seminal vesicles (Fig. 5.21).[44]

Good operative technique also can lead to high rates of postoperative continence. Reduced blood loss has

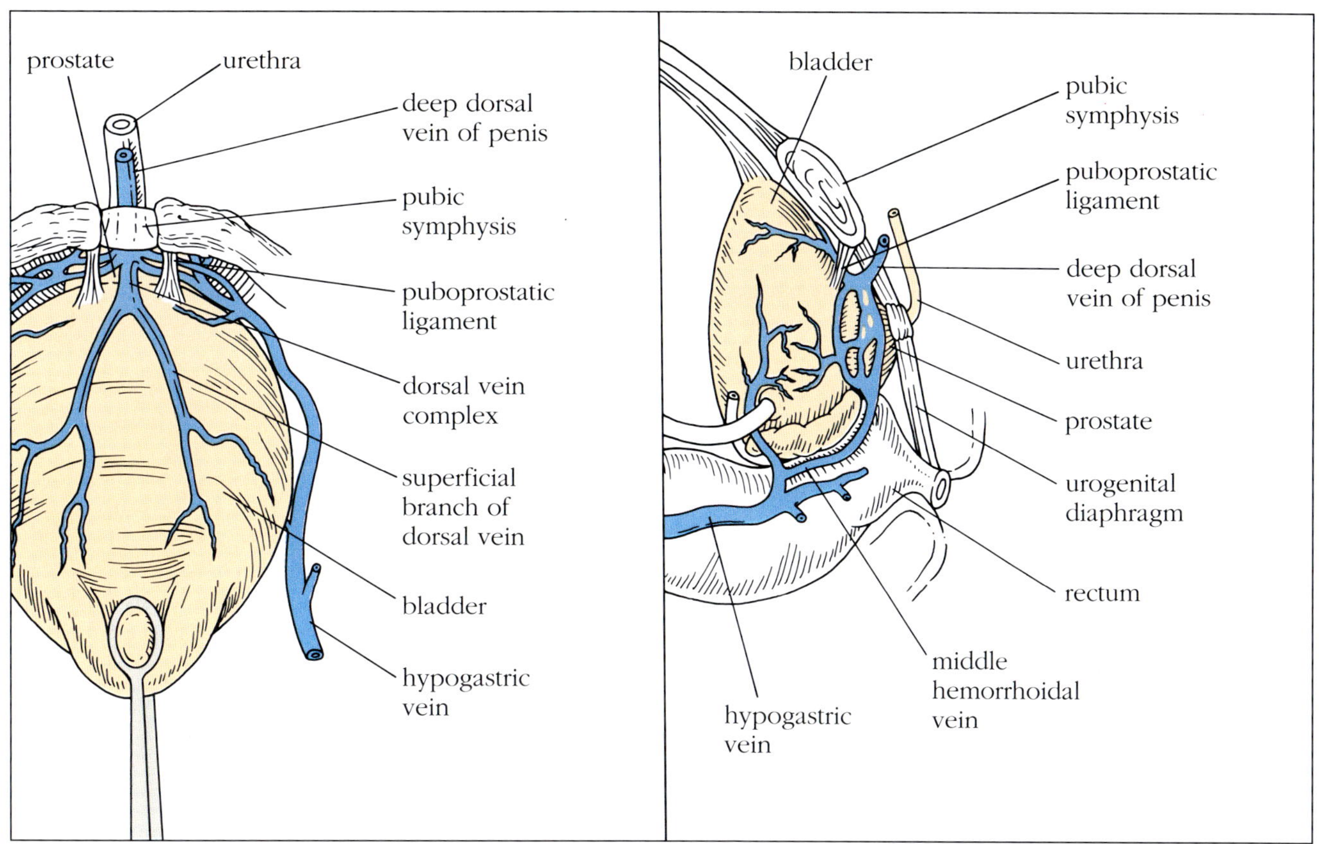

Figure 5.20 The dorsal vein complex can be seen running between the prostate and pubis and medial to the puboprostatic ligaments.

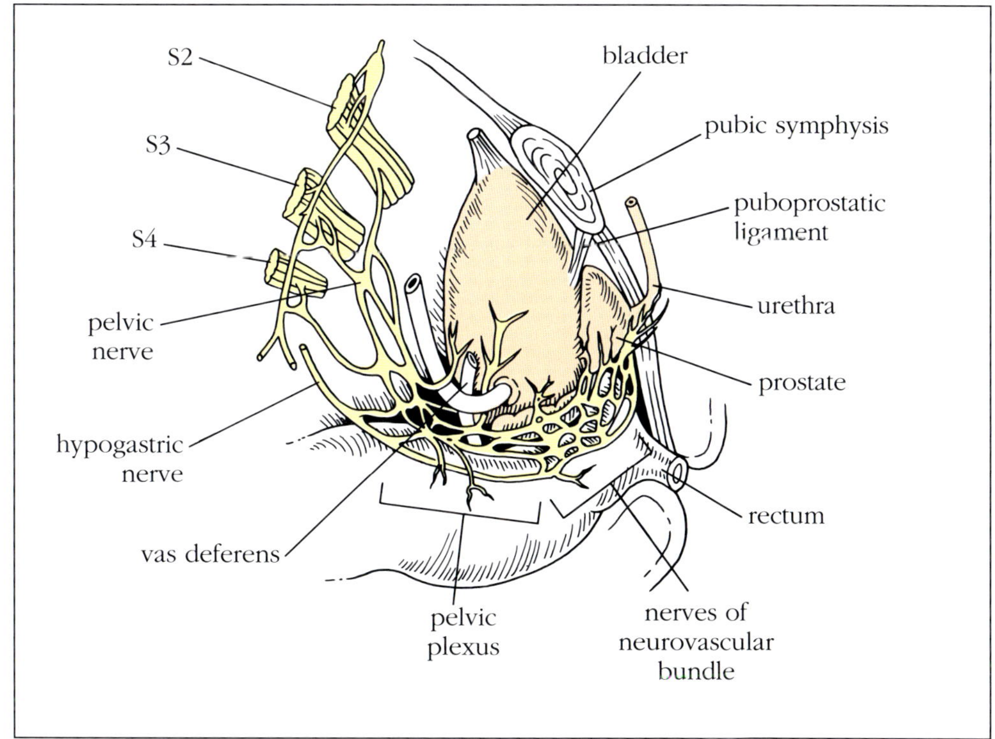

Figure 5.21
The neurovascular
bundle runs
posterolaterally in the
groove between the
rectum and prostate.

given surgeons good visualization at the apex of the prostate for the purpose of anatomic division of the urethra. Preservation of the membranous urethra is essential to postoperative continence. Overzealous attempts to preserve continence that risk leaving the prostatic apex behind are to be avoided, since this area is involved with cancer in a significant percentage of cases. The apex was involved in 75% of posterior zone cancers in one study.[45]

After ligating and dividing the dorsal vein complex, the junction of the urethra and the prostatic apex is visualized. A plane between the neurovascular bundles and the membranous urethra is made and a right angle clamp or umbilical tape is used to isolate the urethra. The anterior

urethral wall is incised at the prostatic apex, and the Foley catheter is delivered through the urethrotomy and clamped and divided. The Foley catheter can then be used for traction on the prostate (Fig. 5.22). The posterior wall of the urethra is then incised at the apex. The rectourethralis muscle can then be bluntly dissected from the rectum in the midline without difficulty. Lateral attachments of the prostate may then be ligated and divided, with care taken to avoid injuring the neurovascular bundles.

The seminal vesicle and vas are usually dissected via a posterior approach. The apex of the prostate is pulled cephalad by traction on the Foley catheter. Denonvilliers' fascia is divided transversely at the junction of the prostate

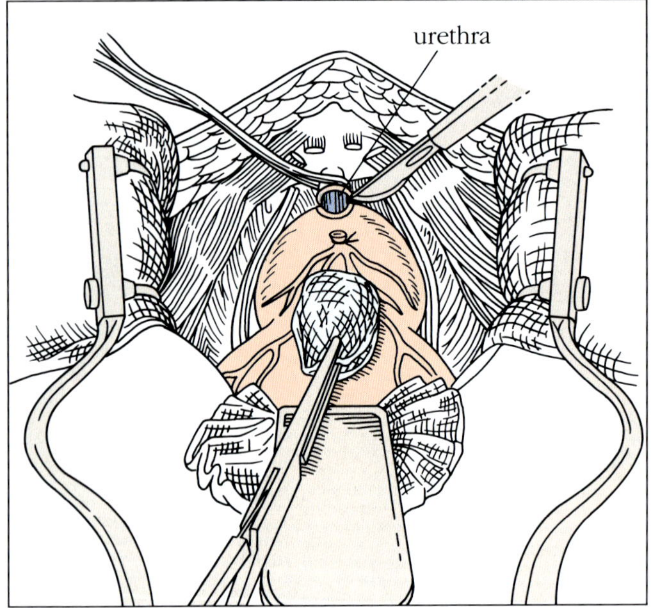

Figure 5.22 Apical dissection. The urethra is incised anteriorly and the Foley catheter is delivered through the urethrotomy. The catheter may then be used for traction, and the posterior urethra is incised. A sponge stick and posterior retraction facilitate dissection of the apical structures.

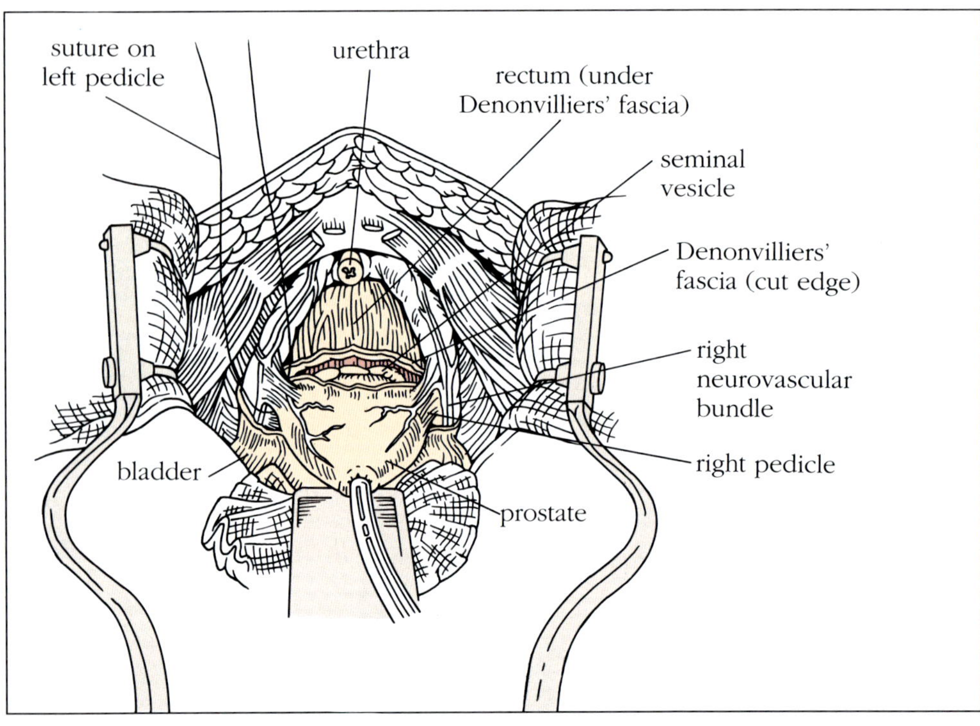

Figure 5.23 Incision of Denonvilliers' fascia posteriorly. This permits dissection of the ampullae of the vasa and the seminal vesicles.

and seminal vesicles using electrocautery (Fig. 5.23). The seminal vesicles may then be bluntly dissected out, though the vessels usually found at the tips of the seminal vesicles should be clipped or ligated and divided. Likewise, the ampulla of the vas is clipped or ligated and divided.

Then the junction of the bladder and prostate is divided anteriorly using electrocautery. The prostatovesicular incision is grasped with Allis clamps. The Foley catheter is delivered and then the ureteral orifices are identified prior to transecting the posterior bladder wall. Intravenous indigo carmine (1 ampule) can aid in identification of the ureteral orifices (Fig. 5.24). After the posterior bladder wall is transected with electrocautery, only the lateral pedicles remain. They are ligated and divided, and care is taken to avoid injuring the neurovascular bundles. After the prostate and seminal vesicles are removed, only the reconstruction of the bladder neck and urethral anastomosis remain.

After transecting the urethra, the chief technical difficulty is obtaining good exposure of the urethral stump to place anastomotic sutures. The membranous urethra's retropubic location is both difficult to visualize and difficult for suture placement. There are several techniques to aid in the placement of these sutures, and each has its advantages and disadvantages. The first method involves direct pressure on the perineum to elevate the urethral stump. This requires placing the patient in a low lithotomy position, including the perineum in the sterile field, and having an assistant use a sponge stick or other device to place pressure on the perineum during this crucial aspect of the operation (Fig. 5.25).[46] A second method involves using a type of urethral sound called a Roth suture guide. The guide has a broad tip with grooves for suture placement. When used, it is passed through the urethra and positioned so that the tip of the guide is showing at the opening of the urethral stump. The Roth suture guide serves two main functions. First, with gentle pressure, it acts to elevate the urethral stump cranially into view in the pelvis. Second, there are grooves in the suture guide that aid in the passing of sutures through the urethra (Fig. 5.26).[47] A third method involves transecting the anterior portion of the urethra and placing sutures before transecting the posterior aspect of the urethra. The advantage of this technique is that the prostate provides traction to keep the urethra in view: no extra step is required to expose the urethral stump. Care must be taken during the remainder of the operation so these preplaced sutures are not disturbed

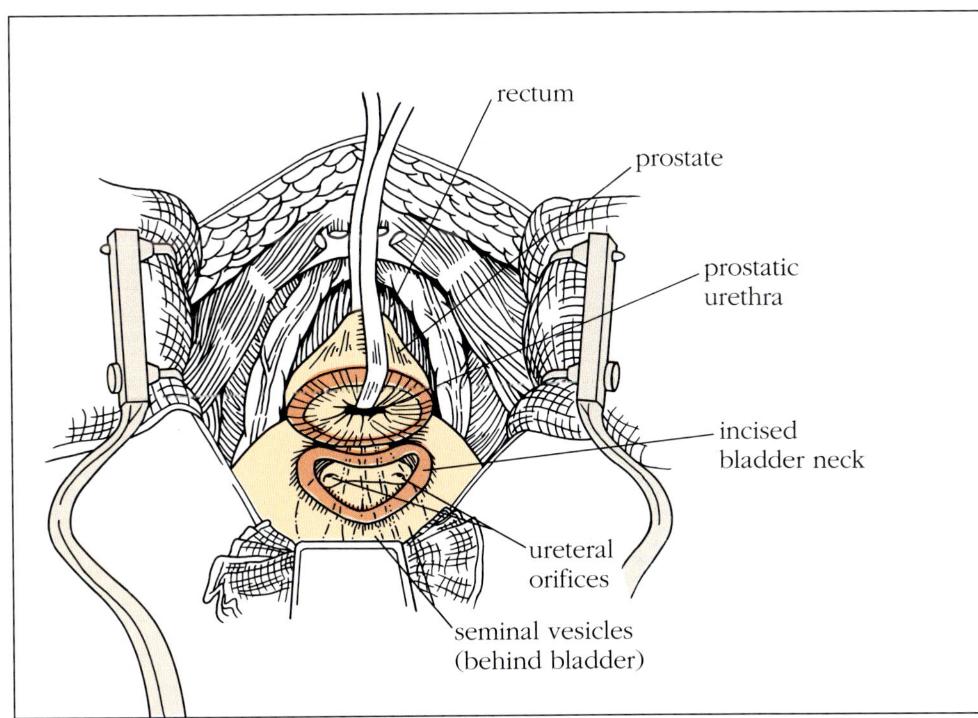

Figure 5.24
Identification of the ureteral orifices and transection of the posterior bladder wall. Intravenous indigo carmine helps in the location of the orifices.

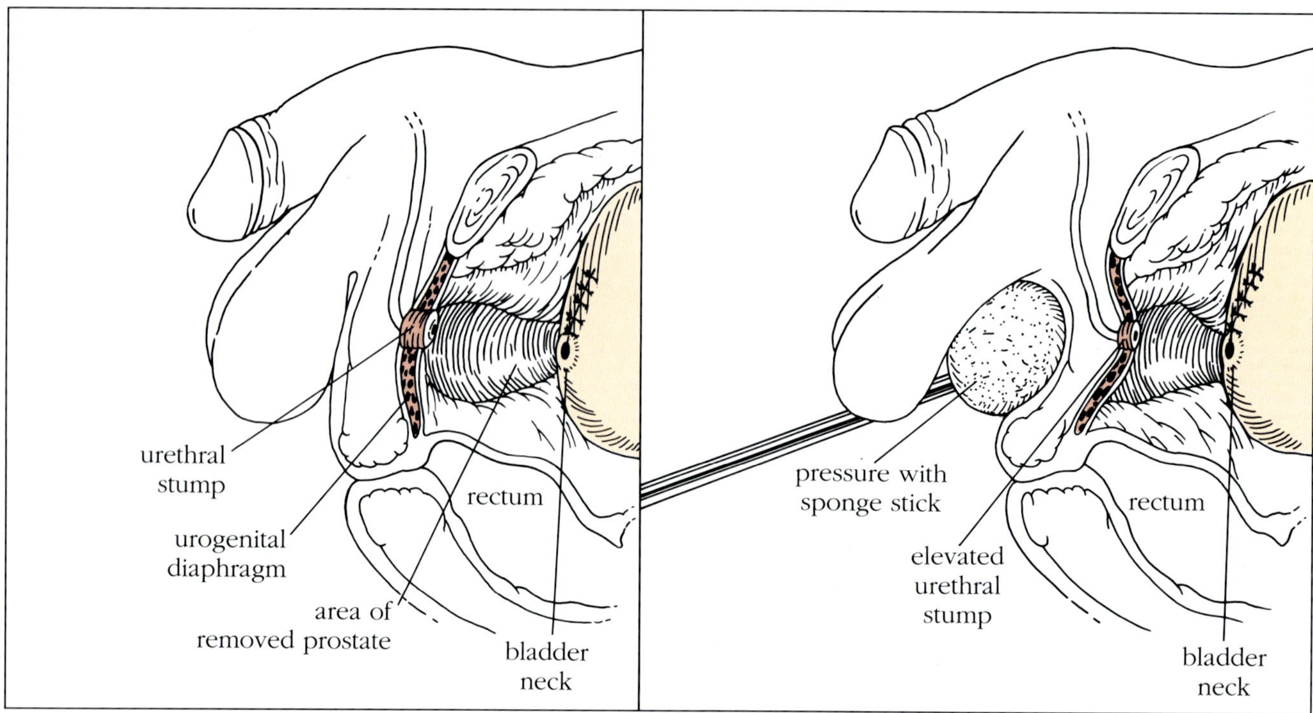

Figure 5.25 Perineal pressure elevates the urethral stump, moving it within the pelvis.

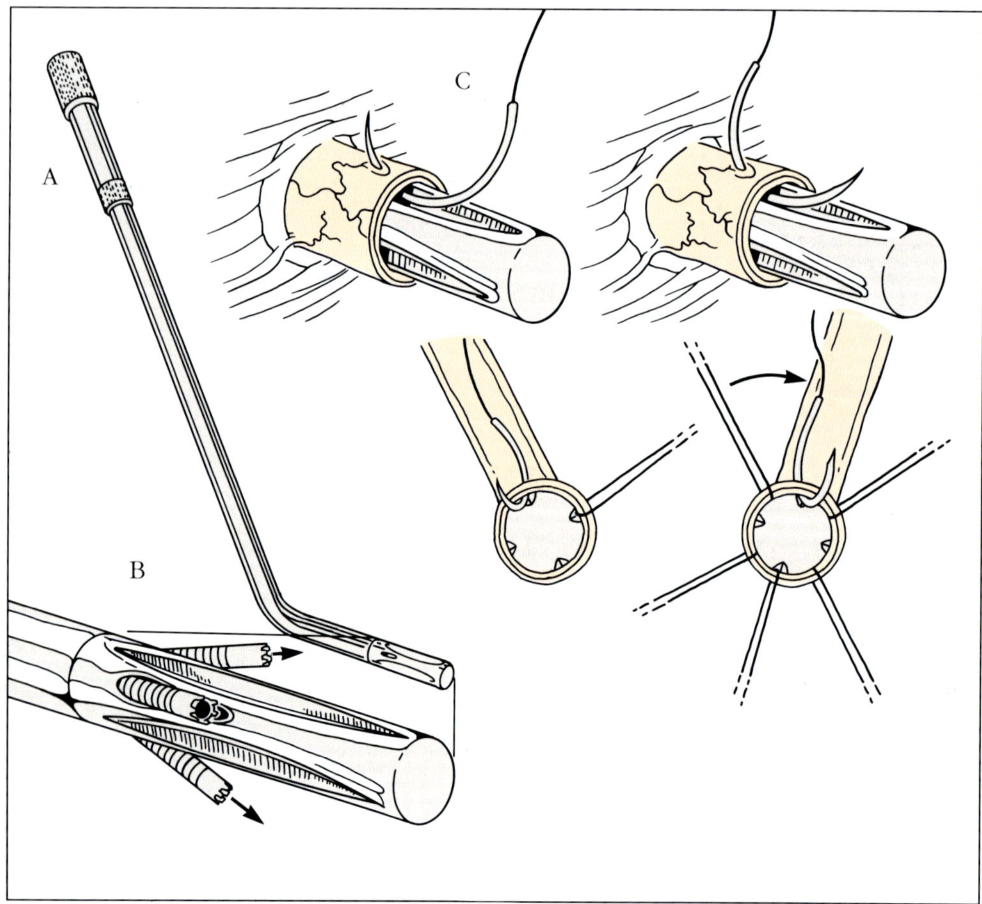

Figure 5.26 The Roth suture guide (Greenwald Surgical). **A** The Roth suture guide is similar to a standard urethral sound, but it has an un-tapered grooved tip. **B** Retractable spring-loaded graspers now allow fixation and more efficient eversion of the urethral stump. **C** Note how the grooved tip helps to place the urethral sutures in either direction.

(Fig. 5.27).[48] A fourth method involves traction on a Foley catheter while the balloon is partially inflated in the urethra. A Foley catheter is passed through the urethra and a silk suture is tied to the eyelet of the catheter. The catheter then is retracted within the urethra so the tip barely shows within the stump, and the balloon is inflated just enough (3 to 5 mL) to fix the catheter in place in the bulbous urethra. Subsequent traction on the silk suture will elevate the urethra into view. Care must be taken to avoid overinflating the balloon and damaging the urethra (Fig. 5.28). The method one uses to place sutures is largely a matter of preference.

Another complication of radical prostatectomy that can be avoided with good technique is postoperative bladder neck contracture. The main causes of bladder neck contracture appear to be lack of mucosal apposition at the urethrovesical anastomosis and excessive bleeding from the dorsal vein complex. Techniques to control the

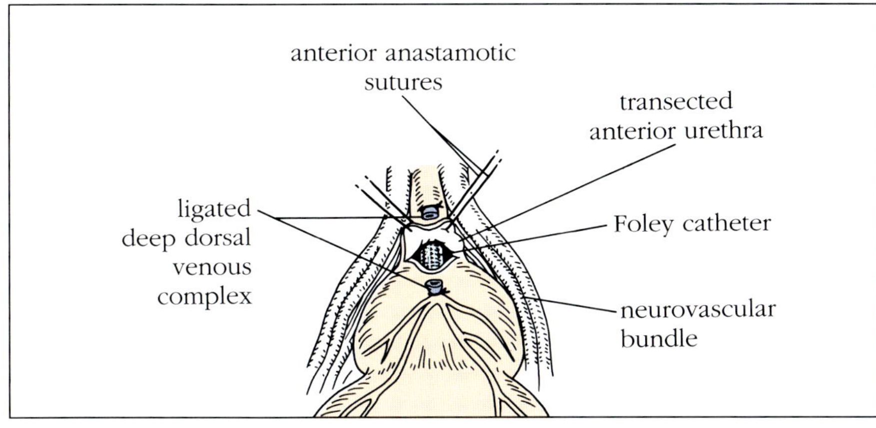

Figure 5.27 Sutures may be "preplaced" in the urethral stump prior to removing the prostate. Care is needed during the rest of the procedure, if this technique is used, to avoid tearing the urethra.

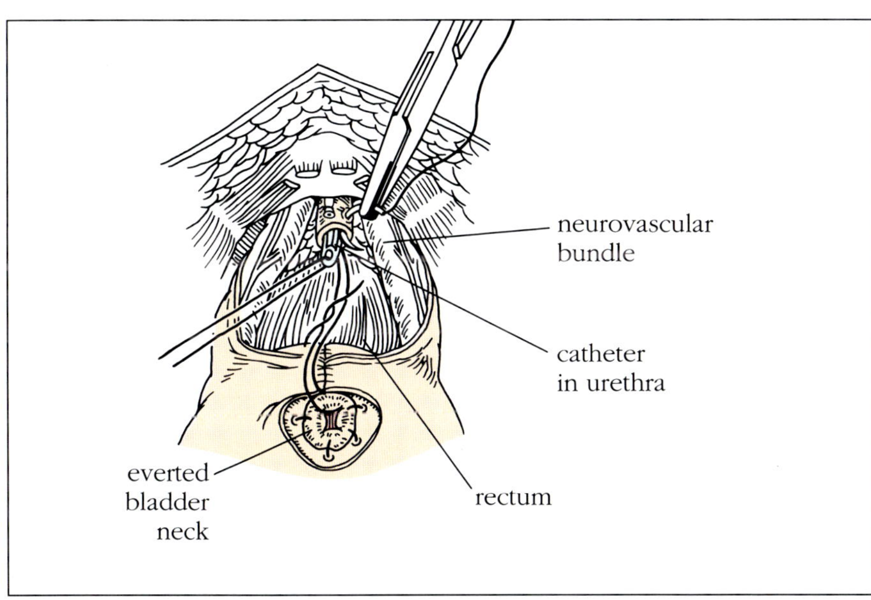

Figure 5.28 Foley balloon urethral traction. Gentle inflation (3 to 5 mL sterile water) of a Foley balloon in the urethral stump allows traction on a silk suture passed through the eye of the catheter. The urethral stump is elevated into view and four sutures are placed in an "outside-in" fashion. After the catheter is passed through the urethra and into the bladder the anastomosis is completed.

dorsal vein complex have been described above. Ligatures should be made of absorbable material and trimmed short, as they may otherwise fall into the urethrovesical anastomosis and cause stone formation and obstruction. Obtaining mucosal apposition at the urethrovesical anastomosis requires first that the bladder neck be closed to a size similar to that of the urethra. A "tennis racket" closure is usually used to bring the bladder neck down to a size of about 30 Fr with 2-0 chromic catgut (Fig. 5.29). The bladder mucosa should be everted at the vesical orifice with four or more absorbable 4-0 chromic catgut sutures. Next, placing four or more anastomotic sutures through the bladder neck and urethra will allow accurate apposition of mucosal surfaces at the anastomosis (Fig. 5.28). Most surgeons use a 20 to 22 Fr Foley catheter with 15 mL of sterile water in the balloon, anticipating that the anastomosis will contract further in size after the catheter is removed. A closed suction drain is also placed in the pelvis prior to closure.

Radical Perineal Prostatectomy

The concept underlying radical prostatectomy is constant regardless of approach, but the perineal exposure has four unique aspects. 1) The patient should be placed in the exaggerated lithotomy position, so as best to expose the perineum (Fig. 5.30A). 2) Lowsley retractors aid in manipulation of the prostate during prostatectomy. At the start of the operation, a curved Lowsley retractor can be used in the urethra to lever the prostate down towards the perineal incision. Once the membranous urethra has been divided from the prostatic apex, the straight Lowsley retractor can be used to retract the prostate in order to dissect around it. 3) No ligation of the dorsal vein complex is required, since the entire dissection occurs posteri-

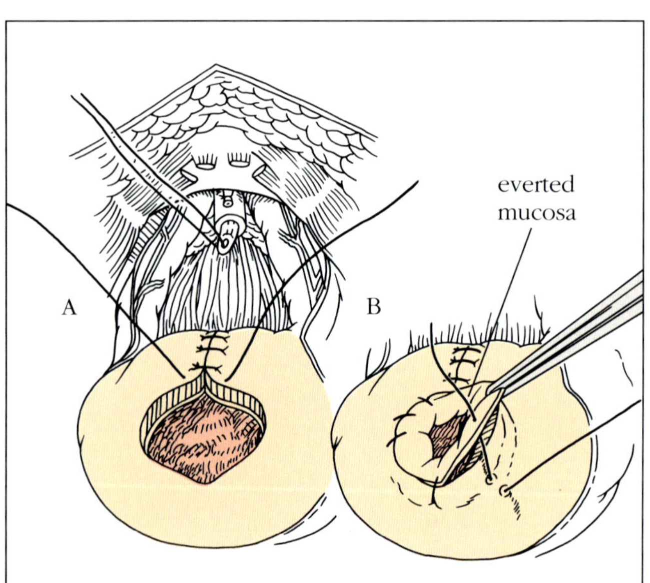

Figure 5.29 **A** Closure of the bladder neck. The bladder neck is closed posteriorly in a "tennis racket" fashion until the bladder opening is about 30 Fr. Either interrupted or running sutures can be used, employing 2-0 absorbable suture. **B** The bladder mucosa is everted to cover the edges of the detrusor muscle with 4-0 chromic catgut. This helps ensure mucosa-to-mucosa apposition of the urethra and bladder neck.

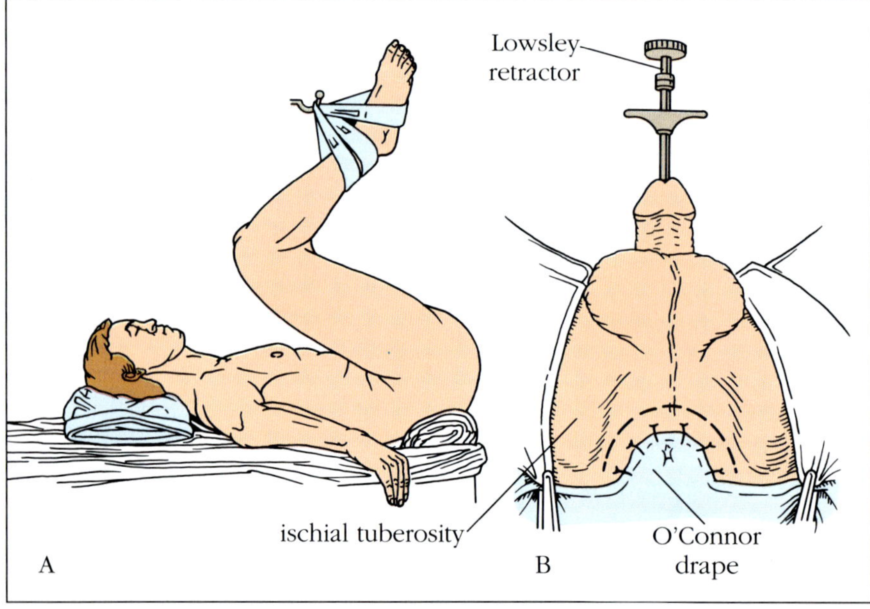

Figure 5.30 Perineal prostatectomy. The patient is placed in the exaggerated lithotomy position **A** and an arched incision is made in the perineum between the ischial tuberosities **B**.

or to this complex. 4) Nerve sparing is performed by taking care to sweep the neurovascular bundle laterally, particularly where it is closest to the prostate—at the apex and at the junction of prostate and seminal vesicles.[40,49]

A transverse perineal incision is made laterally, curving posteriorly towards the ischial tuberosities (Fig. 5.30B). The ischiorectal fossa is developed on each side and the central tendon is dissected out bluntly and divided (Fig. 5.31). Pressure on the curved Lowsley retractor in the bladder helps elevate the prostate, and the prostatic apex is identified. Then the rectourethralis muscle is bluntly divided while developing a plane between Denonvilliers' fascia and the rectum (Fig. 5.32). Attention is turned to the prostatic apex, where the urethra is dissected out and the lateral tissues and neurovascular bundles are preserved. The posterior wall of the urethra is cut and the Lowsley retractor exposed. The Lowsley retractor is then removed, and the anterior urethral wall transected. A straight Lowsley retractor may then be placed in the prostatic urethra to aid in the remainder of the dissection (Fig. 5.33). Blunt and sharp dissection is used to free the prostate from the anteriolateral fascia, which contains the dorsal

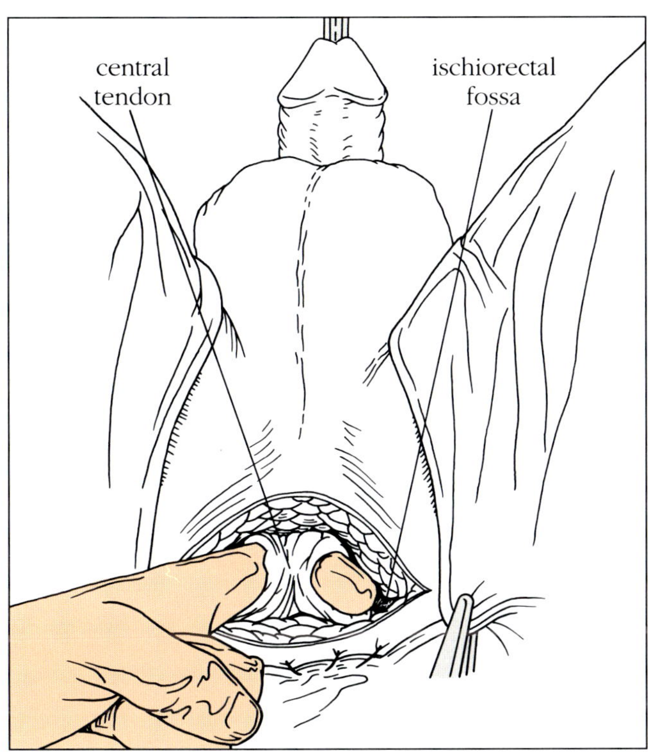

Figure 5.31 After the ischiorectal fossa is opened, the central tendon is exposed.

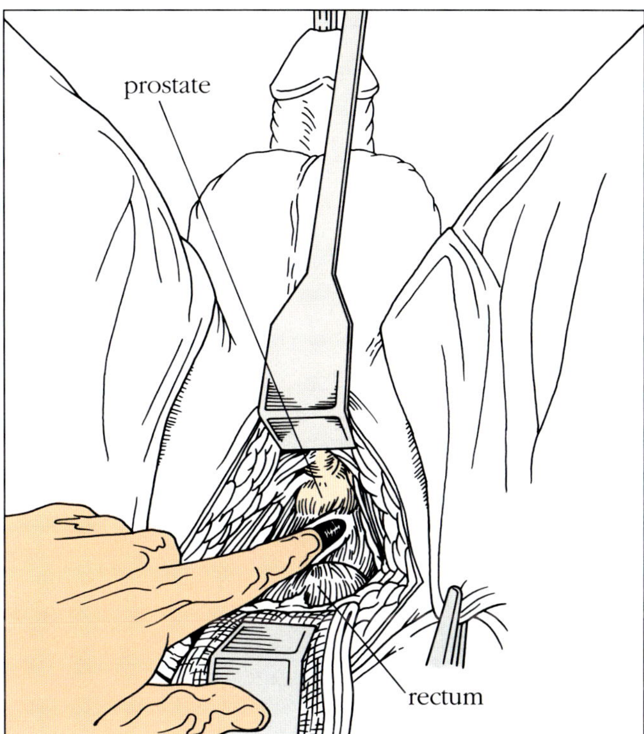

Figure 5.32 A plane is bluntly developed between the rectum and Denonvilliers' fascia.

Figure 5.33 After the urethra is transected, a straight Lowsley retractor is passed into the prostate.

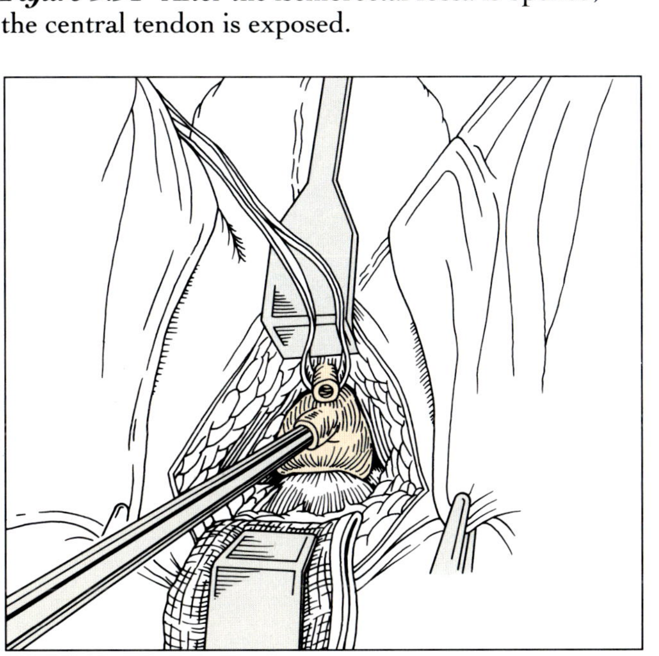

vein complex and the neurovascular bundles. Once the bladder is exposed, the anterior bladder wall is divided where it joins the prostate. The ureteral orifices are identified; 5 mL of intravenous indigo carmine can be helpful in this. The straight Lowsley retractor is best replaced by a Penrose drain looped through the prostatic urethra for traction (Fig. 5.34). The posterior bladder wall is transected, and the seminal vesicles and vas are dissected and removed with the prostate (Fig. 5.35). The bladder neck and urethral anastomoses are performed as in the retropubic approach after a 22 Fr Foley catheter is passed through the urethra (Fig. 5.36). A Penrose drain is left in place.

Postoperative Care

Most patients are hospitalized postoperatively for 3 to 5 days for the perineal approach and 5 to 7 days for the retropubic prostatectomy. Typically there is a 1 to 2 day postoperative ileus with the retropubic approach. Patients ambulate starting the first postoperative day. The Foley catheter is left in place for 2 to 3 weeks and is removed at the first postoperative office visit.

Complications

The main complications of radical prostatectomy are excessive bleeding, infection, incontinence, impotence, and rectal injury. Excessive bleeding (transfusion of more

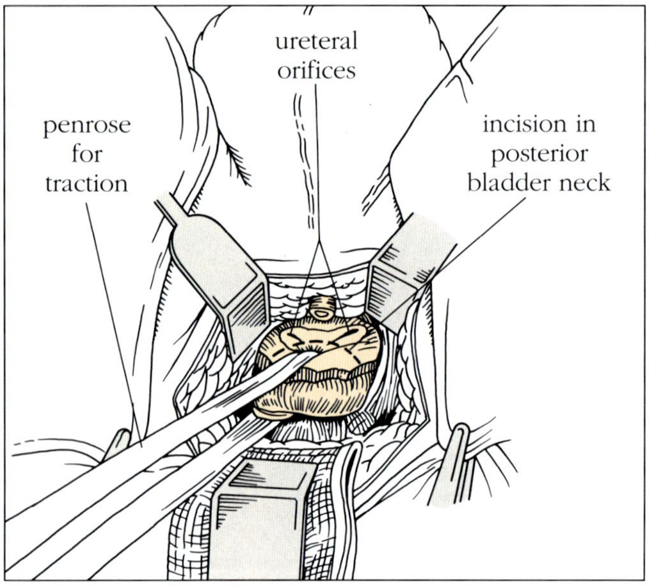

Figure 5.34 After the anterior bladder wall has been incised, a Penrose drain is used to retract the prostate posteriorly.

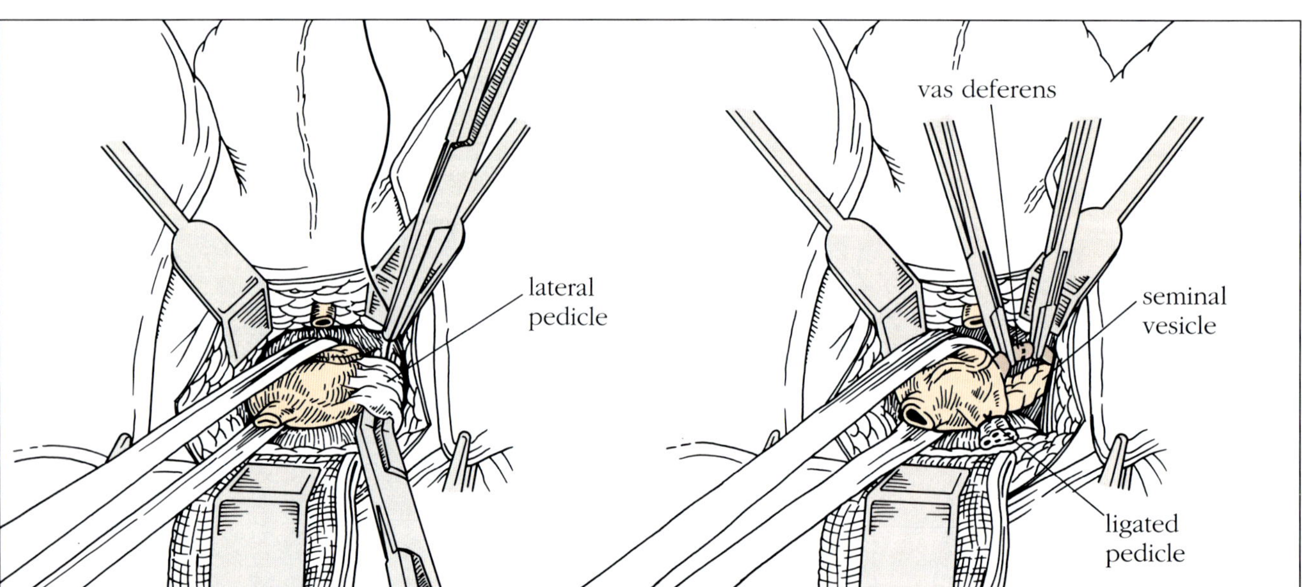

Figure 5.35 The lateral pedicles are ligated and the seminal vesicles and vasa are dissected.

than three units of blood) occurs in 2% of retropubic cases as reported by Walsh, with an average blood loss of 400 to 500 mL. Postoperative continence occurs in 93% of cases, while mild stress incontinence requiring a pad in the underwear occurs in 7% of cases. No patients in Walsh's series were totally incontinent. The average time to achieve continence is 3 weeks, with virtually all patients dry by 6 months. Postoperative potency occurs in more than 70% of patients undergoing retropubic prostatectomy who were potent preoperatively and whose neurovascular bundles were spared. Potency rates are also a function of age, with younger patients having a more favorable prognosis. Potency may return gradually within a year. More experience with the potency-sparing perineal approach is needed before its ability to preserve erectile function can be determined. In the absence of previous pelvic radiation or surgery, rectal injury is rare (1%). Bladder neck contractures are also rare (less than 1%) since the introduction of bladder mucosa eversion, as are wound infections (less than 1%).[50]

RADIATION THERAPY

Radiation therapy has several applications in the treatment of prostatic cancer. Radiation therapy can be used as primary treatment of localized disease in the prostate. Also, radiation therapy can be adjuvant treatment for pathologic stage C prostate cancer (after radical prostatectomy) or as palliative treatment in patients with widespread disease. Radiation therapy can alleviate pain from bony metastases as well as relieve ureteral obstruction.

The main techniques used are external beam radiation therapy and seed implantation (brachytherapy).

EXTERNAL BEAM RADIATION THERAPY

The chief technical difficulty with external beam radiation therapy of the prostate, as with external beam radiation therapy to other areas of the body, is delivering the radiation to the prostate while sparing the surrounding tissue. In most protocols, the goal is to deliver 6000 to 7000 cGy to the prostate and 4000 to 5000 cGy to pelvic lymph nodes. The patient's therapy is planned using plain radiographs and/or CT scans. Often, contrast in the bladder and rectum is used to identify the exact position of the prostate. Standard treatment involves four fields, with portals crafted to deliver the radiation as precisely as possible to the prostate and pelvis. For an example of radiation portals see Figure 5.37.[34]

A new application of external beam radiation therapy is postoperative adjuvant radiotherapy for patients after radical prostatectomy. Because of surgical lymph node dissection, the adjuvant treatment is delivered only to the prostate bed and the dose is usually around 5000 cGy. There are not enough long-term data about these patients to determine whether their overall survival has improved, but recent studies indicate that the incidence of local cancer recurrence is reduced. In patients with pathologic stage C disease, the recurrence rate 5 years postoperatively is reduced from approximately 25% to 5% with the addition of external beam radiation therapy.[51] In another study, patients who had elevated PSA levels after radical

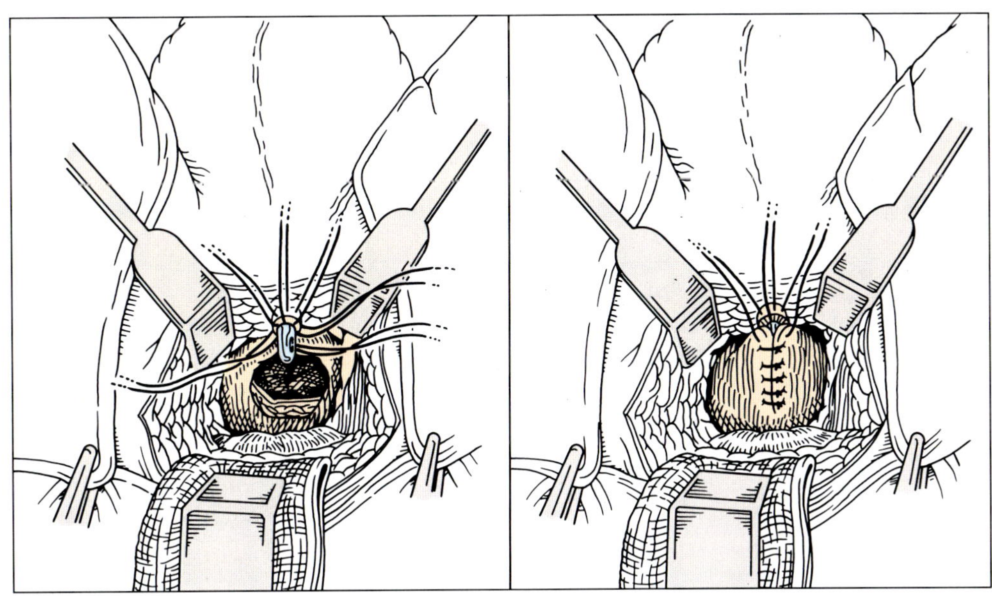

Figure 5.36 Closure of the bladder neck and urethrovesical anastomosis are done as in the retropubic approach with a "tennis racket" closure of the bladder neck and four anastamotic sutures.

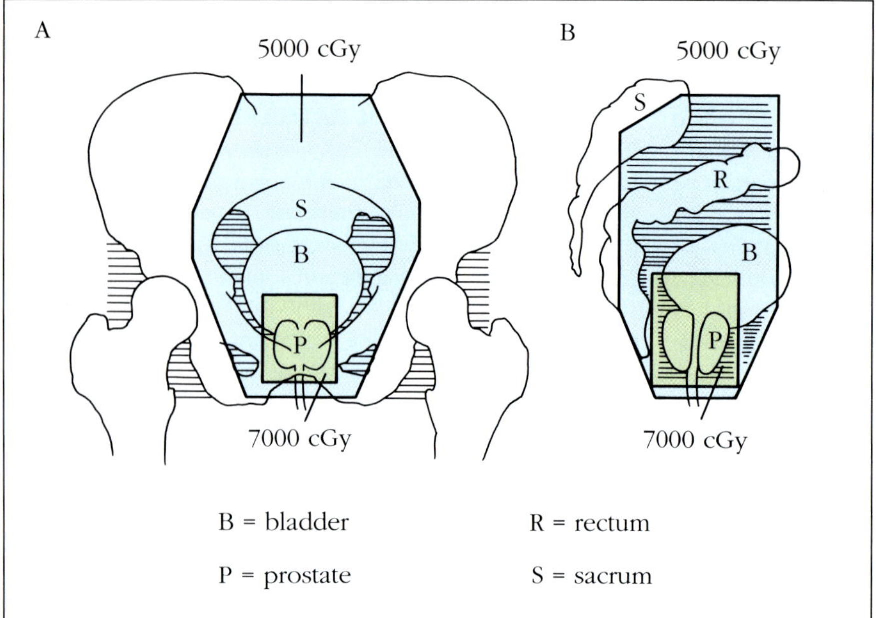

Figure 5.37 Anterior-posterior **A** and lateral **B** portals for definitive external beam radiation therapy for prostate carcinoma.

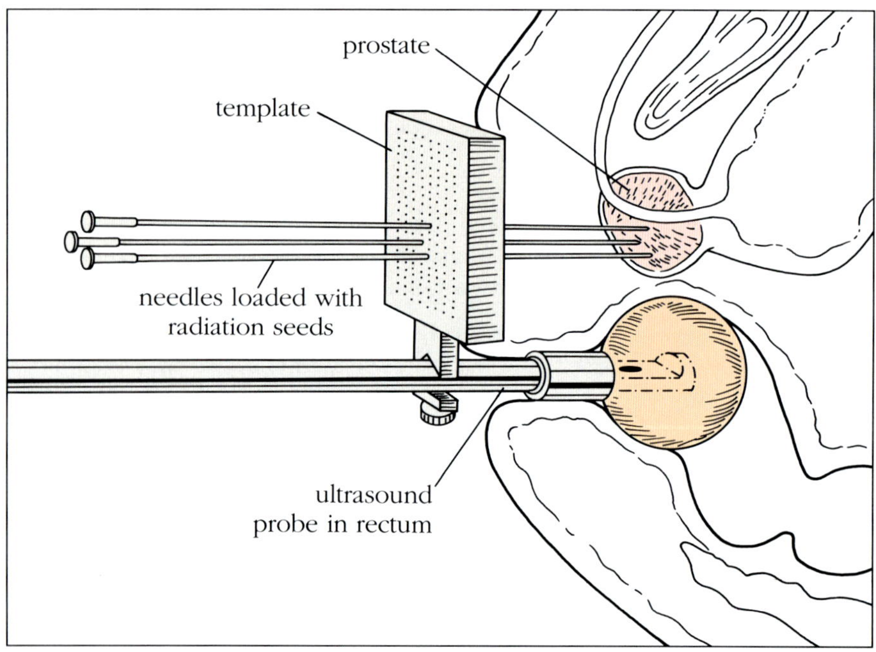

Figure 5.38 Transrectal ultrasound and a perineal template are used to place radiation seeds in the prostate via needles.

prostatectomy were treated with external beam radiation therapy: only one third of the patients treated had reduced postradiation PSA levels.[52] Although only early follow-up data are available, this implies that of patients who have elevated PSA levels after prostatectomy, more have residual prostate cancer distantly than locally.

BRACHYTHERAPY

Brachytherapy treatment of the prostate was popularized by Whitmore and associates at the Memorial Sloan-Kettering Cancer Institute. Implantation of radioactive seeds in the prostate had great popularity in the 1970s. The theoretical appeal of this form of treatment is that high doses of radiation can be delivered to the target tissues without damage to surrounding tissue.[53]

The initial trials used iodine-125 seeds, although other agents have been used, including gold, iridium, and palladium. All patients in Whitmore's series underwent pelvic lymph node dissection at the same time that they had open placement of the seeds. Previous transurethral resection of the prostate made seed placement technically so difficult that it was considered a contraindication. The characteristics of radioactive iodine that make it an ideal agent for brachtherapy are its small radius of tissue penetration and a long half-life. This series revealed two major failures of interstitial brachytherapy of prostate cancer. First, the complication rate was high: as many as 25% of patients experienced complications related to the procedure. Second, local control of prostate cancer was poor, with 50% of the patients having local progression of disease at 5 years. This is a very high rate for patients who are clinically stage B1. Many clinicians felt that the failure of local control was related to inaccurate seed placement, subsequent uneven distribution of radiation, and "cold spots" within the prostate where the cancer remained unradiated.[8,34]

Other interstitial radiotherapy agents either had similarly poor results or long-term follow-up is still pending. Concurrent with the work on iodine-125 were experimental trials of gold seeds. Gold-198 has greater tissue penetration and a shorter half-life compared to [125]I. Therefore, interstitial [198]Au treatment of prostate cancer was supplemented with adjuvant external beam radiation. Results were similar to those with ^{125}I and local control was poor.

Another interstitial radiotherapy agent is iridium-192, which has an extremely short half-life. Instead of open implantation, tubes are placed in the prostate transperineally under manual or ultrasound guidance. Then the iridium is passed through these tubes ("after-loading") and left for hours to days. At the end of treatment, the tubes and the iridium are removed. Long-term follow-up is not yet available, and the immediate complication rate due to local tissue injury and infection is high.

Currently, many centers are participating in trials of ultrasound-guided seed implantation. TRUS is initially used to determine prostatic volume and contour so that computer-assisted calculation of dose and seed placement can be done. Then TRUS is used for a transperineal placement of seeds using a template and needles (Fig. 5.38). Commonly a larger number of low-activity seeds are used compared with previous iodine or gold seed techniques. Also, some centers are using palladium-103, which has a higher dose rate than iodine. Theoretically, this may overcome problems of uneven delivery of radiation within the prostate. Long-term results are as yet unavailable. In conclusion, interstitial radiotherapy of prostate cancer is still considered by many an experimental form of treatment.

Complications

The complications of radiation therapy have been reduced in recent years. The main morbidity of radiation therapy is injury to the gastrointestinal and urinary tracts. Patients can experience diarrhea, gastrointestinal or urinary bleeding, tenesmus, and irritative voiding symptoms. The combined incidence of moderate GI or GU complications is 7% to 9%. Impotence can be a complication of radiation therapy. According to Bagshaw's data, of those patients who are potent before radiation, 86% are potent at 1 year postradiation and 55% are potent at 5 years postradiation. No incontinence results from radiation therapy alone, although incontinence rates with postradiation prostatectomy are dramatically higher.[34,37,54]

PALLIATIVE RADIATION THERAPY

Radiation can be used to palliate painful bony metastases or to treat ureteral obstruction due to tumor. Radiation to bony metastases is only for symptomatic relief of pain and has no effect on survival. Doses of 3000 to 5000 cGy are usually fractionated over 2 to 5 weeks. Complete relief of symptoms occurs in some 40% of patients, with another 35% experiencing partial relief of their pain. Radiation therapy can also be considered for bony lesions in weight-bearing areas (for example, the femoral neck) in order to prevent fracture. The results of palliative radiation therapy for ureteral obstruction due to prostate cancer are less favorable. The best treatment of ureteral obstruction by prostatic cancer is endocrine manipulation, but in patients who have cancer refractory to endocrine treatment, radiation therapy is an option. In dosages of 5000 to 6000 cGy, relief of obstruction occurs in approximately 26% of patients. It should be noted that the survival of patients in this condition is poor, it can take weeks or months for radiation to have any effect, and ureteral obstruction subsequently recurs in some cases. Protocols investigating the systemic administration of strontium-51 for painful bony metastasis are underway.[55]

ENDOCRINE THERAPY

Prostatic tissues have long been known to be responsive to androgen hormones. Normal prostatic tissue, benign prostatic hyperplasia, and carcinoma of the prostate are all generally responsive. The testes produce 95% of circulating testosterone and other androgens, while the adrenal gland produces the remaining 5%. Testosterone is taken up by cells and converted to dihydrotestosterone (DHT) intracellularly by 5α-reductase. DHT then combines with intracellular receptors, is translocated into the cell nucleus, and acts by binding to DNA and regulating DNA transcription (Fig. 5.39). Testosterone broadly promotes prostate cellular hypertrophy as well as proliferation. How altered DNA transcription produces this stimulation of prostate cells has yet to be elucidated. Prostate cancer appears to be heterogeneous, with some cells that respond to hormonal stimulation and others that do not.

Endocrine therapy of prostatic cancer is used mainly to treat metastatic disease, although investigations of adjuvant endocrine treatment for more localized forms of prostatic cancer are ongoing. Endocrine treatment appears to increase overall survival; however, the timing of treatment is controversial. To date, studies appear to show no difference in overall survival between patients treated with hormonal monotherapy immediately upon diagnosis and patients who are treated late for symptomatic disease. With early therapy there is an increased time until progression of disease. There is also a suggestion that early hormonal treatment increases survival in young patients with high-grade tumors, although this is controversial. Delayed treatment has the advantages of avoiding the side effects and expense of treatment until the patient is truly symptomatic.[56] The trend at present is to treat the disease early, at the time of diagnosis. The concept of "total androgen blockade" is discussed below.

Currently there are several options for androgen ablation monotherapy of prostate cancer. Options include orchiectomy, estrogens, luteinizing hormone releasing hormone (LH-RH) agonists, and androgen blockers. A new advance is the use of total androgen blockade. Orchiectomy was the earliest form of hormonal treatment of prostate cancer, and is still the "gold standard." The

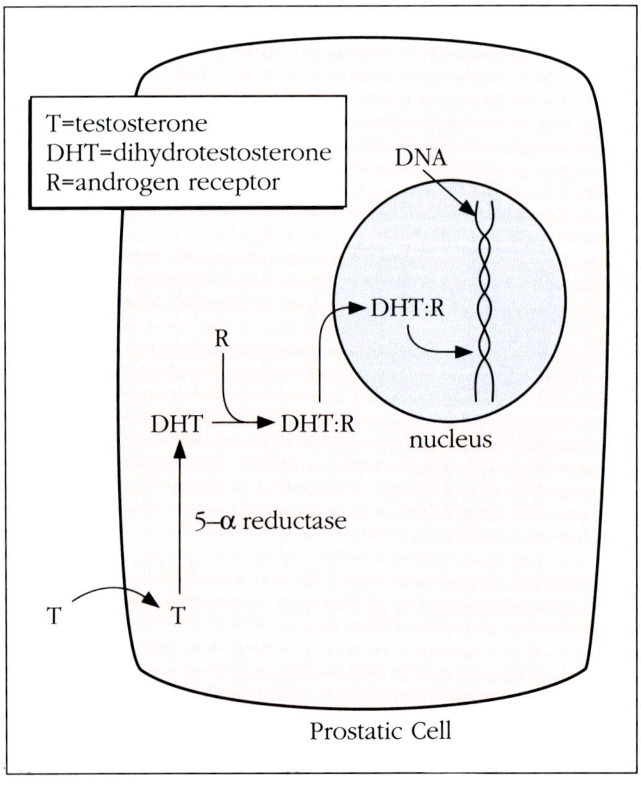

Figure 5.39 Mechanism of action of testosterone. Testosterone is transported across the cell membrane and converted by 5α-reductase to dihydrotestosterone (DHT). DHT binds to an intracellular receptor, translocates into the nucleus, and interacts with DNA to alter transcription.

advantages of orchiectomy are that it is relatively inexpensive and the issue of patient compliance is obviated. Disadvantages are that it is a surgical procedure, albeit a minor one, and there are reports of adverse psychologic effects.

A second option is estrogen therapy, most commonly diethylstilbestrol (DES, 1 mg P.O. t.i.d.). Estrogens work by feedback inhibition of LH-RH secretion and, theoretically, they also have direct toxicity to prostate cancer. The advantages of estrogens are that they are inexpensive and can be taken orally. However, there are many disadvantages of estrogen therapy. The numerous side effects include impotence, loss of libido, gynecomastia, bloating, and pedal edema. There are more serious cardiovascular side effects, including stroke, heart attack, and deep venous thrombosis. The rate of side effects is lowered by lowering the dose of estrogen, but it is not clear that this low dose is an effective treatment since testosterone levels do not reliably become castrate. Due to concerns about the serious side effects, few clinicians currently use estrogen therapy.

LH-RH agonists are a third option. They act by feedback inhibition of LH-RH release and are administered by monthly depot injections. Agents include leuprolide acetate (Lupron) administered IM and gosereline acetate (Zoladex) as a subcutaneous implant. The advantages of this form of treatment are that no surgery is necessary and there are relatively few side effects. The disadvantages are that it is expensive, it requires monthly compliance, and there is a notable flare effect. The flare effect is the predictable rise in LH and circulating testosterone for about the first week after injection of the LH-RH agonists. The increased androgen stimulation of the cancer may cause a worsening of any cancer symptoms initially (such as bone pain, bladder outlet problems, etc). For this reason, LH-RH agonists are contraindicated as the primary monotherapy of spinal cord compression due to prostate cancer.

A fourth option is androgen blockers. These are competitive inhibitors of DHT which act by competing for intracellular receptors. Flutamide (Eulexin) is the most commonly used drug of this class and the only one currently available in the United States (dosage 125 mg, 2 tablets P.O. t.i.d.). The theoretical advantage of androgen blockers is that the action of testosterone is blocked regardless of its testicular or adrenal origin. Also, potency is preserved despite androgen blockade. However, flutamide is not currently approved for monotherapy. The reason is that testosterone levels rise in response to the androgen blocker, and since the blockade is competitive, there is concern that it may be overcome by high testosterone levels. Side effects are important considerations in choosing which type of androgen ablation to use. These are summarized in Figure 5.40.[57]

Another aspect of hormonal therapy is the concept of total androgen blockade. Most hormonal therapies ablate androgens produced by the testis but not adrenal androgens. Historically, surgical adrenal androgen ablation has been attempted by either adrenalectomy or hypophysectomy. These both had high morbidity and little therapeutic benefit. Currently, total androgen blockade can be achieved by employing either orchiectomy or LH-RH agonists in combination with an androgen blocker such as

FIGURE 5.40 *Commonly Reported Side Effects of Hormonal Manipulations for Advanced Prostate Cancer*

	ORCHIECTOMY	DES	LH-RH AGONIST	FLUTAMIDE
Loss of libido	+	+	+	
Impotence	+	+	+	
"Hot flash"	+	+	+	+
Gynecomastia		+		+
Bloating/pedal edema		+		
MI/CVA/DVT		+		
Nausea and vomiting		+		
Flare			+	
Diarrhea				+
Liver dysfunction				+

MI = myocardial infarction; CVA = cerebrovascular accident; DVT = deep venous thrombosis flutamide. Recent studies suggest that there may be as much as a 3 to 7 month improvement in patient survival with total androgen blockade, with even better outcomes in patients treated with early disease.[58] Multiple investigations have been published or are in progress, and more recent studies confirm this finding of improved survival. The disadvantage of total androgen blockade therapy is that it is expensive and may have an increased rate of side effects. Many consider total androgen blockade to be the state-of-the-art treatment for metastatic prostate cancer.

Follow-up After Treatment

After initial treatment, most patients need to be followed every 3 to 6 months. At each follow-up visit, symptoms such as bladder outlet obstruction or bone pain should be sought, DRE performed, and PSA and prostatic acid phosphatase measured. In selected patients, alkaline phosphatase or creatinine measurement, bone scan, or evaluation of bladder outlet obstruction should be done. Serial PSA evaluations may be the best method of following patients with prostate cancer. Progressively rising levels of PSA indicate progression and/or recurrence, either local or distant. Digital rectal exam, transrectal ultrasound, and biopsy when indicated should identify patients with locally recurrent disease. Bone scans can identify many patients with distant disease and should be ordered if clinically relevant.

There are several options for the treatment of locally recurrent prostate cancer. Local recurrence after radical surgery can be treated with radiation therapy (see page 5.25). Adjuvant radiation therapy appears to achieve local control, but whether it improves survival has yet to be seen. After definitive radiation therapy, local recurrence may be treated with salvage radical prostatectomy in some patients, although this is controversial. All studies have shown that after radiation therapy, radical prostatectomy carries significant increases in morbidity: the rates of postoperative incontinence, impotence, and rectal fistula are all much higher after radiation. Consideration of salvage radical prostatectomy requires that these high complication rates be weighed carefully. Hormonal therapy is another option for local disease recurrence.

The treatment of distant recurrence of prostate cancer is more limited. Hormonal treatment, of course, is the mainstay of therapy, as has been discussed above. For patients who have hormone-refractory carcinoma of the prostate, there are currently no good treatment options. Cytotoxic chemotherapy trials have been uniformly unimpressive. There is only a 10% to 15% objective response with any type of chemotherapy tried, and there has been no clear improvement in patient survival. Chemotherapy trials in stage D2 prostate cancer patients who have not had hormonal therapy are particularly difficult to interpret due to the wide range of the natural history of the disease. In studies of patients with stage D2 prostate cancer, 10% survive less than 6 months and 10% survive more than 10 years. Immunotherapy of prostate cancer is still experimental, although there have been some promising reports. Adrenal androgen ablation in hormonally refractory prostate cancer has not been shown to be effective except possibly as a palliative treatment (aminoglutethimide with or without steroids). Estramustine phosphate (Emcyt) may also occasionally provide some palliation but will not prolong survival. Agents under intensive study include suramin, which is thought to interfere with growth factor regulation, and taxol, a microtubule inhibitor. Gene therapy provides additional hope for the future in developing more effective therapy for advanced hormone-refractory prostate cancer.

References

1. Boring CC, Squires TS, Tong T. Cancer statistics, 1993. *CA.* 1993;43:7–26.
2. Scardino PT. Early detection of prostate cancer. *Urol Clin North Am.* 1989;16:635–655.
3. Mettlin C, Jones G, Auerette H, et al. Defining and updating the American Cancer Society Guidelines for the cancer-related checkup: prostate and endometrial cancers. *CA.* 1993;43:42–46.
4. Carter HB, Pearson TD, Metter EJ, et al. Longitudinal evaluation of prostate-specific antigen levels in men with and without prostate disease. *JAMA.* 1992;267:2215–2220.
5. Oesterling JE. PSA leads the way for detecting and following prostate cancer. *Contemp Urol.* 1993;5:60–91.
6. Carter HB, Hamper UM, Sheth S, et al. Evaluation of transrectal ultrasound in the early detection of prostate cancer. *J Urol.* 1989;142:1008–1010.
7. Catalona WJ, et al. Measurement of prostatic specific antigen in serum as a screening test for prostate cancer. *N Engl J Med.* 1991;324:1156–1161.
8. Kozlowski JM, Grayhack JT. Carcinoma of the prostate. In: Gillenwater JY, et al, eds. *Adult and Pediatric Urology.* Chicago, Ill: Yearbook Medical Publishers; 1987:1126–1219.
9. Paulson DF. The prognostic role of lymphadenectomy in adenocarcinoma of the prostate. *Urol Clin North Am.* 1980;7:615–622.
10. Crawford ED, et al. The effect of digital rectal examination on prostate specific antigen levels. *JAMA.* 1992;267:2227–2228.
11. Oesterling JE, Bilharte DL, Tindall DJ. Clinically useful serum markers for adenocarcinoma of the prostate, I: prostatic acid phosphatase. Baltimore, Md: AUA Update; 1991;X:Lesson 17.
12. Chybowski FM, Larson Keller JJ, Bergstralh EJ, Oesterling JE. Predicting radionuclide bone scan findings in patients with newly diagnosed, untreated prostate cancer: prostate specific antigen is superior to all other clinical parameters. *J Urol.* 1991;145:313–318.
13. Rifkin MD, et al. Comparison of magnetic resonance imaging and ultrasonography in staging early prostate cancer. Results of a multi-institutional cooperative trial. *N Engl J Med.* 1990;323:621–626.
14. McSherry SA, Levy F, Schiebler ML, Keef B, Dent GA, Mohler JL. Preoperative prediction of pathological tumor volume and staging clinically localized prostate cancer: comparison of digital rectal examination, transrectal ultrasonography and magnetic resonance imaging. *J Urol.* 1991;146:85–89.

15. Brendler CB, et al. Staging pelvic lymphadenectomy for carcinoma of the prostate: risk versus benefit. *J Urol.* 1980;124:849–854.

16. Rifkin MD, Dahnert W, Kurtz AB. State of the art: endorectal sonography of the prostate gland. *AJR.* 1990;154:691–700.

17. Rifkin MD, Alexander AA, Pisarchick J, Matteucci T. Palpable masses in the prostate: superior accuracy of US-guided biopsy compared with accuracy of digitally guided biopsy. *Radiology.* 1991;179:41–42.

18. Rifkin MD, Sudakoff GD, Gomella LG, Alexander AA. Color doppler ultrasound of the prostate. *J Urol.* 1992;147:321A.

19. Gomella LG, Kozminski M. Laparoscopic lymphadenectomy for staging prostate cancer. *Contemp Surg.* 1992;40:11–15.

20. Winfield HN, Donovan JF, See WA, Loening SA, Williams RD. Urological laparoscopic surgery. *J Urol.* 1991;146:941–948.

21. Elder JS. Laparoscopy and Fowler-Stephens orchiopexy in the management of the impalpable testis. *Urol Clin North Am.* 1989;16:399–411.

22. Leadbetter GW, Gillenwater JY. Urology. *JAMA.* 1991;265:3175–3176.

23. Paulson DF. A close look at the conduct of pelvic lymph node dissection in prostate cancer. *Contemp Urol.* 1991;3:23–33.

24. Winfield HN. Suddenly, urology takes up the laparoscope. *Contemp Urol.* 1991;3:70–80.

25. Scheussler WW, Vanciallie TG, Reich H, Griffith DP. Transperitoneal endosurgical lymphadenectomy in patients with localized prostate cancer. *J Urol.* 1991;145:988–991.

26. Winfield HN, See WA, Donovan JF, Loening SA, Williams RD. A new cancer staging technique: laparoscopic pelvic node dissection. *J Urol.* 1991;145:215A.

27. Chodak GW, Levine LA, Gerber GS, Rustalis DB. Safety and efficacy of laparoscopic lymphadenectomy. *J Urol.* 1992;147:126A.

28. Clayman RV, Griffith DP, Kavoussi LR, Schuessler W, Winfield HN. Laparoscopy: tips on technique. *Contemp Urol.* 1991;3(1):23–30.

29. Kozminski M, Gomella LG, Stone NN, Sosa E. Laparoscopic urologic surgery: outcome assessment. *J Urol.* 1992;147:127A.

30. Catalona WJ. Prostate cancer. *Curr Probl Surg.* 1990;24:394–461.

31. Morgan WR, Lieber MM. Pelvic lymphadenectomy. In: Crawford ED, Das S, eds. *Current Genitourinary Cancer Surgery.* Philadelphia, Pa: Lea and Febiger; 1990:162–170.

32. Lieskowsky G, Skinner DG, Weisenburger T. Pelvic lymphadenectomy in the management of carcinoma of the prostate. *J Urol.* 1980;124:635–638.

33. Catalona WJ, Scott WW. Carcinoma of the prostate. In: Walsh PC, et al, eds. *Campbell's Urology.* Philadelphia, Pa: WB Saunders Co; 1986:1463–1534.

34. Goffinet DR, Bagshaw MD. Radiation therapy of prostate carcinoma. In: Crawford ED, Das S, eds. *Current Genitourinary Cancer Surgery.* Philadelphia, Pa: Lea and Febiger; 1990:552–562.

35. Lepor H, Kimball AW, Walsh PC. Cause-specific actuarial survival analysis: a useful method for reporting survival data in men with clinically localized carcinoma of the prostate. *J Urol.* 1989;141:82–84.

36. Paulson DF, et al. The Uro-oncology Research Group: radical surgery versus radiotherapy for adenocarcinoma of the prostate. *J Urol.* 1982;128:502–504.

37. Schellhammer PF, El-Maudi AM. A local failure and related complications after definitive treatment of carcinoma of the prostate by radiation treatment or surgery. *Urol Clin North Am.* 1990;17:835–851.

38. Kabalin JN, Hodge KK, McNeal JE, Freiha FS, Stamey TA. Identification of residual cancer in the prostate following radiation therapy: role of transrectal ultrasound guided biopsy and prostatic specific antigen. *J Urol.* 1989;142:326–331.

39. Weldon VE, Tavel FR. Potency sparing radical perineal prostatectomy: anatomy, surgical technique, and initial results. *J Urol.* 1987;137:225A.

40. Resnick MI. Radical perineal prostatectomy redux. *Contemp Urol.* 1991;3:44–53.

41. Drago JR, et al. Radical nerve-sparing prostatectomy: the first 30 patients treated with epidural anesthesia. *J Surg Oncol.* 1989;40:182–184.

42. Walsh PC. Radical prostatectomy, preservation of sexual function: cancer control, the controversy. *Urol Clin North Am.* 1987;14:663–673.

43. Reiner WG, Walsh PC. Anatomical approach to the surgical management of the dorsal vein and Santorini's plexus during radical retropubic surgery. *J Urol.* 1979;121:198–200.

44. Walsh PC. Radical retropubic prostatectomy with reduced morbidity: an anatomic approach. *NCI Monogr.* 1988;7:133–137.

45. Lee F, Torp-Pedersen ST, Siders DB. Use of transrectal ultrasound in diagnosis, guided biopsy, staging, and screening of prostate cancer. *Urology.* 1989;33(suppl):7–10.

46. Lang PH. Properly applied perineal pressure improved pelvic exposure of the membranous urethra area. *Contemp Urol.* 1990;2:12.

47. Roth RA. An improved expanded tip urethral suture guide for use in radical prostatectomy. *J Urol.* 1991;146:390–391.

48. Leiskovsky G. Preparing the urethra during radical prostatectomy. *Contemp Urol.* 1991;3(5):13.

49. Paulson DF. The surgical technique of radical perineal prostatectomy. Baltimore, Md: AUA Update; 1986;V:Lesson 38, 1–8.

50. Peters PC. Complications of radical prostatectomy and lymphadenectomy. *Urol Clin North Am.* 1988;15(2):219–221.

51. Montie JE. Significance and treatment of positive margins or seminal vesical invasion after radical prostatectomy. *Urol Clin North Am.* 1991;17:803–812.

52. Hudson MA, Catalona WJ. Effect of adjuvant radiation therapy on prostatic specific antigen following radical prostatectomy. *J Urol.* 1990;143:1174–1177.

53. Spaulding JT. Interstitial brachytherapy for prostatic carcinoma. In: Crawford ED, Das S, eds. *Current Genitourinary Cancer Surgery.* Philadelphia, Pa: Lea and Febiger; 1990:201–212.

54. Greskovich FJ, Zagars GK, Sherman NE, Johnson DE. Complications following external beam radiation therapy for prostate cancer: an analysis of patients treated with and without staging pelvic lymphadenectomy. *J Urol.* 1991;146:798–802.

55. Miskin S, Catalona WJ. Ureteral obstruction from prostatic carcinoma: response to endocrine and radiation therapy. *J Urol.* 1977;118:733–736.

56. Trachtenberg J. Hormonal management of Stage D carcinoma of the prostate. Baltimore, Md: AUA Update; 1990; IX:Lesson 30.

57. Smith JA, Jr. New methods of endocrine management of prostatic cancer. *J Urol.* 1987;137:1–10.

58. Crawford ED, et al. A controlled trial of leuprolide with and without flutamide in prostatic carcinoma. *N Engl J Med.* 1989;321:419–424.

CHAPTER 6

Management of Testis Cancer

Richard S. Foster

John P. Donohue

Testicular tumors are the most common solid tumor in males between the ages of 15 and 40. Of all testis tumors, 97% to 98% are of germ cell origin. Seminoma is the most common histologic type, representing approximately 40% of cases in patients with normal testicular descent. After seminoma, the primary cell types include embryonal carcinoma, teratocarcinoma, and teratoma. Choriocarcinoma is the least common single histologic type. Mixed tumors (tumors of more than one primary histologic type) represent approximately 25% in most series.

Several clinical entities have been associated with testis cancer. These include cryptorchidism, history of trauma, and infertility. The presence of cryptorchidism increases the risk of developing testis cancer by approximately seven to thirty-five times. Trauma is not thought to be a causative factor but is acknowledged to be an indication for examination of the testicle. Infertile men have a higher incidence of carcinoma in situ of the testis, which is known to be a predisposing factor for the development of invasive carcinoma.[1] Similarly, patients diagnosed with testis cancer have been found to have abnormal semen analyses about 60% of the time.[2]

Because most primary testicular tumors are of germ cell origin, this chapter will concentrate solely on these types of tumors. Germ cell testicular cancer is now a highly curable neoplasm. Advances in both surgical and medical oncology have led to an extremely good prognosis for most patients who present with germ cell testicular tumors.

Initial Presentation

Testicular cancer most commonly presents with scrotal enlargement. Patients characteristically complain of a sensation of fullness or heaviness in the scrotum, with actual pain being uncommon. These scrotal masses are usually discovered by a sexual partner. Metastatic testicular cancer presents as back pain, abdominal mass, hemoptysis, and/or adenopathy (neck or supraclavicular).

If physical examination discloses the scrotal enlargement to be secondary to an intrinsic solid testicular mass, the appropriate treatment is immediate radical inguinal orchiectomy. Careful attention should be paid on physical examination to a subtle change in consistency of the testis itself. Small tumors may present in this fashion.

Sudden appearance of a hydrocele in a young patient may mask the diagnosis of testicular tumor. Hydroceles in young patients may be secondary to tumor or epididymitis. If the testis cannot be palpated because of a large hydrocele in a young patient, scrotal ultrasonography is extremely useful in delineating anatomy.

Treatment

Testis cancer is curable surgically even after metastasis has occurred. Therefore, it is reasonable to attempt to limit the sites of metastasis to one lymphatic drainage area. The appropriate treatment for a solid intratesticular mass in a young man is radical inguinal orchiectomy because the chance of cross-contamination of inguinal lymphatics during the surgical procedure is thereby minimized. An inguinal incision is made, and the cord and testis are mobilized up through the incision. Since scrotal and inguinal lymphatic drainage is to the inguinal nodes and testicular lymphatic drainage is to the retroperitoneal nodes, tumor spillage in the scrotal or inguinal areas is minimized.

SEMINOMA
Low-Stage Seminoma

Pathologic analysis of the radical orchiectomy specimen reveals pure seminoma in roughly 40% of cases. If blood samples for assay of serum markers (β-HCG and α-fetoprotein) have not been drawn, they are drawn at this time. Roughly 10% of patients with seminoma have elevations of serum HCG.[3] Conversely, an elevation in serum α-fetoprotein excludes the diagnosis of seminoma; these patients are treated as nonseminomas despite a pathologic diagnosis of seminoma.

Radiographic staging is done with CT scans of the abdomen and chest. Bipedal lymphangiography is still used in some centers but is limited by low sensitivity (75% to 80%) and specificity (10% false-positive rate).

The staging system used most commonly in seminoma is the Royal Marsden staging system. In this system patients with stage I have evidence of testis disease only, stage II includes abdominal disease, stage III supradiaphragmatic but nodally confined disease, and stage IV extranodal involvement of lung, bone, or viscera. Stage II disease can be further classified by the amount of retroperitoneal disease (IIA less than 2 cm, IIB 2 to 5 cm, IIC greater than 5 cm).

CLINICAL STAGE I   About 80% of patients who present with pure seminoma are found to be clinical stage I. The traditional treatment of patients in this situation has been radiotherapy. Doses typically range around 2500 cGy; acute morbidity is extremely low and includes mild nausea. Long-term morbidity is minimal except for the small chance of developing a secondary malignancy. Some patients experience oligospermia, but with modern shielding techniques recovery of spermatogenesis is usually the rule. An illustration of the radiation portal for a left-sided seminoma is shown in Figure 6.1.

Many series of patients with clinical stage I seminoma treated with radiotherapy have documented an excellent long-term prognosis.[4,5] More than 95% of patients will achieve long-term survival. Although some have advocated supradiaphragmatic radiation for these patients, review of the pattern of relapse and the ability of subsequent chemotherapy to salvage these patients argues against the routine use of supradiaphragmatic radiation.[6]

Since most (60% to 80%) of these patients have pathologic stage I disease and since effective salvage therapy (chemotherapy) exists, various investigators have advocated observation after orchiectomy as an alternative to radiotherapy in patients who present with clinical stage I seminoma.[7] Patients who subsequently develop radiographically identifiable disease are then treated with chemotherapy. This approach must be compared to the highly effective, low-morbidity treatment of radiotherapy. In addition, it is now recognized that observation in clinical stage I seminoma requires long-term follow-up compared to primary treatment with radiotherapy.

CLINICAL STAGE II Small amounts of retroperitoneal metastasis are managed very effectively with abdominal radiotherapy. Of patients treated in this fashion, 80% to 90% will be cured.[8] It is apparent that increasing amounts of abdominal disease diminish the ultimate cure rate with radiotherapy. Since these patients are usually cured with chemotherapy, high-volume retroperitoneal disease is usually treated with a platinum-based protocol. The volume of retroperitoneal disease at which the change should be made from radiotherapy to chemotherapy is not known. However, patients with very large abdominal masses (greater than 10 cm) have an extremely high relapse rate after radiotherapy alone, and chemotherapy should be the prime treatment in such cases. Patients with bulky abdominal disease treated with primary chemotherapy have a greater than 90% chance of cure.

High-Stage Seminoma

Approximately 90% of patients who present with clinical stage III seminoma and are treated with cisplatin-based chemotherapy can expect to be cured. Therefore, cisplatin-based chemotherapy is clearly the treatment of choice for this group.

The unusual patient who presents with stage IV seminoma will do less well with chemotherapy. Only 50% to 60% of these patients obtain complete remission with cisplatin-based chemotherapy.[9] Therefore, these rare poor-risk patients are candidates for investigational protocols.

An area of controversy regarding high-stage seminoma involves the use of surgery to resect residual radiographic abnormalities after chemotherapy. Some groups recommend biopsy or resection of residual radiographic abnormalities after chemotherapy if the residual disease measures 3 cm or more.[10] These investigators argue that

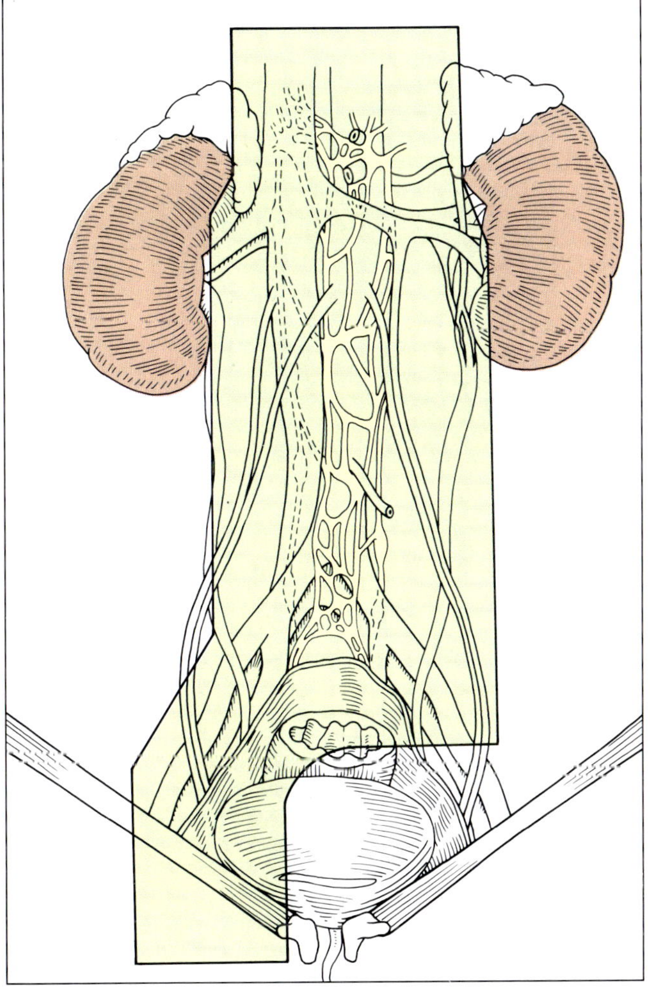

Figure 6.1 Radiation portal for a left-sided seminoma. For a right-sided tumor the iliac portal would be on the right.

if the mass is greater than 3 cm, the probability of finding something other than fibrosis in the resected tumor is high. Other centers manage residual radiographic abnormalities differently. At Indiana University these patients are observed, since the Indiana experience shows only a 10% incidence of significant pathologic findings in seminoma patients subjected to postchemotherapy retroperitoneal lymphadenectomy (RPLND).[11] Also militating against routine exploration in this setting is the intense desmoplastic reaction that usually occurs in the retroperitoneum after metastatic seminoma is treated with cisplatin-based chemotherapy.

NONSEMINOMA

If the diagnosis after radical inguinal orchiectomy is nonseminoma, clinical staging is performed. This includes determination of serum α-fetoprotein and β-HCG along with abdominal and chest CT scanning. The clinical staging system used at Indiana University is depicted in Figure 6.2.

FIGURE 6.2 *Nonseminoma: Clinical Staging*

Stage A   No radiographic disease
Markers normal (or decaying normally)

Stage B   Retroperitoneal radiographic disease

Stage C   Chest radiographic disease

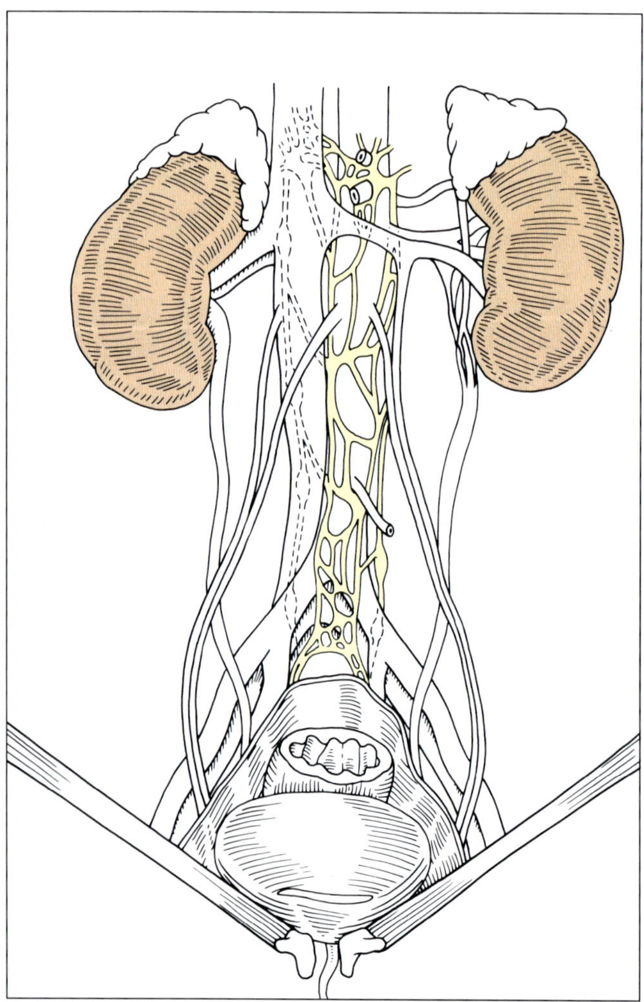

Figure 6.3 Anatomy of the retroperitoneum.

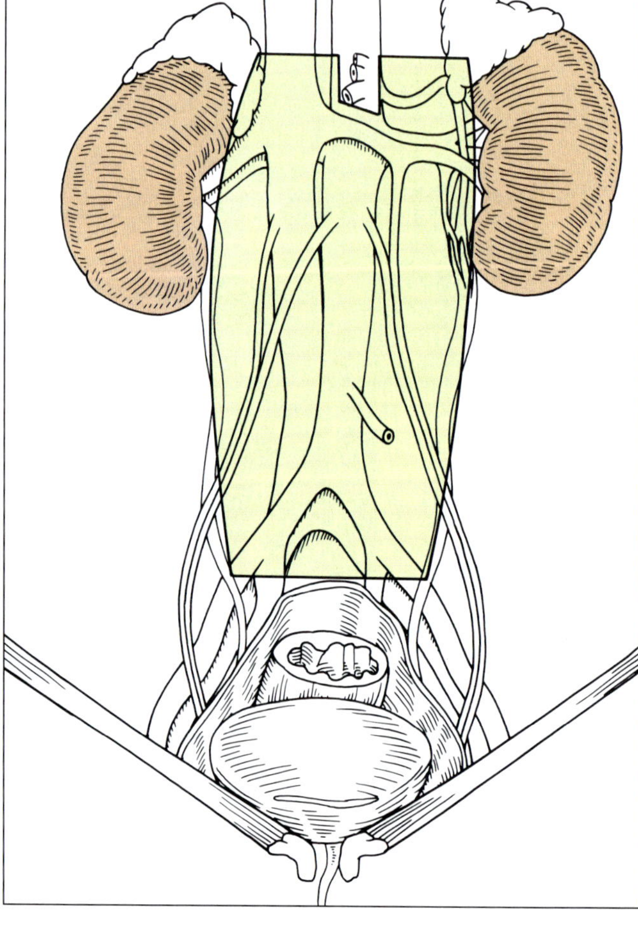

Figure 6.4 The traditional full bilateral suprahilar dissection template.

Clinical Stage A

Approximately 70% of patients who present with clinical stage A nonseminoma are in fact pathologic stage A. The traditional approach to clinical stage A nonseminoma has involved radical retroperitoneal lymphadenectomy. The reasons for proceeding with RPLND are twofold. First, patients who are in fact pathologic stage B are defined early in the course of the disease, so rational assignment of treatment options can be carried out. In addition, 50% to 70% of patients with low-volume retroperitoneal metastasis who undergo RPLND are cured without the necessity of subsequent chemotherapy.

In the traditional full bilateral RPLND technique,[2] all lymphatic tissue is removed en bloc from the bifurcation of the common iliacs to the crus of the diaphragm, from ureter to ureter (Fig. 6.3). The "split-and-roll" technique is used with division of all lumbar arteries and veins to obtain a complete en bloc removal of all lymphatic tissue

(Figs. 6.4–6.6). The morbidity of this procedure was low, with the exception of the universal loss of emission/ejaculation because retroperitoneal sympathetics were removed along with lymphatic tissue.

In an effort to diminish the incidence of anejaculation after RPLND, mapping studies were performed. These studies showed that in patients with small amounts of metastasis the sites of metastasis were highly predictable.[13] In a patient with a right-sided primary tumor, the likely areas of metastasis were shown to be the precaval and interaortocaval zones, and for a patient with a left-sided primary, the likely sites of metastasis were shown to be the upper and mid left periaortic zones. These observations, along with the desire to limit the morbidity of the procedure, led to the adoption of the so-called modified dissections. These procedures use the same surgical principles as the traditional full bilateral dissection, but limit the template of removal of lymphatic tis-

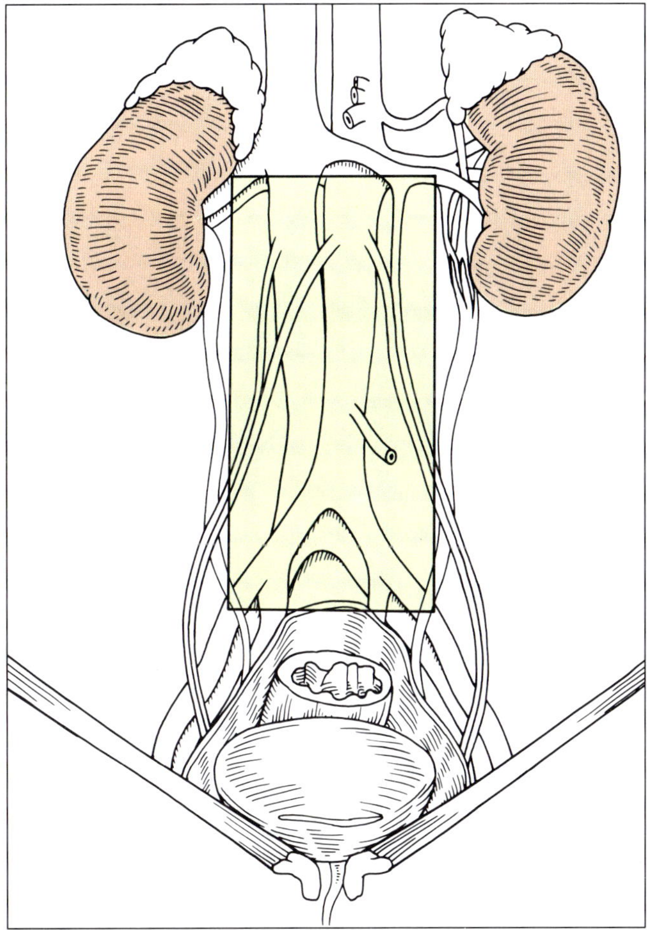

Figure 6.5 The full bilateral template.

sue. These modified dissections preserve emission/ejaculation in approximately 60% to 70% of patients with right-sided primaries and 30% to 40% of patients with left-sided primaries (Figs. 6.7, 6.8). Other investigators have subsequently limited the template of dissection even more and have obtained higher rates of emission/ejaculation,[2,14] approximately 80% to 90% of patients.

The next step in the evolution of surgical therapy for low-stage nonseminoma was the development of the nerve-sparing RPLND.[15] As experience with retroperitoneal surgery increased, it became apparent that the sympathetic efferent fibers emanating from the sympathetic chain and passing distally to the preaortic plexus could be identified reliably from patient to patient. Dissection of these fibers, although tedious, can be carried out prospectively, with subsequent resection of lymphatic tissue. Although sparing these fibers unilaterally preserves emission/ejaculation in most patients, bilateral sparing preserves emission/ejaculation in more than 99% of patients. This procedure therefore employs prospective nerve-sparing followed by en bloc resection of lymphatic

tissue, corresponding roughly to the modified templates. Our review of the experience with this technique has shown that both the staging and the therapeutic aspects of the procedure are preserved despite the prospective dissection of sympathetic nerves. Nerve-sparing RPLND therefore has maintained the efficacy of the procedure while eliminating its major source of morbidity: nerve-sparing techniques now enable emission/ejaculation to be preserved more than 99% of the time.

The surveillance strategy for management of patients with clinical stage A nonseminoma arose in an effort to eliminate the major source of morbidity of RPLND, the loss of emission/ejaculation. After the development of cisplatin-based chemotherapy it became apparent that patients who had low- or moderate-volume metastatic disease could be cured most of the time with chemotherapy alone. Consequently, various investigators adopted a strategy of close observation in patients who presented with clinical stage A nonseminoma.[16] Patients with pathologic stage A disease were therefore spared an RPLND, and the hope was to salvage all patients with pathologic

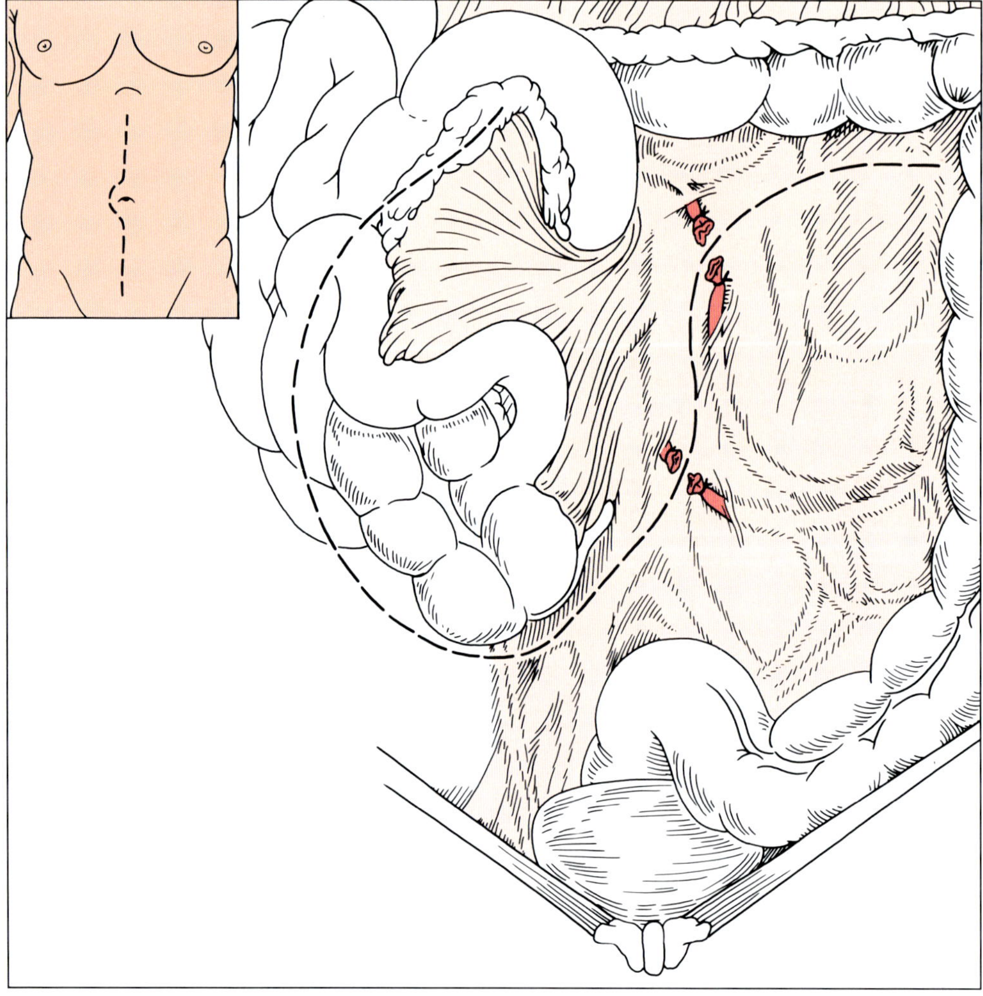

Figure 6.6 The posterior peritoneal incision for a full bilateral RPLND.

stage B disease who subsequently developed obvious radiographic disease with chemotherapy.

Results of surveillance protocols from various institutions around the world have shown cure rates of around 96%. It is apparent, however, that not all patients with pathologic stage B disease who develop radiographic abnormalities on CT scanning are salvaged with platinum-based chemotherapy. On the other hand, more than 99% of patients with low-volume retroperitoneal disease who are managed with an up-front RPLND are curable (although subsequent chemotherapy is necessary in some patients).[17]

At present, attempts are being made to define the cohort of patients presenting with clinical stage A nonseminoma for whom the surveillance strategy is destined to fail. If it were possible to select patients with a high risk of being pathologic stage B, a more rational assignment of therapy could be carried out, with an ultimate reduction in overall morbidity. Although various parameters such as vascular invasion and embryonal histology portend a higher risk of metastasis, more accurate predictors are needed.[16] The surveillance strategy has attempted to maintain

the efficacy of treatment but to minimize its morbidity. It clearly reduces morbidity in some patients but has not proven as effective a form of treatment as immediate RPLND. Our present approach is to individualize treatment, presenting each patient with his options and attempting to determine the best therapy for the individual.

Patients who present with clinical stage A nonseminomatous testis cancer are now advised of treatment options. Surveillance is appealing because it spares unnecessary surgery in the 70% of patients who are pathologic stage A. However, these patients must be informed that the ultimate chance of dying of testis cancer may be higher with surveillance as now practiced. The benefits of immediate RPLND must also be presented: there is precision in disease staging and subsequent treatment requirements are defined, there is therapeutic benefit if the nodes are positive, there is ease of follow-up since retroperitoneal relapse is extremely rare (postoperative CT scans are not routinely performed), and, finally, if relapse occurs it is curable in more than 99% of patients.

Relapse after RPLND occurs in the lungs or serologically.[17] Both of these areas are easy to monitor with chest

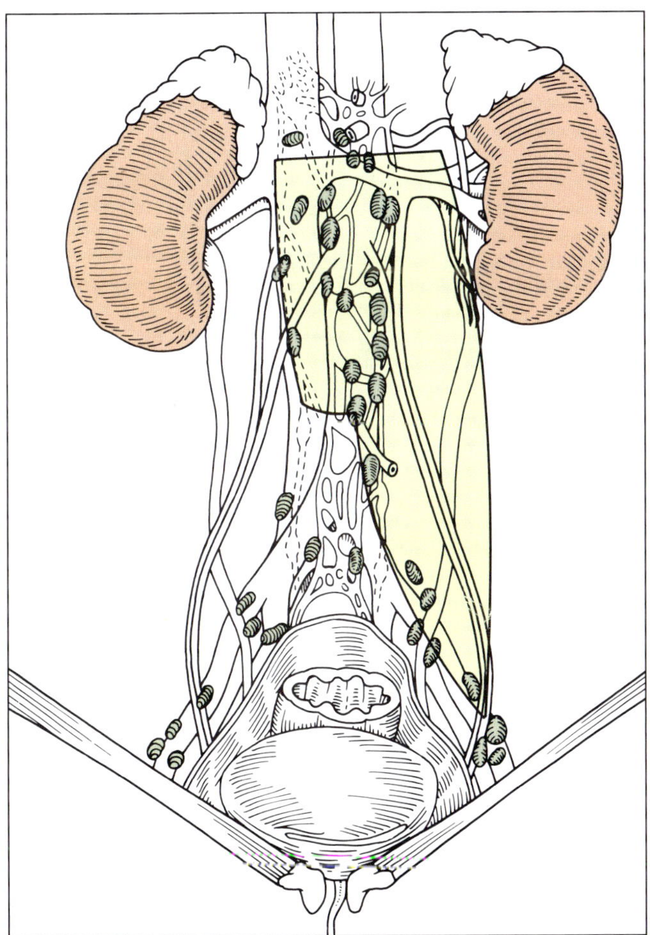

Figure 6.7 The template for a left-sided nerve-sparing RPLND for low-stage disease.

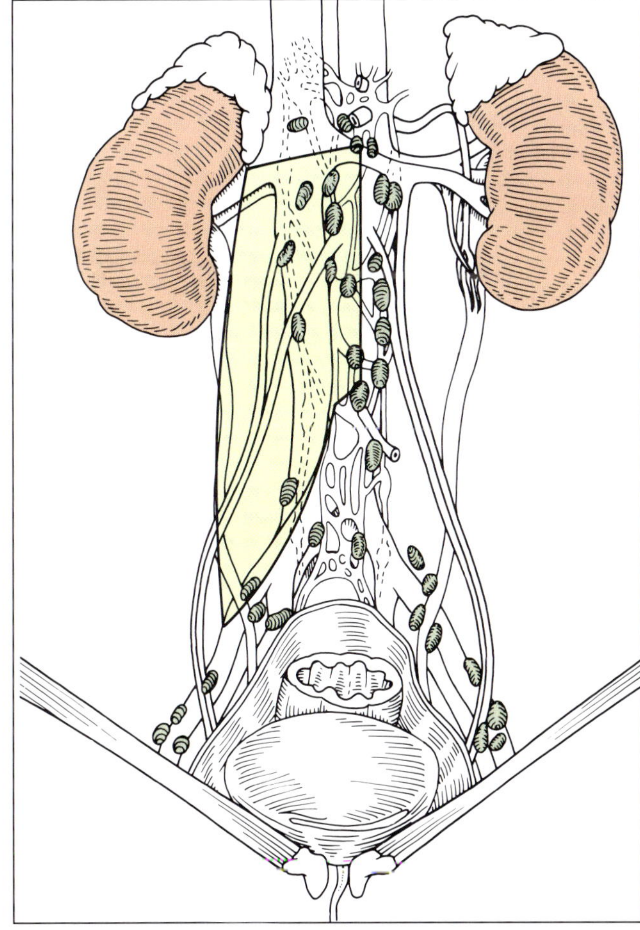

Figure 6.8 The template for a right-sided nerve-sparing RPLND for low-stage disease.

radiographs and determination of serum markers. Chemotherapy rescue with minimal pulmonary disease is almost universal.[18] On the other hand, the efficacy of chemotherapy salvage in patients presenting with both retroperitoneal and pulmonary disease (the relapse form using surveillance) is not as reliable.

Nonseminoma Clinical Stage B

Clinical stage B nonseminoma has traditionally been treated with RPLND. The relapse rate after RPLND in patients in this situation is directly related to the volume of retroperitoneal disease resected. About 30% of patients with microscopic disease relapse. In patients with moderate-volume disease the relapse rate is approximately 40% to 50%. In patients with high-volume retroperitoneal disease the relapse rate is high. Therefore, these patients are usually treated with primary chemotherapy.

If no gross disease is palpated in the retroperitoneum at the time of RPLND, a nerve-sparing RPLND is performed. Mapping studies have shown that when microscopic disease is present in these patients it is confined to the template of dissection.[13] If gross retroperitoneal disease is palpated the traditional approach has been full bilateral RPLND with consequent loss of emission and ejaculation. Nerve-sparing approaches in this context are now beginning to be used.[19] Which of these patients are best served by a nerve-sparing approach rather than a traditional full bilateral RPLND is unclear at present but is an area of active investigation.

Since 30% to 50% of patients with pathologic stage B disease relapse after RPLND, the question of whether or not to administer adjuvant chemotherapy has been raised. A randomized study showed no difference in survival between administration of two courses of cisplatin-based chemotherapy after RPLND versus three or four courses of chemotherapy at relapse.[20] Therefore, the present policy is to individualize the treatment of the patient with pathologic stage B disease after RPLND. These patients are presented with options and elect either observation with treatment of three courses of chemotherapy at relapse or two courses of chemotherapy immediately after RPLND. A qualification to this policy is that patients who are deemed to be poorly compliant should probably receive two adjuvant courses after RPLND.

The results of RPLND in pathologic stage B nonseminomatous testis cancer at Indiana University are depicted in Figure 6.9. The overall survival rate is extremely good. Note should be made of the excellent survival in both the nonadjuvant arm and the adjuvant arm.

An alternative approach to treatment of pathologic stage B disease involves the use of primary cisplatin-based chemotherapy.[21] Various series have shown chemotherapy in this setting to be effective, although 20% to 30% of patients require postchemotherapy RPLND for residual radiographic abnormalities. Some groups have advocated a more careful selection of patients for chemotherapy in this setting, in an attempt to decrease the number of patients who require postchemotherapy

FIGURE 6.9 *Primary RPLND in Pathologic Stage B (1979–1989)*

	NO.	RELAPSE	SURVIVAL	DEATHS
No adjuvant	49	18	96%	2
Adjuvant	59	0	98%	1
Totals	108	18	97%	3

Three deaths: one cancer, one chemotherapy, one post-operative complication

RPLND. The benefits and morbidity of RPLND compared to primary chemotherapy in clinical stage B disease have been the subject of much debate. We recommend that therapy should be tailored to the individual patient and that the morbidities of the two treatments be compared.

Nonseminoma Clinical Stage C

Patients who present with clinical stage C or high-volume clinical stage B disease are candidates for cisplatin-based chemotherapy. Since the initial report in 1977 of cisplatin-based chemotherapy in testis cancer, various modifications to the chemotherapeutic regimen have been made.[22] Although a detailed discussion of these modifications is beyond the scope of this chapter, some generalizations can be given. Many well-done studies have enabled investigators to maintain the efficacy of therapy while minimizing its morbidity. Chemotherapeutic agents commonly employed in testis cancer are listed in Figure 6.10.

Standard therapy for "good-risk" metastatic testis cancer patients now involves three courses of cisplatin, VP-16, and bleomycin. It is now clear that maintenance chemotherapy after induction chemotherapy is not necessary. Patients with disseminated testis cancer classified as "poor-risk" include those with high volumes of metastatic disease, high elevations of tumor markers, extragonadal primary lesions, and visceral organ involvement.[23,24] These patients are treated aggressively with four courses of chemotherapy and are candidates for investigational trials.

Patients with "good-risk" disseminated testis cancer enjoy complete remission rates higher than 95%. Only 60% to 70% of patients with "poor-risk" disease experience complete remissions.

Postchemotherapy RPLND

Patients who undergo cisplatin-based chemotherapy for disseminated disease sometimes experience a partial remission. These patients have normalization of serum markers but persistent radiographic disease. Postchemotherapy RPLND is therefore performed. After removal of the residual tumor, one of three histologic diagnoses may be seen: fibrosis/necrosis, teratoma, or active carcinoma.

Removal of fibrosis/necrosis is not therapeutic. Predicting which patients have only fibrosis/necrosis is very difficult. Needle biopsies or samplings of the tumor are not adequate because these masses are typically heterogeneous. One group of patients in whom prediction of the pathologic entity of fibrosis is possible consists of those who had no teratoma in the orchiectomy specimen and who experience normalization of serum markers along with a greater than 90% reduction in the volume of radiographic tumor.[25] These patients at Indiana University are now followed expectantly, since virtually all have fibrosis/necrosis pathologically. They are, however, a highly select group.

The second pathologic entity found in postchemotherapy RPLND is teratoma. Teratoma is a benign tumor,

FIGURE 6.10 *Chemotherapeutic Agents Used in Testis Cancer*

	MECHANISM OF ACTION	TOXICITY
Cisplatinum	DNA crosslinking	Nephrotoxicity Ototoxicity Nausea and vomiting
Etoposide (VP-16)	Topoisomerase II inhibitor	Myelosuppression
Bleomycin	DNA cleavage	Pulmonary fibrosis Skin toxicity
Vinblastine	Mitotic inhibitor	Myelosuppression Ileus
Ifosfamide	Alkylating agent	Hemorrhagic cystitis

although it continues to enlarge if not resected. It is not chemosensitive and is a predictor of subsequent recurrence with sarcoma or carcinoma. Therefore, resection at postchemotherapy RPLND is mandatory. It is also clear that patients who have had multiple recurrences of ter-atoma have a higher chance of eventually presenting with sarcoma at each subsequent recurrence.[26] Hence, low-volume teratoma should be resected if at all possible.

Finding carcinoma in the resected material is an indication for additional chemotherapy. In this group of

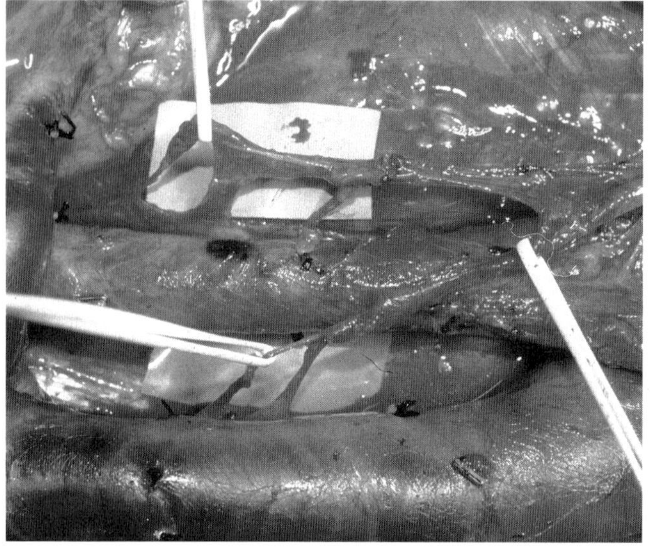

Figure 6.11 Intraoperative photo of a full bilateral RPLND with bilateral preservation of sympathetic efferents. This patient presented with clinical stage B3 disease, received chemotherapy, and subsequently underwent postchemotherapy nerve-sparing RPLND.

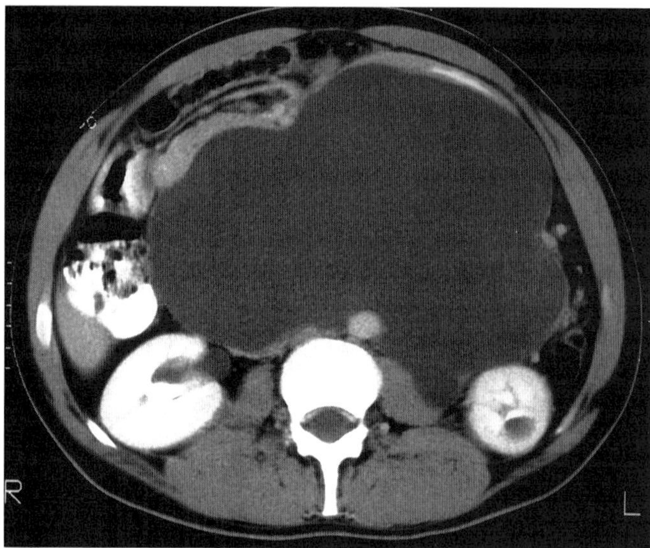

Figure 6.12 Residual retroperitoneal teratoma after platinum-based chemotherapy for stage C nonseminomatous testis cancer.

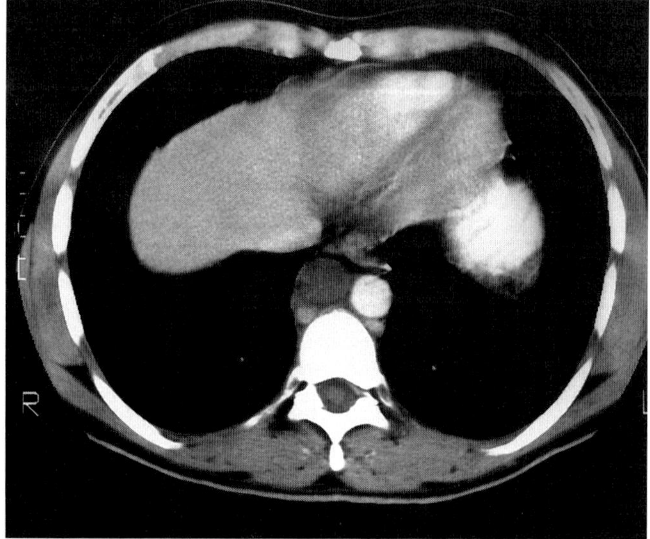

Figure 6.13 Residual right retrocrural tumor after primary chemotherapy for disseminated testis cancer.

patients the survival rate is 60% to 70%, if postchemotherapy RPLND is complete and two subsequent courses of chemotherapy are administered.[27]

The technique of postchemotherapy RPLND has been described.[12] Briefly, a full bilateral RPLND is performed after division of lumbar arteries and veins. Sympathetic fibers are removed, although in carefully selected patients nerve-sparing techniques are now used (Fig. 6.11). The surgical approach is dictated by the site of disease. Retroperitoneal disease can be resected via a transperitoneal approach (Fig. 6.12). Mediastinal and retrocrural disease is usually approached thoracoabdominally or by thoracotomy (Fig. 6.13). It should be stressed that postchemotherapy RPLND is by and large a vascular procedure. The surgeon who embarks on postchemotherapy RPLND should be thoroughly familiar with techniques of hemostasis (Fig. 6.14).

The morbidity associated with postchemotherapy RPLND is greater than that for primary RPLND performed in patients with clinical stage A or stage B disease. Various factors account for this increased morbidity. Pulmonary toxicity associated with bleomycin has made fluid management difficult in some of these patients. Pulmonary function must therefore be monitored very closely, and patients undergoing postchemotherapy RPLND are routinely managed overnight in the intensive care unit.

Conclusion

The therapy of germ cell testicular cancer continues to evolve. Central to the progress in this disease will be cooperation between medical and surgical oncologists. Better selection of patients for various therapies, minimization of therapy-associated morbidity, and development of better therapy for patients with poor-risk disease are active areas of investigation.

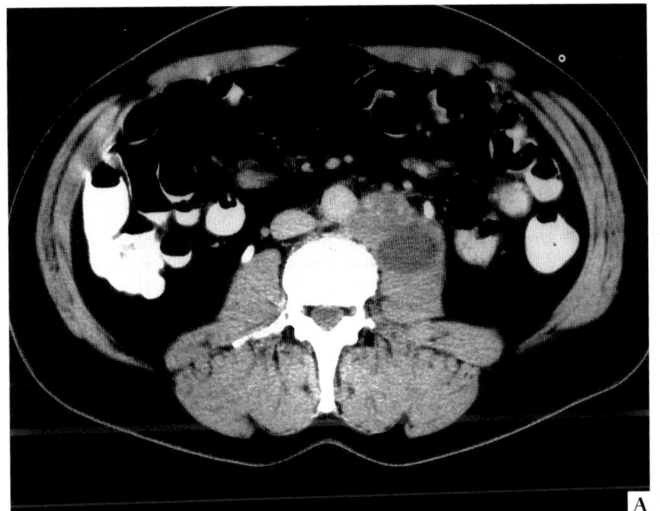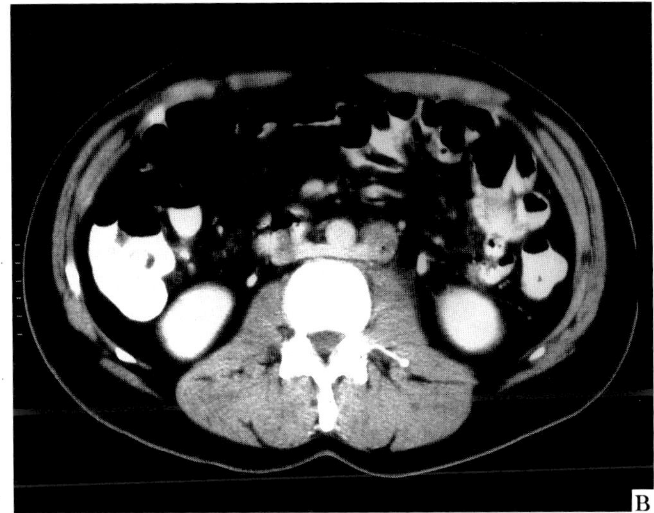

Figure 6.14 A,B Residual left periaortic fibrosis after primary chemotherapy for high-volume retroperitoneal disease. Note retroaortic left renal vein involved with tumor.

References

1. Skakkebaek N. Carcinoma in situ of the testis: frequency and relationship to invasive germ cell tumors in infertile men. *Histopathology*. 1978;2:157.

2. Lange P, Chang W, Fraley E. Fertility issues in the therapy of nonseminomatous testicular tumors. *Urol Clin North Am*. 1988;15:237.

3. Javadpour N, McIntire K, Waldman T, et al. The role of alpha fetoprotein and human chorionic gonadotropin in seminoma. *J Urol*. 1978;120:687.

4. Van der Werf–Messing B. Radiotherapeutic treatment of testicular tumors. *Int J Radiat Oncol Biol Phys*. 1976;1:235.

5. William B, McGowan D. Seminoma of the testis: a 22 year experience with radiation therapy. *Int J Radiat Oncol Biol Phys*. 1985;11:1769.

6. Calman F, Peckham M, Hendry W. The pattern of spread and the treatment of metastases in testicular seminoma. *Br J Urol*. 1979;51:154.

7. Oliver R. Limitations to the use of surveillance as an option in the management of stage I seminoma. *Int J Androl*. 1987;10:263.

8. Gregory C, Peckham M. Results of radiotherapy for stage II testicular seminoma. *Radiother Oncol*. 1986;6:285.

9. Einhorn L, Williams S, Loehrer P, et al. Phase III study of cisplatin dose intensity in advanced germ cell tumors (GCT): a Southeastern and Southwestern Oncology Group Protocol. *Proc Am Soc Clin Oncol*. 1990;9:132.

10. Motzer R, Bosl G, Heelan R, et al. Residual mass: an indication for further therapy in patients with advanced seminoma following systemic chemotherapy. *J Clin Oncol*. 1987;5:1064.

11. Schultz S, Einhorn L, Conces D, et al. Management of post-chemotherapy residual mass in patients with advanced seminoma: Indiana University experience. *J Clin Oncol*. 1989;7:1497.

12. Donohue J. Retroperitoneal lymphadenectomy: the anterior approach including bilateral suprarenal-hilar dissection. *Urol Clin North Am*. 1977;4:509–521.

13. Donohue J, Zachary J, Maynard B. Distribution of nodal metastases in nonseminomatous testis cancer. *J Urol*. 1982;128:315.

14. Pizzocaro G, Salvioni R, Zanoni F. Unilateral lymphadenectomy in intraoperative stage I nonseminomatous germinal testis cancer. *J Urol*. 1990;144:287.

15. Donohue J, Foster R, Rowland R, Bihrle R, Jones J, Geier G. Nerve-sparing retroperitoneal lymphadenectomy with preservation of ejaculation. *J Urol*. 1990;144:287.

16. Freedman L, Parkinson M, Jones W, et al. Histopathology in the prediction of relapse of patients with state I testicular teratoma treated by orchidectomy alone. *Lancet*. 1987;2:294.

17. Donohue J, Thornhill J, Foster R, et al. Primary retroperitoneal lymph node dissection in clinical stage A nonseminomatous germ cell testis cancer: a review of the Indiana University experience (1965–1989). Submitted to *Br J Urol*.

18. Einhorn L, Williams S, Loehrer P, et al. Evaluation of optimal duration of chemotherapy in favorable prognosis disseminated germ cell tumors. *J Clin Oncol*. 1989;7:387.

19. Wahle G, Donohue J, Foster R. Nerve-sparing RPLND after primary chemotherapy for testicular carcinoma. NC Section of AUA, Phoenix AZ, November, 1991.

20. Williams S, Stablein L, Einhorn L, et al. Immediate adjuvant chemotherapy versus observation with treatment at relapse in pathological stage II testicular cancer. *N Engl J Med*. 1987;317:1433.

21. Logothetis C, Swanson D, Dexeus F, et al. Primary chemotherapy for clinical stage II nonseminomatous germ cell tumors of the testis: a followup of fifty patients. *J Clin Oncol*. 1987;5:906.

22. Einhorn L, Donohue J. Cis-diaminedichloroplatinum, vinblastine, and bleomycin combination chemotherapy in disseminated testicular cancer. *Ann Intern Med*. 1977;87:293.

23. Birch R, Williams S, Cone A, et al. Prognostic factors for favorable outcome in dissemiated germ cell tumors. *J Clin Oncol*. 1986;4:400.

24. Ozols R, Diesseroth A, Javadpour N, et al. Treatment of poor prognosis nonseminomatous testicular cancer with a "high dose" platinum combination chemotherapy regimen. *Cancer*. 1983;51:1803.

25. Donohue J, Rowland R, Kopecky K, et al. Correlation of computerized tomographic changes and histologic findings in 80 patients having radical retroperitoneal lymph node dissection after chemotherapy for testis cancer. *J Urol*. 1987;137:1176.

26. Loehrer P, Hvi S, Clark S, et al. Teratoma following cisplatin-based combination chemotherapy for nonseminomatous germ cell tumors: a clinicopathologic correlation. *J Urol*. 1986;135:1183.

27. Nichols C, Gupta S, Loehrer P, et al. Outcome in patients with residual germ cell cancer after post chemotherapy surgery. *Proc Am Soc Oncol*. 1987;6:100.

CHAPTER 7

Carcinoma of the Penis

Hugh A. G. Fisher

Squamous cell carcinoma of the penis accounts for more than 95% of all penile malignancies. It is a relatively rare disease in the United States, accounting for less then 1% of all cancers and cancer deaths in men. The incidence is 0.1 to 0.2 cases per 100,000 males, and the most common age at presentation is during the seventh decade of life. The incidence is higher in uncircumcised and nonwhite populations. The highest global incidence occurs in Central and South American countries. Carcinoma of the penis is almost nonexistent in Jews, who practice early circumcision.

The presence of the foreskin, combined with phimosis and poor hygiene, is the most common predisposing factor for development of penile carcinoma. Whereas men who have been circumcised during infancy rarely develop penile carcinoma, delayed circumcision offers only slight protection against the subsequent development of carcinoma. Phimosis is present in 50% to 75% of patients with penile cancer. The closed space under the foreskin may allow accelerated carcinogenesis associated with chronic balanoposthitis. There is increasing evidence of the relationship of human papilloma virus (HPV) to squamous cell carcinoma of the penis. HPV types 16, 18, and 33 have been implicated.[1]

Clinical Presentation

Penile cancer most often develops on the glans penis or prepuce. The skin of the shaft of the penis is rarely the first site of disease. The tumor begins as a small nodule or nonhealing ulcer (Fig. 7.1). Erythroplasia of Queyrat, described in 1911, represents carcinoma in situ and appears as a red, velvety, well-marginated lesion on the glans or foreskin (Figs. 7.2, 7.3). Verrucous carcinoma (giant tumor of Buschke-Lowenstein) appears papillary and may be a variant of condyloma acuminatum. This lesion can destroy adjacent tissues by direct extension but does not metastasize. Rarely, complete destruction of the penis

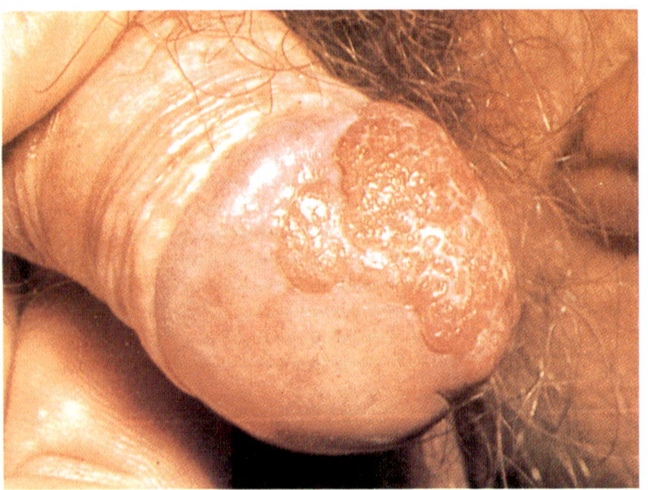

Figure 7.1 Squamous cell carcinoma of the glans penis.

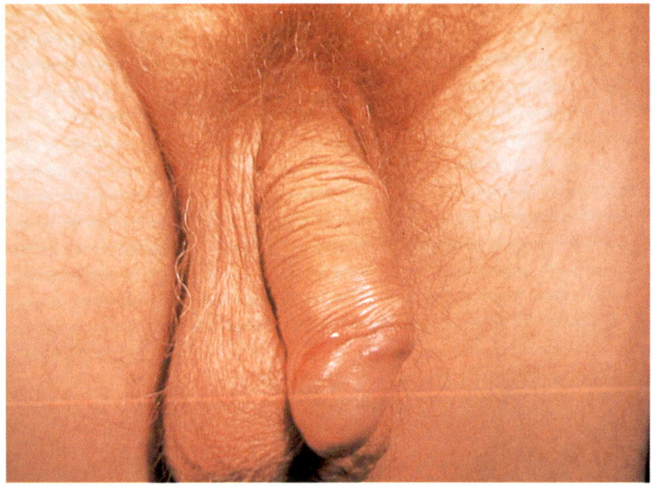

Figure 7.2 Velvety red skin lesion of erythroplasia of Queyrat (carcinoma in situ).

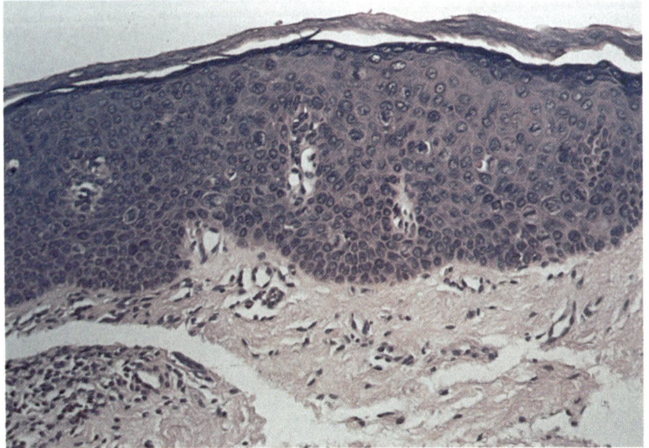

Figure 7.3 Carcinoma in situ, microscopic appearance.

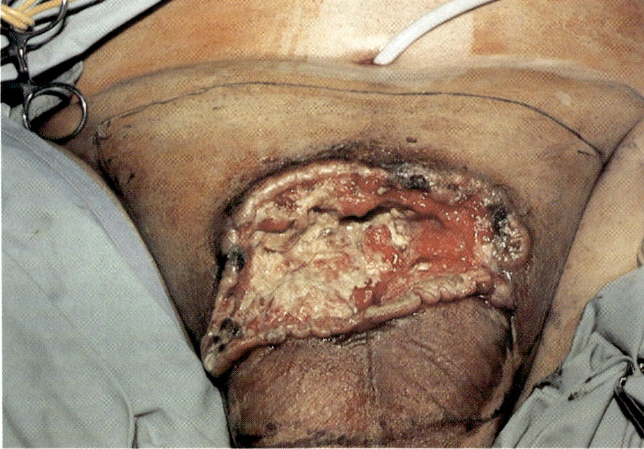

Figure 7.4 Complete destruction of the penis by invasive squamous cell carcinoma.

occurs with invasive squamous cell carcinoma (Fig. 7.4).

Secondary infections are common, resulting in a foul-smelling discharge that typically emanates from beneath the phimotic prepuce (Fig. 7.5). Inguinal adenopathy is palpable in approximately 40% to 60% of patients at presentation. Although these nodes are the first sites of metastatic disease, inflammatory nodal disease is common and only 50% actually contain tumor. Presentation with metastatic disease to distant sites such as lung, bone, and liver is unusual.

Staging

The clinical staging system proposed by Jackson in 1966 has been widely adopted (Fig. 7.6).[2] According to this system lesions on the foreskin and glans penis are grouped in stage I. Tumors involving the shaft or corpora are classified as stage II, and those with proven inguinal nodal metastases are stage III. Stage IV includes inopera-

ble regional nodal disease or distant metastases. Although survival is directly related to the Jackson stage assignment (Fig. 7.7),[3] this classification fails to separate superficial from invasive lesions in stage I, and therefore there are subsets within this patient population that have excellent survival rates and other subsets that have a relatively high incidence of nodal disease. Fifty-eight percent of tumors are pathologically stage I, 13% are stage II, 25% are stage III, and 4% are stage IV at diagnosis.[3]

The TNM system, proposed by the International Union Against Cancer (Fig. 7.8) in 1982 and modified in 1988,[4] is more precise and recognizes depth of invasion as an important prognostic variable regardless of location. Therefore, carcinoma in situ and noninvasive lesions (Tis,TA) are separate classifications, and invasive tumors involving the glans penis are recognized as more ominous lesions (T2). Regional lymph node involvement is subclassified by location, number, and bilaterality. Unfortunately, the majority of publications in the litera-

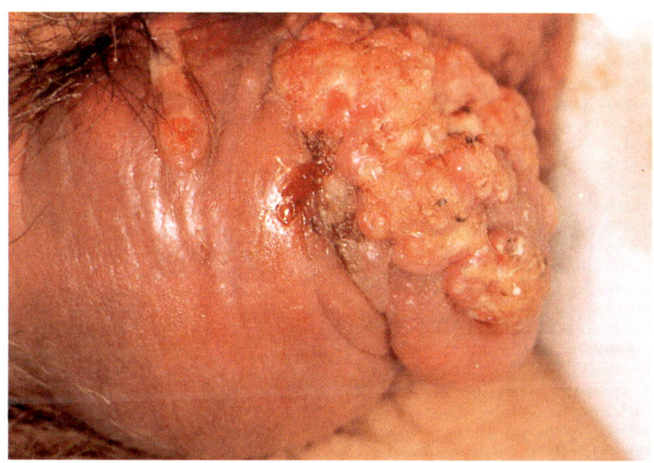

Figure 7.5 Squamous cell carcinoma associated with phimosis and secondary infection.

Stage I	Tumor limited to glans penis and/or prepuce
Stage II	Invasion into shaft or corpora; negative nodes
Stage III	Tumor confined to penis with proven regional nodal disease
Stage IV	Invasion from shaft with inoperable regional nodal disease or distant metastases

STAGE	NO. CASES	SURVIVAL (%)
I	434	65
II	212	42
III	164	27
IV	30	0

ture preceded the TNM system, although current retrospective reviews use it more often. This system has definite advantages over the Jackson staging system and should be applied by all physicians treating penile cancer. It is imperative for the pathologist who examines the primary specimen to measure the depth of invasion into underlying subepithelial tissue or corpora, to facilitate accurate staging and to guide treatment.

Management of the Primary Lesion

Lesions involving the prepuce that are noninvasive and not located near the coronal sulcus can be adequately treated by circumcision. Lesions near the coronal sulcus and those that involve the glans penis and distal shaft usually require partial penectomy with a 2-cm margin proximal to the tumor (Fig. 7.9). The technique of partial penectomy is shown in Figures 7.10 to 7.14. After application of a tourniquet to the base of the penis, a circumferential incision is made 2 cm proximal to the lesion (Fig. 7.10). Buck's fascia is incised and the superficial dorsal vein is ligated and divided. The corpora cavernosa are transected vertically with a scalpel (Fig. 7.11). The corpus spongiosum and urethra are divided 1 cm distal to the corpora cavernosa and spatulated dorsally (Fig. 7.12). The cut edges of the corpora cavernosa are approximated with horizontal absorbable mattress sutures (Fig. 7.13). The spatulated urethra is sutured to the skin to form a wide-caliber neomeatus. A catheter is left indwelling (Fig. 7.14).

The rate of recurrence after partial penectomy with negative margins is less than 10%. In most cases upright urination is possible, and sexual function may be preserved. Extension of tumor onto the proximal penile shaft may require total penectomy to obtain adequate margins.

FIGURE 7.8 *TNM Classification of Penile Carcinoma*

PRIMARY TUMOR (T)

TX	Primary tumor cannot be assessed
T0	No evidence of primary tumor
Tis	Carcinoma in situ
TA	Noninvasive verrucous carcinoma
T1	Tumor invades subepithelial connective tissue
T2	Tumor invades corpus spongiosum or cavernosum
T3	Tumor invades urethra or prostate
T4	Tumor invades other adjacent structures

REGIONAL LYMPH NODES (N)

NX	Regional lymph nodes cannot be assessed
N0	No regional lymph node metastasis
N1	Metastasis in a single, superficial, inguinal lymph node
N2	Metastasis in multiple or bilateral, superficial, inguinal lymph nodes
N3	Metastasis in deep inguinal or pelvic lymph node(s), unilateral or bilateral

DISTANT METASTASES (M)

MX	Presence of distant metastasis cannot be assessed
M0	No distant metastases
M1	Distant metastases

FIGURE 7.9 *Management of the Primary Lesion of Penile Carcinoma: Treatment Options*

SURGERY
Circumcision
Excision
Mohs micrographic surgery
Partial penectomy
Total penectomy

RADIATION THERAPY
External beam
Brachytherapy–interstitial iridium

LASER
Carbon dioxide
Neodymium:YAG

CHEMOTHERAPY
Topical
Systemic

CRYOSURGERY

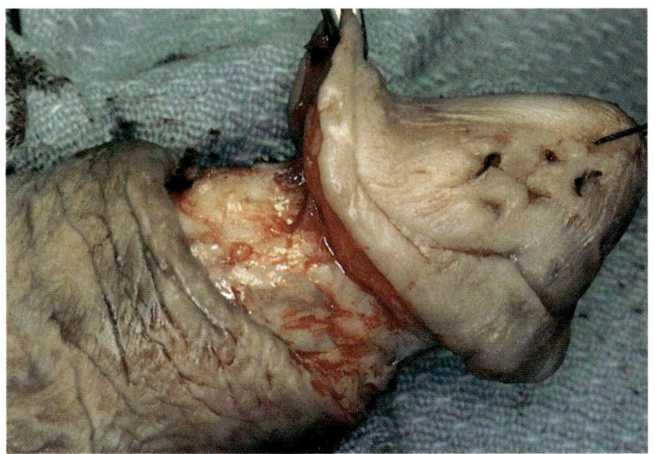

Figure 7.10 Partial penectomy. A circumferential skin incision is made proximal to the glans penis.

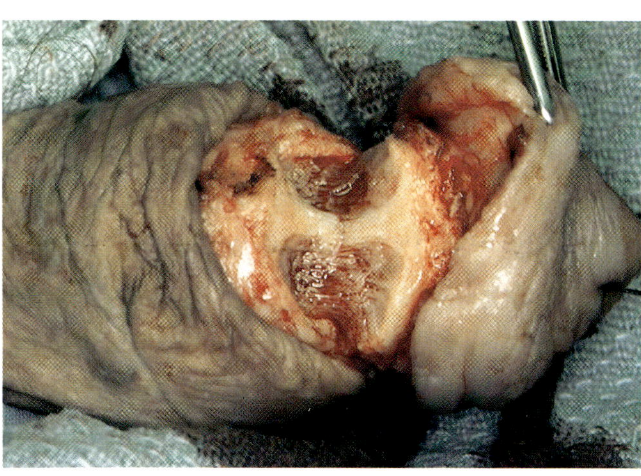

Figure 7.11 Partial penectomy. The corpora cavernosa are transected vertically.

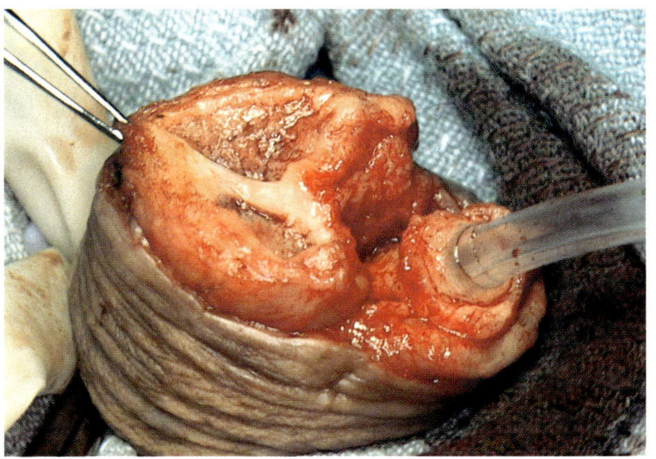

Figure 7.12 Partial penectomy. The corpus spongiosum and urethra are divided 1 cm distal to the corpora cavernosa and spatulated dorsally.

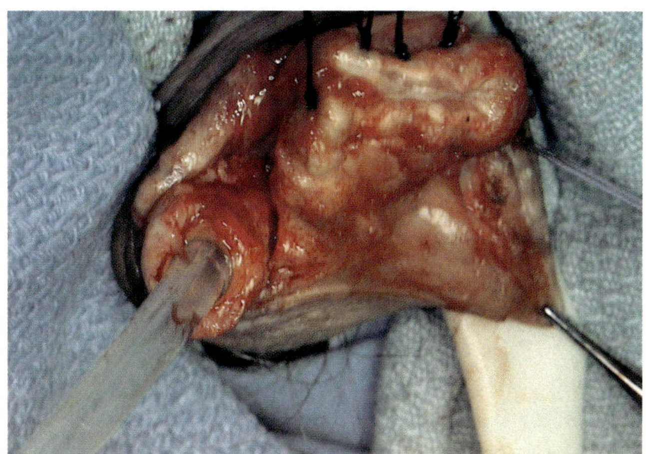

Figure 7.13 Partial penectomy. Corpora cavernosa are closed with absorbable horizontal mattress sutures.

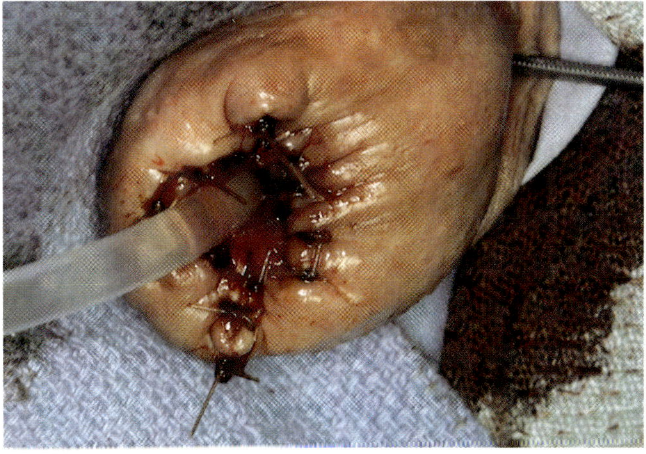

Figure 7.14 Partial penectomy. Spatulated urethra is sutured to skin edges to form wide-caliber neomeatus.

In this situation, a perineal urethrostomy is created from the proximal urethra. The scrotum and its contents are usually preserved.

The use of alternatives to partial or total penectomy to achieve total tumor ablation with an improved cosmetic result is possible in select cases. Mohs micrographic surgery removes the primary tumor in thin layers, with careful mapping of the tissue and frozen section guidance.[4] This technique may produce cancer-free margins with a superior cosmetic result. It is best applied to lesions less than 1 cm in diameter. However, considerable scarring and deformity of the glans penis may occur, and secondary plastic reconstruction of the distal penis may be necessary.

Both CO_2 and Nd:YAG lasers have been successfully employed for control of stage Tis and T1 tumors. Small, superficial or minimally invasive lesions are ideal for these techniques, but it is important to perform deep biopsies for accurate staging. For more extensive T1 or T2 lesions, the local recurrence rate is 10% to 15% with the CO_2 laser, inferior to treatment with partial penectomy.[6] Using the Nd:YAG laser in T1, T2, and some T3 lesions, Kriegmair et al. reported recurrence in only 2 of 28 patients who were followed for 5 years. Careful case selection is mandatory to achieve optimal results with penis-sparing laser surgery.

Radiation therapy administered by external beam or brachytherapy has been successfully used to control small penile lesions and may allow cosmetic and functional preservation of the penis. However, the failure rate is approximately 5% to 62%, depending on the size and depth of invasion of the lesion. Complications from the radiation, including urethral stricture disease, occur in up to 30% of patients, and evaluation of the irradiated site for recurrence may be difficult.[8] With the use of lasers and Mohs micrographic surgery, radiation would seem to be a less attractive treatment option.

Management of Regional Nodes

Penile cancer spreads in a predictable pattern, with inguinal nodes as the primary landing site for metastases. Detailed anatomic studies have demonstrated that: 1) primary drainage from the foreskin involves the superficial inguinal nodes; 2) the glans penis and the urethra drain mainly into the superficial system but occasionally directly into the deep inguinal lymph nodes and rarely directly into the iliac nodes; and 3) the corpora cavernosa also drain primarily into the superficial and deep inguinal nodes.[9] The lymphatic channels of the penis anastomose freely along the penile shaft so that bilateral involvement and crossover metastasis are not uncommon. Rouviere and associates[9] divided the superficial inguinal nodes into zones related to the saphenofemoral junction and venous branches (Fig. 7.15). Zones 2, 3, and 5 contain nodes that most frequently drain penile structures.[10]

Proper evaluation and management of the regional lymph nodes are keys to successful treatment of penile cancer. Forty percent to 60% of patients have palpable inguinal adenopathy at presentation before treatment of the primary lesion. However, only 50% of palpable nodes harbor tumor. The remainder are inflammatory, secondary to infection of the penile primary lesion. Conversely, 20% of patients with nonpalpable nodes at presentation with Jackson clinical stage I or II have positive lymph nodes when prophylactic lymph node dissection is performed. There is no doubt that lymph nodes which remain palpable 4 to 6 weeks after treatment of the primary lesion despite antibiotic therapy require definitive evaluation. Controversy exists concerning the methods of lymph node evaluation and the extent of lymph node dissection that is necessary to achieve optimal diagnostic and therapeutic efficacy. Controversy also exists concerning the need for prophylactic lymph node dissection versus close observation when lymph nodes are not palpable.

Survival is directly related to the presence or absence of lymph node metastases. In the absence of such metastases, two thirds of patients will survive for 5 years, in contrast to only 27% after lymph node metastasis occurs. However, complete excision of involved lymph nodes by superficial and deep inguinal lymphadenectomy may be curative in 20% to 80% of patients and is dependent on the number of lymph nodes involved and the presence of bilateral disease.[11] Involvement of more than two nodes by tumor has an adverse effect on survival.[12]

deKernion[13] reported that nodes were involved in 17 of 25 (68%) patients with invasive primary tumors (clinical stage II). McDougal et al.[14] noted that six of nine patients with clinical stage II disease had clinically undetectable nodal metastases at the time of immediate adjunctive inguinal lymph node dissection and that five of the six patients (83%) survived for 5 years. These results are superior to those achieved in patients with clinically and pathologically positive nodes who undergo immediate or delayed therapeutic lymph node dissections (Fig. 7.16).[12,15–17] The above data suggest that early lymph node dissection for high-risk patients may produce a survival advantage. In a patient population that is notoriously unreliable regarding follow-up visits, the opportunity for cure may be lost in the 20% of patients who have occult inguinal metastases at presentation.

Attempts have been made to identify patients at high risk for lymph node involvement who might benefit from early lymph node dissection. Pathologic features of the primary tumor specimen that correlate with higher incidence of lymph node involvement are depth of invasion below the epithelial surface, tumor grade, and presence of vascular invasion. Pettaway et al.[18] noted that 94% of patients with positive nodes had depth of invasion greater than 0.5 cm in the primary specimen, but that none of patients with well-differentiated lesions and mini-

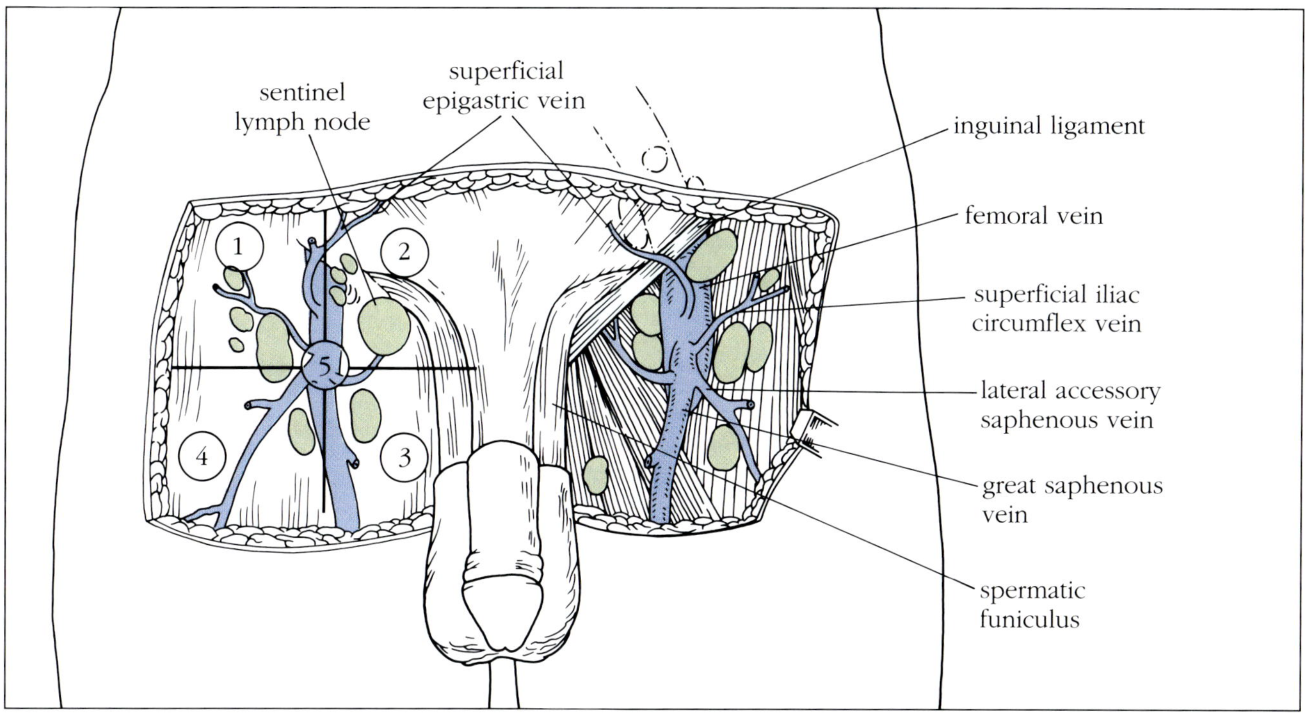

FIGURE 7.15B *Zonal Classification of Superficial Lymph Nodes, Right Groin*

Zone 1 Nodes located around the superficial circumflex iliac vein
Zone 2 Nodes located in the superomedial area around the superficial epigastric
and superficial external pudendal vein
Zone 3 Nodes located inferomedially around the greater saphenous vein
Zone 4 Nodes inferolateral around the lateral accessory saphenous vein
Zone 5 Saphenofemoral junction

Zones 2, 3 and 5 drain penile structures most frequently

Figure 7.15 **A** Inguinal anatomy and location of sentinel node. **B** Zonal classification of superficial lymph nodes, right groin.

FIGURE 7.16 *Five-Year Survival of Patients Undergoing Immediate or Delayed Therapeutic Lymphadenectomy With Palpable Nodes*

		SURVIVAL (%)	
AUTHOR	**YEAR**	**Immediate**	**Delayed**
Ekstrom and Edsmyr	1958	32	50
Baker et al.	1976	59	61
Johnson and Lo	1984	57	13
Fraley et al.	1989	66	8

mally invasive disease had lymph node metastases. Fraley et al.[17] reported that one of 19 patients with well-differentiated tumor, 15 of 19 patients with moderately differentiated tumor, and all of 16 patients with poorly differentiated tumor developed nodal metastases. The analysis of DNA ploidy by flow cytometry has not proven to be a superior predictor of lymph node metastases when compared with conventional pathologic features.[18]

The principal drawback to the application of complete superficial and deep inguinal node dissection for all patients with penile cancer has been the attendant morbidity of the procedure. Historically, the rate of wound infection, sloughing of skin flaps, phlebitis, pulmonary embolism, and chronic scrotal and lower extremity edema has been prohibitively high, with one or more events occurring in more than 50% of patients.[19] However, improvements in perioperative care and modifications of the procedure have reduced the morbidity significantly with negligible mortality (see below).[20] CT scanning of the abdomen, pelvis, and groin will help to rule out iliac or paraaortic lymph node involvement and should be used, along with palpation, to detect enlarged inguinal nodes. Alternate methods of groin node evaluation include fine needle aspiration and sentinel lymph node biopsy. Aspiration cytology requires a palpable lymph node or one visualized on imaging studies. Scappini et al.[21] noted excellent correlation between aspiration cytology after penile or pedal lymphangiography and lymphadenectomy specimens. This technique is useful in determining the need for iliac lymph node dissection before inguinal node dissection when inguinal lymph nodes are palpable, but it lacks the accuracy to detect microscopic involvement reliably in clinically normal nodes.

In 1977, Cabanas[22] introduced the concept of sentinel node biopsy. After detailed studies of the lymphatic drainage of the penis, he concluded that the primary landing site for carcinoma was in the lymph nodes located superiorly and medially to the saphenous bulb within 1 cm of the superficial epigastric vein (see Fig. 7.16). This lymph node can be sampled with minimal morbidity through a small incision parallel to the inguinal ligament. In 15 patients with a positive sentinel node and in whom a deep inguinal lymph node dissection was performed, 12 had no other lymph node involvement. In addition, in patients with a negative sentinel node biopsy, deeper nodes were uniformly negative. Ninety percent of patients with negative lymph nodes lived for 5 years. Ten percent of patients were lost to follow-up and were therefore considered failures for statistical purposes. In contrast to these favorable results, other investigators have reported later development of deep inguinal or iliac metastases in patients with negative sentinel node biopsies.[23,24] These reports have dampened the enthusiasm for the sentinel node biopsy technique.

Therefore, all patients with palpable lymph nodes should undergo thorough lymph node assessment by modified superficial and deep inguinal dissection, accompanied by iliac dissection when inguinal nodes are involved. In the case of impalpable nodes, modified lymphadenectomy should be performed in patients with invasive disease (stages T1–T3) and should be considered in patients with poorly differentiated primary tumors or those who exhibit vascular invasion.

Technique of Ilioinguinal Lymphadenectomy

Patients undergoing ilioinguinal lymphadenectomy are placed on a liquid diet and are given enemas the evening before surgery. Prophylactic antibiotics are infused before the procedure. Pneumatic compression stockings are used intraoperatively and for several days postoperatively until the patient is ambulatory. Low-dose subcutaneous heparin can be used but must be weighed against the possibility that it might promote lymphocele formation.

A variety of incisions have been used for ilioinguinal lymphadenectomy (Fig. 7.17). In cases of palpable aspiration-positive lymph nodes, or when CT scan is suspicious for iliac node involvement, the iliac dissection precedes the inguinal dissection. Although the prognosis is usually poor with iliac node involvement, the extent of nodal involvement has been poorly documented and survival with minimal pelvic disease has been reported in a small number of patients.[22] The iliac nodes are readily accessible through a midline extraperitoneal incision. Alternatively, laparoscopic techniques can be employed. A modified lymph node dissection is advisable, with preservation of lymphatics surrounding and lateral to the external iliac artery to reduce lower extremity edema. The other boundaries of the dissection are the hypogastric artery superiorly, the obturator nerve and vessels posteriorly, and the femoral canal, which lies medial to the femoral vein and posterior to the inguinal ligament, inferiorly. The inferior boundary of the iliac dissection will join with the deep inguinal dissection. When inguinal node metastases are documented at the time of presentation of the primary tumor, a bilateral iliac dissection should be performed. Suction drains are placed in the node dissection areas.

The incision for inguinal node dissection can be made above or below the groin crease, which lies several centimeters below the inguinal ligament. The advantage to a supragroin crease incision is that the subcutaneous tissue is thicker, which allows improved vascularity of the superior and inferior tissue flaps. Satisfactory exposure to the limits of dissection is possible through this incision, and access to the iliac nodes is possible if a separate midline incision is not used.

Figures 7.18 through 7.23 demonstrate the technique of complete superficial and deep inguinal node dissection through a supragroin crease incision in a patient with palpable aspiration-positive inguinal nodes. The incision, 8

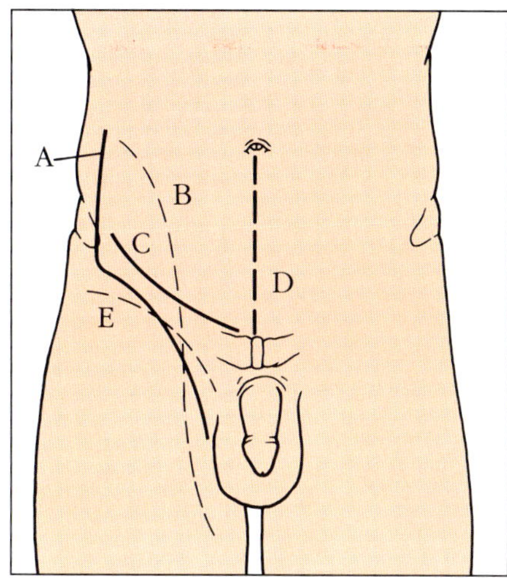

Figure 7.17 Possible incisions for ilio-inguinal lymphadenectomy.

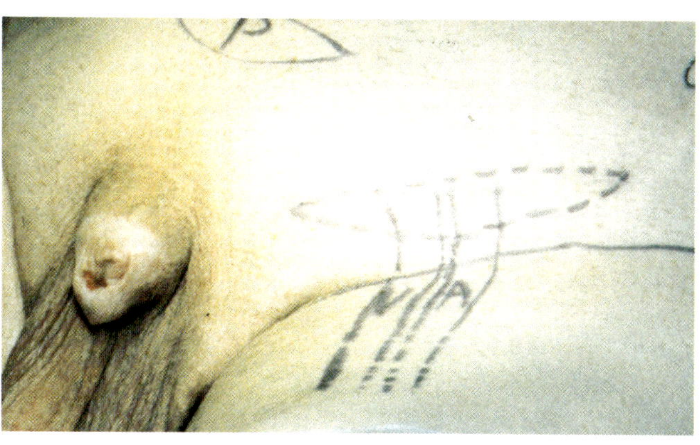

Figure 7.18 Technique of inguinal lymphadenectomy for a node-positive patient.

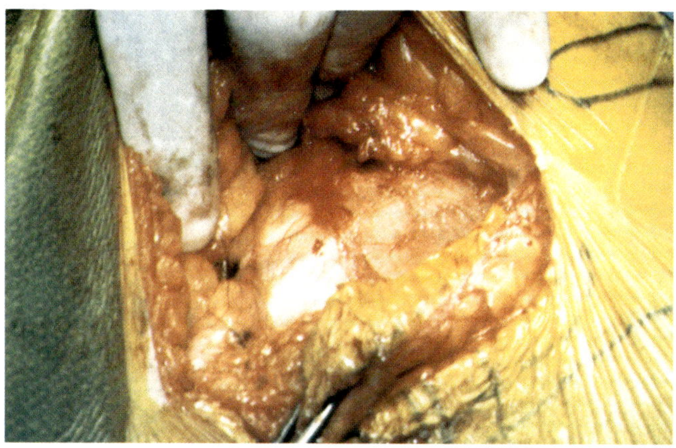

Figure 7.19 Inguinal lymphadenectomy. The upper flap is developed to the external oblique aponeurosis starting just beneath Scarpa's fascia.

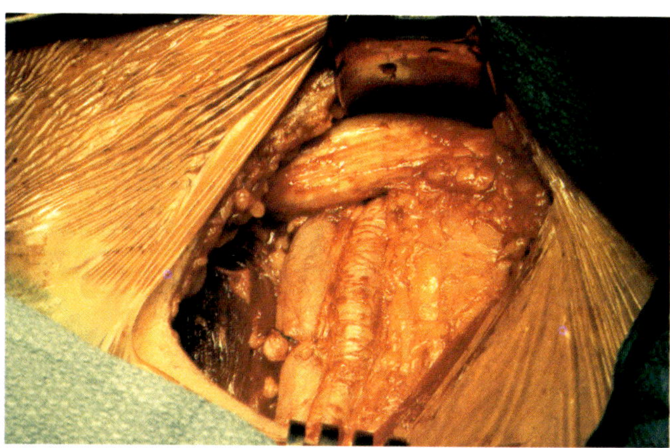

Figure 7.20 Inguinal lymphadenectomy boundaries of dissection. Superior: external oblique aponeurosis. Lateral: sartorius muscle. Medial: adductor muscle of thigh. Inferior: apex of femoral triangle.

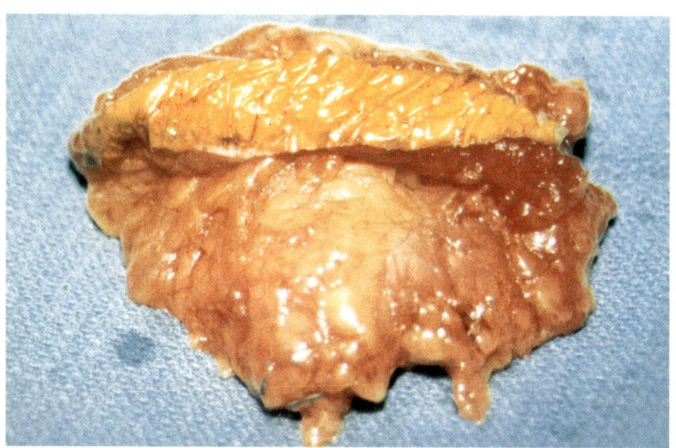

Figure 7.21 Inguinal lymphadenectomy specimen including superficial and deep nodes.

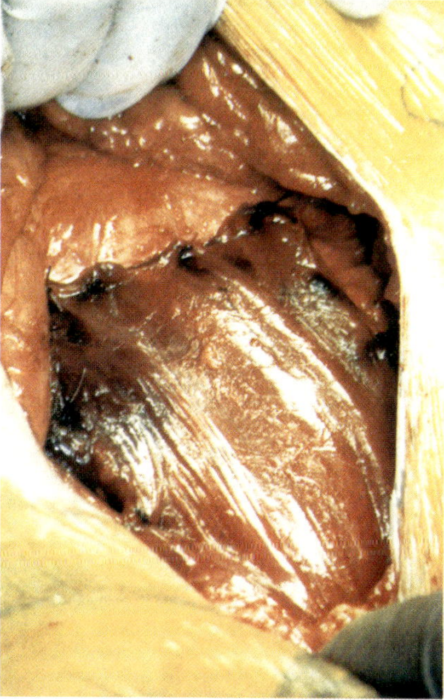

Figure 7.22 Inguinal lymphadenectomy. The sartorius muscle is transposed over the femoral artery and vein.

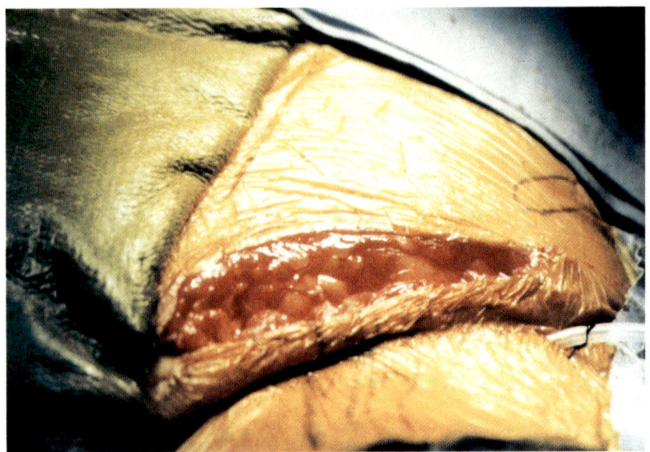

Figure 7.23 Inguinal lymphadenectomy. The tension on the skin edges is relieved by advancing and suturing flaps to underlying muscle with chromic sutures.

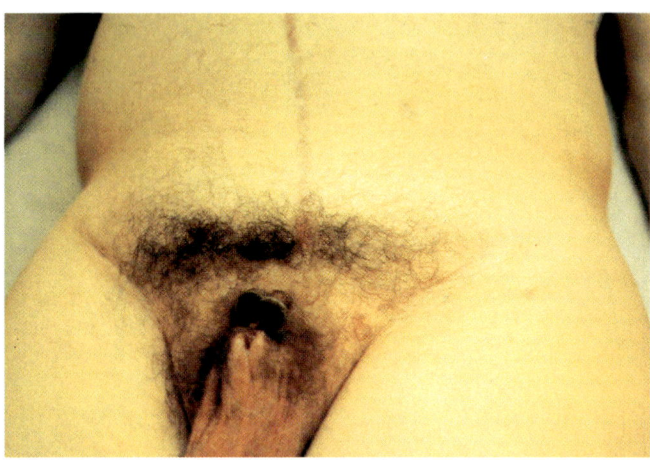

Figure 7.24 Wound appearance 2 months after lymphadenectomy.

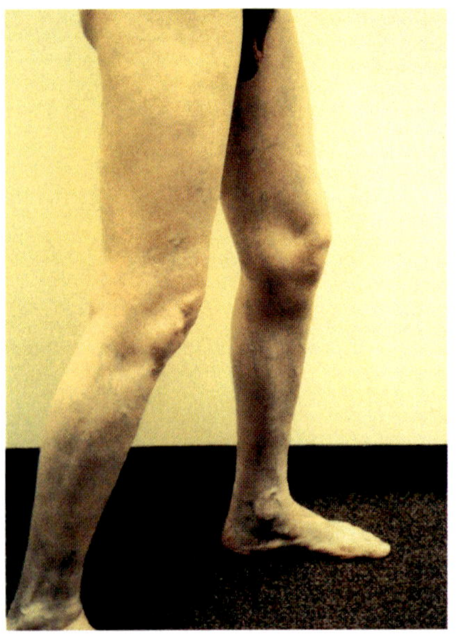

Figure 7.25 Absence of peripheral or scrotal edema.

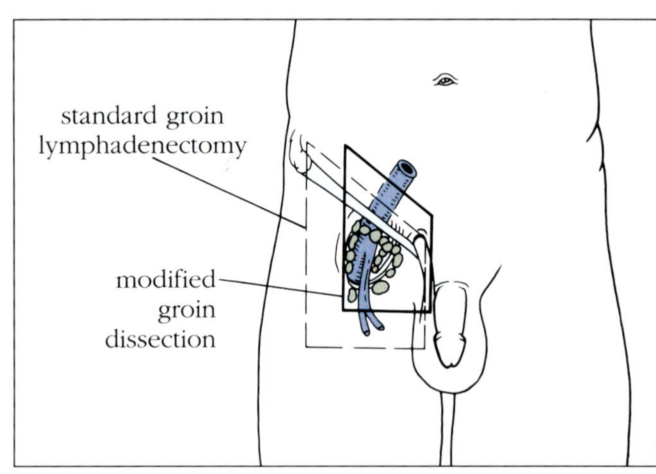

Figure 7.26 Comparison of the boundaries of standard groin lymphadenectomy with modified groin dissection.

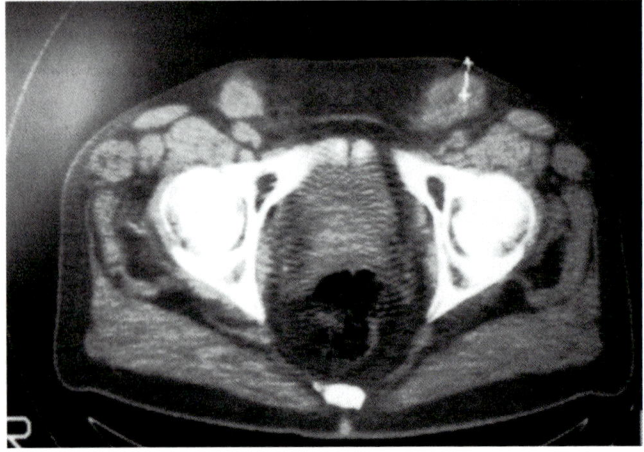

Figure 7.27 CT scan of bulky inguinal adenopathy prior to two cycles of neoadjuvant chemotherapy using cisplatin and 5-fluorouracil.

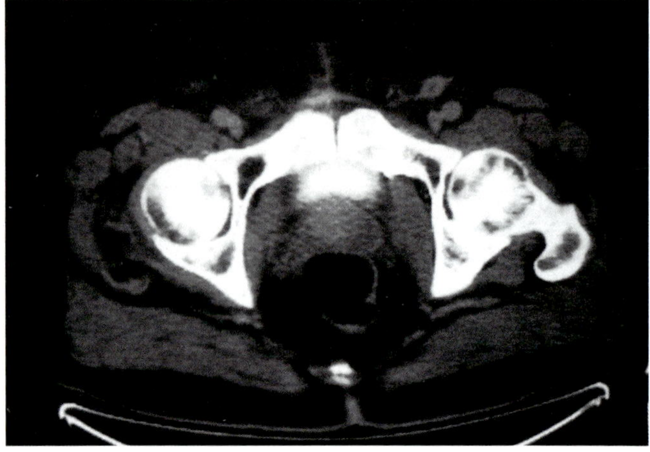

Figure 7.28 CT scan of inguinal nodes after neoadjuvant chemotherapy (same patient as Figure 7.27) indicates significant reduction in node size.

to 10 cm in length, is made 2 cm above the groin crease and parallel to the inguinal ligament. An ellipse of skin at highest risk for slough is removed from directly over the involved nodes (see Fig. 7.19). The incision is deepened to expose Scarpa's fascia. An upper flap is developed obliquely just below Scarpa's fascia to expose the external oblique aponeurosis for a distance of 5 cm. This results in a well-vascularized thick upper flap. Venous tributaries are ligated with fine silk sutures and the tissue beneath Scarpa's fascia is meticulously ligated with 3-0 plain or 4-0 chromic ties. The spermatic cord is identified at the external inguinal ring and all tissue overlying the cord at the base of the penis is ligated with absorbable sutures and divided (see Fig. 7.19)

A thick lower flap is developed in similar fashion, beginning just beneath Scarpa's fascia and above the major lymphatic channels from the lower extremity. The inferior boundary of the dissection is the apex of the femoral triangle formed by the sartorius and adductor muscles. Lymphostasis is obtained with absorbable ligatures. Cautery is used sparingly. The superficial fascia of the thigh is exposed, directly beneath which lies the saphenous vein medially. The fascia lata overlying the adductor muscle and the sartorius muscle are divided to expose the surface of the muscles. The femoral vessels are identified at the inferior margin of the fossa ovalis. The femoral sheath overlying the vessels is incised and the anterior surface of the vessels is exposed. The lymph node package is then tractioned upwards and dissection proceeds superiorly, sweeping all lymphatic tissue off the vessels to the inguinal ligament. With bulky positive nodes, the saphenous vein must be excised and ligated or oversewn at the saphenous bulb. Dissection then proceeds from lateral to medial, ending medially to the femoral vein in the femoral canal where the dissection meets the corresponding iliac dissection from above. Figure 7.20 shows the completed standard dissection. Note that the exposure is excellent, even with a supragroin crease incision. Figure 7.21 shows the excised lymph node specimen.

The sartorius muscle is dissected bluntly from its enveloping fascia and transected at its origin from the anterior superior iliac spine. A suture is placed at the point of transection. Care must be taken to preserve the blood supply to the sartorius, which enters posteriorly. The sartorius muscle is then transposed over the femoral vessels and attached to the inguinal ligament with 2-0 chromic sutures (see Fig. 7.22).

A Jackson-Pratt suction drain is placed above the sartorius muscle and beneath the skin flaps. Tension on the skin edges is relieved by advancing and suturing the skin flaps to the underlying muscles with chromic sutures (see Fig. 7.23).

The patient remains at bedrest with legs elevated for 2 to 3 days postoperatively. Figures 7.24 and 7.25 demonstrate excellent wound healing and absence of scrotal or lower extremity edema 3 months postoperatively. I have used this technique successfully in 12 patients with minimal morbidity, no mortality, and local recurrence in only one patient. Alternatively, complete superficial and deep inguinal node dissection can be performed through an incision beneath the groin crease. Comparable results may be achievable with a thick flap technique.

Catalona[20] modified the boundaries of the standard dissection for patients with nonpalpable nodes or minimal nodal involvement. The lateral border of the dissection is the lateral border of the femoral artery (Fig. 7.26). The saphenous vein is preserved and the sartorius muscle is not transposed to cover the femoral vessels. Wound complications and lower extremity edema were minimized. Based on the likelihood of sampling the nodes most frequently involved by penile cancer, this dissection appears to be a satisfactory compromise between the sentinel lymph node biopsy and the standard inguinal dissection for diagnosis and treatment of minimal nodal disease.

Neoadjuvant Chemotherapy

Ilioinguinal lymphadenectomy to remove bulky nodes has been associated with increased morbidity and a poor survival rate. Neoadjuvant chemotherapy has been employed in the hope of improving margins of dissection and of reduction of the morbidity of the procedure.[25] Figures 7.27 and 7.28 demonstrate response in a patient with bulky lymphadenopathy who was treated with two cycles of cisplatin (100 mg/m^2) and continuous infusion of 5-fluorouracil (1000 mg daily $\times$ 5 days), with marked reduction in size of nodes. In four patients thus treated, two had no tumor in the lymphadenectomy specimen and the patients are alive without recurrence up to 5 years postoperatively. Pizzocaro[26] also achieved partial responses in three of five patients treated with 12 weekly courses of vincristine, bleomycin, and methotrexate, who were without disease at 20 to 72 months after lymphadenectomy.[26]

Bulky inguinal lymphadenopathy may require wide excision with coverage by use of a myocutaneous flap. Figures 7.29 through 7.32 show a patient with bulky adenopathy who did not respond to neoadjuvant chemotherapy and who underwent wide excision with a rectus abdominis myocutaneous flap for coverage. He experienced minimal lower extremity edema, possibly because of enhanced lymph drainage through the flap itself. Iliac nodes were not involved by tumor.

Treatment of Locally Advanced and Metastatic Penile Cancer

Metastatic penile cancer is almost universally fatal. However, several chemotherapeutic agents, alone or in combination, have produced objective responses with prolongation of survival. The best-studied agents are cisplatin, bleomycin, and methotrexate. Cisplatin as a single agent produced objective responses in 15% to 23% of treated patients. Bleomycin as a single agent showed activity in approximately 45% of patients; partial responses were noted in 8 of 13 patients (61%) treated with methotrexate.[27] Using the combination of these three agents, Dexeus et al.[28] reported a 72% response rate in 14 patients with inoperable or metastatic squamous cell carcinoma of the male genital tract. These results are superior to single-agent chemotherapy. Larger experiences comparing drug regimens are necessary.

Conclusion

Penile cancer is a rare but potentially fatal disease. Proper management depends on the location and stage of the primary lesion. Conservative measures for treatment of the primary lesion are indicated when the lesion is small or superficial, or is located on the prepuce. The local recurrence rate after conservative treatment with simple excision, Mohs micrographic surgery, or laser therapy is higher for invasive lesions, and partial penectomy must be strongly considered.

Noninvasive lesions (stages Tis, TA) metastasize to inguinal nodes rarely, regardless of size. Patients with noninvasive tumors or those with minimally invasive (stage T1), low-grade lesions can be safely followed after treatment of the primary lesion with palpation of the inguinal nodes at 2- to 3-month intervals for 3 years, then every 3 to 4 months in years 4 and 5. CT scans at 6-month intervals may help to detect change in small nodes. If inguinal metastases occur, complete ilioinguinal lymphadenectomy is indicated.

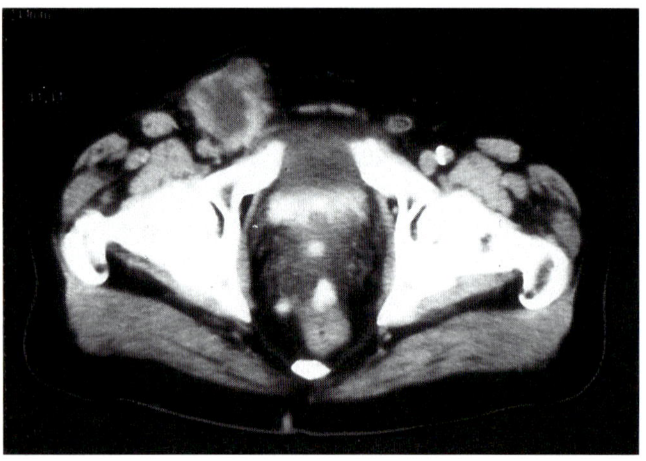

Figure 7.29 CT scan of bulky inguinal adenopathy not responsive to neoadjuvant chemotherapy.

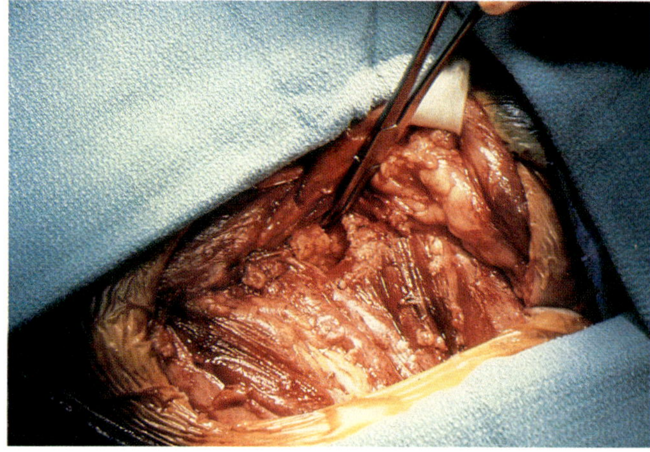

Figure 7.30 Wide excision of inguinal nodes with resection of inguinal ligament.

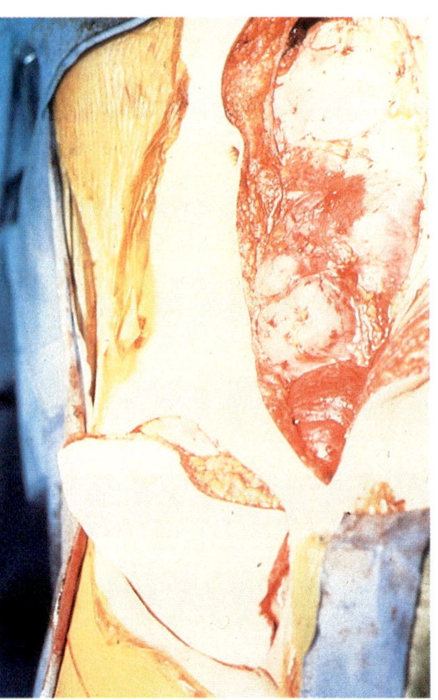

Figure 7.31 Left rectus abdominis myocutaneous flap is rotated and fashioned to cover large defect.

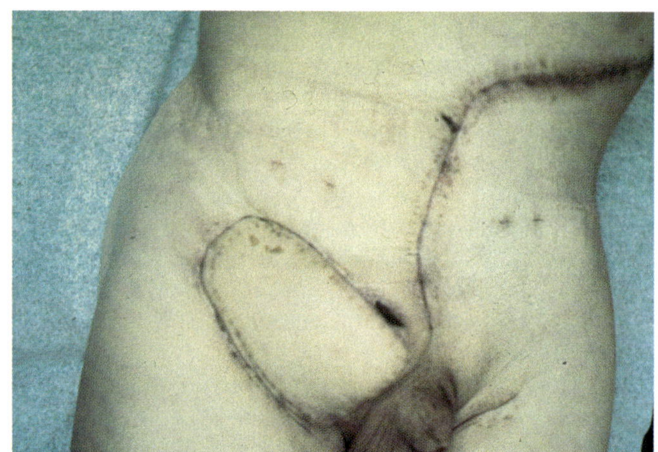

Figure 7.32 Wound appearance 6 weeks postoperatively.

Patients with moderately or poorly differentiated tumors that invade the subepithelial tissue (stage T1), or those with lesions that invade the glans, corpora cavernosa, or urethra (T2, T3), regardless of grade, should undergo modified inguinal lymphadenectomy to rule out occult metastatic disease when inguinal nodes are clinically negative. Delayed therapeutic lymphadenectomy may be curative, but only in cases of minimal disease. All patients with palpable inguinal nodes that persist after treatment of the primary lesion and 4 weeks of antibiotic therapy (potential stage III, any N+) must undergo definitive evaluation. Modified lymphadenectomy allows excision of the superficial and deep inguinal nodes at highest risk for metastatic involvement, without significant morbidity. If inguinal nodes are positive, a complete dissection, including iliac lymphadenectomy, is recommended.

References

1. Barrasso R, Brux J, Croissant O, Orth G. High prevalence of papillomavirus-associated penile intraepithelial neoplasia in sexual partners of women with cervical intraepithelial neoplasia. *N Engl J Med.* 1987;317:916–923.

2. Jackson SM. The treatment of carcinoma of the penis. *Br J Surg.* 1966;53:33–35.

3. Sufrin G, Huben R. Benign and malignant tumors of the penis. In: Gillenwater JY, Grayhack JT, Howards SS, Duckett SW, eds. *Adult and Pediatric Urology.* 2nd ed. St. Louis, Mo: CV Mosby; 1991:1648–1681.

4. Union International Contre le Cancer (UICC): *TNM Atlas: Illustrated Guide to the TNM/pTNM Classification of Malignant Tumors.* 3rd ed. New York, NY: Springer-Verlag: 1989:232–244.

5. Mohs FE, Snow SN, Messing EM, et al. Microscopically controlled surgery in the treatment of carcinoma of the penis. *J Urol.* 1985;133:961–966.

6. Bandieramonte G, Santoro O, Boracchi P, et al. Total resection of glans penis surface by CO_2 laser microsurgery. *Acta Oncol.* 1988;27:575–578.

7. Kriegmair M, Rothenberger KH, Spitzenpfeil R, et al. Neodymium-YAG laser treatment for carcinoma of the penis. *J Urol.* 1990;143:351A. Abstract 650.

8. Schellhammer P, Jordan CH, Schlossberg SM. Tumors of the penis. In: Walsh P, Stamey T, eds. *Campbell's Urology.* 6th ed. Philadelphia, Pa: WB Saunders Co; 1992:1264–1298.

9. Rouviere H; Tobin MT, trans. *Anatomy of the Human Lymphatic System.* Ann Arbor, Mich: Edward Brothers; 1938.

10. Daesler EH, Anson BJ, Reimann AF. Radical excision of the inguinal and iliac lymph glands: a study based upon 450 anatomical dissections and upon supportive clinical observations. *Surg Gynecol Obstet.* 1948;87:679.

11. Srinivas V, Morse MJ, Herr HW, et al. Penile cancer: relation of extent of nodal metastasis to survival. *J Urol.* 1987;137:880–882.

12. Johnson DE, Lo RK. Management of regional lymph nodes in penile carcinoma. *Urology.* 1984;24:308–311.

13. deKernion JB, Tynberg P, Persky L, et al. Carcinoma of the penis. *Cancer.* 1973;32:1256–1262.

14. McDougal WS, Kirchner FK, Edwards RH, et al. Treatment of carcinoma of the penis: the case for primary lymphadenectomy. *J Urol.* 1986;136:38–41.

15. Ekstrom T, Edsmyr F. Cancer of the penis: a clinical study of 229 cases. *Acta Chir Scand.* 1958;115:25–45.

16. Baker BH, Spratt JS, Perez-Mesa C, et al. Carcinoma of the penis. *J Urol.* 1976;116:458–461.

17. Fraley EE, Zhang G, Manivel C, Nichans GA. The role of ilioinguinal lymphadenectomy and significance of histological differentiation in treatment of carcinoma of the penis. *J Urol.* 1989;142:1478–1482.

18. Pettaway CA, Stewart D, Vuitch F. Penile squamous carcinoma: DNA flow cystometry versus histopathology for prognosis. *J Urol.* 1991;145(suppl):367A. Abstract 618.

19. Johnson DE, Lo RK. Complications of groin dissection in penile cancer. *Urology.* 1984;24:312–314.

20. Catalona WJ. Modified inguinal lymphadenectomy for carcinoma of the penis with preservation of saphenous veins: technique and preliminary results. *J Urol.* 1988;140:306–310.

21. Scappini P, Piscioli F, Pusiol T, Hofstetter A, Rothenberger K, Luciani L. Penile cancer: aspiration biopsy cystology for staging. *Cancer.* 1986;58:1526–1533.

22. Cabanas RM. An approach for the treatment of penile carcinoma. *Cancer.* 1977;39:456–466.

23. Wespes E, Simon J, Schulman CC. Cabanas' approach: is sentinel node biopsy reliable for staging of penile carcinoma? *Urology.* 1986;28:278–279.

24. Perinetti EP, Crane DC, Catalona WJ. Unreliability of sentinel lymph node biopsy for staging penile carcinoma. *J Urol.* 1980;124:734–735.

25. Fisher HAG, Barada J, Horton J, Von Roemeling R. Neoadjuvant therapy with cisplatin and 5-fluorouracil for stage III squamous cell carcinoma of the penis. *J Urol.* 1990;143:352A. Abstract 653.

26. Pizzocaro G, Piva L. Adjuvant and neoadjuvant vincristine, bleomycin and methotrexate for inguinal metastases from squamous cell carcinoma of the penis. *Acta Oncol.* 1988;27:823–824.

27. Eisenberger M. Chemotherapy for carcinoma of the penis and urethra. *Urol Clin North Am.* 1992;19:333–338.

28. Dexeus FH, Logothetis CJ, Sella A, et al. Combination chemotherapy with methotrexate, bleomycin, and cisplatin for advanced squamous cell carcinoma of the male genital tract. *J Urol.* 1991;146:1284–1287.

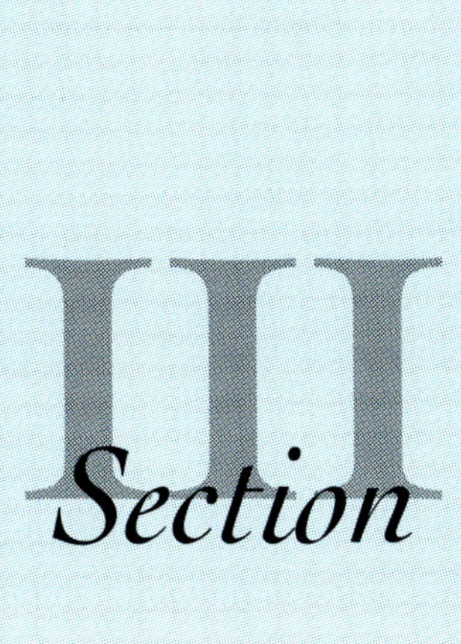

Section III

Neurourology

William D. Steers, editor

CHAPTER 8

Hydronephrosis and Urinary Obstruction in Children

Craig A. Peters

Hydronephrosis and urinary obstruction represent one of the largest diagnostic categories in urology and are associated with a wide range of severity and outcome. The consequences of urinary obstruction range from neonatal death with pulmonary insufficiency to incidentally discovered minimal hydronephrosis in young adults. It is this enormous spectrum of severity and clinical presentation that provides the clinician with an ongoing challenge and source of interest in the diagnosis and management of these conditions. The prenatal diagnosis of hydronephrosis through ultrasound has significantly affected the timing, clinical presentation, and management of this condition. It has also provided new insights into the natural history and pathophysiology of congenital obstruction. Because of the sensitivity of ultrasonographic techniques, however, a large number of these cases are of minimal to moderate severity and have taxed the clinician with the question of the necessity or appropriateness of surgical intervention.

Although controversy exists regarding appropriate treatment of lesser degrees of obstruction, the basic principles of management of hydronephrosis serve as a useful foundation in the evaluation of new approaches to managing these problems. Fundamentally the goals remain to protect renal function, permit normal renal growth and development in the child, and prevent complications from hydronephrosis. The complications include pain, infection, hematuria, and calculi. The importance of a thorough evaluation remains paramount, and in all cases this should be focused on a careful assessment of both anatomy and function of the entire urinary tract. It is important to recognize that all hydronephrosis does not represent obstruction. In some instances this raises the challenge of discriminating between nonobstructive and obstructive hydronephrosis, but it also includes hydronephrosis in the setting of significant vesicoureteral reflux.

At present the diagnosis and management of hydronephrosis and obstruction in children are distinct in the prenatal and postnatal periods. These will be dealt with separately, although it is clear that they are part of a continuum; all prenatal evaluation must be coupled to postnatal evaluation.

Prenatal Period

DIAGNOSIS

Ultrasound evaluation has permitted the early identification of numerous congenital uropathies in the developing fetus, the most common of which is hydronephrosis, representing approximately 50% of all uropathies identified. In large population series the overall incidence of uropathies is approximately 0.1% to 0.2%. Prenatal ultrasound is very sensitive at detecting interfaces between fluid and tissue, which enables it to define with great structural accuracy even minor degrees of hydronephrosis in utero. The earliest detection of such conditions has been reported at 13 or 14 weeks of gestation, with most being identified on a regular basis between 16 and 18 weeks of gestation.[1] Ultrasonographic evaluation is extremely sensitive but is less specific in its diagnostic capacity. The major diagnoses identified with consistency include ureteropelvic junction obstruction, duplex systems with polar hydronephrosis, ureterovesical obstructions with megaureter, and bladder outlet obstruction resulting from posterior urethral valves.[2] Vesicoureteral reflux is being identified more commonly during the fetal period and can be demonstrated sonographically as hydronephrosis or hydroureteronephrosis.[3] Occasionally this fluctuates between examinations or during the course of a single examination. Prenatal distinction between obstruction and reflux can be difficult.

Ureteropelvic junction obstruction is the most common entity identified prenatally and is usually unilateral.[4] When bilateral involvement is seen the degree of hydronephrosis may be asymmetric (Fig. 8.1). The important feature to note with a presumed ureteropelvic junc-

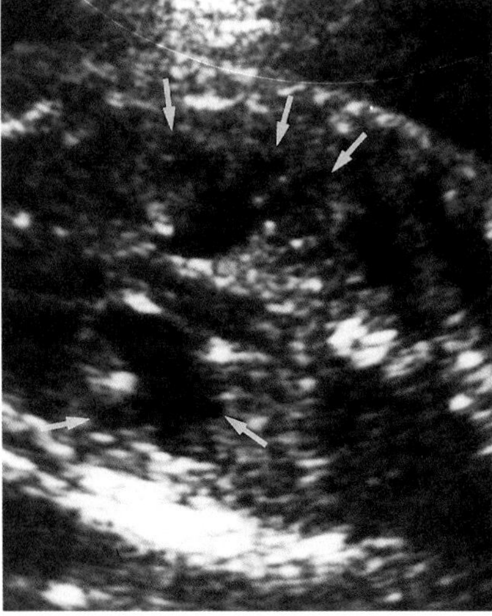

Figure 8.1 Prenatal ultrasonographic view of bilateral moderate hydronephrosis. Caliectasis is present (arrows). The ureters are not seen to be dilated. The degree of hydronephrosis is symmetric in this case.

tion obstruction is caliectasis, which suggests a greater severity of obstruction than if no caliectasis is present. It is important to assess and follow the renal parenchymal echotexture. Increased echogenicity indicates cortical microcysts associated with renal dysplasia and suggests a poor functional outcome for that kidney. Perinephric fluid collections may be identified. These have been seen to be progressive and to cause compression of the affected kidney to the point of producing parenchymal involutions. Postnatally, a small, nonfunctional kidney is seen in what had previously appeared to be a simple ureteropelvic junction obstruction.

Identification of a dilated ureter suggests ureterovesical obstruction, bladder outlet obstruction, or vesicoureteral reflux. The degree of bladder distention and bladder wall thickness can be useful in differentiating these conditions. In posterior urethral valves (Fig. 8.2) the bladder wall is often quite thickened, although the degree of bladder distention is often not so great as is seen with massive bilateral reflux, the so-called megacystis-megaureter syndrome. In all cases of posterior urethral valves and most cases of megacystis-megaureter, one should confirm that the fetus is male.

Prenatal evaluation of the urinary tract must be integrated with an assessment of the overall condition of the fetus, particularly with regard to associated CNS or cardiovascular abnormalities. The status of the amniotic fluid must be assessed and followed, particularly with the possibility of total urinary tract obstruction.

The aim of prenatal ultrasonographic evaluation is to assess the degree of hydronephrosis, indirectly assess the renal consequences, assess the effect on amniotic fluid, and identify the anatomic level of obstruction and associated significant fetal anomalies (Fig. 8.3). This evaluation should permit a broad prognostic categorization, such as a normal outcome, an outcome that would probably require surgical intervention in the postnatal period, or a likelihood of severe renal or pulmonary complications in the immediate postnatal period. Within this latter group exists another group of severe obstructive uropathies in which little likelihood of any salvageable renal function is anticipated. It is on the basis of the initial ultrasonographic evaluation that subsequent management and evaluation are determined.

In the setting of presumed total urinary obstruction, usually due to bladder outlet obstruction with associated oligohydramnios, the risk of respiratory failure and neonatal death is extremely high.[6] However, when this situation develops later in gestation with previous documentation of normal amniotic fluid, the likelihood of a respiratory death is reduced. With early gestational presentation, more invasive evaluation may yield a more accurate prognosis and help determine if invasive intervention in utero to prevent neonatal death should be performed. The primary aim of invasive evaluation is an assessment of renal salvageability. If no significant renal function can be expected to develop with in utero decompression, the likelihood of reversing the pulmonary consequences of severe bladder outlet obstruction is low. This can be assumed if ultrasonographic evaluation demonstrates bilateral dysplastic changes, as manifested by increased renal parenchymal echogenicity. Evaluation is carried out by aspiration of fetal bladder or ureteral urine and then sampling of freshly accumulated urine. This permits an estimate of urine production as well as biochemical and electrolyte analyses of the newly produced urine, which can be correlated with renal salvageability. In cases where urinary sodium is below 100 mg/dL and urinary osmolarity is below 210 mOsm/dL the likelihood of salvageable renal function is good.[7,8] Other urinary indicators of the status of the fetal kidney are being developed, but at present none has been thoroughly tested.

MANAGEMENT

Prenatal diagnosis is an intervention in and of itself. Careful observation of the affected fetus with subsequent

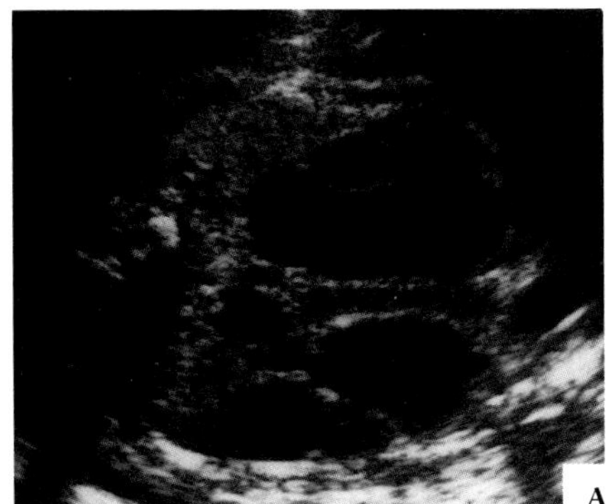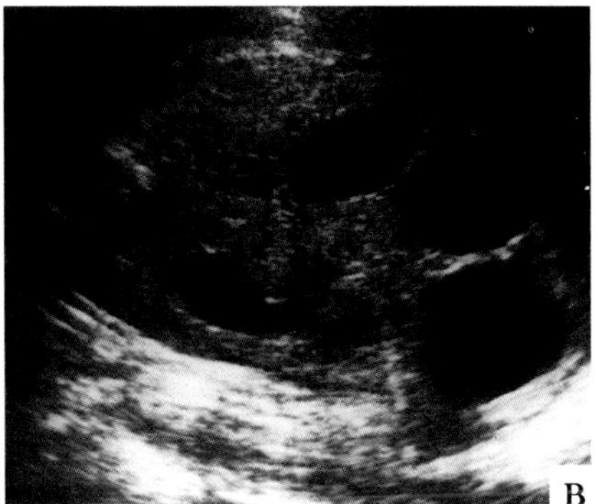

Figure 8.2 **A** Prenatal ultrasonographic view of massive bilateral hydronephrosis in a male fetus. The dilated, urine-filled spaces are the tortuous ureters. **B** View of the bladder in the same fetus, with a thickened wall. The bladder is not massively distended. This boy was found to have posterior urethral valves.

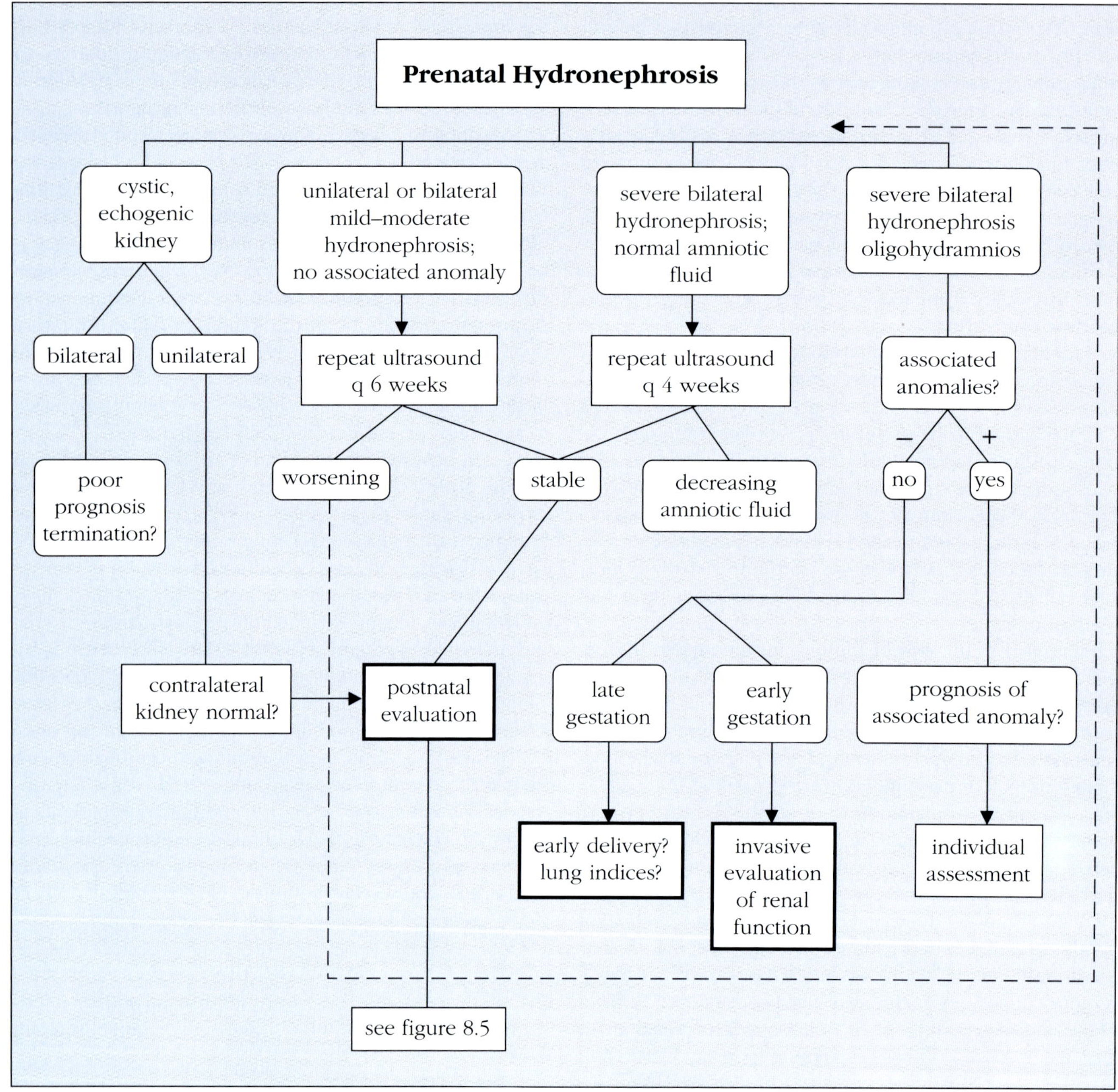

Figure 8.3 Algorithm for the evaluation and treatment of prenatal hydronephrosis.

prenatal ultrasound examinations is usually the most appropriate management. The aim of observational management is to identify changes such as the development of oligohydramnios, fetal growth retardation, or alteration in fetal well-being. The anatomic appearance of the urinary tract is followed, including renal echogenicity and size, the development of extrarenal fluid collections, changes in the degree of hydronephrosis, and bladder wall thickness. The degree of hydronephrosis in a fetus has been seen to change with time and usually increases as an absolute measure over gestational age.[2] This is most likely due only to renal growth and does not reflect an increase in the severity of obstruction. If marked changes take place, increasing obstruction or decreasing compensation for obstruction may be occurring. In most cases of unilateral hydronephrosis, however, this would not change the management scheme. This period of observation is often very reassuring to the mother of the fetus, as it confirms the overall well-being of the child and its kidneys. This is also an opportunity to establish a relationship with the urologist who will be supervising the postnatal evaluation.

The second management option is that of early delivery of the fetus with congenital hydronephrosis. This is seldom necessary, and rarely in the setting of unilateral hydronephrosis or in the absence of total urinary obstruction. In more severe instances of total urinary obstruction, oligohydramnios may develop later in gestation, sometime after 27 or 28 weeks, and the question of early delivery is raised. A balance must be drawn between normal lung development that is ongoing until near term and the progressive effect of obstruction on the kidneys. It is impossible to quantify exactly the relative effects of these two elements. However, it has become evident from clinical experience that in a fetus with recent-onset oligohydramnios from obstruction, delivery after 34 weeks of gestation is not associated with significant respiratory complications. It is unclear whether lungs exposed to oligohydramnios for a longer period of time are even benefited by further time in utero, since the normal relationship between the kidneys and lungs has been disrupted. Presumably, the increased duration of the obstruction imposed on the kidneys will have a deleterious effect on kidney development and function. This suggests that if pulmonary compromise can be minimized, earlier delivery in the setting of total urinary obstruction with oligohydramnios may be appropriate. This requires a careful review of the situation by a combined team of obstetricians, perinatologists, and pediatric urologists. If lung maturation has been maximized in utero and can be augmented somewhat by exogenous steroid or surfactant therapy, earlier delivery may be of some benefit in terms of preserving renal function.

In extreme situations where total urinary obstruction, usually caused by posterior urethral valves, is identified early in gestation, in utero urinary decompression may be appropriate.[9] The time period for this consideration at our center has ranged from 16 to 22 weeks of gestation. At present, the rationale for such intervention is based on the identification of a high rate of newborn death with total urinary obstruction and oligohydramnios before 22 weeks. Experimental evidence suggests that in utero decompression of the obstructed urinary tract permits more normal lung growth and development. Anecdotal clinical evidence also supports this.[8,10] If evaluation suggests salvageable renal function, consideration of in utero shunting is warranted. Indications include bilateral hydronephrosis with probable bladder outlet obstruction due to posterior urethral valves, oligohydramnios developing early in gestation, evidence of salvageable renal function on the basis of renal parenchyma and fetal urinary electrolytes, and informed consent. Contraindications include twin pregnancy, life-threatening associated anomalies, renal dysplasia, or poor-prognosis urinary electrolytes.

An alternative that should be discussed with the family in such cases is termination of pregnancy. It must be recognized that even with completely successful prenatal decompression, the possibility remains for significant pulmonary as well as renal functional impairment, producing a living child with severe medical problems. The legal status of termination of pregnancy in the United States continues to evolve.

In utero percutaneous shunting has now supplanted open fetal surgery for accomplishing satisfactory urinary decompression in utero.[11] Shunt placement is performed with ultrasound guidance. A trocar needle is passed through the fetal abdomen and bladder after traversing the maternal abdomen, uterine wall, and membranes. Within this trocar a modified double-J drainage catheter is passed. Satisfactory in utero decompression can be achieved in most situations with percutaneous placement of a vesicoamniotic shunt. In some instances more than one placement effort is needed. The criteria for a successful decompression include resolution in whole or part of the upper tract hydronephrosis and sustained persistence of the amniotic fluid. After an in utero shunting procedure, careful observation of shunt function, as well as fetal and maternal well-being, is important. Premature labor may occur and must be treated aggressively.

Delivery of the child with a prenatal shunt should be under controlled conditions, usually by caesarean section and with the availability of complete intensive care and imaging facilities. The timing of evaluation can be based on the respiratory status of the newborn, but in most cases some form of urinary decompression is required for the postnatal period.

Postnatal Period

In all cases of prenatally detected hydronephrosis the primary aim postnatally is to prevent complications related to the obstruction (predominantly infection) and to establish the appropriate diagnosis by a carefully performed elective evaluation. The nature and timing of postnatal evaluation for prenatally detected hydronephrosis depend on the presumed severity of the obstruction. Prophylactic antibiotics are recommended until the evaluation is complete. Unilateral obstruction does not require immediate evaluation in most cases. Too early an evaluation may actually underestimate the severity of obstruction owing to the physiologic oliguria in the newborn (Fig. 8.4). In cases of possible bladder outlet obstruction or bilateral ureteral obstruction, evaluation should be performed more promptly, depending largely on the condition of the newborn. The guidelines reviewed below are appropriate for most newborns with prenatally detected hydronephrosis.

WHOM TO EVALUATE

With prenatal identification of significant numbers of children with hydronephrosis, a particularly difficult problem has been the selection of those children who will require postnatal evaluation. In children with clinical presentations such as infection or pain, hydronephrosis is usually detected by evaluation of particular symptoms. Initially, all children who had prenatal hydronephrosis of virtually any degree were evaluated during the postnatal period by various modalities. Many of these children had normal evaluations, and attempts are being made to identify those children prospectively. This has been difficult, largely because of the difficulty in quantifying the degree of prenatal hydronephrosis as well as the inadequacy of many studies in defining precisely the pre- or postnatal condition of the urinary tract.

With severe hydronephrosis this is usually not a difficult decision. With minor degrees of pelvic dilatation, now frequently seen with high-resolution prenatal ultrasound, however, it is difficult to assess the risks of obstructive renal impairment (Fig. 8.5). Gestational age at diagnosis must be considered. Mandell et al.[2] have attempted to do this and have found a cutoff point of 10 mm of pelvic dilatation after 30 weeks of gestation to be a useful threshold for selecting patients warranting postnatal examination. It must be recognized that any such arbitrary limit will have a certain incidence of missing clinically significant cases. Some children evaluated postnatally, using such a threshold, will have normal results. Other criteria that would prompt evaluation are associated significant congenital anomalies, indistinct anatomic definition prenatally, and the presence of prenatal caliectasis, suggesting a more significant degree of obstruction.

In the past, initial identification of hydronephrosis in children has been prompted by a clinical problem such as infection, pain, hematuria, hypertension, or azotemia. Incidental diagnosis in association with nonurologic evaluation also occurs. We have seen isolated instances of affected siblings of children with obstructive uropathies. Although this is widely recognized to exist with vesicoureteral reflux, it is less well characterized with regard to ureteropelvic junction obstruction or ureterovesical junction obstructions.

EVALUATION

The principal aim of postnatal evaluation is to obtain an accurate assessment of the anatomy and function of the entire urinary tract. Both parameters must be completely evaluated and are not mutually exclusive within any single diagnostic study. All diagnostic studies can provide information regarding some element of each, albeit indirectly in some instances. The modalities used for delineating the anatomy and function of the urinary tract include

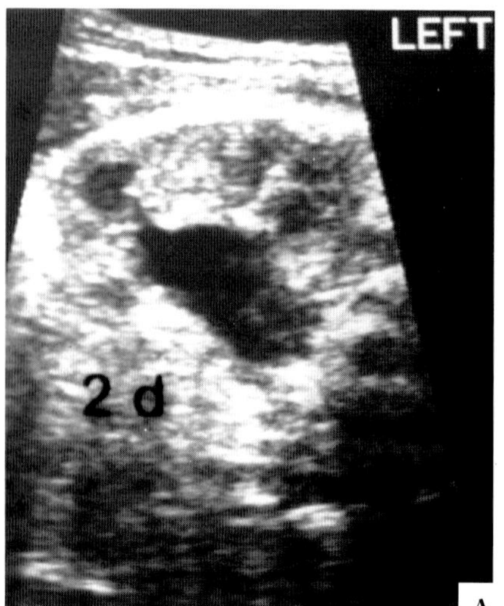

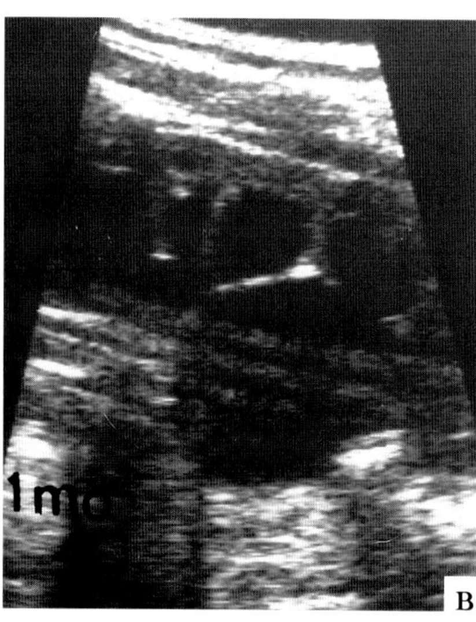

Figure 8.4 **A** Second-day postnatal ultrasound of child with prenatally detected hydronephrosis. There is minimal pelvic dilatation and no caliectasis. **B** Ultrasound of the same child, same kidney at 1 month of age, showing significant pelvicaliectasis associated with a ureteropelvic junction obstruction. Early postnatal ultrasound examinations of the kidneys may be inaccurate because of the physiologic oliguria of the newborn.

ultrasound, intravenous urography, radionuclide renal scanning, cystography, antegrade pyelography with pressure perfusion studies, and cystoscopy with retrograde pyelography. Selection of the appropriate method depends on the clinical situation, the degree of relative invasiveness of each procedure, and the type of information that must be obtained to make a clinical decision. A realistic understanding of what each study can provide is important in permitting the clinician to select the correct diagnostic evaluation efficiently.

Ultrasound provides a readily available, noninvasive assessment of renal, ureteral, and bladder structure, with indirect assessment of renal function and bladder function. The structural detail obtainable with ultrasound is excellent, including separation of duplex systems and identification of calyceal or ureteral dilatation and the presence of a ureterocele. With skillful use the ectopic insertion of a dilated ureter or even the presence of posterior urethral valves, as manifested by a dilated posterior urethra, can be identified. Increased echo texture of the

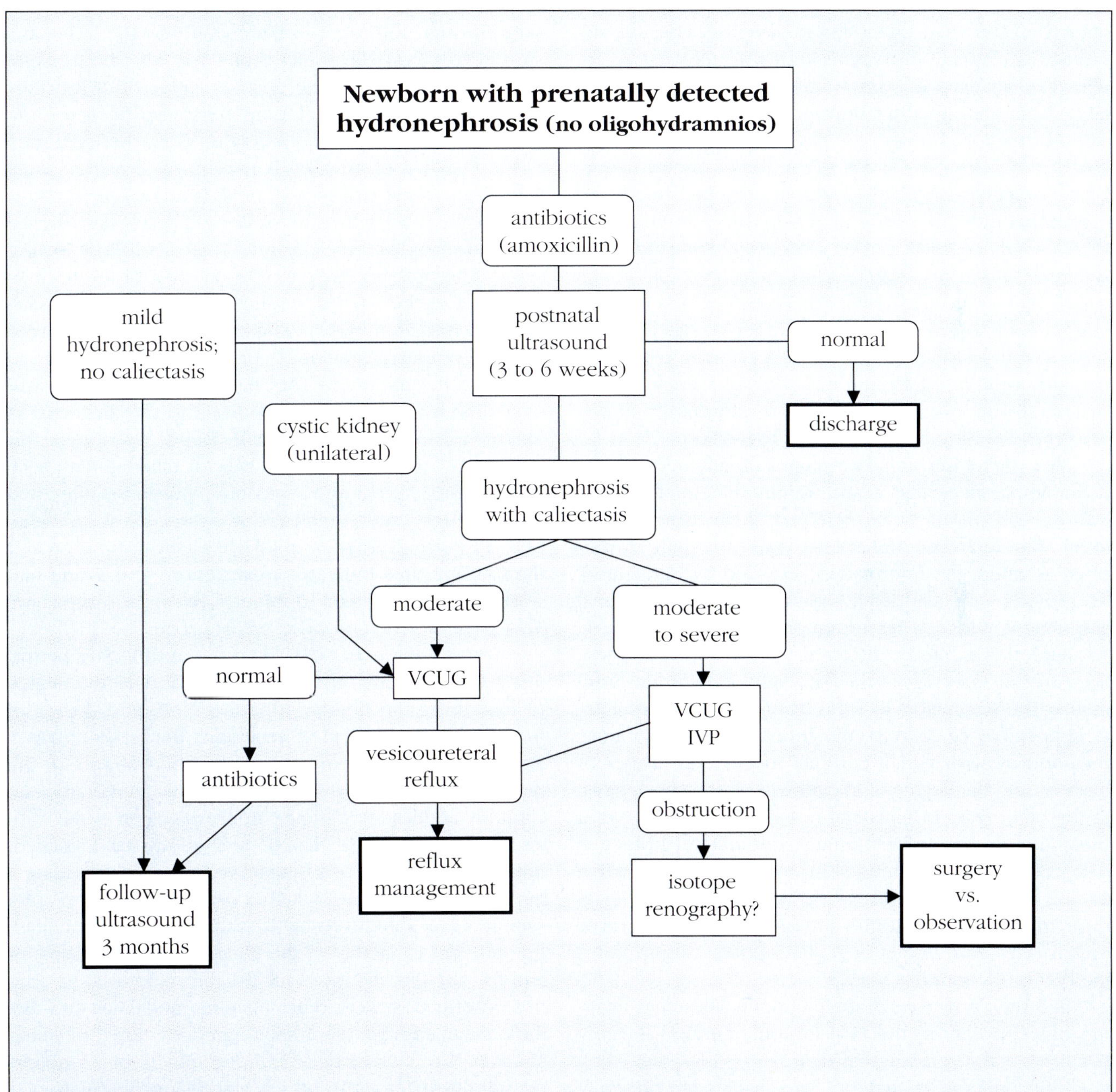

Figure 8.5 Algorithm for the evaluation and treatment of a newborn with prenatally detected hydronephrosis.

renal parenchyma suggests some degree of structural damage with concomitant functional impairment.[12] Preser-vation of the sonolucent medullary pyramids in the newborn is a good indicator of a relatively normal kidney, structurally and presumably functionally. More recently, pulse-flow duplex Doppler ultrasound has permitted quantification of renal vascular resistance, and initial reports have shown this to be elevated in obstruction. The correlation of this finding with functional parameters in obstruction remains to be characterized. Ureteral function can be assessed with ultrasound by observing the activity of ureteral peristalsis with real-time imaging. Very often the obstructed ureter can be seen to peristalse vigorously, a clinical observation known to most surgeons, who can observe this phenomenon on the operating table. This finding is not universally considered to indicate obstruction, however. It has been reported that the absence of peristalsisis is a better indicator of obstruction. Bladder emptying is readily assessed with ultrasound, and catheterization for postvoid residual can be avoided. Bladder wall thickness can be assessed, particularly in the setting of posterior urethral valves, which are often suggested by marked thickening. The presence of a ureterocele is usually apparent on a bladder image and will serve to focus further investigation. A carefully performed pediatric urinary ultrasound can provide a great deal of structural and inferential functional information and is usually the starting point for further evaluation.

More direct functional imaging is usually necessary to define impairments that would warrant release of obstruction or, in extreme cases, removal of the affected segment. The anatomic details provided by such studies often augment the information provided by ultrasound. To provide anatomic detail with a qualitative functional assessment, intravenous urography (IVU) is necessary. Although this is often considered merely a structural test, the careful observer can make useful functional judgments. The parameters to focus on include the symmetry of appearance of contrast, the concentration of contrast, the rapidity with which contrast reaches the ureter or bladder, and the degree of impairment of drainage relative to the other side. In unilateral disease, the presence of a presumed normally functioning contralateral kidney is important in making judgments regarding the relative severity of obstruction (just as it is with radionuclide imaging). In complex anatomic situations, such as ectopic ureteroceles and ureters or partial ureteral duplications, the IVU is of enormous benefit.

Recently, however, diuretic radionuclide renal imaging has supplanted the IVU in some centers, largely because of the quantitative data it provides regarding renal function and drainage.[13] Three agents are presently used for radionuclide renal imaging: DMSA, DTPA and, more recently, MAG-3 (Fig. 8.6). Each of these radionuclide tracers provides slightly different information. DTPA and MAG-3 are essentially equivalent except for the greater specificity of MAG-3. DMSA scanning provides an accurate assessment of relative renal function as well as a structural image of the functioning renal mass and of any areas of focal renal scarring. In significant obstruction DMSA scanning may overestimate the degree of function. Diuretic renography with agents such as DPTA or MAG-3 has become extremely popular in the assessment of childhood obstruction, particularly in cases of neonatal hydronephrosis with prenatal diagnosis. This method can provide an estimate of relative function. The rapidity of passage through the renal parenchyma into the collecting system (the cortical transit time) may also be a useful parameter in assessing the relative degree of obstruction. More sophisticated calculations have also been used to provide information on obstruction (i.e., the extraction factor).[14] When obstruction is present the tracer accumulates in the renal pelvis. A diuretic is administered to the child at the point when the obstructed pelvis has reached maximal filling, and the rapidity of tracer washout is measured. The time taken to excrete one half of the tracer is calculated as the one-half washout time ($t_{1/2}$) and is usually expressed in minutes. This number is often derived from a computer-generated curve with extrapolation to the one-half time point. The shape of the washout curve over time may be equally important in the diagnosis of obstruction. When it was initially being developed, this study was compared with a variety of other studies, such as intravenous urography, pressure-perfusion studies, and clinical history, and parameters of obstruction were identified. In current usage a one-half washout time greater than 20 minutes indicates obstruction, and a one-half washout time less than 10 minutes rules out obstruction. This leaves a generous indeterminate zone.

Controversy exists regarding the appropriate performance of the study, including such factors as the degree of hydration, the timing, administration, and dosing of furosemide, the method of generating the washout curve, and the relative importance of residual counts in the pelvis. Many variations on the "textbook" curve are seen clinically and lead to difficulty in interpretation of the studies. The clinical use of diuretic renography has increased, presumably because of its attractive feature of providing a number that determines whether or not obstruction is present. It is important to recognize the source of the number, the inherent variability in the generation of that number, and the fact that the bases for the threshold used to diagnose obstruction were other imaging modalities and that these parameters have not been rigorously tested in young children. We consider diuretic renography to be an adjunct technique for cases in which significant obstruction is thought to exist, and its results are integrated with findings from other imaging modalities. Particular caution should be exercised when diuretic renography is used in young children, less than 1 month to 6 weeks of age, because of the functional immaturity of the kidney. As usual, clinical judgment must be a significant component of the decision-making process in children with hydronephrosis.

Pressure-perfusion studies are an alternate and adjunctive way of assessing the degree of upper tract outflow obstruction. These are usually combined with antegrade radiologic imaging of the upper tract anatomy and are based on assessment of pressure and flow relationships in the upper urinary tract. The technique of constant flow described by Whitaker has been widely used in adult and pediatric urology.[15] This method infuses a constant amount of fluid and measures the pressure gradient between the upper urinary tract and the bladder with a drainage catheter in place. Pressures greater than 20 cm H_2O with a flow of 10 mL/min are considered diagnostic of obstruction. As with diuretic renography, the indeterminate area (between 15 and 20 cm H_2O) is often the subject of question. Controversy exists as to the clinical usefulness of the Whitaker test in children, particularly because of the necessity for a percutaneous renal puncture. Again, the basis for comparison and validation of the study remains uncertain, especially in the very young infant. An alternate pressure-perfusion study has been described by Mitchell and others[16] in which a constant pressure is maintained and the amount of flow necessary to sustain that pressure is assessed. Both studies are single-point estimates of the pressure-flow relationship of a given system. The clinical utility of pressure-perfusion studies in small children remains to be established.

Cystography is an important part of the assessment of hydronephrosis in children. Vesicoureteral reflux must be considered a possible contributor to prenatally detected hydronephrosis and in older children who present with infection and hydronephrosis. Identification of associated bladder pathology, such as posterior urethral valves, ureterocele, diverticula or ureteral ectopia, or inadequate emptying, is important. For specific anatomic delineation the radiographic VCUG remains the gold standard and in small infants can be performed without significant difficulty. Radionuclide cystography is the most efficient means for follow-up of vesicoureteral reflux. However, the comparability of anatomic detail and grading of reflux between radionuclide cystography and radiographic VCUG is imprecise. It is essential for voiding to occur with concurrent imaging; a static cystogram is inadequate for evaluating hydronephrosis in a child.

Cystoscopy with or without retrograde pyelography remains a useful diagnostic tool in certain instances. If

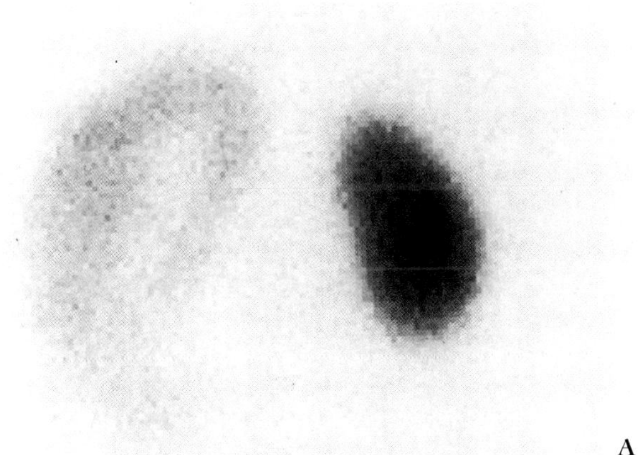

A

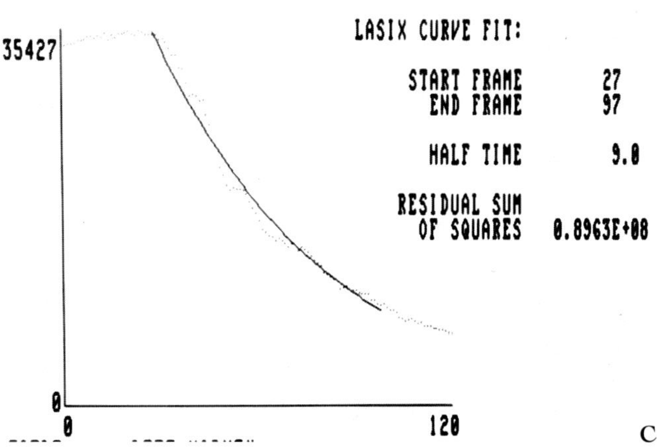
C

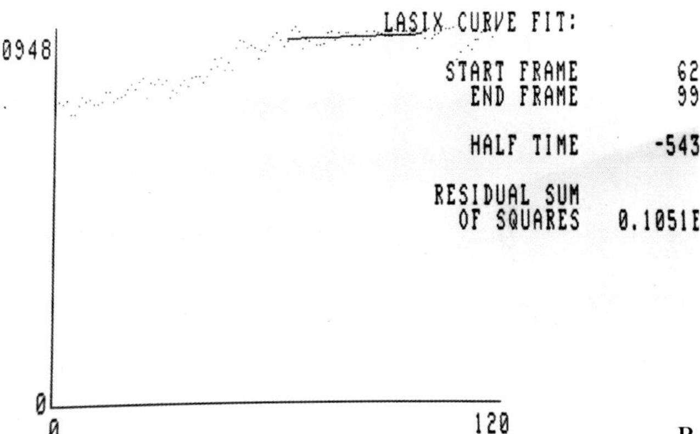

B

Figure 8.6 Isotope renography in the infant with hydronephrosis. **A** DMSA scan of child with unilateral hydronephrosis detected prenatally. There is diminished left renal function (33% of total renal function) and evidence of hydronephrosis (posterior view). **B** Diuretic phase of MAG-3 isotope renogram, showing markedly abnormal washout curve from the left kidney with diminished function. The amount of pelvic tracer continues to rise rather than to decline after diuretic administration. **C** After surgical correction of the left UPJ obstruction, the washout curve has improved significantly, with a $t_{1/2}$ of 9 minutes. Functional fraction has not significantly changed.

ureteral visualization has not been achieved with upper tract studies, retrograde pyelography is important for delineation of the anatomic location of obstruction as well as its extent. Even in infants this can be achieved with minimal trauma to the ureters by using a cutoff 3 Fr ureteral catheter gently placed to occlude the ureteral orifice. Less than 1 mL of contrast is usually adequate to fill the ureter and characterize the point of obstruction. Although it is unusual to find other areas of obstruction with ureteropelvic junctions, the clinical utility of identifying those few cases is extremely high. In complex anatomic situations with duplications or ectopia, retrograde pyelography may be the only way to delineate the anatomy clearly. Cystoscopy may be the only means of confirming the ectopic location of ureteral orifices, the relationship of diverticula to ureteral orifices, and the anatomic state of the bladder and posterior urethra.

In unusual situations, percutaneous drainage of a hydronephrotic segment with "nonfunction" on imaging studies may provide the ability both to describe the anatomy and to assess salvageability with temporary decompression. This should be accompanied by a specific plan of action, since the placement of a percutaneous drainage tube invariably introduces infection. This commits the urologist to either removal of the affected segment or correction of the obstruction.

Renal functional assessment is important in the evaluation of hydronephrosis, particularly at the more severe end of the spectrum. This is usually done with an estimation of glomerular filtration rate (GFR) using a creatinine clearance study. Estimation of GFR by a simple serum creatinine measurement and body weight may be useful in mild to moderate degrees of hydronephrosis but may not accurately assess GFR in more severe cases of impaired renal function. The other aspects of renal function, particularly concentrating ability, are also important, as many children with moderate to severe hydronephrosis have impaired concentration of urine. This inability to concentrate may further aggravate the effect of an obstruction by constantly subjecting that system to high fluid volumes. Assessment of concentrating ability with a fasting urine and serum osmolarity determination may identify children who require further evaluation. Screening tests of obstructive damage using renal tubule enzyme levels in the urine have been suggested as clinically useful and may identify children with more subtle degrees of damage, possibly in an early and reversible period.

Evaluation of the child with hydronephrosis can be considered complete when a clear image of urinary tract anatomy and an estimation of relative function of the renal components have been achieved. It is both difficult and injudicious to attempt any surgical intervention before such an assessment has been completed. Any management scheme, including nonoperative management, should also be based on a complete evaluation.

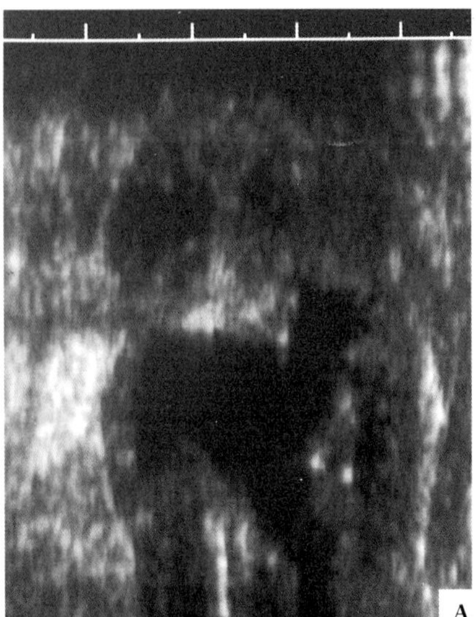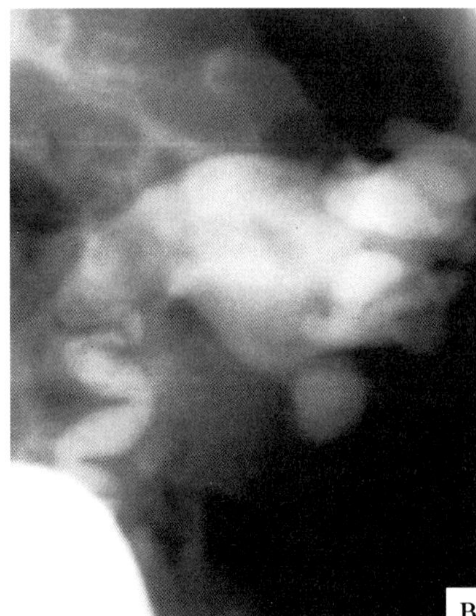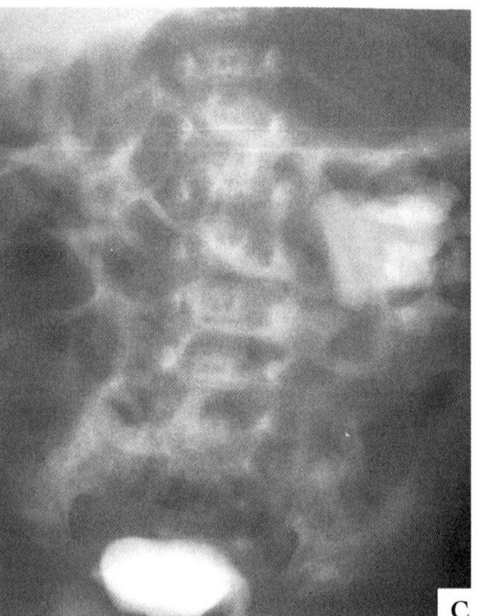

***Figure 8.7* A** Postnatal ultrasound of boy with prenatal hydronephrosis, showing lower pole hydronephrosis of moderate degree. **B** Voiding cystourethrogram in this boy demonstrating grade 4 to 5 lower pole reflux. No evidence of valves was seen. **C** Delayed film of VCUG in this boy, showing delay in drainage of the refluxing lower pole system, suggesting an element of obstruction at the ureteropelvic junction.

MANAGEMENT

The principal aim of the management of any child with hydronephrosis is to prevent obstructive renal damage and complications associated with hydronephrosis and obstruction, including infection, pain, and hematuria. In children this cannot be considered simply as a maintenance of function but must permit as much renal growth and development as possible. Renal functional capacity increases rapidly during the first 2 years of life, and during this time the kidney appears to be particularly sensitive to obstructive and infectious damage. There is much evidence to suggest that earlier repair of obstructions permits the most normal renal growth and development.[17] It is known that infections early in life have a greater tendency to produce renal scarring than those in later life. The controversy about the appropriateness of invasive intervention of presumed obstruction rests on the threshold of obstruction beyond which impairment of normal renal growth and development occurs. That threshold has not been identified and cannot be reliably predicted with available clinical studies. The clinician must carefully balance the risks and benefits of surgical intervention with this uncertainty regarding the long-term outcome of any individual case of hydronephrosis with obstruction. "Conservative" management may require surgical correction to protect the child's potential for renal growth and development.

Antibiotic prophylaxis is a critical element in the protection of the child with a presumed urinary obstruction, particularly in preventing urosepsis with associated obstruction, the most acute and threatening complication. The child with obstruction and infection may present with profound sepsis, including shock, disseminated intravascular coagulation, and hemodynamic failure. Such potentially life-threatening conditions emphasize the importance of preventing infections, particularly in the context of urinary obstruction. Until a specific diagnosis or treatment has been undertaken, antibiotic prophylaxis is a safe and effective means of preventing life-threatening infection. In the neonatal period we use amoxicillin preparations, 50 mg/d, as our routine prophylactic agent. Sulfa preparations are avoided until 3 months of age because of the risk of jaundice in the young child. At that age, however, we usually recommend a change to a trimethoprim-sulfa combination if long-term prophylaxis will be needed. It is important to initiate antibiotic prophylaxis on the first day of life in prenatally detected cases, until the specific nature of the condition can be identified and managed.

Although hydronephrosis is usually suggestive of obstruction when detected prenatally, occasionally it represents vesicoureteral reflux. Reflux and obstruction can coexist, and this represents a more threatening situation than either one alone (Fig. 8.7). This situation is particularly common with ectopic ureters located near the bladder neck. Reflux with obstruction is unusual in primary obstructive megaureters but may also be seen with ureteropelvic junction obstruction.[18] Reflux and obstruction at the level of the ureterovesical junction may also coexist with posterior urethral valves. Reflux is common in posterior urethral valves. Although obstruction at the UVJ may be due to a primary intrinsic abnormality, it is more often due to the effects of bladder wall thickening on the distal ureter and its function. Management of the primary condition is the critical factor in these patients. In most cases hydronephrosis represents an obstructive process, but it is essential for the contribution of vesicoureteral reflux or bladder dysfunction to be considered and identified.

The management of hydronephrosis in children is specific to the underlying anatomy and will be reviewed on the basis of the primary entity that produces the hydronephrosis. These primary entities include ureteral ectopia, ureterocele, posterior urethral valves, and ureteral obstructions (ureteropelvic and ureterovesical junction obstructions).

Ureteral Ectopia

Ureteral ectopia produces hydronephrosis because of an ectopic location of the ureteral orifice that produces obstruction. This is most common in boys in whom the orifice is located at the level of the bladder neck or enters into the ejaculatory or prostatic duct system. This can occur with vesicoureteral reflux and is often associated with significant functional impairment of the renal segment. These boys typically present with urinary infection. In girls, ureteral ectopia is often associated with continuous urinary incontinence rather than hydronephrosis. Ectopia into the bladder neck, upper vagina, or uterus usually produces hydronephrosis, often associated with a poorly functioning segment of a duplex system (Fig. 8.8). It is unusual for a hydronephrotic upper pole associated with an ectopic ureter to have sufficient function to warrant preservation but, if indicated, this can be accomplished with an upper to lower pole ureteropyelostomy or ureteroureterostomy. In general, these cases are best managed with upper pole partial nephrectomy and subtotal ureterectomy. In the absence of reflux it is not necessary to remove the entire ureter. This can usually be performed in a single operation through one incision. In cases of significant reflux the entire ureter should be removed, with care being taken to avoid injury to the lower pole ureter. When the ureter is ectopic into the bladder neck, care is necessary to avoid injury to the sphincter mechanism. With careful removal of this segment, the child is usually free of further infections or complications.

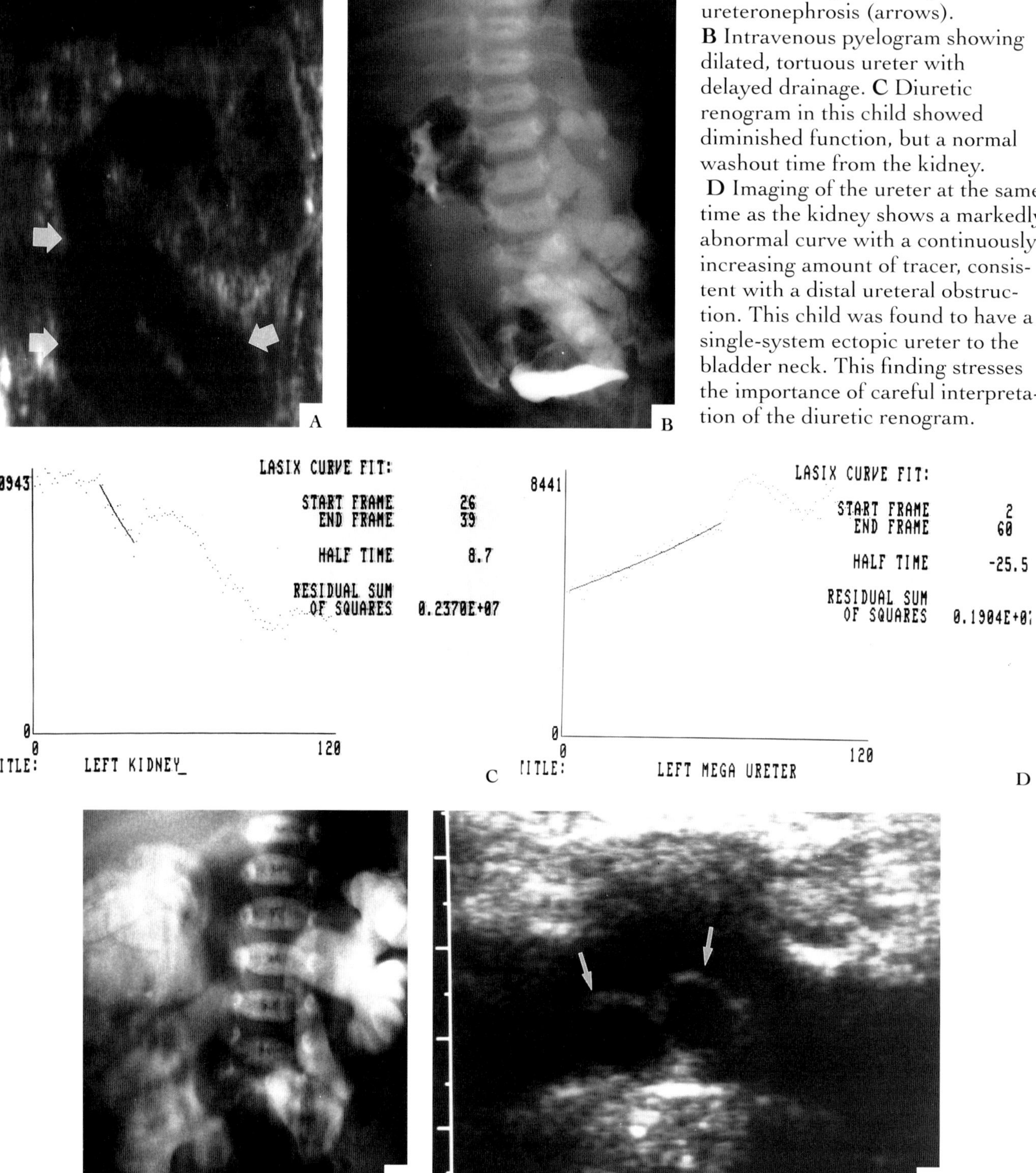

Figure 8.8 **A** Postnatal ultrasound in a newborn girl with hydro-ureteronephrosis (arrows). **B** Intravenous pyelogram showing dilated, tortuous ureter with delayed drainage. **C** Diuretic renogram in this child showed diminished function, but a normal washout time from the kidney. **D** Imaging of the ureter at the same time as the kidney shows a markedly abnormal curve with a continuously increasing amount of tracer, consistent with a distal ureteral obstruction. This child was found to have a single-system ectopic ureter to the bladder neck. This finding stresses the importance of careful interpretation of the diuretic renogram.

Figure 8.9 **A** Intravenous pyelogram in a newborn boy with bilateral hydroureteronephrosis detected prenatally and confirmed postnatally. Bilateral high-grade obstruction is evident. Adequate IVPs can be obtained in the very young. VCUG did not show evidence of posterior urethral valves but confirmed the diagnosis suggested by ultrasonography. **B** Ultrasonographic demonstration of bilateral ureteroceles in this boy, with single-system obstructing ureteroceles (arrows). He had a slightly elevated creatinine level (0.8 mg/dL) and underwent transurethral incision of ureteroceles at 3 weeks of age. This has provided complete decompression without reflux.

Ureterocele

Management of hydronephrosis associated with a ureterocele depends on the anatomy of the ureterocele (Fig. 8.9), the presence or absence of associated reflux, the presence or absence of obstruction of the lower pole segment in a duplex system, and the function of the affected and contralateral renal segments. In most cases ureteroceles are associated with a duplex system and the status of the lower pole becomes an important factor in management. The ureterocele is often associated with a poorly functioning upper pole segment and a relatively normal lower pole. Upper pole partial nephrectomy with subtotal ureterectomy and decompression of the ureterocele is usually curative. However, up to one half of these patients require repair of the ureterocele within the bladder to prevent infectious complications of the lower pole resulting from either reflux or creation of a diverticulum.[19] When the upper pole segment has salvageable function, options include a proximal ureteroureterostomy with decompression of the ureterocele or a distal repair, resecting the ureterocele and reimplanting both ureters in a common sheath. Transurethral incisions of the ureterocele to permit decompression, without inducing reflux into that segment, have recently been gaining in popularity.[20] This approach has specific applicability in the neonate, particularly when obstruction of a functioning segment is present (Fig. 8.10). With an appropriate incision one can assess the functional capability of the affected renal segment and provide decompression of both segments. On rare occasions this management is sufficient, but usually it requires later procedures, either within the bladder or with partial nephrectomy of the nonfunctioning segment. In few other situations is a meticulous preoperative evaluation of more importance than with ureterocele.

Posterior Urethral Valves

Posterior urethral valves is one of the most important diagnostic entities that produces hydronephrosis in newborn boys, and it remains a significant cause of long-term morbidity related to bladder dysfunction and renal failure. Early recognition and treatment of such valves should reduce this long-term morbidity.[21,22] Although prenatal diagnosis has reduced the incidence of uremic and septic newborns with posterior valves, such cases

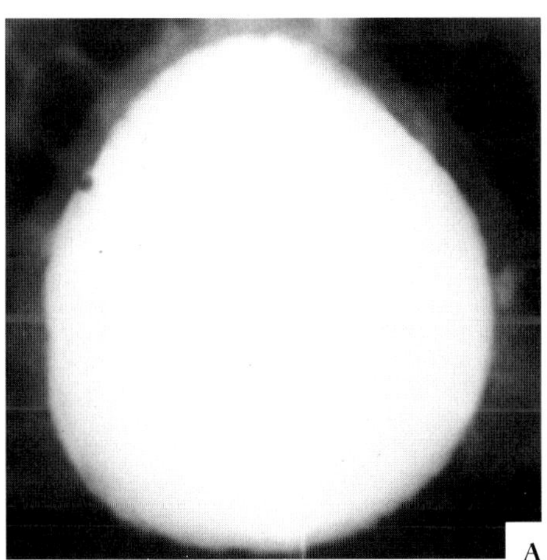

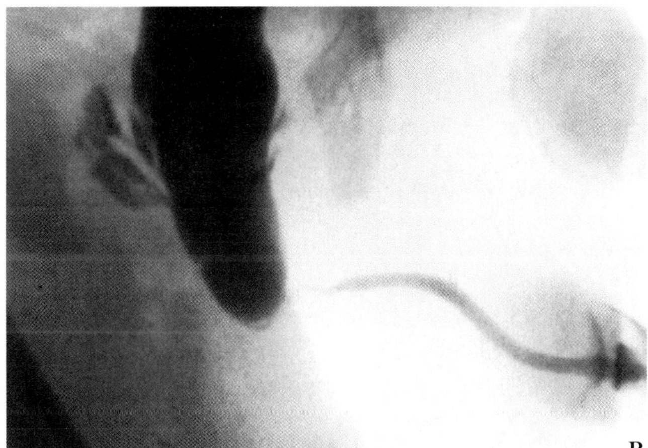

Figure 8.10 **A** VCUG of a 2-week-old boy with posterior urethral valves, showing markedly thickened bladder wall and trabeculation. **B** Posterior urethra in this boy, showing the typical appearance of posterior urethral valvular obstruction. This boy had been seen to have only mild to moderate bilateral hydronephrosis on prenatal ultrasound examinations. **C** The same boy after valve resection.

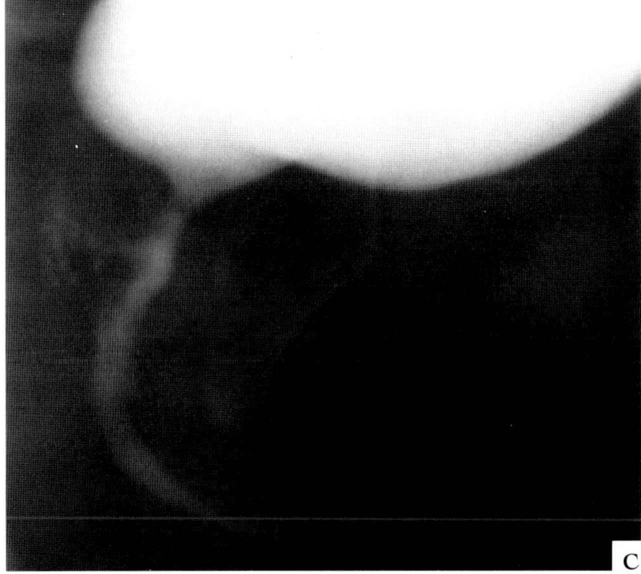

still occur. These children may not have a history of a weak or dribbling stream but present with sepsis, failure to thrive, a palpable bladder, and hydronephrosis. Ultrasound examination reveals a thick-walled bladder that may not be markedly distended. The specific diagnosis and identification of the valves is made on voiding cystography (see Fig. 8.10), which also provides information about the condition of the bladder. Initial catheter drainage provides an estimate of the effect of valve ablation alone on upper urinary tract hydronephrosis and on renal function.

When the response to catheter drainage is positive, as is usual, valve ablation will be sufficient initial management. However, if the upper tracts do not drain with a bladder catheter, concern for relative ureterovesical obstruction, usually due to the thick-walled bladder, must be entertained. Rarely, the bladder is so severely affected that upper tract urinary diversion becomes necessary. With currently available instrumentation, primary valve ablation can be performed in all but the smallest newborns and premature infants. In those children a bladder diversion with a vesicostomy is the most appropriate initial means of management. After valve ablation, upper tract decompression can be anticipated and monitored. The vesicoureteral reflux that is frequently present with these valves often resolves spontaneously. Renal function should be followed and can be expected to increase with age or to remain stable in older children.

If the upper urinary tract remains hydronephrotic after valve ablation, if anticipated growth of renal function with age does not occur, or if derangements of renal function do not resolve, upper urinary tract reconstruction must be considered. It is absolutely critical to recognize the potential contribution of bladder dysfunction to persistent hydronephrosis in posterior urethral valves. A noncompliant, hypertonic bladder (the "valve bladder") (Fig. 8.11) is often the cause of persisting upper tract dilatation in boys with previously resected valves.[23] It may be difficult to determine the most appropriate management in such children, augmentation cystoplasty versus ureteral

reconstruction including tapering and reimplantation of the dilated ureters. A combined approach may ultimately be the most successful. It is important to integrate urodynamic evaluation with structural evaluation in such situations.

Long-term follow-up of renal function is essential in these children and a measured creatinine clearance (rather than simply serum creatinine) is our preferred indicator of overall renal function. Determinations concerning the need for more aggressive interventions early in life are based on renal functional assessments. It is often reported in the literature that a serum creatinine level less than 0.8 mg/dL within the first year of life in a boy with valves suggests a favorable renal prognosis. We have followed several children with low serum creatinine and reduced measured creatinine clearance (less than 25 mL/min/m^2). All of these boys have ultimately progressed to end-stage renal failure. It is important that in such boys the clinician should not be falsely reassured by the serum creatinine, a relatively insensitive measure of renal functional reserve.

Ureteropelvic Junction Obstruction

Obstruction at the ureteropelvic junction is one of the most common causes of hydronephrosis in children.[24] This is particularly true for those detected prenatally, and it is on this specific condition that some of the most controversial and difficult questions regarding the management of obstructive hydronephrosis have been focused. Two anatomic anomalies can lead to ureteropelvic junction obstruction. The most common is an anatomic narrowing or stenosis of the proximal ureter just at or below the ureteropelvic junction; this is characterized histologically by disordered muscle and collagen bundles in the ureteral wall.[25] There may be associated kinking or distortion of the ureter at this point. The second, much less common anomaly is a lower pole renal vessel that creates a kinking and compression of the ureter against the pelvis. The degree of hydronephrosis varies widely, from minimal dilatation of the pelvis without calyceal dilatation to giant hydronephrosis that may extend across the mid-

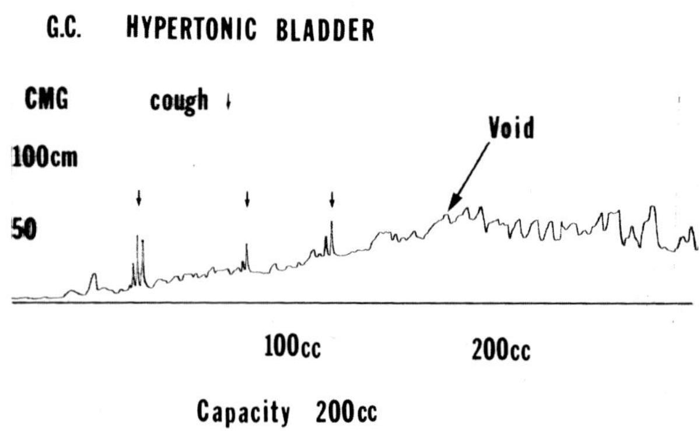

Figure 8.11 Cystometrogram of a boy with posterior urethral valves (resected several years previously) and hydronephrosis. This shows a high-pressure, noncompliant, small-capacity bladder, typical of the "valve bladder."

line and is often associated with minimal to very poor renal function. Prenatal ultrasound has demonstrated this enormous range, and much of the current difficulty in determining the need for surgical therapy rests on the large number of mild and asymptomatic cases now identified (Fig. 8.12). The long-term functional implications of these conditions are unknown.

The clinical presentation of ureteropelvic junction obstruction has previously been that of pain, infection, hematuria, or an incidental finding on imaging studies. The majority of these cases are now detected prenatally with various degrees of prenatal hydronephrosis. These children are asymptomatic and in many ways present a different clinical situation than the symptomatic cases. The fact that adults can be found to have significant ureteropelvic junction obstructions without a prior history of signs or symptoms confirms the fact that this entity can remain asymptomatic for long periods and, in many cases,

is associated with significant renal damage. Identifying those at risk for that ultimate outcome is a challenge.

In a child with symptoms compatible with ureteropelvic junction obstruction, ultrasound is often the most effective initial imaging modality. Hydronephrosis without hydroureter but with a normal bladder study is strongly suggestive of UPJ obstruction. This should be confirmed with a functional imaging study, either an IVP or a diuretic renal scan. The IVP has the advantage of providing better anatomic detail, whereas the radionuclide study provides relative quantitative information regarding function as well as drainage. The latter is particularly useful for long-term follow-up. In clear-cut cases of significant high-grade obstruction, however, either study or both are appropriate. During the evaluation it is important to look for the anatomy of the distal ureter and the possibility of a secondary level of obstruction. In moderate to severe cases the ureter can be imaged with a small amount of contrast

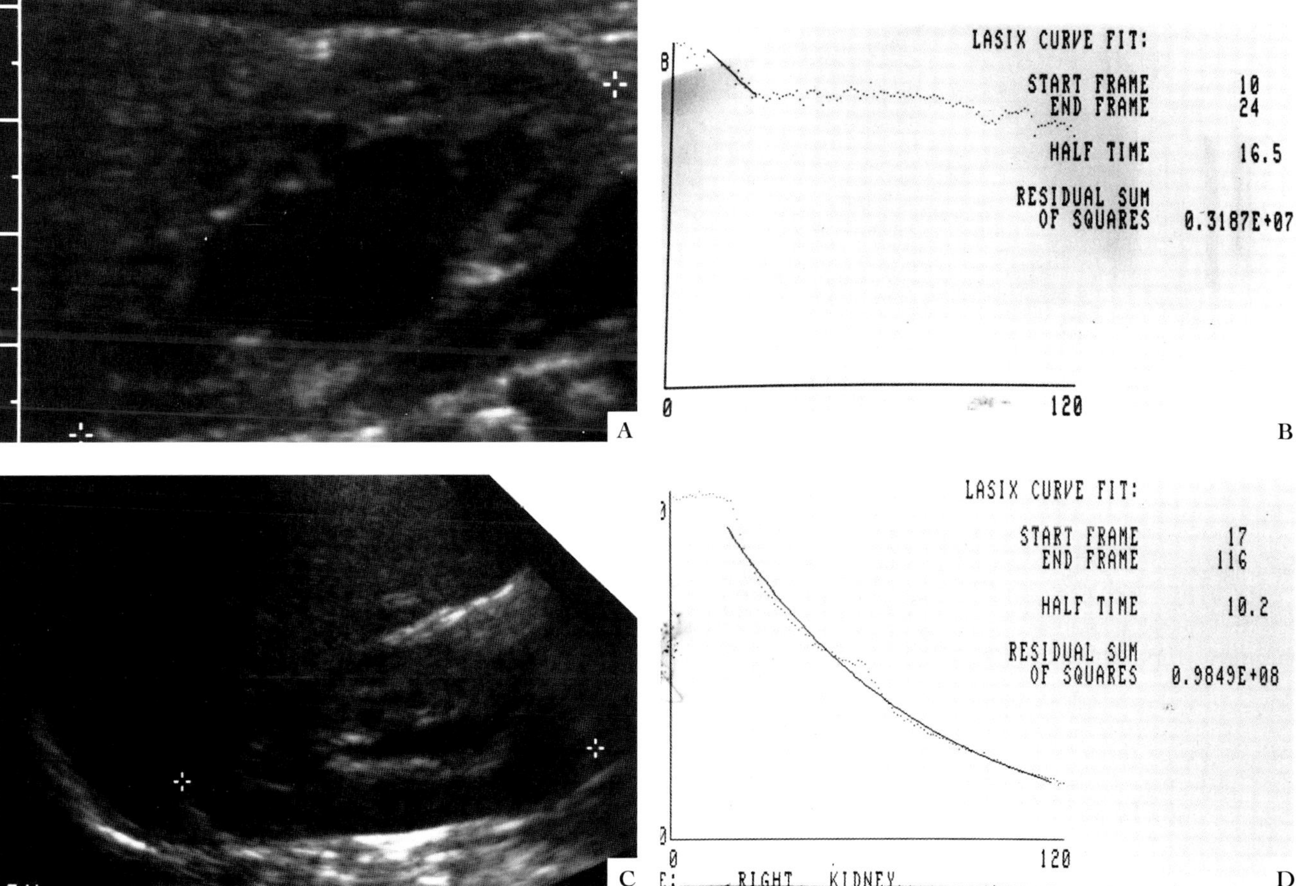

Figure 8.12 **A** Postnatal ultrasonographic view of kidney in a newborn boy with unilateral hdronephrosis. No ureteral dilation was seen. **B** MAG-3 diuretic renogram at 1 month of age, showing abnormal "washout" curve. Although the calculated $t_{1/2}$ was 16.5 minutes, the curve is indicative of obstruction and has a high residual count of tracer. **C** Postoperative ultrasound showing almost complete resolution of hydronephrosis and normal parenchyma. **D** Postoperative MAG-3 renogram with a normal washout curve and $t_{1/2}$ of 10.2 minutes.

dye that trickles by the obstruction, yet in the more profound cases the entire distal ureter may not be visualized. Although controversial, our recommendation is that the distal ureter associated with ureteropelvic junction should be imaged at one time point before definitive surgical correction. It is unlikely that significant associated pathology will be identified, but in the unusual case where it is the information will be of enormous benefit. Associated conditions include ureteral folds, plications, and a distal primary obstructive megaureter. Such a finding could significantly alter the surgical management. If radionuclide scan is used to the exclusion of intravenous pyelography, we recommend retrograde studies just before definitive surgery. These should not be performed separately because of the possibility of infection, and they must be done atraumatically to prevent edema at the ureterovesical junction.

Voiding cystourethrography is appropriate as an adjunctive imaging test in patients who have presented with infection. There is seldom any question about the appropriateness of surgical intervention, given a symptomatic presentation of ureteropelvic junction obstruction.

Asymptomatic neonates with prenatally detected hydronephrosis comprise a large segment of patients with ureteropelvic junction obstruction and present a significant clinical challenge in evaluation and recommendations for therapy. After postnatal confirmation of the hydronephrosis we assess the need for further imaging on the basis of degree of hydronephrosis. When massive dilatation is present further evaluation is appropriate, as it is in the presence of caliectasis. Although lesser degrees of hydronephrosis may not have significant obstruction, it is always safer to have an evaluation of the functional status of the kidney, even if only as a baseline for follow-up. At some point a cutoff must be made beyond which imaging other than ultrasound is not performed. This is usually in a kidney with mild dilatation of the pelvis and no caliectasis, with full and normal-appearing renal parenchyma, including sonolucent medullary pyramids. The degree of dilatation should not exceed 10 mm in a full-term child. There should not be any ureteral dilatation. In cases more severe than this, however, we recommend an intravenous pyelogram as well as VCUG to rule out associated reflux.

The IVP provides a relative functional assessment of the condition of the kidney, as well as anatomic delineation of the point of obstruction and the distal ureter. We then recommend an adjunctive renal scan to provide a baseline measurement of function and drainage; this is useful whether or not surgery is ultimately performed. We have seen discrepancies in interpretation between the IVP and radionuclide renography, but as yet no specific pattern of disagreement has been identified. The IVP and diuretic renogram are complementary and mutually supportive rather than mutually exclusive techniques. The integration of these various diagnostic tests remains the principal clinical challenge.

Factors that prompt us to recommend surgical repair are those indicating that some functional impairment has occurred, even if it has not been specifically documented by differential function on the renal scan. The scan provides an estimate of glomerular filtration rate, with a significant degree of variation in accuracy. GFR may not be as impaired as concentrating ability, for example. The latter can be determined by lesser concentration of contrast agent on the intravenous pyelogram. The relative rate of appearance, as compared with the presumably normal contralateral kidney, of the contrast in an IVP suggests a higher grade of obstruction. Effacement of the medullary pyramids and parenchymal thinning on ultrasound or IVP are strong indications of significant renal damage. Impairment of growth over a period of follow-up, documented ultrasonographically, is a strong indication of a significant obstructive process. A high residual volume of tracer in the pelvis of a hydronephrotic system suggests significant obstruction, despite the calculation of a normal washout time. When the presence of reflux is documented, it is essential to drain the bladder with a catheter to prevent a falsely poor washout or a falsely high functional estimate resulting from refluxed bladder tracer.

Despite the controversy and relative uncertainty about long-term functional effects of mild to moderate obstruction, a clinical decision must be made regarding management of each case. Our perspective is that when surgical repair can be performed with minimal morbidity and complications, such an approach will obviate the need for continued follow-up and will minimize the chances of functional damage. This approach has significant implicit responsibilities.

Observational therapy of ureteropelvic junction obstruction carries the responsibility of ensuring long-term follow-up to protect the child and the developing renal function.[26] A single episode of serious infection can produce significant damage to a partially obstructed system. An abrupt change in the severity or effect of obstruction can cause irreversible renal damage unless it is detected promptly. The duration of follow-up remains undefined, since the true natural history of these conditions is unknown. If an observational approach to management is undertaken, periodic monitoring of the status of the hydronephrosis and renal function is necessary. Isotope renal scans are well suited to this and provide relatively comparable quantitative assessments of both function and drainage. Concurrent ultrasonography is helpful to give a physical picture of the degree of hydronephrosis, renal parenchymal thickness, and growth. Periodic cultures are important. The duration of antibiotic therapy remains unknown. We have chosen to continue antibiotics, particularly in girls, until essentially all caliectasis has resolved. When a significant change occurs in the functional status or the degree of hydronephrosis, recommendation for surgical repair is appropriate.

Surgical management of the ureteropelvic junction obstruction can be performed at any age.[27,28] We have performed many such operations in infants without a significant incidence of complications. The overall functional and anatomic results are satisfactory. The specifics of surgical management are described elsewhere, but we have learned the importance of minimizing intraoperative manipulation of the ureteropelvic junction after the dismembering of the narrowed segment (Fig. 8.13). A number of cases have been seen in which this area of obstruction seems to be a kinking and folding of the ureter with adventitial bands constricting the ureter against the dilated pelvis. On occasion, a crossing lower pole vessel is the cause of obstruction. Avoiding devascularization of the proximal ureter during mobilization reduces the risks of postoperative stenosis. Minimizing handling during the procedure reduces postoperative edema with transient obstruction. We do not routinely use nephrostomy or stenting tubes. A Foley catheter is often left in the bladder for 1 to 3 days. Drainage of the surgical area is also necessary.

In cases where the ureter has not been visualized preoperatively with an intravenous pyelogram, we perform a retrograde ureterogram and pyelogram to ensure that no distal obstruction or anatomic abnormality is present. Such abnormalities are unusual but would change our surgical approach and would prompt placement of a nephrostomy tube in certain instances. Postoperative monitoring includes a functional study at 1 month postoperatively and a follow-up IVP or diuretic renogram at 4 to 6 months. After this we use ultrasonography to follow the resolution of hydronephrosis. Although there is still controversy as to the specific indications for ureteropelvic junction repair in infancy, it is clear that the notable improvement in washout times and the resolution of hydronephrosis suggest the preoperative presence of obstruction. The relatively crude functional studies presently available do not demonstrate impairment, nor therefore improvement, but in our view a conservative approach that emphasizes conservation of renal function remains the most appropriate.

Ureterovesical Junction Obstruction

Obstruction of the distal ureter at the ureterovesical junction is termed *primary obstructive megaureter* (Fig. 8.14). This condition occurs secondary to previous surgery or bladder dysfunction as well, and a megaureter may also show reflux. The simple obstructed megaureter, however,

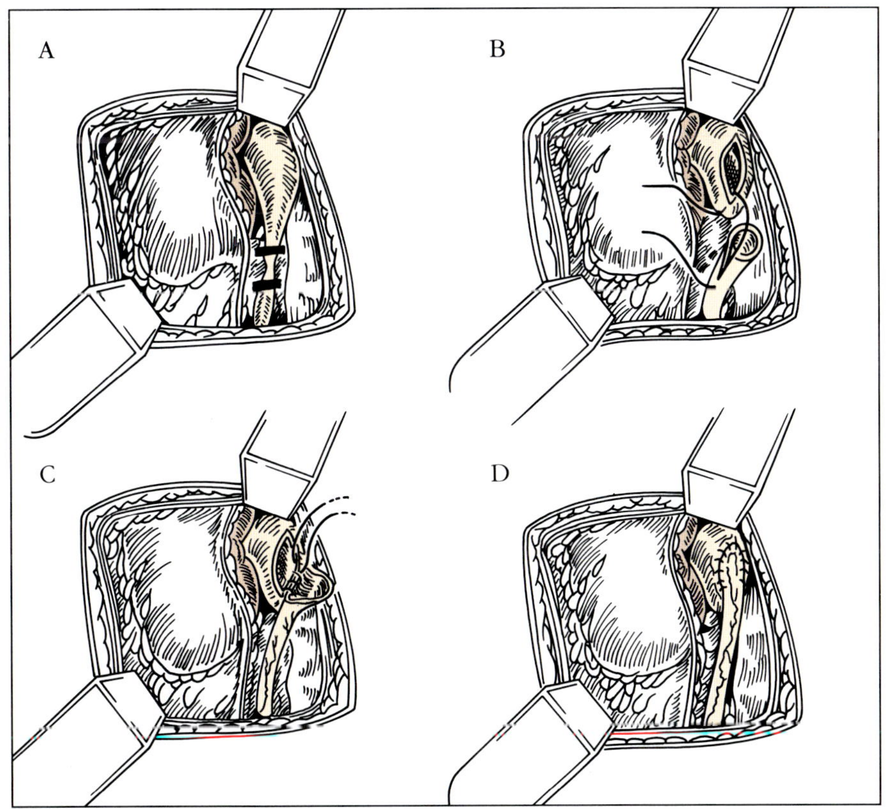

Figure 8.13 Diagram of surgical correction of ureteropelvic junction using a dismembered pyeloplasty. **A** The left pelvis and upper ureter are exposed from a posterior approach. The ureter is minimally mobilized. Bold lines indicate the lines of transection. **B** The obstructive segment has been removed and the ureter spatulated along a line facing the renal pelvis. **C** The posterior wall of the ureteropelvic anastomosis is being closed. **D** The completed repair with a wide-open ureteropelvic anastomosis. No nephrostomy tubes are used in routine cases.

is being identified prenatally and is more of a challenge, in determining the need for surgical intervention, than ureteropelvic junction obstruction. It is clear that the wide range in severity and the possibility of spontaneous resolution are true phenomena. Previous series of older children probably represented selected cases with infection or complications and were a subgroup of the patients now being identified prenatally. Many of the same issues pertain to ureterovesical obstructions as to ureteropelvic obstructions, in terms of the necessity for careful functional and anatomic evaluation. Because of the large-capacity system including both a dilated pelvis and ureter, the assessment of obstruction can be an even greater problem. These children can have complications, particularly those caused by infection, which will prompt a more aggressive treatment approach. Ureteral dilatation and hydronephrosis in the presence of a significant infection are not diagnostic of obstruction. Many of these children will show resolution of what was presumably toxic hydronephrosis due to paralysis of the smooth musculature from the bacterial infection. Careful assessment after complete resolution of the infection is necessary. During the acute episode it is important to confirm that high-grade obstruction is not present by either an IVP or isotope renography. In some instances these children require emergency decompression.

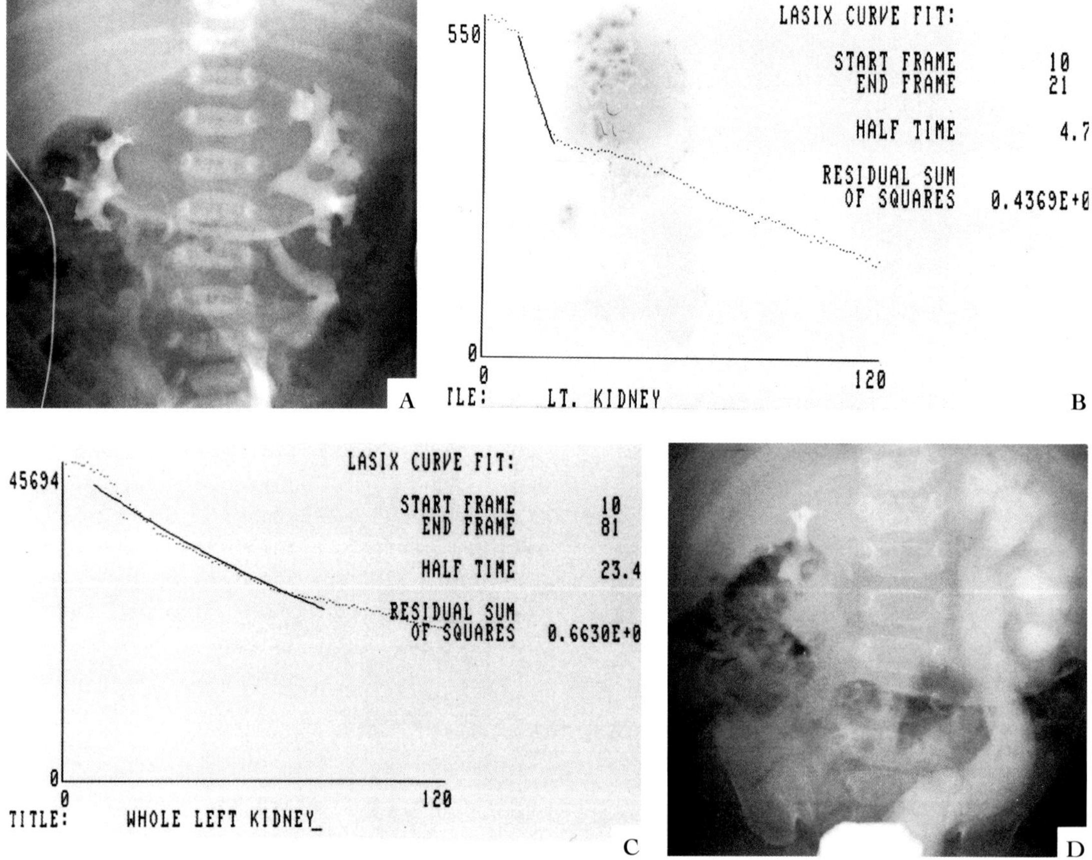

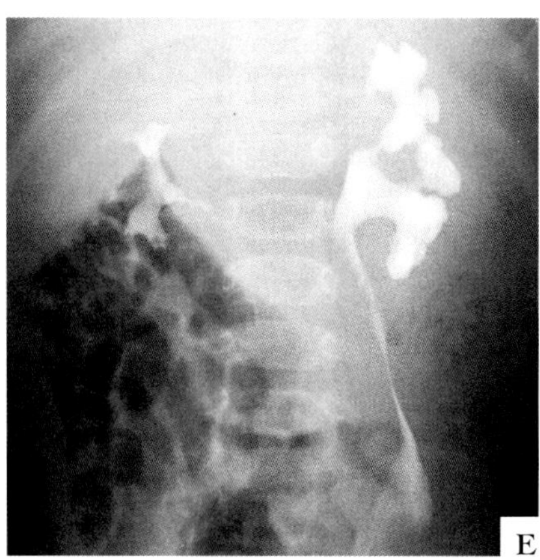

Figure 8.14 **A** IVP of a boy with hydroureteronephrosis shortly after an episode of urosepsis. A very mild ureterovesical junction obstruction is suggested. **B** Diuretic renogram (MAG-3) at the same time as the IVP, confirming the absence of obstruction, with a $t_{1/2}$ washout time of 4.7 minutes. Note the biphasic nature of the curve. Follow-up ultrasound 5 months later showed markedly increased hydronephrosis, and **C** a MAG-3 renogram showed an obstructive pattern with a $t_{1/2}$ of 23.4 minutes. **D** IVP also demonstrated evidence of obstruction with a dilated, tortuous, poorly draining megaureter. **E** Postoperative IVP (6 weeks) shows prompt function and drainage of the affected system.

The point of obstruction in primary megaureter has been described as an aperistaltic segment of distal ureter at the bladder wall. Histologically, this shows disordered collagen and muscle bundles. The presumed pathophysiologic mechanism is that dysfunctional peristalsis produces a functional obstruction; the subsequent ureteral dilatation impairs the efficiency of further urine transmission. Cases of spontaneous improvement in significant dilatation have been well documented, but at present it is difficult to determine which cases will resolve spontaneously and which will not.[29] Any child with evidence of markedly delayed drainage with functional impairment and significant dilatation should undergo surgical repair. In other children an observational approach can be elected, with the same considerations as noted above and with careful monitoring and antibiotic coverage.

If surgical management is elected, this can be performed in infancy with minimal complications.[30] Surgical repair of the megaureter is associated with a greater incidence of complications than repair of ureteropelvic junction obstructions. A number of alternative surgical techniques have been developed for this procedure. For a massively dilated ureter, excisional tapering of the ureter with reimplantation is probably the most effective (Fig. 8.15). Others have recommended an infolding or plication technique for this repair. The latter tends to produce a more bulky ureter to be reimplanted. We usually stent tapered ureters for 5 to 7 days and obtain a functional study at 1 month postoperatively. These children need a follow-up cystogram or radionuclide cystogram to make sure that no reflux is present. Postoperative reflux may occur in approximately 10% to 12% of cases, but with observation over the subsequent year the vast majority of these resolve spontaneously and do not require sec-

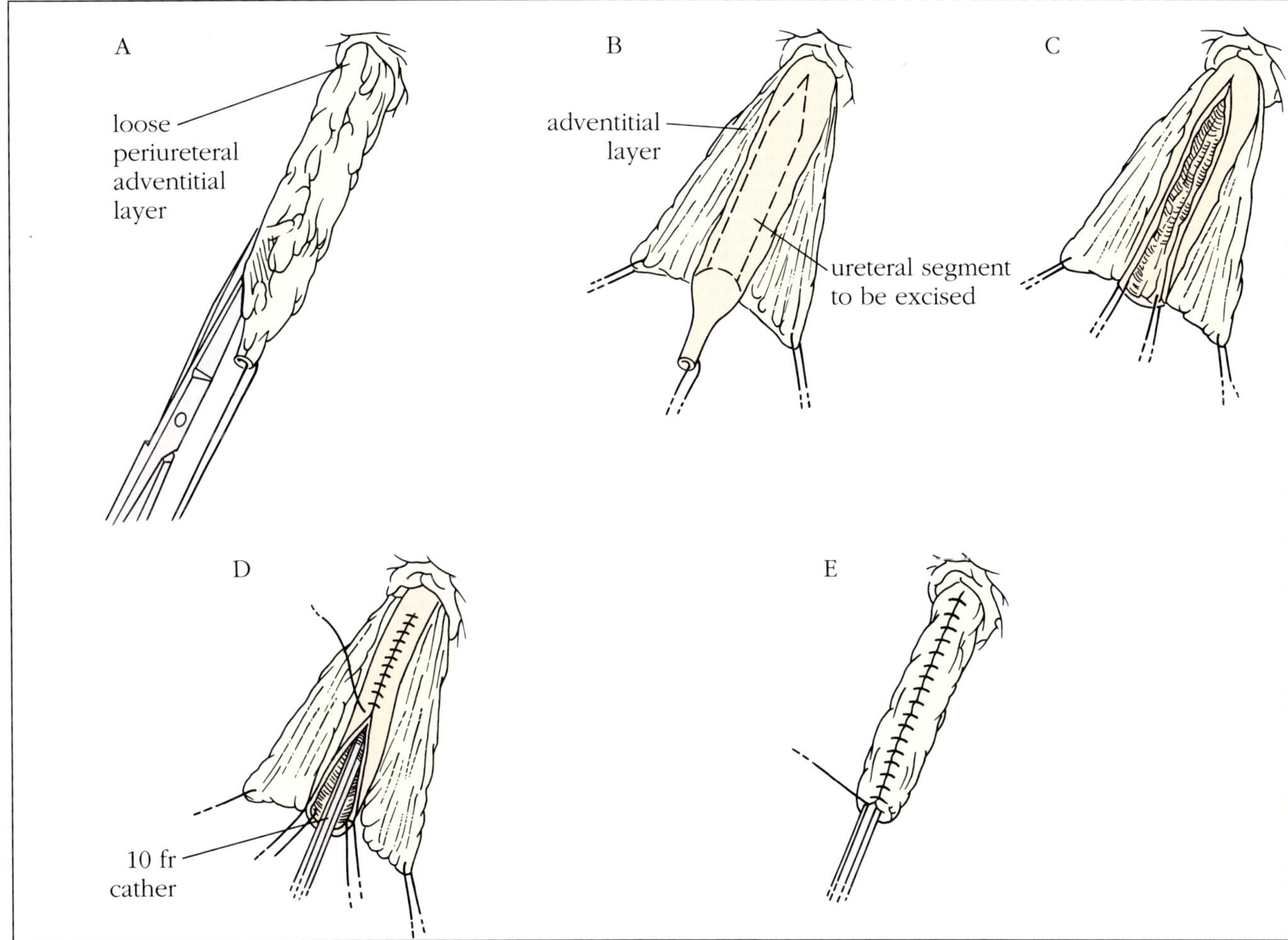

Figure 8.15 Diagram of the surgical tapering of a dilated obstructed megaureter. **A** The ureter has been fully mobilized, leaving a loose layer of adventitial tissue surrounding the ureter. **B** This is bluntly dissected from the area of the ureter to be excised. **C** The anterolateral segment of ureteral wall has been excised. This segment is the watershed of ureteral vasculature. **D** The ureter is being reapproximated over a 10 Fr catheter using a running suture line of absorbable suture. **E** Completed tapering, ready for reimplantation into the bladder as in a routine ureteral reimplantation.

ondary operations. Obstructions of repaired megaureters are a risk and may require endoscopic stenting and dilatation or even secondary reoperation if this is not effective. The usual surgical principles of meticulous attention to maintaining the ureteral vasculature are just as important with megaureter repair as with ureteropelvic junction repair.

Conclusion

The management of hydronephrosis in children has changed significantly with ultrasonography, which has identified an expanded population of children with asymptomatic hydronephrosis of unclear significance. The identification of this new patient population has emphasized the critical importance of obtaining a careful anatomic and functional assessment of the hydronephrotic urinary tract. It has served to focus attention on the functional consequences of congenital obstruction and the significant need for a better understanding of the natural history of these conditions. The cornerstone of management of these children is the recognition that the basic goal is to protect the child's capacity for renal function and that hydronephrosis is an indicator of increased risk for renal damage from either obstruction or infection. Although observational management is appropriate in certain instances, recognition of the responsibility implicit within this is of critical importance. Similarly, surgical management of the neonate with hydronephrosis obligates the surgeon to be familiar with the surgical repair of delicate anatomic structures and the attendant complications. In any evaluation of hydronephrosis the entire urinary tract must be included, from the urethra to the kidney. Hydronephrosis does not always indicate that obstruction is present but always requires that the possibility of obstruction be considered. Hydronephrosis is not a normal condition and, regardless of the management scheme, it requires careful monitoring.

References

1. Bellinger MF, Comstock CH, Grosso D, Zaino R. Fetal posterior urethral valves and renal dysplasia at 15 weeks gestational age. *J Urol.* 1983;129:1238–1239.
2. Mandell J, Blyth BR, Peters CA, Retik AB, Estroff JA, Benacerraf BR. Structural genitourinary defects detected in utero. *Radiology.* 1991;178:193–196.
3. Scott JE. Fetal ureteric reflux. *Br J Urol.* 1987;59:291–296.
4. Bosman G, Reuss A, Nijman JM, Wladimiroff JW. Prenatal diagnosis, management and outcome of fetal uretero-pelvic junction obstruction. *Ultrasound Med Biol.* 1991;17:117–120.
5. Benacerraf BR, Peters CA, Mandell J. The prenatal evolution of a nonfunctioning kidney in the setting of obstructive hydronephrosis. *J Clin Ultrasound.* 1991;19:446–450.
6. Nakayama DK, Harrison MR, de Lorimier, AA. Prognosis of posterior urethral valve syndrome presenting at birth. *J Pediatr Surg.* 1986;21:43–45.
7. Glick PL, Harrison MR, Golbus MS, et al. Management of the fetus with congenital hydronephrosis, II: prognostic criteria and selection for treatment. *J Pediatr Surg.* 1985;20:376–387.
8. Harrison MR, Ross N, Noall RA, de Lorimier AA. Correction of congenital hydronephrosis in utero, I: the model: fetal urethral obstruction produces hydronephrosis and pulmonary hypoplasia in fetal lambs. *J Pediatr Surg.* 1983;18:247–256.
9. Manning FA. Fetal surgery for obstructive uropathy: rational considerations. *Am J Kid Dis.* 1987;10:259–267.
10. Crombleholme TM, Harrison MR, Langer JC, et al. Early experience with open fetal surgery for congenital hydronephrosis. *J Pediatr Surg.* 1988;23:1114–1121.
11. Nicolini U, Rodeck C, Fisk N. Shunt treatment for fetal obstructive uropathy. *Lancet.* 1987;2:1338–1339.
12. Estroff JA, Mandell J, Benacerraf BR. Increased renal parenchymal echogenicity in the fetus: importance and clinical outcome. *Radiology.* 1991;181:135–139.
13. Kass E, Fink-Bennett D. Contemporary techniques for the radioisotopic evaluation of the dilated urinary tract. *Urol Clin North Am.* 1990;17:273–289.
14. Heyman S, Duckett J. Extraction factor: an estimate of single kidney function in children during routine radionuclide renography with 99m-technetium diethylenetriaminepentaacetic acid. *J Urol.* 1988;140:780–783.
15. Whitaker R. The Whitaker test. *Urol Clin North Am.* 1979;6:529–539.
16. Woodbury P, Mitchell M, Scheidler D, Adams M, Rink R, McNulty A. Constant pressure perfusion: a method to determine obstruction in the upper urinary tract. *J Urol.* 1989;142 (part 2):632–635.
17. King LR, Hatcher PA. Natural history of fetal and neonatal hydronephrosis. *Urology.* 1990;35:433–438.
18. Lebowitz RL, Johan BG. The coexistence of ureteropelvic junction obstruction and reflux. *Am J Radiol.* 1982; 140:231–238.
19. Kroovand RL, Perlmutter AD. A one-stage surgical approach to ectopic ureterocele. *J Urol.* 1979;122:367–369.
20. Rich MA, Keating MA, Snyder HM III, Duckett JW Jr. Low transurethral incision of single system intravesical ureteroceles in children. *J Urol.* 1990;144:120–121.
21. Hendren WH. Posterior urethral valves in boys: a broad clinical spectrum. *J Urol.* 1971;106:298–307.
22. Johnston JH, Kulatilake AE. The sequlae of posterior urethral valves. *Br J Urol.* 1971;43:743–748.
23. Peters CA, Bolkier M, Bauer SB, et al. The urodynamic consequences of posterior urethral valves. *J Urol.* 1990;144(part 2):122–126.
24. Brown T, Mandell J, Lebowitz RL. Neonatal hydronephrosis in the ultrasound era. *AJR.* 1987;148:959–963.
25. Hanna MK, Jeffs RD, Sturgess JM, Baskin M. Ureteral structure and ultrastructure, II: congenital ureteropelvic junction obstruction and primary obstructive megaureter. *J Urol.* 1976;116:725–730.
26. Ransley PG, Dhillon HK, Gordon I, Duffy PG, Dillon MJ, Barratt TM. Postnatal management of hydronephrosis diagnosed by prenatal ultrasound. *J Urol.* 1990;144(part 2): 584–587.
27. Bernstein GT, Mandell J, Lebowitz RL, Bauer S, Colodny AH, Retik AB. Ureteropelvic junction obstruction in the neonate. *J Urol.* 1988;140(part 2):1216–1221.
28. Hendren WH, Radhakrishnan J, Middleton AW Jr. Pediatric pyeloplasty. *J Pediatr Surg.* 1980;15:133–144.
29. Keating M, Escala J, Snyder H, Heyman S, Duckett J. Changing concepts in management of primary obstructive megaureter. *J Urol.* 1989;142(part 2):636–640.
30. Peters CA, Mandell J, Lebowitz RL, et al. Congenital obstructed megaureter in early infancy: diagnosis and treatment. *J Urol.* 1989;142:641–645.

CHAPTER 9

The Neurogenic Bladder

Steven A. Kaplan

The purpose of this chapter is to provide the reader with a clear understanding of the basic mechanisms that underlie the physiology of micturition. The lower urinary tract is very well suited for its primary function, the storage and timely expulsion of urine. The storage function of the bladder is largely based on its ability to increase in volume, up to a point, with little or no change in intravesical pressure. The sphincter action of both the vesical neck and proximal urethra maintains continence despite the wide range in intravesical pressures that occurs during ordinary physical activity.

Neurophysiology of Normal Voiding

Micturition is a complex series of finely tuned and integrated neuromuscular events that involve many neurologic pathways (Fig. 9.1). Final integration of these events occurs in the rostral pons in an area known as the pontine micturition center.[1]

The micturition reflex is an event characterized by relaxation of the urinary sphincter, opening of the bladder outlet, and contraction of the detrusor muscle, all occurring in a coordinated fashion. As the bladder fills with urine, intravesical pressure remains low and fairly constant (normal compliance).[1] Electrical activity of the external urethral sphincter gradually increases as the bladder distends. The bladder neck remains closed throughout this period and remains so except during voiding. During voiding there is relaxation of the external urethral sphincter, a concomitant fall in urethral pressure, and the onset of a detrusor contraction. Voiding can be voluntarily interrupted by contraction of the external urethral sphincter (Fig. 9.2).

Although primarily centered in the rostral brain center, the micturition reflex is dependent on other neurologic components, specifically the sacral cord somatic and parasympathetic nerves, as well as on thoracolumbar sympathetics.[1,2] Briefly, voluntary control of micturition involves several suprapontine pathways. Interruption of these pathways results in loss of control of the micturition

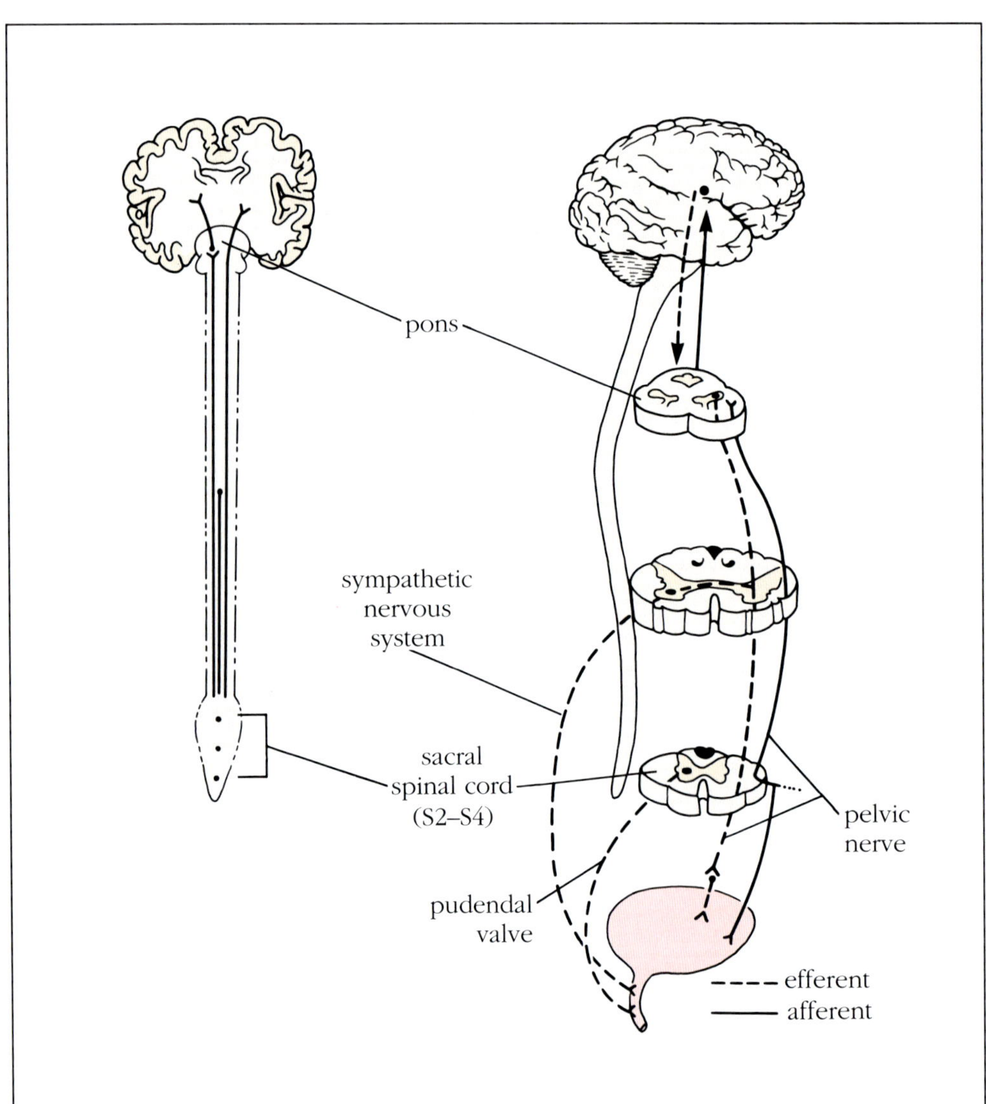

Figure 9.1 Neurologic pathways in micturition.

reflex. The "integration center" for both the sacral and pontine micturition centers is within the rostral brain stem. When these supraspinal tracts are injured (i.e., spinal cord injury or multiple sclerosis), detrusor–external sphincter dyssynergia (DESD) ensues. Voluntary control of the external urethral sphincter is coordinated with direct cortical pathways between the pudendal nucleus and cerebral cortex (see Fig. 9.1).

Sympathetic autonomic pathways have two roles in modulation of micturition. First, the α-adrenergic system prevents premature bladder contractions by affecting the parasympathetic synapse. Second, maintenance of vesical tone is modulated by sympathetic nerve fibers. In summary, sympathetic nerves aid in modulation of urine storage. This suggests that these systems are "at rest" during voiding.

The role of the sympathetic nervous system in voiding is controversial. Modulation of reflex activity affecting micturition is an important function of the intramural neuronal network. α-Adrenoreceptors of the sympathetic system mediate the storage of urine in two ways. The first action is by closure of both the proximal urethra and the bladder neck; the second action is by inhibition of neural transmission between the pre- and postganglionic parasympathetic nerves.

The sacral micturition center is composed of both afferent and efferent parasympathetic "pelvic" pathways and pudendal pathways. These are located between S-2 and S-4. Neurologic lesions that affect this pathway, such as in diabetes, may impair bladder contractility. Neurologic lesions that interrupt any of these nerve pathways cause voiding dysfunction. Injury to pathways connecting the "sacral micturition center" and the brain stem invariably results in DESD. This is of particular importance to urologists because untreated DESD patients are at high risk for serious urologic complications such as hydronephrosis, vesicoureteral reflux, infection, and stones.[3] Neurologic lesions that interfere with the sacral reflex arc, such as diabetic neuropathy and herniated lumbar discs, may cause a constellation of voiding symptoms such as decreased bladder sensation and incomplete bladder emptying.[4]

The primary parasympathetic nerve involved in micturition is the pelvic nerve. Its primary neurotransmitter at both the pre- and the postganglionic synapses is acetylcholine. However, recent reports suggest the presence of noncholinergic, nonadrenergic receptors at the postganglionic synapse.[5] The pelvic nerve nucleus is located in the intermediolateral cell column of the second, third, and fourth segments of the sacral spinal cord.[6] Afferent

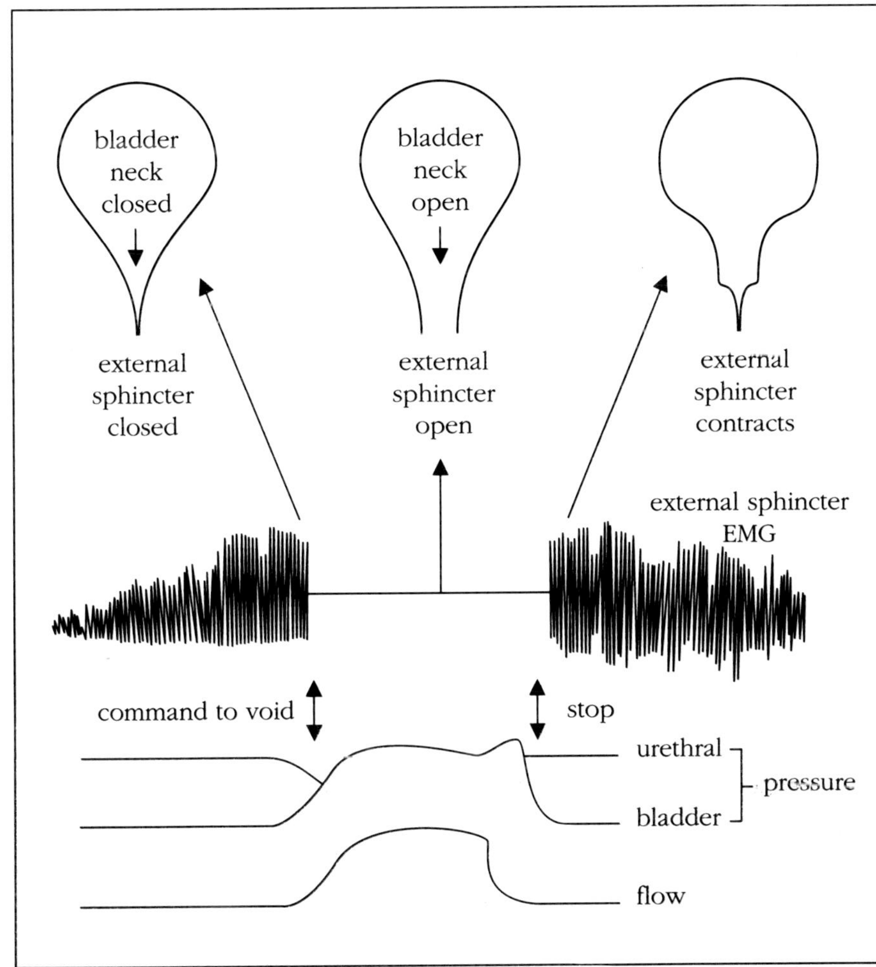

Figure 9.2 A representation of the neurologic events that occur during storage of urine, bladder emptying, and sudden interruption of the voiding stream. Note that during micturition detrusor (bladder) pressure is greater than urethral pressure, with electrical silence of the EMG.

fibers are projections of dorsal spinal root ganglion axons. Of note is that there is evidence in some species that some of the afferent fibers are also located in the ventral root.[7] Afferent fibers establish many synapses after leaving the posterior root ganglion. Among these synapses are the pelvic nucleus in the intermediolateral area, the dorsal horns that ascend ipsilaterally, and the dorsal horns that cross the midline and ascend the contralateral spinothalamic tract. It is believed that the afferent fibers of the pelvic nerve are most important for initiating voiding.[8] Impulses from tension receptors in the bladder wall are transmitted by small-diameter Aδ and C fibers. Bladder afferents contain substance P, vasoactive intestinal polypeptide (VIP), and other neuropeptides. In patients with lower spinal cord lesions, Crowe et al.[9] reported a decrease in the density of VIP, calcitonin gene-related peptide, and substance P. These substances are associated with both parasympathetic and sensory nerve function. In contrast, there was little change in the density of neuropeptide Y (NPY) or somatostatin-immunoreactive nerves, which are associated with sympathetic nerve function. The minimal change in NPY may refute the concept that lower motor neuron lesions lead to "adrenergic overgrowth." Although NPY inhibits electrically induced, tetrodotoxin-sensitive smooth muscle contractions in the normal bladder, these nerves may have a compensatory stabilizing effect in patients with lower motor nerve lesions.

Detrusor contractions can be caused by either administration of acetylcholine or electrical stimulation of the pelvic nerve.[10] However, the bladder contraction induced by electrical stimulation cannot be completely blocked by atropine, unlike the detrusor contraction elicited by administration of acetylcholine. This "atropine-resistance" phenomenon has been recognized for many years, and recent evidence suggests that it is related to a noncholinergic, nonadrenergic neurotransmitter (NANC).

Vasopressin has been described as having a putative neuromodulatory role in the lower urinary tract. Holmquist et al.[11] studied the effects of arginine vasopressin (AVP) in isolated bladder and urethral preparations of both rabbits and humans. AVP binding sites were located in both the circular and longitudinal smooth muscle cell layers as well as in the submucosa of the rabbit bladder. In contrast, there were no AVP binding sites in human bladders. In the rabbit bladder and urethra, AVP-induced bladder contractions could be antagonized noncompetitively by a selective antagonist, A16. In contrast, A16 had no effect on electrical stimulation. These results suggest that AVP is an unlikely NANC transmitter, although its relatively high concentration suggests a possible modulatory role. Its effects in humans remain doubtful.

Tachykinins are a family of neuropeptides present in the urinary bladder. These peptides exert a variety of effects, including smooth muscle contraction, vasodilation, and facilitation of neurotransmitter release. These effects are mediated by the activation of three distinct receptor types: NK-1, NK-2, and NK-3. In humans, only the NK-2 receptor is biologically active. Maggi et al.[12] reported on the effects of (βAla8)-neurokinin A[4–10], a selective NK-2 tachykinin receptor agonist, in rat and guinea pig bladder strips. Their results indicate that this substance has a facilatory effect on micturition and that it induces significant contractions. The potential clinical applicability of this drug is in patients with either impaired or absent detrusor contractions.

The first event in the micturition reflex is relaxation of the external urethral sphincter. This is caused by cessation of efferent pudendal nerve firing.[1] At the same time sympathetic activity is suppressed, which results in cessation of the inhibitory effects of sympathetic stimulation. Therefore, the combination of neural impulses across the pelvic ganglion and efferent postganglionic firing results in a detrusor contraction. Finally, inhibition of vesical neck stimulation allows opening of the urethra (see Fig. 9.1).

Spinal cord injury, transverse myelitis, multiple sclerosis, and myelodysplasia, all of which can interrupt this "long routed micturition reflex," usually lead to uncoordinated micturition.[1] Control over the micturition reflex is accomplished by poorly understood neural pathways connecting different parts of the brain with the pontine micturition center. Suprapontine neurologic lesions, such as cerebrovascular accident, tumor, Parkinson's disease, and normal-pressure hydrocephalus, usually result in loss of control over the micturition reflex.[1]

Physiology of Voiding

The behavior of the normal bladder is dependent on both active and passive properties. Collagen, elastin, and resting smooth muscle are the elements mainly responsible for the passive properties of the bladder. In contrast, the active behavior of the bladder is determined by the contractile elements of smooth muscle. Elasticity has been defined as that property of a material which determines the tendency of the stressed material to return to its unstressed geometrical configuration; viscosity is that property of a material which tends to retard deformation of the stressed material. Elasticity can be measured by the change in wall tension as the bladder is stretched. In a cystometrogram bladder pressure and volume are measured. When pressure and volume are plotted against each other the relationship is not linear, indicating that physical properties other than elasticity are involved.

The response of the bladder to stretch is dependent on a number of factors, including the duration of stretch, the rate at which it is stretched, and hysteresis. When the bladder is stretched rapidly, detrusor pressure and wall tension are great, but if the bladder is stretched to a new length and that length is maintained, pressure falls. Therefore, during a cystometrogram, the faster the filling rate, the higher the rise in pressure. *Hysteresis* refers to a property of the bladder in which the tension–length or pressure–volume relationship is dependent on the conditions that existed prior to the strain, i.e., the degree of filling. In theory, if the bladder is filled and emptied at a constant rate, each phase will have a different pressure–volume curve. However, recent studies in whole rabbit bladders have revealed that peak isovolumetric pressure after electrical stimulation remains the same regardless of the method of filling or the rapidity of emptying.[13]

Compliance refers to the ability of the urinary bladder to fill at relatively low intravesical pressure. Patients with lower motor neuron lesions secondary to pathologic spinal cord conditions are at particular risk for developing poor compliance.[14] In a retrospective analysis of 489 patients with spinal cord injury, poor bladder compliance was noted in 54 (11%) of patients. The majority of these had injuries of the sacral cord.

Pathophysiology of Lower Urinary Tract Symptoms

On the basis of urinary tract physiology, it is useful to classify lower urinary tract dysfunction into one of three groups: bladder filling and storage problems, bladder emptying problems, and combinations of the two.[1] Accurate diagnosis of a problem depends on careful assessment of the patient's history, physical examination, laboratory studies, and urodynamic assessment. Bladder symptoms are characterized as either irritative or obstructive. Irritative symptoms include urinary frequency, urgency, urge incontinence, nocturia, dysuria, and a constant feeling of suprapubic discomfort, pain, or urge to void. Obstructive symptoms include urinary hesitancy, decreased size and force of the stream, a feeling of incomplete bladder emptying, postvoid dribbling, overflow incontinence, and total urinary retention. Symptoms described by the patient are often unreliable predictors of underlying pathology and should serve only as a guideline for directing further diagnostic evaluation. The most remediable cause of urinary bladder symptoms is urinary tract infection, and no patient should be further evaluated until infection has been excluded by urinalysis and appropriate cultures. If hematuria is noted on routine urinalysis where infection has been excluded, evaluation of the kidneys and upper tracts by either intravenous pyelography or ultrasonography and cystoscopy is mandatory to exclude neoplastic conditions or urolithiasis.

Screening urodynamic evaluation should be performed on any uninfected patient with persistent bladder symptoms that do not respond to empiric treatment. For most patients, an accurate diagnosis can be obtained by cystometry, estimation of urinary flow rate, postvoid residual urine volume and, in selected cases, voiding cystourethrography. More sophisticated studies, such as sphincter electromyography, urethral pressure profilometry, and combined video/urodynamic studies, are necessary only in patients with persistent diagnostic and therapeutic problems that have not been answered by the screening procedures.[14] Cystometry is performed by filling the bladder with gas or liquid while recording the detrusor pressure, bladder volume, and sensations of first urge and severe urge to void. Cystometry is most useful for detecting involuntary bladder contractions (Fig. 9.3).

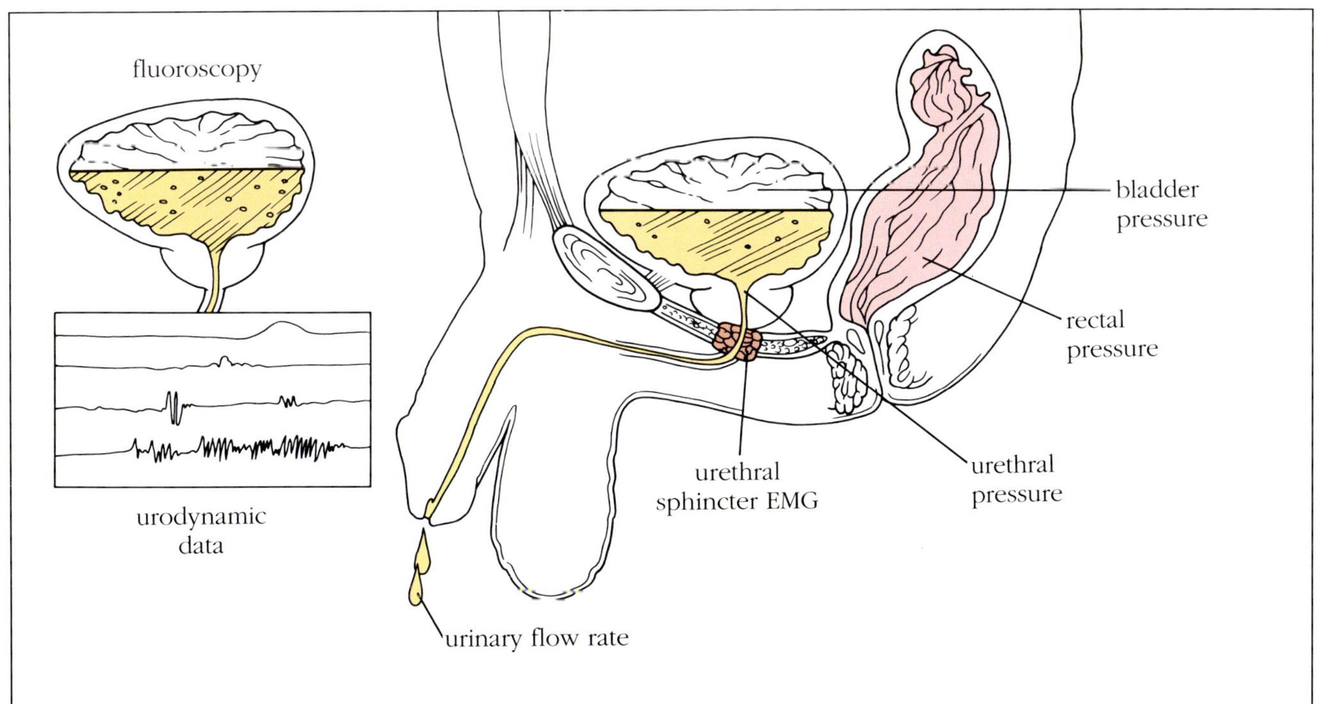

Figure 9.3 The components of synchronous video/pressure/flow urodynamics.

Urinary flow rate can be measured electronically with commercially available flowmeters, or the examiner can simply watch the patient void. Reduced urinary flow suggests either bladder outlet obstruction or impairment of bladder contractility.[64]

URINARY FILLING AND STORAGE PROBLEMS
Involuntary Detrusor Contractions

The most common cause of irritative voiding symptoms is involuntary detrusor contractions, defined as a sudden nonvolitional rise in bladder pressure. The many etiologies of involuntary bladder contractions can be classified as neurologic, those secondary to long-term bladder out-

let obstruction, or idiopathic. Involuntary bladder contractions caused by neurologic disorders are categorized as detrusor hyperreflexia. In the absence of a neurologic lesion the condition is termed detrusor instability.

Involuntary detrusor contractions are treated according to cause (Fig. 9.4). When they are secondary to bladder outlet obstruction, relief of the obstruction usually leads to their cessation. When no obstruction is present, the "gold standard" of therapy has been anticholinergic medication such as propantheline bromide. Other agents used include musculotropic agents, which act directly on smooth muscle distal to the cholinergic receptor. Oxybutynin (Ditropan) has strong musculotropic proper-

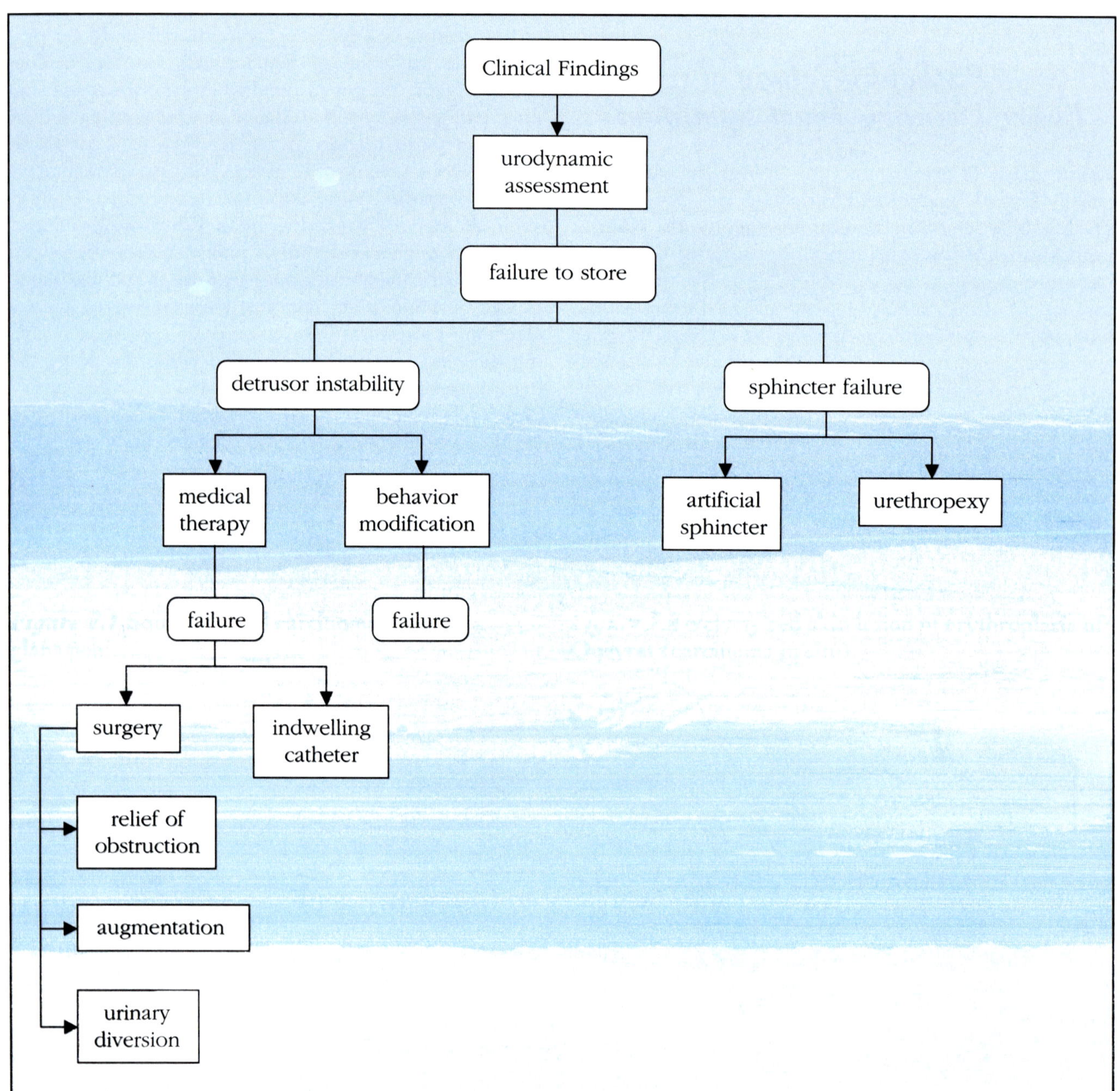

Figure 9.4 Treatment algorithm for patients with storage dysfunction.

ties together with moderate anticholinergic properties. There have been reports comparing the clinical efficacy of propantheline with that of oxybutynin. Gajewski and Awad found that 5 mg t.i.d. of oxybutynin was superior to 15 mg t.i.d. of propantheline in patients with detrusor hyperreflexia.[15] The use of intravesical instillation of oxybutynin has been reported but awaits further clinical trials.[16] Other agents reported include calcium channel antagonists, potassium channel openers, prostaglandin inhibitors, β-adrenergic agonists, and tricyclic antidepressants. Many patients also require intermittent self-catheterization to empty the bladder. Other therapeutic modalities presently under investigation include behavior modification, functional electrical neural stimulation (transcutaneously, percutaneously, or by direct stimulation of nerve roots), surgical "denervation procedures" such as cystolysis, and operations designed to increase bladder capacity, such as ileocecal augmentation cystoplasty.

Small-Capacity Bladder

Normal bladder capacity ranges from 300 to 500 mL. Therefore, irritative voiding symptoms occur with low-capacity bladders, defined as 200 mL or less. The two most common etiologies of a "pathologically" reduced bladder capacity are active infection or involuntary detrusor contractions. Other causes include scarring from tuberculosis, radiation, or interstitial cystitis. Patients with small bladders void frequently to prevent the discomfort brought on by a full bladder.

It is very difficult to distinguish "idiopathic sensory urge" (i.e., urinary frequency, urgency, and occasional urge incontinence in the absence of intrinsic lower urinary tract disease) from a pathologically reduced bladder. Both tuberculosis and interstitial cystitis exhibit characteristic cystoscopic changes; however, these are not present in all patients. Repeating the cystoscopic examination under high (above T-6) spinal or general anesthesia may be useful, since the bladder capacity of patients with detrusor fibrosis remains small, whereas in those with idiopathic sensory urgency it is normal.

Therapy of symptomatic small-capacity bladders is directed at the underlying pathophysiology. All patients with sensory urge should undergo diagnostic cystoscopy and any suspicious lesions should be biopsied, since one of the most important diagnostic entities to rule out is transitional-cell carcinoma in situ of the bladder. This condition may be overlooked unless routine bladder biopsies are obtained, even when there are no overt cystoscopic lesions. Balloon hydrodistention with a specially designed catheter (Helmstein) can be used under anesthesia to distend a bladder with a capacity of less than 400 mL. The catheter is introduced into the bladder under high epidural anesthesia and the balloon is inflated to the volume needed to achieve a balloon pressure equal to the systolic blood pressure, usually a volume of 500 to 1000 mL. The bladder is left in this distended state

for 4 hours while fluid is added or removed from the balloon as necessary to maintain the desired pressure. This treatment has proven effective in over 60% of patients, but there have been reports of intraoperative bladder rupture in 5% of cases. The rupture is usually retroperitoneal and can be treated by leaving an indwelling vesical catheter for 5 to 7 days and administering broad-spectrum antibiotics.

If hydrodistention fails, surgical augmentation cystoplasty can be attempted, with the goals of increasing bladder capacity and lowering intravesical pressure. A segment of bowel is isolated with its vascular pedicle intact and is anastomosed to the dome of the bladder. In some instances it may be necessary to excise most of the diseased bladder and anastomose the bowel to the remaining trigone. Supravesical diversion should be reserved for patients who either are not amenable or do not respond to hydrodistention or augmentation cystoplasty.

Sensory Urgency

Sensory urgency comprises a constellation of symptoms characterized by urinary frequency and urgency, often accompanied by suprapubic pain and discomfort or a constant urge to void, all without any overt urodynamic abnormalities. These symptoms can usually be reproduced at relatively low bladder volumes. At the time of these symptoms no bladder contractions are evident on cystometry and bladder capacity is normal under anesthesia. Diagnostic misnomers for this symptom complex have included "urethral syndrome," "trigonitis," and "interstitial cystitis." Patients with idiopathic sensory urgency void frequently, not because of involuntary detrusor contractions or infection but simply because it hurts too much if they *don't* void.

Therapy directed at curing infection or alleviating involuntary bladder contractions is doomed to failure. Empiric therapy in this group of patients is also unsuccessful and, in fact, may exacerbate the condition. Patients develop secondary psychologic symptoms and are often thought to have a primary psychiatric etiology for their symptoms; there is no absolute way to distinguish patients with primary psychopathology from those who have developed secondary psychiatric symptoms because of their "incurable bladder condition." However, regardless of the underlying etiology, structured behavior modification seems to be the most practical approach for these patients.

SPHINCTER ABNORMALITIES
Stress Incontinence

This describes involuntary voiding or leaking when the patient coughs, sneezes, or strains. In women it is almost always caused by abnormal descent of the proximal urethra when the patient increases intraabdominal pressure. The etiology is seconsary to unequal transmission of the increased intraabdominal pressure to the bladder and urethra. Leakage occurs when the intravesical pressure exceeds the intraurethral pressure. The sphincter itself is relatively normal; it is capable of maintaining a watertight seal but cannot withstand the effects of increased pressure. Therefore, any operation designed to prevent descent of the proximal urethra (the suspension operations) is almost uniformly successful in effecting a cure.

Sphincter Failure

This describes a condition in which the sphincter cannot maintain a watertight seal and leakage therefore occurs at the slightest provocation. Sphincter failure almost always is the result of neurologic injury or secondary to multiple previous surgeries.[17] Neurologic injury to either the sympathetic chain or the pudendal nerve (such as in an abdominoperineal resection) may result in sphincter

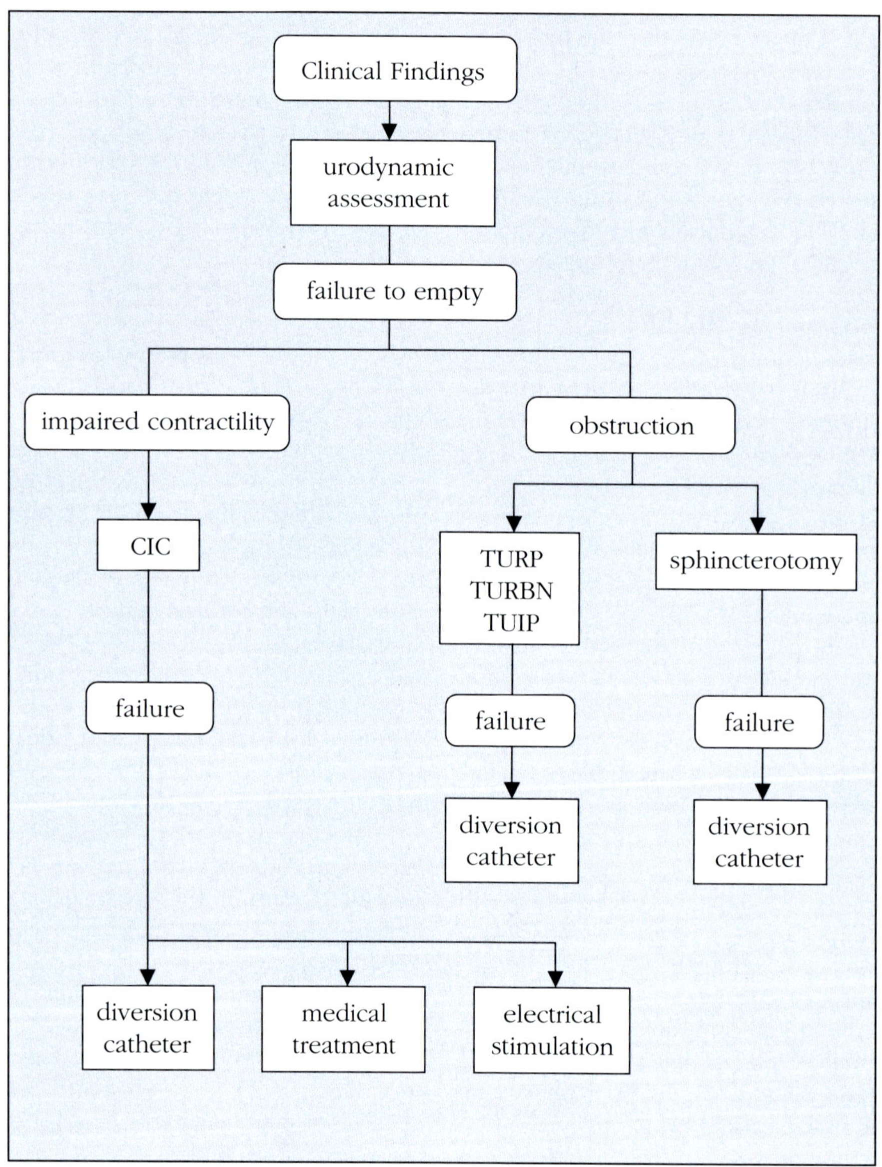

Figure 9.5 Treatment algorithm for patients with emptying dysfunction.

incontinence. The standard procedures described above to alleviate stress incontinence have no role in the management of these patients. However, the creation of a pubovaginal sling in women has met with almost universal success. In men, the insertion of an artificial urinary sphincter has met with some success. Other procedures described include the injection of substances such as Teflon or collagen around the urethra. Preliminary results have been encouraging, although careful patient selection is required.[18]

BLADDER EMPTYING PROBLEMS
Impairment of Bladder Contractility

Poor bladder emptying is secondary to either bladder outlet obstruction or impaired detrusor contractility (Fig. 9.5). Although poor detrusor contractions may be attributable to myogenic, neurogenic, or psychologic origin, it is not possible at present to distinguish between these origins with current tests. However, most neurologic causes of detrusor abnormalities are associated with other neurologic deficits. For example, a neurologic lesion that affects the second through fourth segments of the sacral spinal cord usually results not only in detrusor areflexia but also in perianal anesthesia, poor anal tone, absent voluntary control of the anal sphincter, and absence of the bulbocavernosus reflex.

The most effective therapy in this group of patients, regardless of the etiology of impaired contractility, is intermittent clean self-catheterization (CIC), timed to empty the bladder regularly and prevent periods of overdistention. A reasonable regimen is to perform CIC approximately every 6 hours, with highest priority given to accomplishing the catheterization on schedule.

The rationale for using acetylcholine-type agents is that a significant portion of bladder contractility is mediated by muscarinic cholinergic receptors. The classic agent used has been bethanechol chloride. However, despite its widespread use, bethanechol chloride has achieved disappointing results in reported trials.[19]

The use of electrical stimulation has met with variable results. This can be done either directly to the bladder or nerve roots or via transurethral intravesical electrotherapy. The most encouraging results have come from the work of Tanagho and Schmidt, who have combined dorsal rhizotomy and ventral root stimulation.[20]

Bladder Outlet Obstruction

Outlet obstruction caused by an enlarged prostate is the most common cause of voiding dysfunction in older men. Approximately 10% to 15% of men 50 years of age will require a definitive procedure for prostatism by the age of 80. The pathognomonic diagnosis for bladder outlet obstruction is a poor uroflow in the presence of an adequate detrusor contraction (greater than 45 cm H_2O).

Relief of the obstruction usually leads to resolution of the patient's symptoms. Prostatectomy has always been the primary therapy. The procedure is generally well tolerated, with a mortality rate of 0.2%, but recently there has been an explosion in the urologic literature regarding alternative methods for relief of bladder outlet obstruction. These include use of medications, balloon dilatation of the prostatic urethra, hyperthermia, laser prostatectomy, and insertion of intraprostatic coils. These have met with variable success, and long-term studies are needed to assess their efficacy. In women, the diagnosis of bladder outlet obstruction is very difficult to make and usually requires the use of sophisticated video/urodynamic techniques to delineate precisely both the site and the nature of the obstruction.[22]

Bladder neck obstruction also occurs and can be either primary or secondary. Primary bladder neck contraction is probably caused by either abnormal contraction of the vesical neck during voiding or failure of the vesical neck to open. The bladder neck usually appears normal during cystoscopic visualization, so diagnosis may not be made. Transurethral bladder neck incision is usually curative. This procedure can be done at the 5 o'clock and/or the 7 o'clock position. The reported incidence of retrograde ejaculation is between 15% and 50%.[21] α-Sympathetic blocking agents and urethral dilatation have been reported to be effective, but this has not been our experience. Secondary bladder neck obstruction is almost always secondary to surgery for prior incontinence, resulting in scarring, and must be treated surgically.

Urethral meatal stenosis is an uncommon cause of bladder outlet obstruction but is commonly overdiagnosed. Most urethral meatal "strictures" diagnosed by calibrating the size of the meatus are found on urodynamic testing not to cause obstruction. Empiric urethral dilatation or meatoplasty is common, even though there is no evidence in the literature to support their efficacy. Of greater importance is the potential harm that these procedures may cause, since these operations may themselves result in either bladder outlet obstruction or urinary incontinence by causing fibrosis of the urethra.

Urinary Storage and Emptying Problems

Detrusor–external sphincter dyssynergia (DESD) describes involuntary contraction of the external urethral sphincter during an involuntary detrusor contraction (Fig. 9.6). It is seen in patients with neurologic lesions of the suprasacral spinal cord.[22] Despite the outlet obstruction caused by the contracting external sphincter, women with this condition, in contrast to men, are at little risk for developing urologic complications unless they are treated with an indwelling catheter.[3] Their main problem is incontinence that is very difficult to manage. The optimal therapy is a combination of relaxation of the detrusor with anticholinergic medication and intermittent self-catheterization.

In men who are unable to catheterize, the next course of management is external sphincterotomy. This is done by making a transurethral incision from the bladder neck and extending it distally beyond the external urethral sphincter.

The procedure renders the patient incontinent and prevents the high intravesical pressures associated with DESD. If this fails, augmentation cystoplasty with continent vesicotomy and closure of the vesical neck probably offers the best alternative to supravesical urinary diversion.

Patients with areflexic or low-compliant bladders and sphincter incontinence usually have conditions associated with parasympathetic, sympathetic, and pudendal denervation. This can be caused by a variety of conditions, including spinal cord infarction, myelodysplasia, and prior radical pelvic surgery (abdominoperineal resection of the rectum or radical hysterectomy). Treatment of these patients is very difficult. On occasion, intermittent self-catheterization will suffice if the bladder is emptied often enough that incontinence does not occur. Patients with bladder neck denervation will occasionally respond to α-sympathetic stimulation, either alone or in combination with β-blockade. Once rendered continent, the bladder can be emptied by intermittent self-catheterization. Sometimes it is necessary to create a pubovaginal sling and then manage the patient with intermittent self-catheterization.

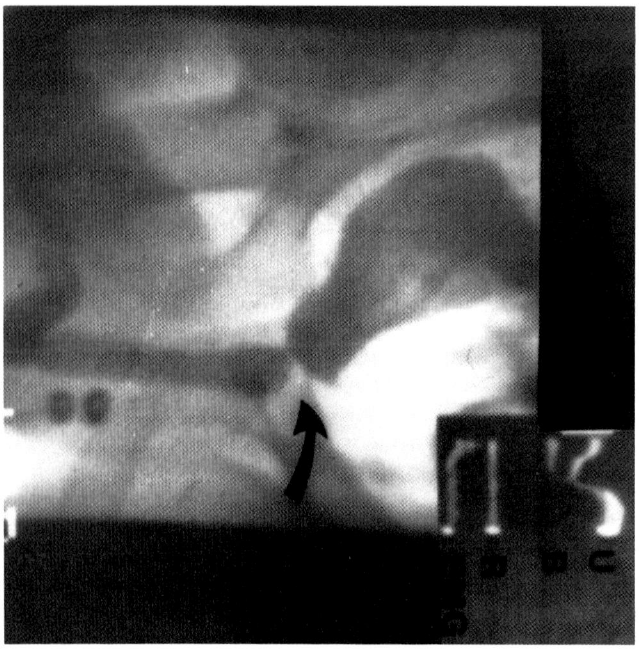

Figure 9.6 Urodynamic and radiographic representation of detrusor–external sphincter dyssynergia. Note that during sustained involuntary bladder contraction (B) there is maximal EMG activity. There is minimal passage of contrast beyond the contracted external urethral sphincter. (U = urethral pressure)

References

1. Blaivas JG. The neurophysiology of micturition: a clinical study of 550 patients. *J Urol.* 1982;127:958–962.
2. deGroat WC, Booth AM, Krier J, et al. Neural control of the urinary bladder and large intestine. In: Chandler BM, Koizumi K, Sato A, eds. Amsterdam: Elsevier Biomedical Press; 1979:2–45.
3. Blaivas JG, Barbalias GA. Detrusor external sphincter dyssynergia in men with multiple sclerosis: an ominous urologic condition. *J Urol.* 1984;131:94–97.
4. McGuire EJ, Wagner FC Jr. The effects of sacral denervation on bladder and urethral function. *Surg Gynecol Obstet.* 1980;144:343–344.
5. Elbadawi A. Neuromorphologic basis of vesicourethral function, I: histochemistry, ultrastructure, and function of intrinsic nerves of the bladder and urethra. *Neurourol Urodyn.* 1982;1:3–7.
6. Yamamoto T, Satomi H, Ise H, et al. Sacral spinal innervation of the rectal and vesical smooth muscles and the sphincteric striated muscles demonstrated by the horseradish peroxidase method. *Neurosci Lett.* 1978;7:41–42.
7. Coggeshall RE. Law of separation of function of the spinal roots. *Physiol Rev.* 1980;60:716–720.
8. deGroat WC, Kawatani M. Neural control of the urinary bladder: possible relationship between peptidergic inhibitory mechanisms and detrusor instability. *Neurourol Urodyn.* 1985;4:285–288.
9. Crowe R, Moss HE, Chapple CR, et al. Patients with lower motor spinal cord lesion—a decrease of vasoactive intestinal polypeptide, calcitonin gene-related peptide and substance P, but not neuropeptide-Y and somatostatin-immunoreactive nerves in the detrusor muscle of the bladder. *J Urol.* 1991; 145:600–604.
10. Brindley GS. Control of the bladder and urethral sphincters by the surgically implantable electrical stimulators. In: Chisolm GD, Williams DF, eds. *Scientific Foundations in Urology.* Chicago, Ill: Year Book; 1982:464–470.
11. Holmquist F, Lundin S, Larsson B, et al. Studies on binding sites, contents, and effects of AVP in isolated bladder and urethra from rabbits and humans. *Am J Physiol.* 1991; 261:R865–874.
12. Maggi CA, Giuliani S, Santicioli P, et al. Facilitation of reflex micturition by intravesical administration of (beta-Ala-8)-neurokinin-A (4-10), a selective NK-2 tachykinin receptor agonist. *J Urol.* 1991;145:184–187.
13. Kaplan SA, Blaivas JG, Brown WC, et al. Parameters of detrusor contractility, I: the effects of electrical stimulation, hyseteresis and bladder volume in an in-vitro whole rabbit bladder model. *Neurourol Urodyn.* 1991;10:1:53–59.
14. Kaplan SA, Chancellor MB, Blaivas JG. Bladder and sphincter behavior in patients with spinal cord injury. *J Urol.* 1991; 146:113–117.
15. Gajewski A, Awad A. Oxybutynin versus propantheline in patients with multiple sclerosis and detrusor hyperreflexia. *J Urol.* 1986;133:403.
16. Wein AJ. Practical uropharmacology. *Urol Clin North Am.* 1991;18:269.
17. McGuire EJ, Lytton B. Pubovaginal sling procedure for stress incontinence. *J Urol.* 1978;119:82–84.
18. Appell RA. Injectables for urethral incompetence. *World J Urol.* 1990;8:208–211.
19. Finkbeiner AE. Is bethanechol chloride clinically effective in promoting bladder emptying? *J Urol.* 1985;134:433.
20. Tanagho EA, Schmidt RA. Electrical stimulation in the clinical management of the neurogenic bladder. *J Urol.* 1988;140: 1331–1339.
21. Turner-Warwick R. Bladder outflow obstruction in the male. In: Mundy AR, Stephenson TP, Wein AJ, eds. *Urodynamics: Principles, Practice and Application.* New York, NY: Churchill Livingstone; 1984:183–204.
22. Blaivas JG, Fisher DM. Combined radiographic and urodynamic monitoring: advances in technique. *J Urol.* 1981; 125:541–544.

CHAPTER 10

Diagnosis and Management of Urinary Incontinence

M. Susan Tucker

Urinary incontinence, a symptom or sign of a pathologic process, is simply defined as the involuntary loss of urine. Although no demographic group is spared the risk of developing urinary incontinence, women are affected more commonly than men and the elderly more often than younger persons. The psychosocial consequences of urinary incontinence and the misconception that incontinence is a normal part of aging deter some afflicted patients from seeking medical attention.

Many diagnostic tests are available for the evaluation of urinary incontinence and the types of therapy include medical, behavioral, electrophysiologic, and surgical intervention. At present there is no consensus regarding optimal cost-effective evaluation and treatment for patients with urinary incontinence, but guidelines have been developed by the United States Department of Health and Human Services (Figs. 10.1–10.3).

Pathophysiology and Classification

According to the classification of Dr. Alan Wein, urinary incontinence is a disorder of bladder filling and/or storage and can be either transient or persistent. Persistent incontinence can be caused by detrusor dysfunction, bladder outlet dysfunction, or a combination of the two, resulting from anatomic, psychologic, neuromuscular, or idiopathic etiologies. Common etiologies of transient incontinence include urinary tract infection, vulvovaginal atrophy, over-the-counter or prescription medications, and temporary alteration in mental status or mobility.

Persistent urinary incontinence is classified as urge, stress, overflow, or functional. Urge incontinence, the inability to delay voiding, is caused by an uninhibited bladder contraction. Detrusor instability (DI), uninhibited bladder contraction unrelated to neurologic disease, can

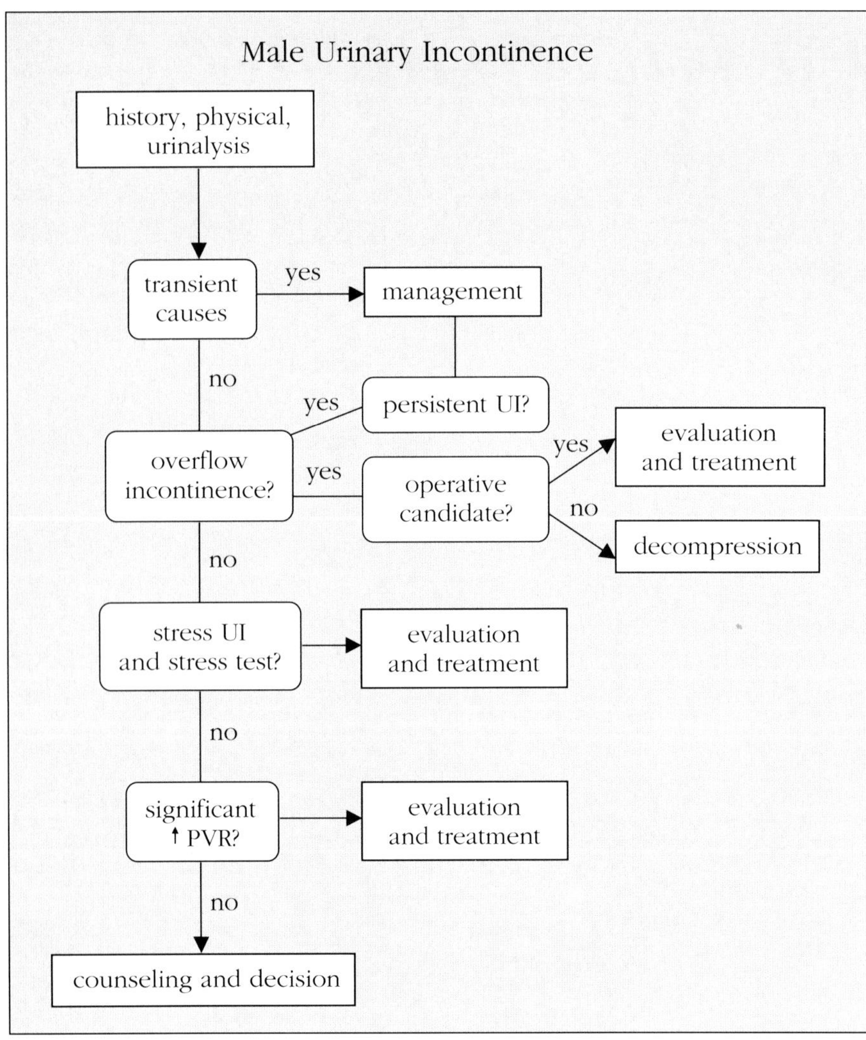

Figure 10.1 Algorithm for management of male urinary incontinence. (Adapted from Urinary Incontinence Guideline Panel, 1992)

result from outlet obstruction or can be idiopathic. The term detrusor hyperreflexia (DH) is used for uninhibited bladder contraction of neurogenic etiology. Urinary stress incontinence can be caused either by inferoposterior bladder neck displacement with an increase in intraabdominal pressure (anatomic stress urinary incontinence) or by functional disorders of the bladder neck and proximal urethra [intrinsic sphincter dysfunction (ISD)]. Overflow incontinence is characterized by the loss of urine from an overdistended bladder and may simulate stress or urge incontinence. It is caused by detrusor dysfunction with or without outlet obstruction. Overflow is usually distinguished from other types of incontinence by the presence of small-volume involuntary loss of urine associated with a large postvoid residual. Functional urinary incontinence is associated with psychologic or physical factors that prevent the patient with a normal urinary tract from getting to a toilet. A patient may be afflicted with more than one type of urinary incontinence; this is referred to as mixed-type urinary incontinence. The most common combination of mixed incontinence is stress with urge incontinence.

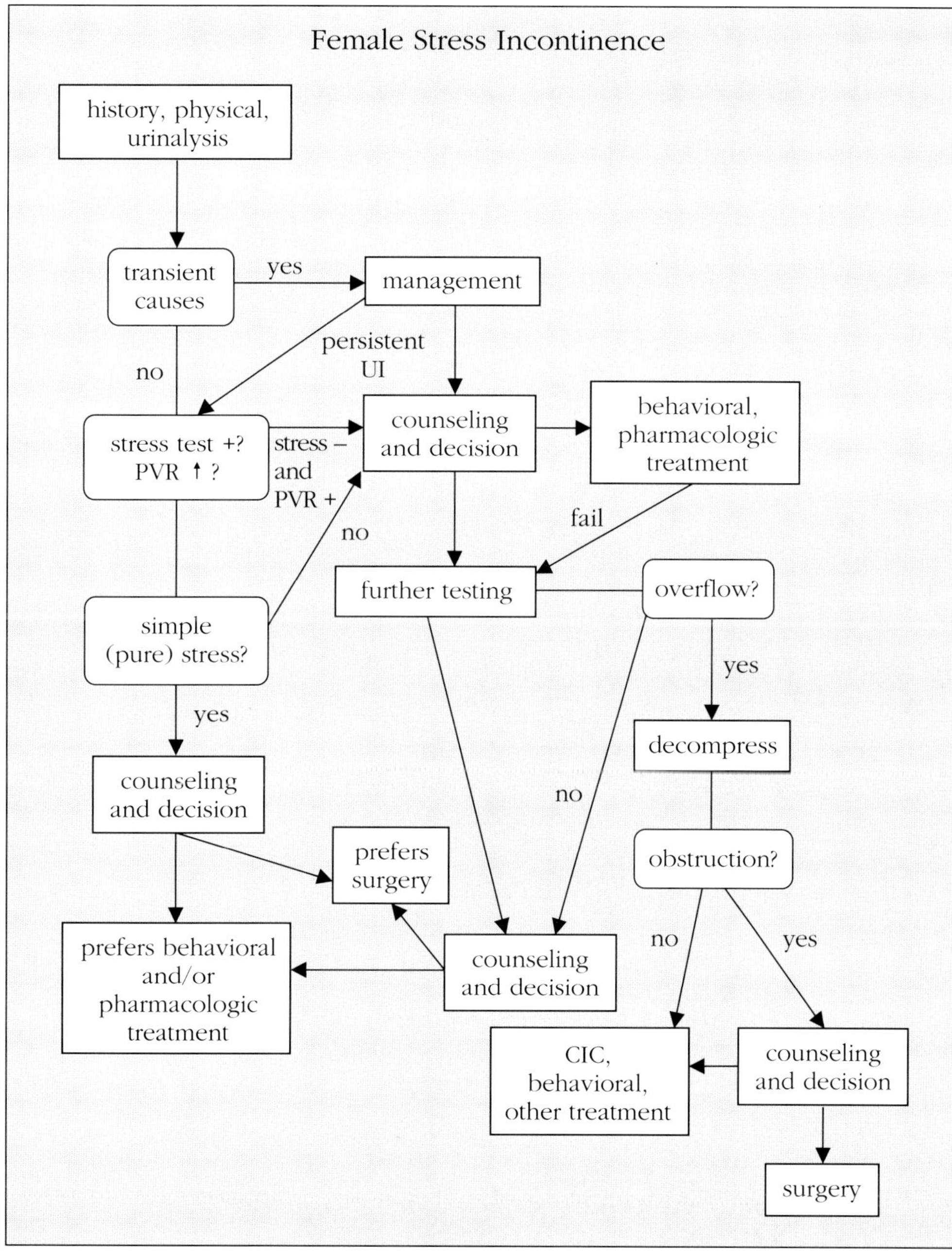

Figure 10.2 Algorithm for management of female stress incontinence. (Adapted from Urinary Incontinence Guideline Panel, 1992)

Screening Evaluation

A screening evaluation for the patient presenting with urinary incontinence consists of objective confirmation of incontinence, type classification, identification of potential causes of transient incontinence, and a risk assessment to determine which patients require further evaluation before a therapeutic trial is undertaken. The desired end point of treatment, comorbidity, and surgical risk must be assessed to provide a cost-effective, minimally invasive work-up that is tailored towards optimal treatment for the individual patient.

The initial evaluation consists of history, physical examination, post-void residual determination, urinalysis, and analysis of a voiding diary (timed intake and voided volume record). Cystoscopy and upper tract imaging studies are selectively indicated for patients with hematuria, renal insufficiency, or severe bladder dysfunction associat-ed with an increased risk for cancer or renal deterioration. Patients with high-pressure uninhibited bladder contractions associated with a high leak pressure or outflow obstruction, and those with conditions associated with decreased bladder compliance, such as previous radiation therapy or radical surgery, require close monitoring for the development of hydronephrosis and renal insufficiency. Video or nonvideo urodynamic evaluation is performed in patients with lower urinary tract symptoms who have 1) failed empiric therapy, 2) suspected neurogenic etiology, 3) risk for hydronephrosis, or 4) confusing symptoms with complex incontinence.

Treatment Options

After the screening evaluation, empiric therapy may be elected in low-risk patients (Fig. 10.4). After urodynamic characterization of a lower urinary tract disorder, medical

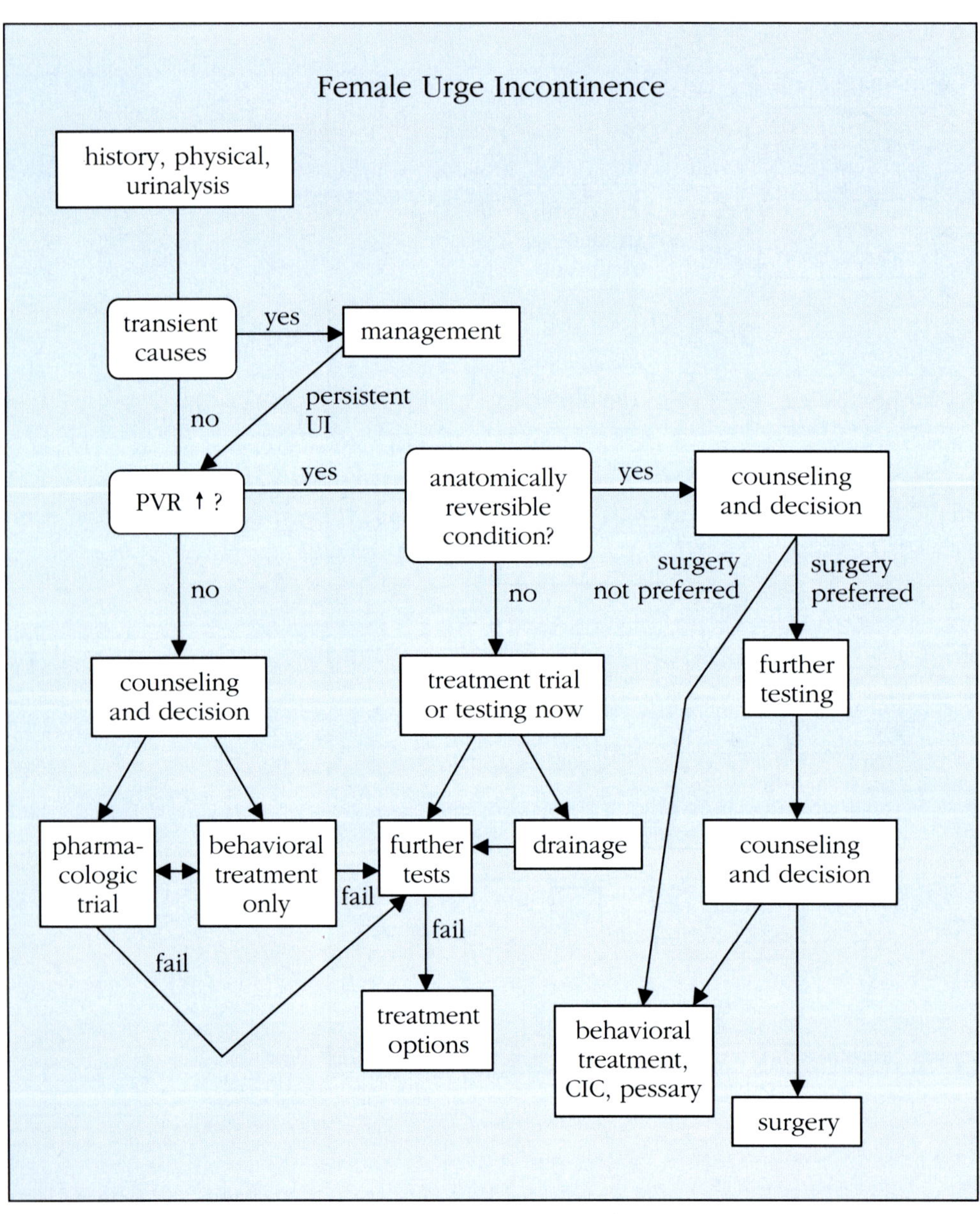

Figure 10.3 Algorithm for management of female urge incontinence. (Adapted from Urinary Incontinence Guideline Panel, 1992)

treatment, behavioral training, electrical stimulation, or surgery may be used (Fig. 10.5). Medical treatment consists of drugs to relax the detrusor (such as anticholinergics, smooth-muscle relaxants, tricyclic antidepressants, calcium channel blockers, potassium channel openers) or increase outlet resistance (α-agonists, tricyclic antidepressants, estrogen). Medication can be administered by the oral, transcutaneous, transvaginal, sublingual, or intrathecal route. Behavioral training consists of bladder drills, timed voiding, pelvic floor exercises (PFE) and, in some patients, biofeedback. Electrical stimulation can be employed transcutaneously, to elicit contraction of the pelvic floor muscles, or via implanted electrodes, which alter bladder sensation or the micturition reflex. Further evaluation of the role of electrical stimulation for the treatment of urinary incontinence is required before these techniques can be generally applied.

When anatomic defects are responsible for urinary incontinence, surgical treatment may be primary or may follow a trial of nonsurgical therapy. Most surgery in this setting is performed on the bladder outlet (e.g., to improve bladder neck competence for stress incontinence or to relieve outlet obstruction). When nonsurgical treatment is contraindicated or fails to lower bladder filling pressures, surgical augmentation of the bladder can be used to improve compliance and improve reservoir function.

STRESS INCONTINENCE

Anatomic stress incontinence occurs when the normally functioning bladder neck is displaced inferiorly during straining. Internal sphincter function fails, with an increase in intraabdominal pressure as the bladder neck secondarily funnels and becomes incompetent. It is important to distinguish a hypermobile, displaced bladder neck that leads to anatomic stress incontinence from a dysfunctional proximal urethra, which is characterized by an open bladder neck at rest and severe, often postural, incontinence. With either disorder, the patient complains of stress urinary incontinence; however, the surgical approach differs for the two conditions. Bladder neck suspension is the procedure of choice for the correction of anatomic stress incontinence, but it seldom cures stress incontinence caused by intrinsic sphincter dysfunction.

The goal of bladder neck suspension is to restore the displaced but normally functioning bladder neck to a stationary retropubic position. Abdominal, vaginal, or combined approaches are effective. The goal of surgery for intrinsic sphincter dysfunction is to compress the normally positioned but abnormally functioning proximal urethra to provide improved sphincter function.

EVALUATION OF THE STRESS-INCONTINENT WOMAN

Preoperative evaluation of the woman with suspected stress incontinence includes history, neurourologic examination, pelvic examination with empty and full bladder, and urinalysis. In the preoperative assessment, stress incontinence should be demonstrated and a determination made regarding displacement versus dysfunction of the internal sphincter. Patients for whom previous inconti-

FIGURE 10.4 *Empiric Treatment for Urinary Incontinence*

TYPE	MEDICAL	BEHAVIORAL
Urge incontinence	Drugs to relax the detrusor	PFE, bladder drills, biofeedback
Stress incontincncc	Drugs to increase outlet resistance	PFE
Overflow incontinence	Clean, intermittent self-catheterization	
Functional incontinence		PFE, bladder drills, biofeedback, bedside commode
Mixed, stress and urge	Drugs to relax detrusor and increase outlet resistance	PFE, bladder drills, biofeedback

PFE = pelvic floor exercises

FIGURE 10.5 *Specific Nonsurgical Treatment for Urinary Incontinence*

URODYNAMIC DIAGNOSIS	MEDICAL	BEHAVIORAL
DI, DH	Drugs to relax the detrusor	All
GSUI (anatomic)	Drugs to increase outlet resistance	All
GSUI (ISD)	Drugs to increase outlet resistance	All
Functional	Drugs to increase outlet resistance	All
Mixed	Drugs to increase outlet resistance	All

nence procedures have failed, those with a history of neurologic disease, and those whose primary complaint is frequency, urgency, or urge incontinence, should be evaluated further, and a urodynamic evaluation considered. Urodynamic evaluation is also performed in patients with suspected disorders of detrusor contractility to assess postoperative risk for urinary retention.

When stress incontinence coexists with urge incontinence the patient should be assessed and the sequence of therapy determined. When urge incontinence is a major problem and when high bladder filling pressures are demonstrated on urodynamic evaluation, medical or behavioral intervention is the initial treatment of choice. After low-pressure bladder filling is proven, surgical augmentation of outlet function can safely follow. The finding of idiopathic detrusor instability with stress incontinence does not preclude primary surgical anatomic repair, since idiopathic detrusor instability often resolves after bladder neck suspension for stress incontinence. If persistent, it can usually be treated postoperatively by medical intervention.

History

A careful history with complete review of urologic, gynecologic, and neurologic systems is recorded. Anatomic stress incontinence is characterized by the loss of urine when intraabdominal pressure is increased. Incontinence that occurs shortly after coughing or a Valsalva maneuver is characteristic of detrusor instability precipitated by stress and is not improved by surgical procedures for stress incontinence.

Over-the-counter medications taken by the patient should be determined and assessed for their potential effects on bladder or urethral function. The patient must also be examined for signs of vaginal prolapse. Symptoms of cystocele, rectocele, or enterocele, such as pelvic pressure, protrusion of a vaginal mass, defecation on digital examination, and other bowel complaints, must be assessed. The patient's sexual activity should be considered on the first visit, as vaginal surgery may be complicated by vaginal foreshortening or loss of volume. When infection is present, the question of bacterial persistence versus reinfection should be explored preoperatively by reviewing the history and the laboratory data.

Physical Examination

On physical examination, a brief neurologic exam—for the presence of an anal wink, assessment of the bulbocavernosus reflex, and sensory examination of low thoracic, upper lumbar, and sacral dermatomes along with lower extremity reflexes, vibratory sensation, and proprioception—is included to screen for neurourologic dysfunction. Bimanual and rectovaginal pelvic examination complete the evaluation for cystocele, rectocele, enterocele, and uterine descensus or vault prolapse. Vulvovaginal atrophy, if present, should be corrected before surgery. Administration of estrogen improves urethral coaptation, reduces irritation, and may improve bladder neck function, occasionally obviating the need for surgery.

Urodynamics

After the physical examination, bedside urodynamic studies can be performed to assess bladder function and to document the presence of stress incontinence. A catheter is placed per urethram, the postvoid residual is measured, and the bladder is gravity-filled through the barrel of a 60 mL catheter-tipped syringe. Uninhibited contractions are seen as a rise of the fluid meniscus in the syringe. Bladder capacity is noted, the catheter is removed, and the patient is asked to cough in the lithotomy position. Hypermobility and inferior displacement of the bladder neck, the defects seen in anatomic stress incontinence, are assessed at rest, during a Valsalva maneuver, and during coughing. When incontinence is demonstrated, a Marshall test is performed to determine if the stress incontinence is relieved by paraurethral vaginal support lateral to the bladder neck. When no incontinence is seen with stress in the lithotomy position, the patient is asked to stand over a towel and cough. If loss of urine occurs in the lithotomy position and on standing, and if the patient loses urine with minimal increases in intraabdominal pressure during Valsalva maneuver, intrinsic sphincter dysfunction (ISD) is probable. (The patient then requires complete assessment of proximal urethral function before any proposed surgery, optimally with videourodynamics and determination of abdominal leak pressure.) To conclude the bedside urodynamic evaluation, the patient may void into a uroflowmeter to screen for disorders of bladder emptying. If a significant abnormality is detected, pressure-flow studies may be indicated. Patients with impaired detrusor contractility sometimes experience prolonged or permanent urinary retention after surgery to correct incontinence.

When multichannel urodynamic studies are performed for stress incontinence, either videourodynamic studies or a VCUG, in addition to a nonvideo study, are helpful. An upright VCUG in the oblique or lateral position with stress views can accurately demonstrate the degree of cystocele and the presence of intrinsic sphincter dysfunction (open bladder neck at rest with postural incontinence). It may also demonstrate urethral abnormalities such as diverticula during voiding. Indications for videourodynamics in patients with stress incontinence include a history of neurologic disease, radiation therapy, radical pelvic surgery, failed prior antiincontinence procedures, a history suggestive of voiding dysfunction that could manifest as postoperative urinary retention, and the presence of confusing symptomatology. A history of occasional urge incontinence in the presence of suspected anatomic stress incontinence may not be confirmed during urodynamic evaluation; this is not an absolute indication for invasive testing. If reflux, high-pressure storage of urine, or outlet obstruction (all risk factors for upper tract deterioration) is suspected, videourodynamic studies should be done before outlet surgery. Poor reservoir function is most often seen in patients who have undergone radical pelvic surgery or radiation therapy and in those with myelodysplasia or other neurologic disease. A bladder neck suspension performed in a patient with high-pressure detrusor instability or poor compliance may increase filling pressures by raising the pressure at which urine leaks across the outlet and thus result in renal insufficiency. Although the patient may be relieved of stress incontinence postoperatively, urge incontinence or silent hydronephrosis may occur. Adjunctive pharmacologic therapy to promote urine storage or surgical procedures designed to improve bladder compliance may be necessary in addition to correction of low outflow resistance.

Surgery for Anatomic Stress Incontinence in Women

Either a transvaginal or a transabdominal procedure can be chosen for the correction of anatomic stress incontinence. When there is associated prolapse, the vaginal approach offers the advantage of simultaneous correction of urethral hypermobility and repair of the prolapse. Vaginal surgery is usually followed by a shorter hospital stay and less postoperative pain. If an augmentation cystoplasty or other abdominal procedure is contemplated, one of the transabdominal suspension procedures is more convenient and may be preferred in the patient without prolapse.

TRANSVAGINAL SURGERY
Operative Preparation
The patient is placed in the dorsal lithotomy position and the hair-bearing area of the proposed incisions is shaved. Prophylactic antibiotics may be given. The vagina, lower

abdomen, and vulva are prepped and draped. A suprapubic tube can be inserted percutaneously into the full bladder or a curved Lowsley tractor can be used to place a 16 Fr Foley catheter through the abdominal wall. If a suprapubic tube is not planned, the patient should be instructed preoperatively in self-catheterization or else an indwelling Foley catheter can be placed, with intermittent voiding trials, until urinary retention resolves. A 16 Fr Foley catheter is placed through the urethra and 10 mL of water used to inflate the balloon. A weighted vaginal speculum is placed and the labia minora are sutured to the labia majora if visualization of the urethra and bladder neck is obscured. An incision site appropriate for the proposed procedure is then selected and the site is infiltrated with injectable saline.

Incisions Used in Vaginal Surgery
Only three basic incisions are used in vaginal surgery: inverted U, anterior midline, and posterior T. The inverted U/bilateral oblique incision or a variant is used for most suspension procedures in patients with minimal, moderate, or no cystocele (Fig. 10.6). The anterior midline/inverted T incision or variant is used for formal cystocele repair with or without bladder neck suspension (Fig. 10.7A). An episiotomy may be performed if poor exposure results from a narrow introitus (Fig. 10.7B). The posterior inverted T incision is used for rectocele and enterocele repair and for sacrospinalis vault suspension. In addition, a superficial triangle of perineal skin is removed when perineorrhaphy is required (Fig. 10.8).

Raz Bladder Neck Suspension
The bladder neck is identified through the anterior vaginal wall by palpation of the Foley balloon when traction is

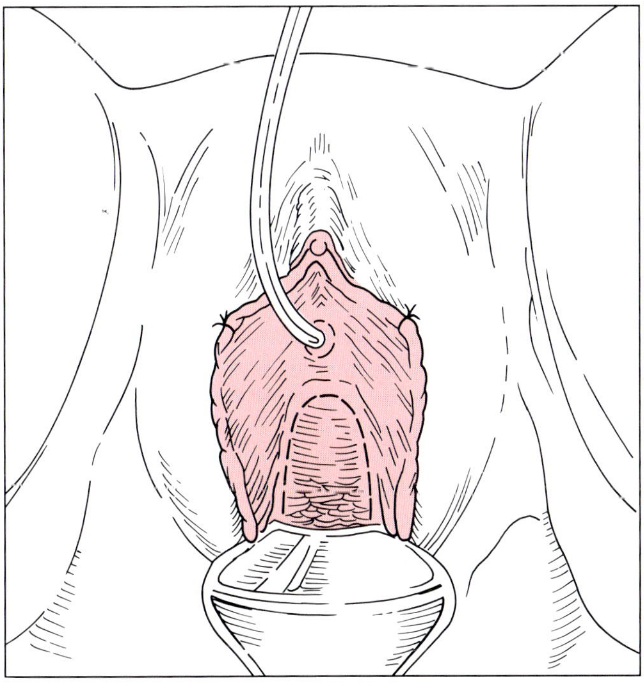

Figure 10.6 Inverted U incision.

applied to the catheter. An Allis clamp is placed midway between the bladder neck and urethral meatus. The clamp is retracted towards the meatus and the proposed bilateral oblique or inverted U incision is infiltrated with saline, then incised (Fig. 10.9A). On each side, two Allis clamps are placed on the lateral margins of the incision for retraction. The superficial urethral fascia is freed from the vaginal wall by spreading dissection with Botcher or Metzenbaum scissors until the pubic bone is encountered (Fig. 10.9B). The scissors are then angled towards the ipsilateral shoulder to perforate the endopelvic fascia and enter the retropubic space. The pubis is freed from the posterior symphysis to the bladder neck with blunt finger dissection. A 4 × 4 sponge is placed in the defect to aid hemostasis. Bilaterally, three passes with a #1 polypropylene suture swedged onto an MO5 or MO6 needle are used to secure the medial edge of the endopelvic fascia (tendinous arc) and the vaginal wall, excluding the epithelium at the level of the bladder neck (Fig. 10.9C). All sutures are placed lateral to the perivesical and periurethral tissues to avoid pain, erosion, or obstruction of the urethra. To correct a small or moderate cystocele, the vaginal wall suture is sequentially placed more proximally (towards the cervix or cuff) or a second proximal suture is

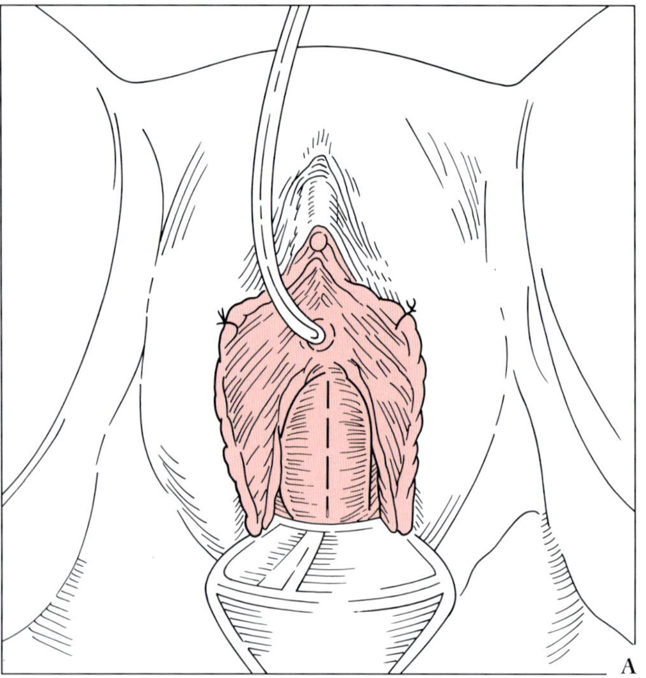

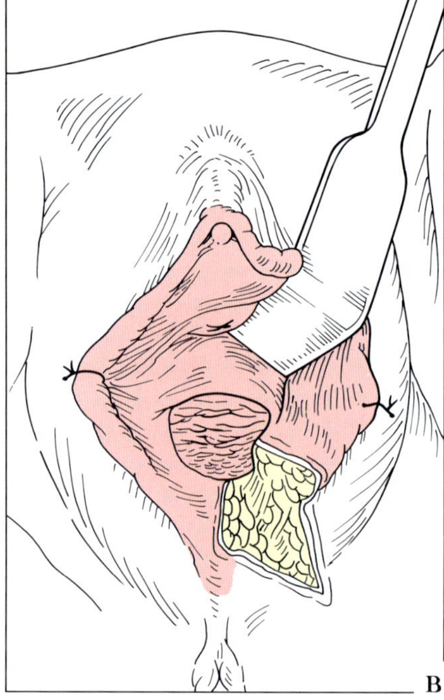

Figure 10.7 **A** Anterior vaginal midline incision. **B** Mediolateral episiotomy.

Figure 10.8 Incision for rectocele repair with perineorrhaphy.

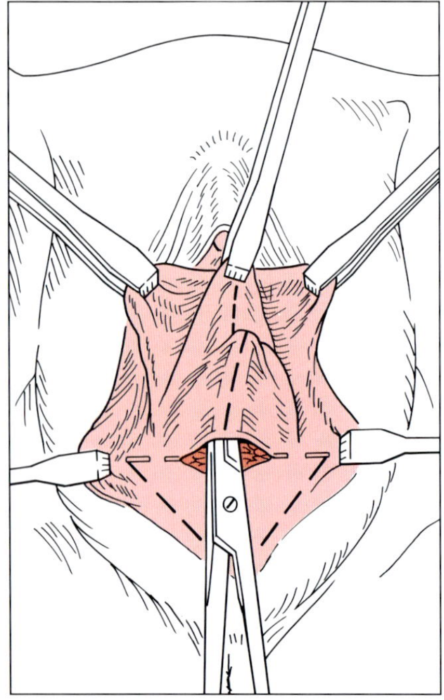

used. The Foley catheter is opened and allowed to drain continuously. The table is then placed in a horizontal position and a transverse 1-inch incision is made over the pubic bone in the midline. The anterior rectus sheath is exposed. By placing the nondominant index finger through the vagina into the retropubic space, the posterior abdominal wall can be contacted just above the symphysis pubis. The Raz needle (double pronged) is passed through the fascia immediately above the symphysis, hugging the periosteum, to contact the index finger in the retropubic space (Fig. 10.9D). The needle is guided by a fingertip through the vaginal incision. On each side the

tails of the polypropylene suture are placed through a separate needle eye. The needle is then withdrawn through the suprapubic wound to transfer the suture, which is secured with a hemostat (Fig. 10.9E).

Indigo carmine is injected intravenously and cystoscopy is performed. The initial bladder effluent should be clear. The urethra is inspected with a 0° lens and the bladder, including the anterior wall, is inspected with a 70° lens. There should be no blue suture in the bladder and no buckling of the epithelium when traction is placed on the suprapubic suture, which would indicate that the suture is placed too deep and must be removed and replaced. If the

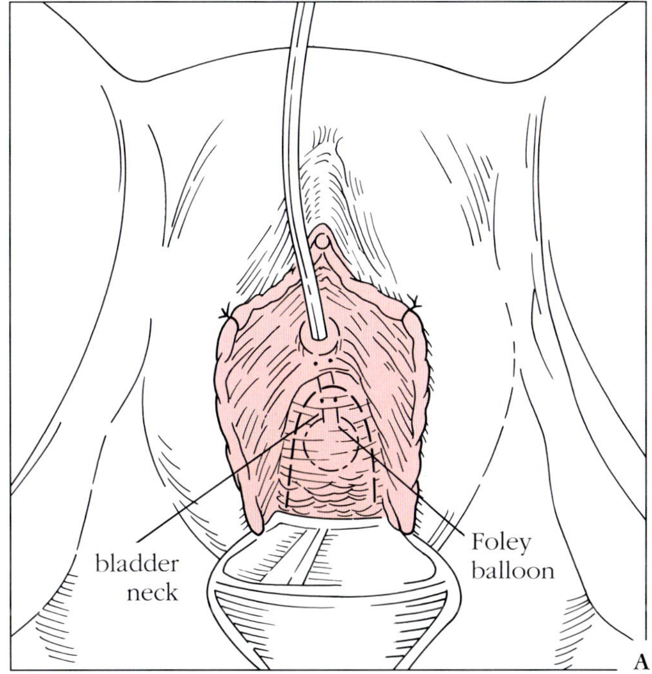

Figure 10.9 **A** Raz bladder neck suspension. Inverted U incision with apex midway between bladder neck and urethral meatus. **B** Isolation of urethropelvic ligament. **C** Vaginal suture placement for correction of urethral hypermobility with moderate cystocele.

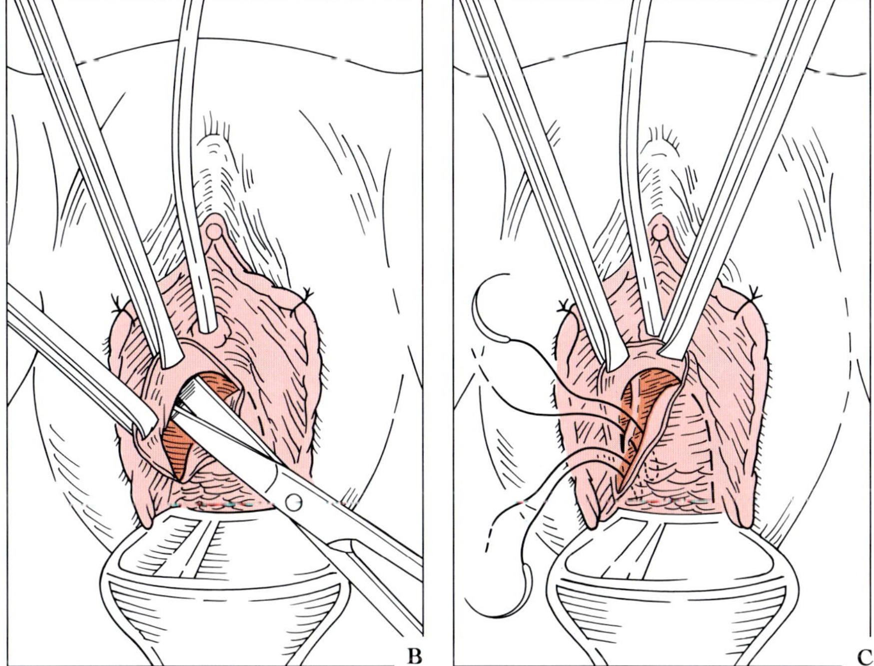

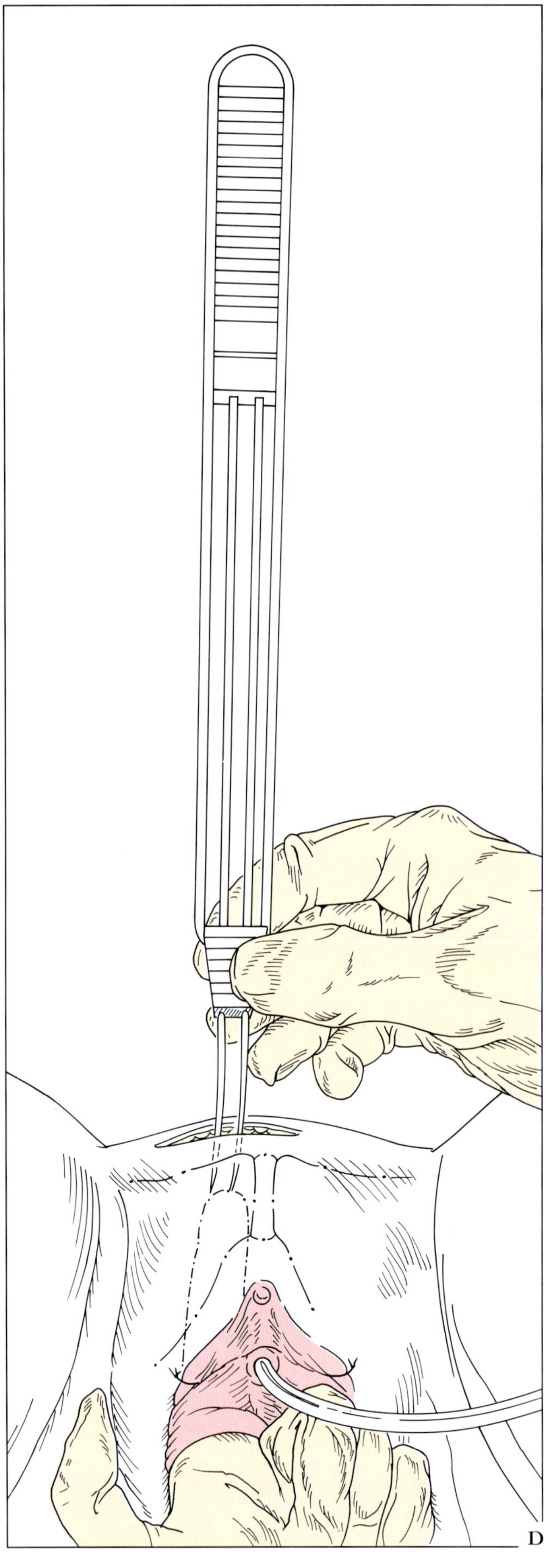

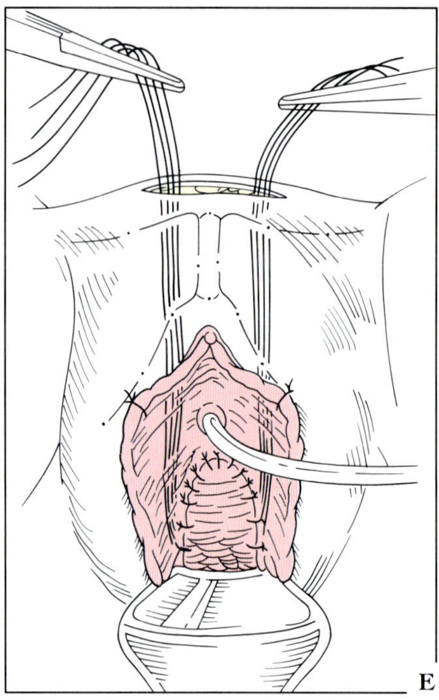

***Figure 10.9
(continued)***
D Placement of
ligature carrier.
E Sutures
transferred,
incision closed.

suture is correctly placed, brisk ureteral efflux is confirmed and bladder neck elevation and closure are observed with minimal tension on the suprapubic sutures.

Each half of the vaginal incision is closed with running absorbable 2-0 or 3-0 sutures. A vaginal pack is placed to elevate the anterior vaginal wall. Without tension the sutures on each side are tied to each other, and one tail of each suture is tied across the midline, if desired.

Endoscopic Bladder Neck Suspension

With the patient prepped and draped in the lithotomy position, bilateral oblique anterior vaginal wall incisions are made after infiltration with injectable saline. A Foley catheter is placed (Fig. 10.10A).

Two small transverse incisions are made an inch above the symphysis and a 15° or 30° angled needle is passed between the ipsilateral incisions adjacent to the bladder neck (Fig. 10.10B). The catheter is then removed and cystoscopy is done to demonstrate proper needle placement outside the bladder wall. The needle is moved to observe indentation of the vesical neck (Fig. 10.10C).

On each side, a #1 polypropylene suture is placed through the eye of the needle and transferred suprapubically. The needle is passed through the same incision, perforating the anterior rectus sheath 1 cm lateral to the first puncture and exiting 1 cm distal to the bladder neck. Cystoscopy confirms the positions. The suture is placed through a 1-cm^2 Dacron pledget used to reinforce the

pubocervical fascia before the free suture is transferred through the anterior rectus sheath (Fig. 10.10D).

Cystoscopy is performed to confirm bladder neck closure. The vagina is closed, a vaginal pack is placed, and the suprapubic sutures are tied under tension. A Foley catheter is placed.

Gittes (No Incision) Pubovaginal Suspension

A #15 blade is used to puncture the skin above the pubic hairline 3 cm lateral to the midline. A Stamey needle with a 30° angulation is advanced through the wound and rectus fascia and hugs the posterior pubis. The surgeon's finger is placed in the vagina, elevating the bladder neck towards the pubis. The Stamey needle is directed towards the finger until the vaginal wall is tented. Once it is confirmed that the vaginal perforation is next to the bladder neck, the needle is advanced through the vaginal wall and out of the introitus.

A #2 permanent monofilament suture (nylon or polypropylene) is threaded into the eye of the Stamey needle. A hemostat is placed on one of the suture tails and the needle is withdrawn suprapubically, advancing the free suture tail through the suprapubic puncture site. A hemostat is applied to the free suprapubic suture tail.

A second pass of the needle is made through the same skin perforation, perforating the rectus fascia 1 cm medial to the first pass. A second vaginal perforation site is selected, 1.5 to 2 cm cephalad or caudad to the first,

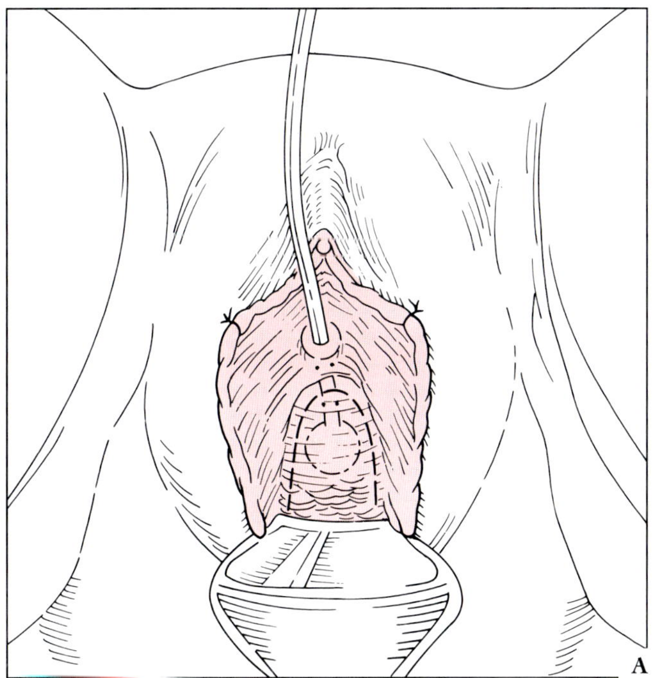

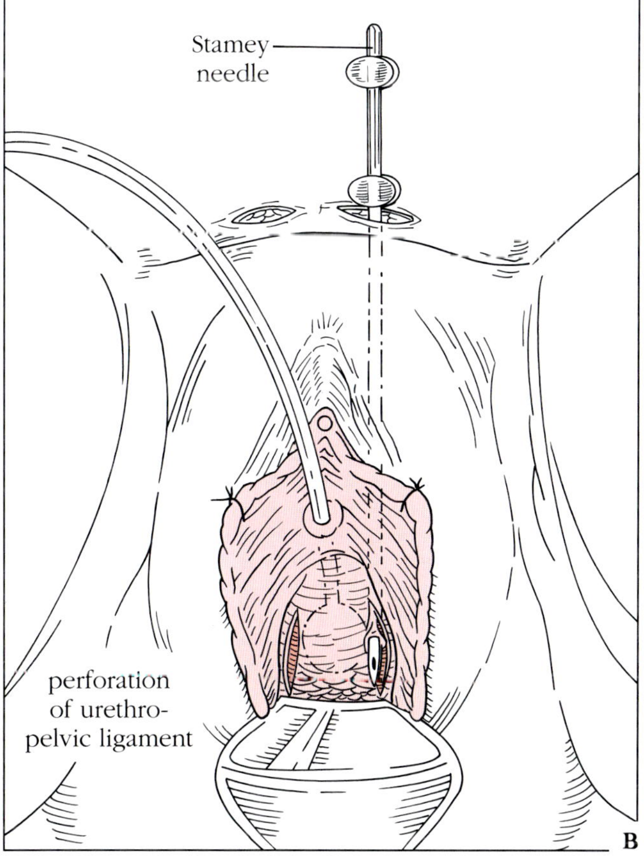

Figure 10.10 Endoscopic BNS. **A** Anterior vaginal wall oblique incisions. **B** Placement of Stamey needle.

and the epithelium is punctured with the Stamey needle. With the needle extending through the introitus, the tagged vaginal suture tail is placed through a #5 or #6 Mayo needle. A full-thickness mattress suture is placed into the vaginal wall between the two vaginal perforations. The Mayo needle is then removed and the free end of the suture is threaded through the Stamey needle and withdrawn through the suprapubic puncture site. The opposite side is secured in an identical manner.

The urethral catheter is removed and cystoscopy is performed, with careful inspection of the urethra, the bladder neck, and the entire bladder wall. Using a 0° lens,

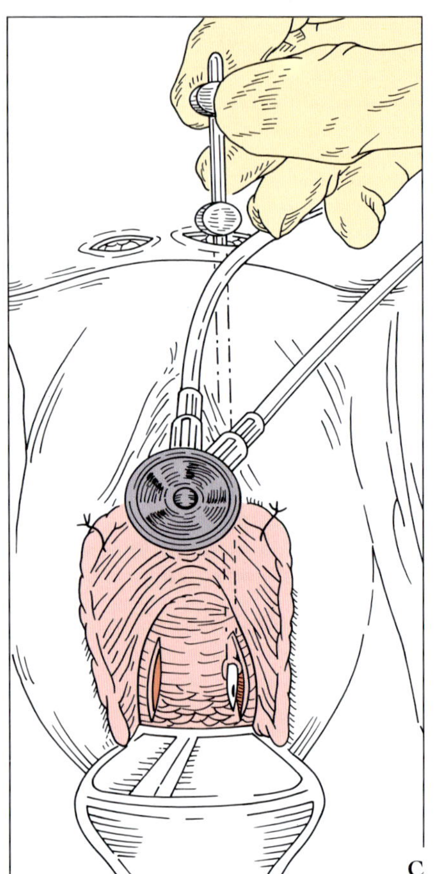

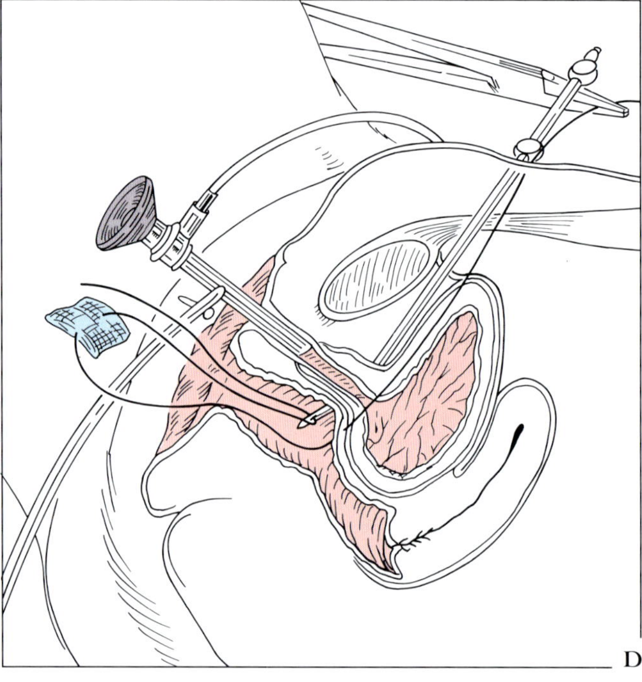

Figure 10.10 (continued) C Cystoscopy with needle movement to ensure placement at vesical neck. **D** Suture and pledget placement.

Figure 10.11 Four-corner suspension. Extension of inverted U incision to the cervix.

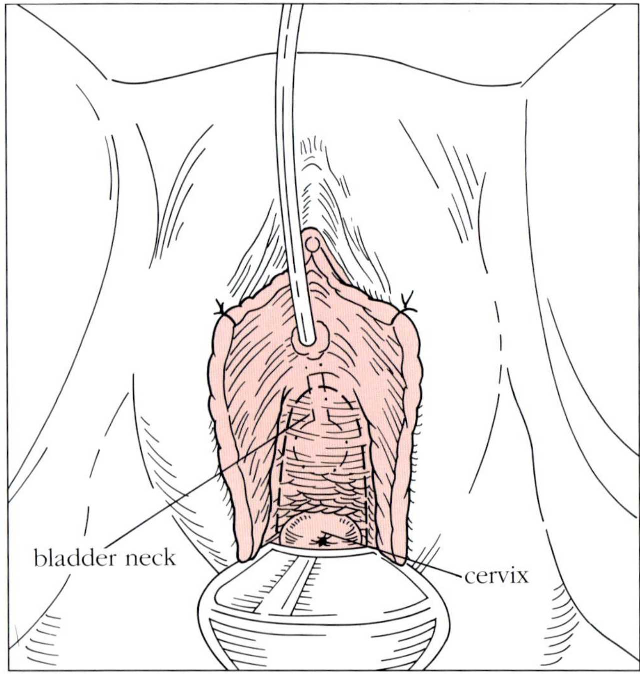

appropriate elevation of the bladder neck should be confirmed by traction on the suprapubic sutures.

The suspension sutures are individually tied with tension and the knots are allowed to retract through the puncture sites. Addison forceps are used to remove tension from the skin edges and a sterile bandage is applied. The permanent mattress suture will penetrate the vaginal wall during the postoperative period and epithelialization of the defect will ensue.

Four-Corner Suspension for Correction of Cystocele with Anatomic Stress Incontinence

The indication for this procedure is a moderate cystocele that extends to or through the introitus with strain. The patient is placed in the dorsal lithotomy position, a suprapubic tube is placed, and a urethral Foley is inserted.

Extended inverted U or bilateral oblique incisions are made in the anterior vaginal wall from the midurethra to the cuff or cervix (Fig. 10.11). The urethropelvic fascia towards the pelvic side wall is dissected and sharp entry into the retropubic space at the level of the bladder neck is performed as in a Raz suspension (see Fig. 10.10). In the patient with prior hysterectomy, two sutures of #1 polypropylene swedged onto a #5 or #6 Mayo needle are placed at the bladder neck and the cuff on each side, respectively, incorporating three helical sections of vaginal wall with pubocervical fascia. The proximal (bladder base or cuff) suture is then placed three times through the residual uterine ligaments—uterosacral and anterior cardinal—located at the lateral edge of the cuff. If the uterus is in situ, the tissue anterolateral to the cervix comprises the proximal support. In both cases, the distal bladder neck suture is identical to the Raz suspension suture, incorporating three sections of the tendinous arc and urethropelvic ligament as well as the vaginal wall and pubocervical fascia.

The sutures are transferred through the suprapubic incision with a double-pronged needle near the midline. Cystoscopy is performed to ensure brisk efflux from the ureteral orifices, elevation of the bladder neck with traction on the sutures, and absence of bladder perforation.

The vagina is closed with absorbable suture, a vaginal pack is placed, and the ipsilateral sutures are tied to each other—optimally, across the midline. The suprapubic wound is closed.

VAGINAL SURGERY FOR PROLAPSE

The urologist must evaluate each incontinent female patient for prolapse. Significant prolapse, even if asymptomatic, is repaired at the time of surgery for urinary incontinence. Complete evaluation for cystocele, uterine descensus, vault prolapse, enterocele, and rectocele is required. This ensures that the patient does not have to undergo multiple surgeries for the sequential repair of preexisting prolapse, which is often exaggerated after suspension of the bladder neck.

Cystocele Repair

A cystocele is caused by vaginal herniation of the trigone and posterior bladder wall through attenuated pubocervical fascia. This defect must be repaired when bladder neck suspension is performed, to avoid retention and irritative voiding symptoms resulting from angulation of the trigone and bladder base (Fig. 10.12). Small cystoceles are corrected during a Raz or Burch bladder neck suspension by placing proximal supporting sutures in the vaginal wall and securing them to the anterior rectus sheath or Cooper's ligament. Moderate cystoceles can be repaired by either four-corner bladder suspension or anterior colporrhaphy. Large cystoceles that extend through the introitus at rest require formal midline cystocele repair.

Rectocele Repair

Rectocele repair in the patient undergoing vaginal surgery for urinary incontinence is indicated when a moderate (or larger) rectocele is present. The symptoms caused by a rectocele are usually related to difficulty with defecation. Some women with rectocele require digital pressure on the posterior vaginal wall to facilitate bowel movement. With a large rectocele, a large vaginal mass is noted when the rectum is full. There may be incontinence of flatus when gas collects in the large hernia and the perineal body is too weakened to contain the rectal contents. Some women have no symptoms from even large rectoceles. Nevertheless, the apparent size of a posterior vaginal wall prolapse may increase when a cystocele is repaired or the bladder neck is suspended. It is therefore usually advisable to repair asymptomatic as well as symptomatic rectoceles at the time of other vaginal surgery. The vaginal capacity is sometimes reduced by concomitant anterior and posterior repair, and the sexually active patient must be counseled preoperatively. Occasionally a patient with a moderate, asymptomatic rectocele declines repair for this reason.

The purpose of posterior repair is to achieve a permanent reduction of the rectal hernia. This is accomplished

FIGURE 10.12 *Surgical Correction of Cystocele*

SIZE	DEFECT	TREATMENT
Small	Bladder base to interior pubic ramus with strain	Burch or Raz bladder neck suspension
Moderate	Bladder base to or through introitus at rest	Four-corner suspension
Large	Bladder base through introitus at rest	Anterior colporrhaphy

by plication of the perirectal fascia and the levator ani muscles. A two- to three-layer closure is required.

It is important to differentiate rectocele from enterocele preoperatively, and to repair both simultaneously if they coexist. The length and breadth of the vagina should be preserved. The integrity of the perineal body should also be assessed preoperatively and repaired at the time of rectocele repair if it is deficient. With perineal body attenuation, a gaping introitus with posterior displacement of the anus is noted on physical examination. In such cases perineorrhaphy at the time of rectocele repair is indicated. Suture placement into the rectum must be avoided. A rectal examination at the conclusion of the repair is important to detect intraluminal sutures.

PREOPERATIVE PREPARATION The patient is counseled to begin a high-fiber diet well before surgery. Stool softeners are provided. The evening before surgery, an oil-retention enema is recommended. A Fleet enema is provided for the early morning of surgery. Antibiotics, includ-

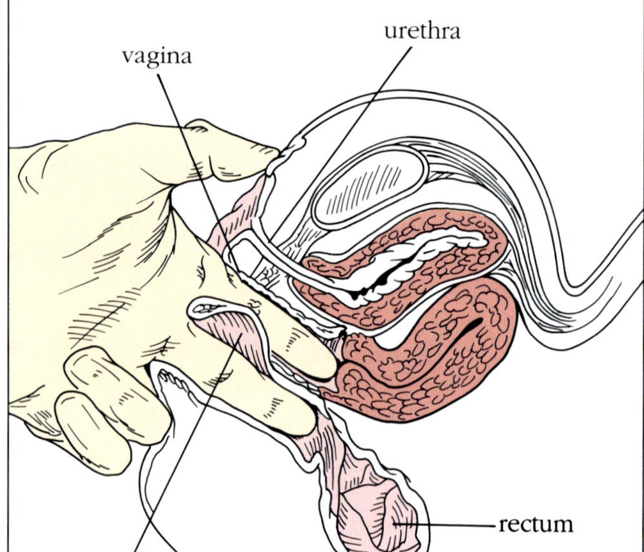

Figure 10.13 Pelvic examination for assessment of rectocele and perineal body evaluation.

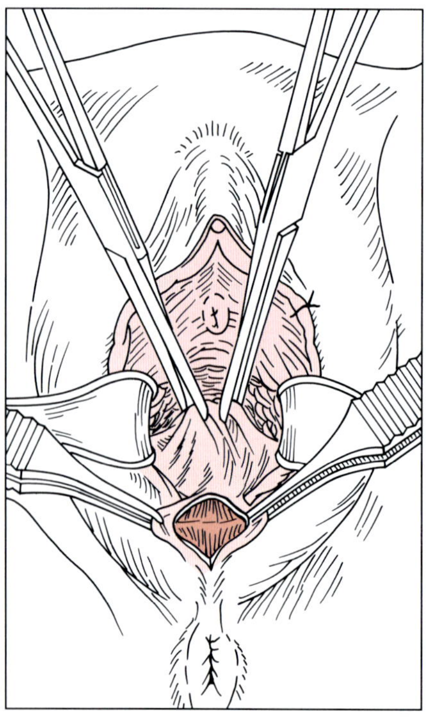

Figure 10.14 Rectocele repair. Dissection of posterior vaginal wall from perirectal fascia.

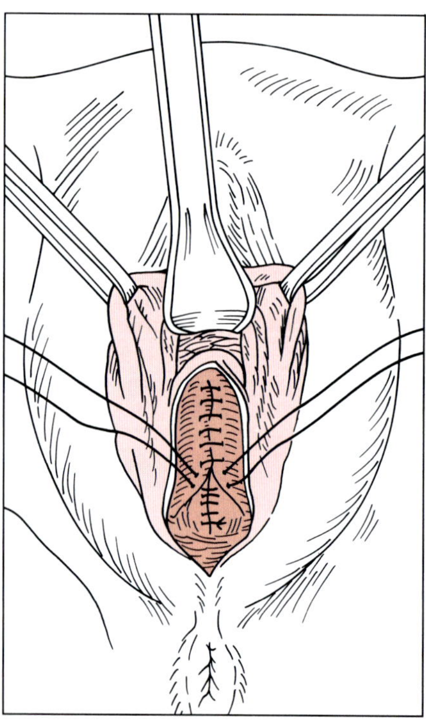

Figure 10.15 Rectocele repair. Following plication of the levator muscles, the redundant vaginal epithelium is resected and the perirectal fascia is approximated.

ing coverage for anaerobes, are given prophylactically and continued for 24 hours postoperatively.

PROCEDURE

Step 1. The patient is placed in the dorsal lithotomy position. A bimanual examination under anesthesia is performed, including assessment of the integrity of the perineal body, the extent of rectocele, and the presence of enterocele (Fig. 10.13).

Step 2. The vagina, perineum, and perirectal areas are then prepped and draped. The labia minora can be secured laterally with sutures. An Allis clamp or suture is placed proximal to the rectocele. Two clamps or marking sutures are placed laterally at the level of the hymeneal ring (see Fig. 10.8).

Step 3. A transverse incision is made at the posterior fourchette between the marking sutures or clamps.

Step 4. With Metzenbaum scissors, a Kelly clamp, or Botcher scissors, a plane is developed between the posterior vaginal wall and the perirectal fascia (the plane of dissection is extremely superficial). A midline vertical incision is then made through the dissected area (Fig. 10.14).

Step 5. A triangle of skin is removed from the perineum, with the base of the triangle at the hymenal ring. Superficial dissection should be used to remove only the skin of the overlying perineal body so that the superficial transverse perineal muscles are not damaged.

Step 6. The perirectal fascia is dissected from the posterior vaginal wall, initially with a scalpel and then by sharp scissor dissection or blunt dissection. This dissection is performed from the posterior fourchette (hymenal ring) to 1 cm proximal to the rectocele, the site of the marking Allis clamp or suture. A spoon, narrow malleable retractor, or finger is used to reduce the rectocele into the rectum, exposing the levator ani muscles. A rectal examination at this point may help to distinguish the levator muscles from the rectal wall.

Step 7. #0 or 2-0 simple sutures are used to bring the levators together from the proximal incision to the level of the hymenal ring. The sutures are then tied in reverse order.

Step 8. Redundant vaginal epithelium is resected, taking care to preserve as much tissue as possible.

Step 9. The perirectal fascia is approximated in the midline with interrupted #0 or 2-0 absorbable suture (Fig. 10.15).

Step 10. To approximate the vaginal epithelium, a long 2-0 or #0 absorbable suture is placed at the apex of the incision and tied equidistant from the ends of the suture. The suture end without the needle is laid beneath the mucosa while the needle is used to approximate the mucosa in the midline (Fig. 10.16A). Running simple sutures are placed to the level of the posterior fourchette. The two ends of suture are then tied together, restoring the normal posterior axis of the vagina (Fig. 10.16B).

Step 11. Interrupted #0 Vicryl sutures are then placed in the bulbocavernosus muscles to reconstruct the perineal body (these muscles are identified at the lateral margins of the residual triangular defect in the perineum). The superficial

perineal muscles are plicated as a second layer (Fig. 10.16C).

Step 12. The running suture used to close the vaginal epithelium continues as a running subcutaneous suture from the reconstructed hymenal ring to the bottom of the triangular incision (Fig. 10.16D).

Step 13. The suture is then run from the base of the perineal body incision to the level of the hymenal ring to close the skin of the perineum in a subcuticular fashion. It is tied to the remaining tail at the posterior fourchette (Fig. 10.16E).

Step 14. Rectal examination is performed to ensure that there are no intraluminal sutures. A vaginal pack can be placed at the surgeon's discretion (Fig. 10.16F).

Transvaginal Enterocele Repair

Enterocele occurs most commonly in women who have undergone hysterectomy. It is caused by prolapse of the peritoneum posterior to the vaginal cuff and can be seen as a posterosuperior vaginal mass. Patients with enterocele may present with an asymptomatic bulge in the vagina, complete eversion of the vagina, or a sense of pelvic pressure. Bowel obstruction from intestinal incarceration in an enterocele is rare. Rectovaginal examination (sometimes with the patient in the standing position) is required to distinguish enterocele from rectocele. The rectal finger is placed at the apex of the rectocele and the vaginal finger is placed at the vault. The patient is asked to strain, and any protrusion between the two fingers occurring with strain is identified as an enterocele.

The purpose of enterocele repair is to resect and ligate the peritoneal hernia sac and to prevent its recurrence. This is accomplished by placing pursestring sutures around the enterocele sac and then reconstructing the levators and uterosacral ligaments to provide support.

As with rectocele repair, it is important to identify and differentiate enterocele from rectocele and to repair them simultaneously. Shortening of the vagina may follow enterocele repair, and the patient should be advised about this possibility. The ureter lies next to the uterosacral ligaments and may be injured during plication. The rectum may be injured when the levators are approximated to reconstruct the vagina after ligation of the enterocele sac. This can be avoided by using a small, malleable retractor over the rectum or depressing it with a finger before suture placement. When enterocele repair is performed simultaneously with rectocele repair, a rectal examination performed at the conclusion of the procedure should include the portion of the rectum posterior to the enterocele repair to detect intraluminal sutures.

PREOPERATIVE PREPARATION   For a large or recurrent enterocele, a bowel prep with GoLYTELY may be given a day before surgery. If a concomitant rectocele repair is planned, enemas should be given in addition to the GoLYTELY. Prophylactic antibiotics are administered.

PROCEDURE   With the patient in the dorsal lithotomy position, a bimanual examination under anesthesia is performed to assess the size of the enterocele and rectocele.

The vagina, perineum, and perirectal and lower abdominal areas are then prepped and draped. Marking sutures are placed at the level of the hymenal ring and a transverse incision is made at the posterior fourchette between the marking sutures. A triangle of perineal skin is then excised as in perineorrhaphy (see Fig. 10.8). A stay suture is placed in the vaginal mucosa overlying the enterocele sac. The rectum is then dissected from the posterior vaginal mucosa by a combination of blunt and sharp dissection (Fig. 10.17). The sac of the enterocele is exposed near the apex of the vagina and is clamped with a fine Allis clamp. The perirectal fascia is dissected from the posterior vaginal wall and the enterocele

sac. A transverse incision is made into the sac, taking care not to injure the peritoneal contents (Fig. 10.18).

The index finger is placed through the sac into the peritoneal cavity and two #0 absorbable pursestring sutures are placed at the neck of the enterocele sac. The patient is then placed in the extreme Trendelenburg position and the abdominal contents are pressed away from the pursestring sutures into the abdomen. The pursestring sutures are sequentially tied (Fig. 10.19). The sac is then amputated, leaving a small cuff protruding caudally.

The uterosacral ligaments anteriorly and the anterior rectal wall posteriorly are visualized and a #0 absorbable suture is placed as follows: right uterosacral ligament →

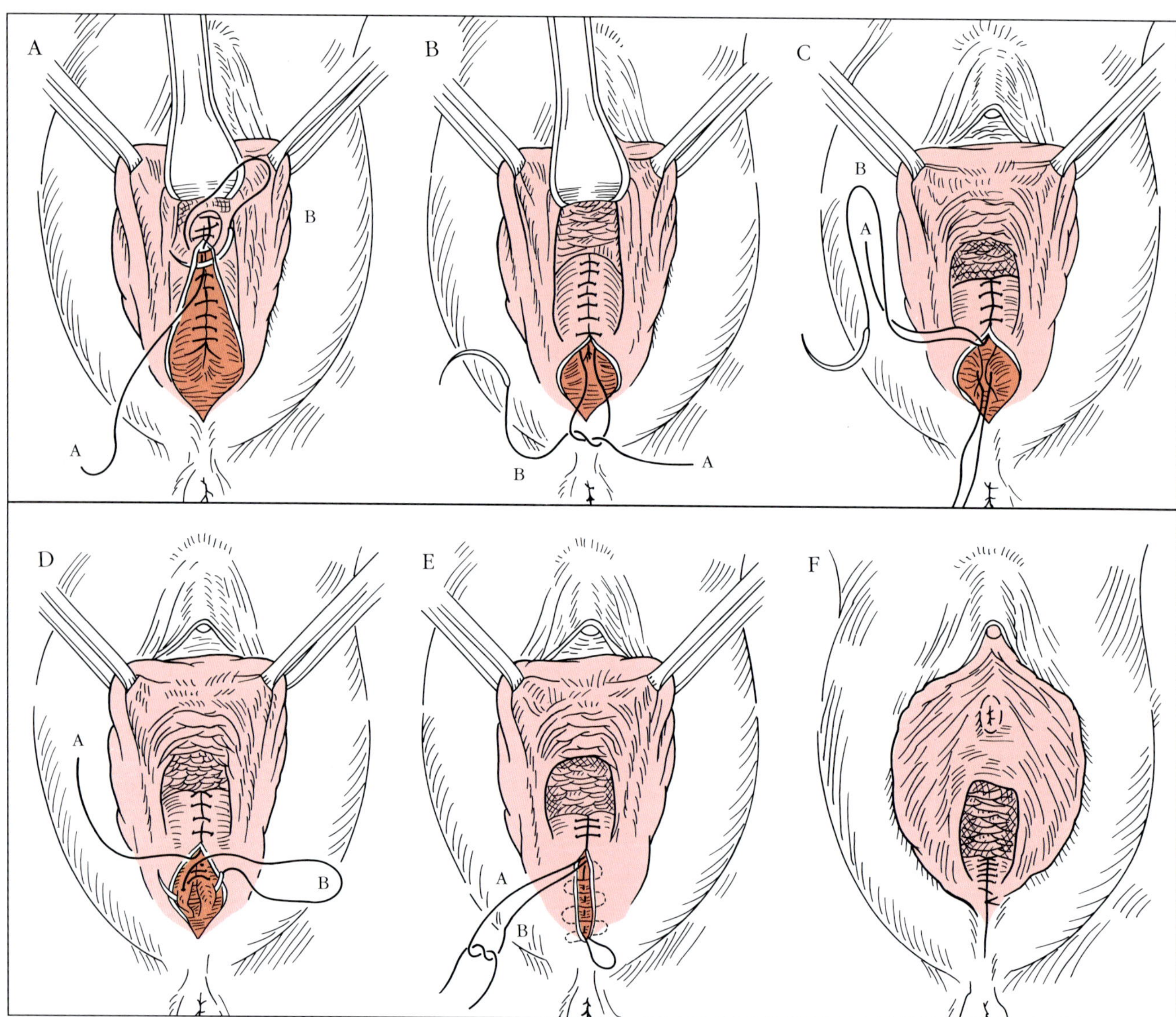

Figure 10.16 Rectocele repair. **A** Approximation of vaginal epithelium with one suture tail laid beneath the closure. **B** Completion of vaginal closure with axis restored. **C** Deep perineal reconstruction. **D** Subcutaneous closure of perineum. **E** Perineal skin approximation. **F** Completed rectocele repair with perineorrhaphy. Note posterior approximation of hymenal ring to avoid "dashboarding" effect.

anterior rectal wall → enterocele → cuff → left uterosacral ligament. The tail of the suture is clamped and two more identical sutures are placed caudally at a spacing of 0.5 cm (Fig. 10.20). The sutures are then tied in the order opposite that in which they were placed, with the most cephalad tied last (Fig. 10.21). The levator ani muscles are then plicated over the rectum, with a narrow malleable retractor placed to protect the rectal wall (Fig. 10.22). If a rectocele is present, it can now be repaired (Fig. 10.23).

Surgical Repair of Vault Prolapse

After hysterectomy some women develop descensus of the vaginal vault. The poorly supported vaginal vault may pro-trude through the vagina and lead to complete vaginal eversion, with the potential for ureteral obstruction (Fig. 10.24). Discomfort and pressure are commonly reported by patients with complete vault prolapse, as well as difficulties with bladder and bowel function and with sexual inter-course. Cystocele, rectocele, and enterocele are commonly present and must be repaired before sacrospinalis fixation or any other procedure is undertaken for vault prolapse.

The purpose of sacrospinalis fixation is to provide permanent support for the vaginal apex while maintaining functional vaginal length. The sacrospinal ligament must be identified with certainty before suture placement. Bleeding, chronic pain from nerve entrapment, or recur-

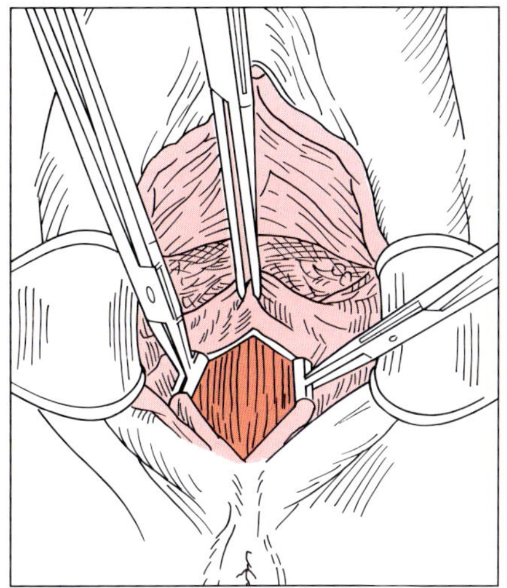

Figure 10.17 Enterocele repair. Dissection of perirectal fascia from posterior vaginal wall.

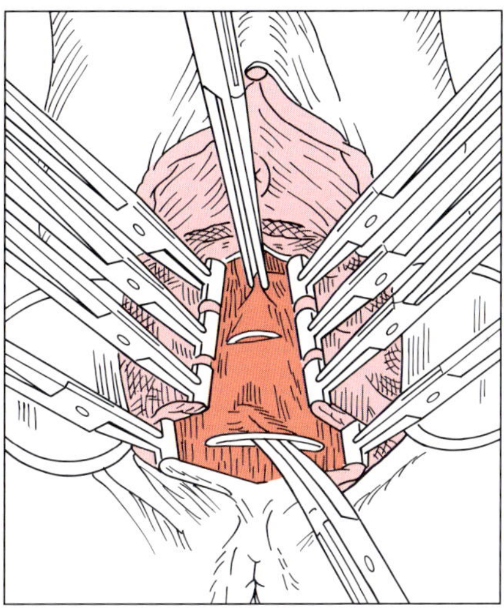

Figure 10.18 Enterocele repair. Identification and dissection of enterocele sac.

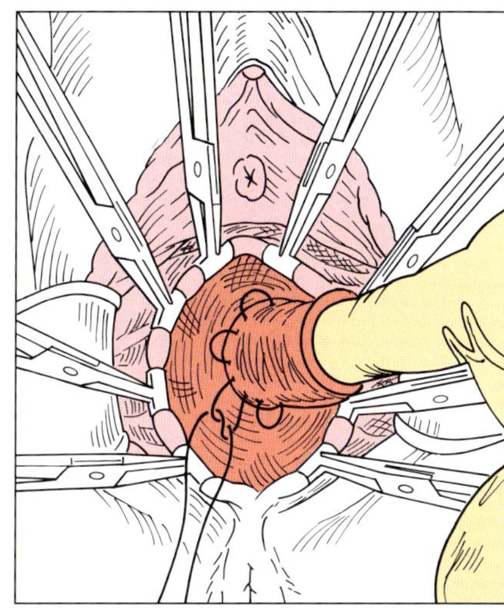

Figure 10.19 Enterocele repair. Placement of pursestring sutures.

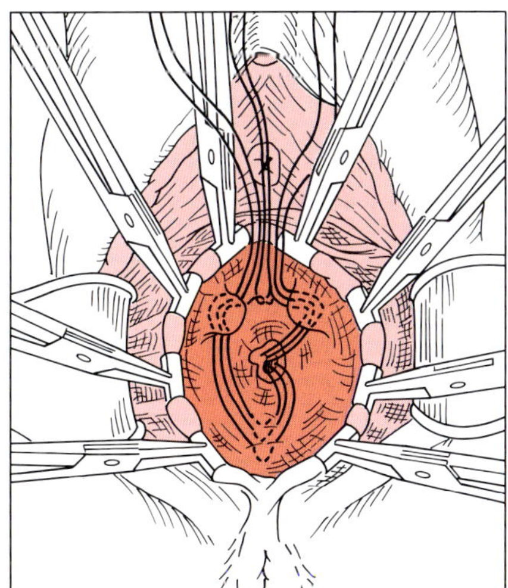

Figure 10.20 Enterocele repair. Deep reconstruction of the vaginal vault.

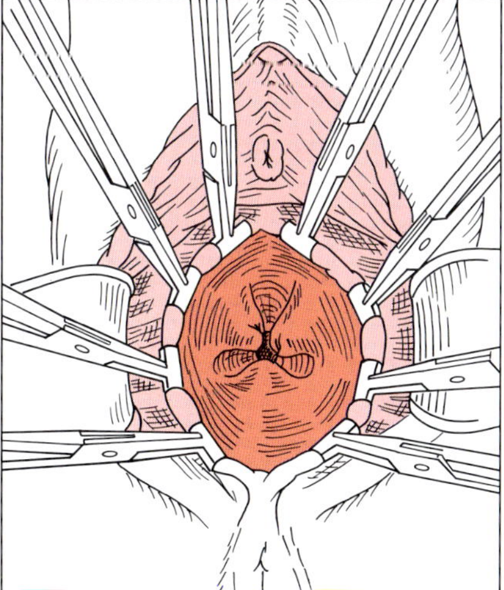

Figure 10.21 Enterocele repair. Deep vault plication sutures are tied.

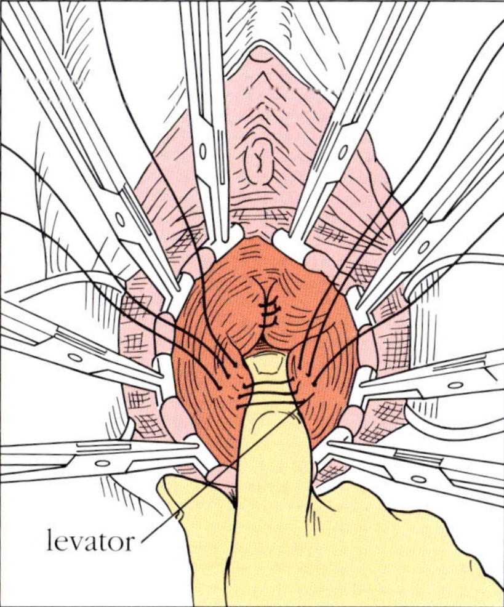

Figure 10.22 Enterocele repair. Approximation of levators.

rent prolapse may result from improper suture placement. In addition, the sutures must be tied securely to ensure that the sacrospinal ligament and the vaginal vault coapt. The vagina is suspended to only one ligament, usually the right, and the patient should be aware that there will be some deviation of the vaginal apex postoperatively.

PREOPERATIVE PREPARATION   This is the same as for rectocele repair.

PROCEDURE   With the patient in the dorsal lithotomy position, the lower abdomen, vagina, and genitalia are prepped and draped into a sterile field. The vault prolapse is reduced and any cystocele repaired (Fig. 10.25).

Marking sutures are placed at the level of the hymenal ring and a transverse incision is made in the posterior fourchette between the marking sutures. A triangle of perineal skin is then excised as in rectocele repair (Fig. 10.26).

The rectovaginal space is dissected from the posterior

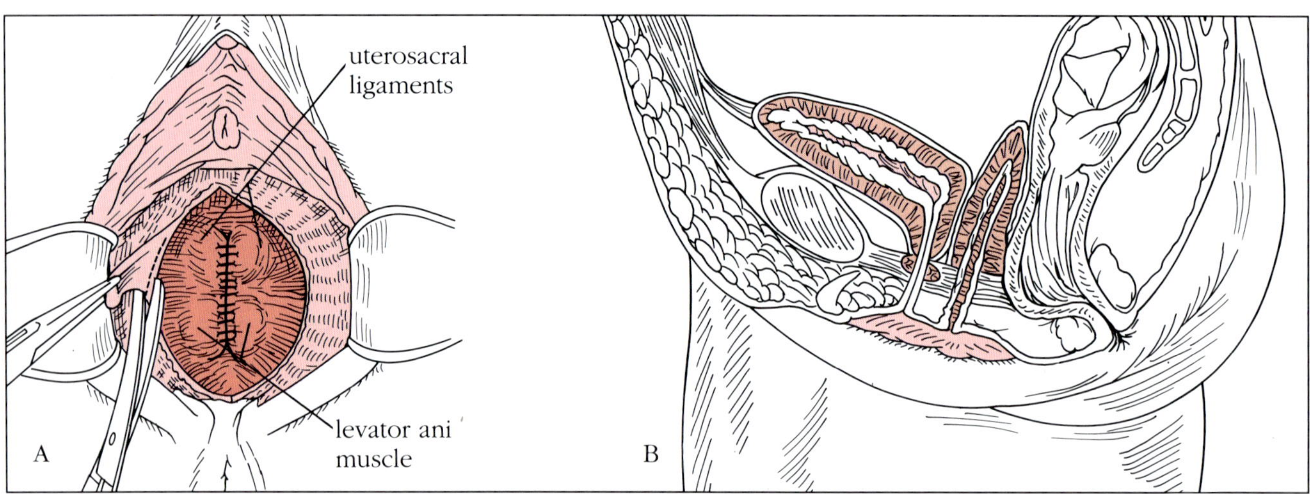

Figure 10.23 Enterocele repair. **A** Completed vault reconstruction. **B** Lateral view of the pelvis following obliteration of the cul-de-sac.

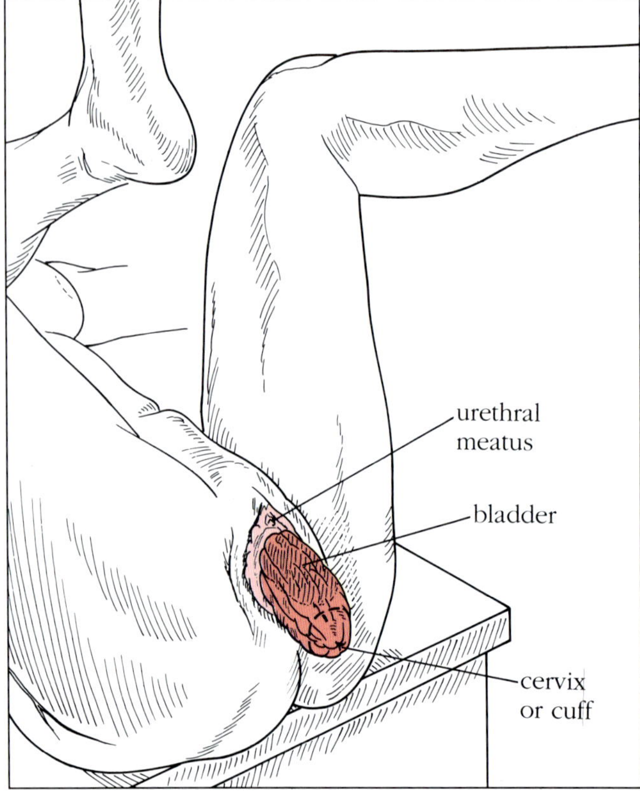

Figure 10.24 Large cystocele with complete vault prolapse.

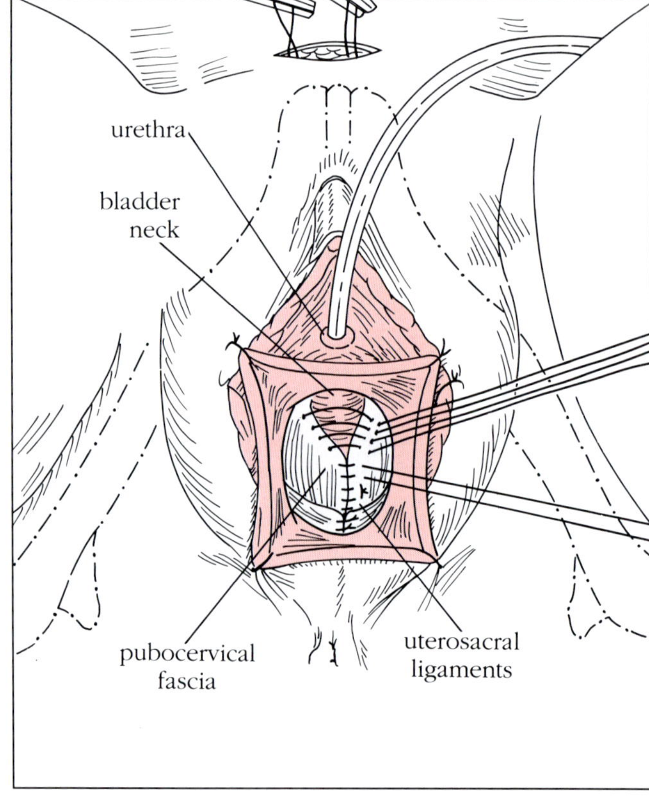

Figure 10.25 Cystocele repair. Uterosacral approximation followed by plication of pubocervical fascia.

vaginal wall by blunt or sharp dissection. The rectal pillars are seen on either side of the rectovaginal septum. The right rectal pillar is perforated bluntly. The posterior vaginal wall is retracted and the pararectal space visualized. With Botcher or Metzenbaum scissors, the pararectal space is perforated to the right of the rectum (Fig. 10.27). The rectum, cardinal ligament, and ureter are retracted anterolaterally to expose the sacrospinal ligament, which runs from the ischial spine to the sacrum. The superficial

areolar tissue overlying the ligament can be removed, but this is not necessary (Fig. 10.28).

With a finger on the ischial spine, a polypropylene suture is placed 1 inch medially to avoid injuring the pudendal vessels and nerve beneath the spine (Fig. 10.29A). A second suture is placed adjacent to the first. Each of the sutures is then placed through the vaginal wall, excluding the epithelium (Fig. 10.29B). These suture tails are tagged with hemostats. Both sutures are then tied,

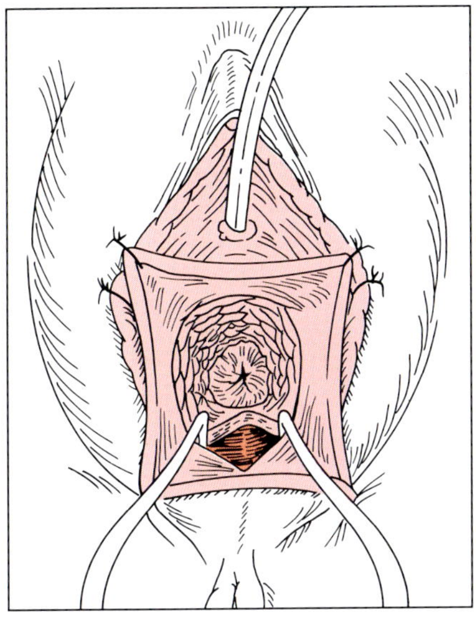

Figure 10.26 Sacrospinalis fixation. Initial incision into posterior fourchette.

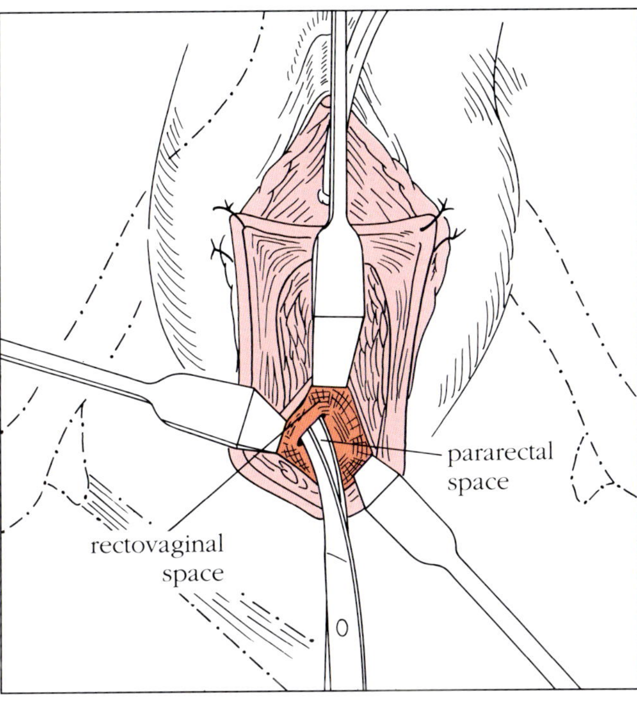

Figure 10.27 Sacrospinalis fixation. Perforation of right pararectal space.

Figure 10.28 Sacrospinalis fixation. Medial retraction of rectum to expose sacrospinal ligament.

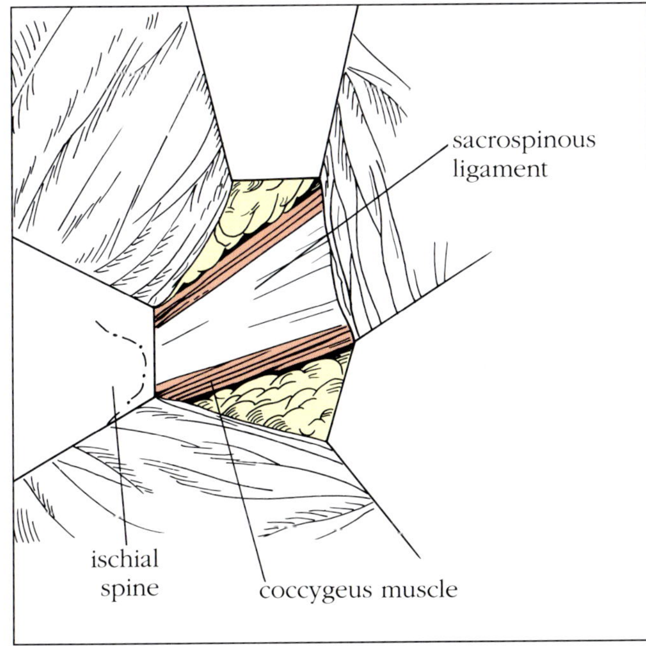

while making sure that the vagina is in contact with the sacrospinal ligament (Fig. 10.29C).

The rectocele is then repaired. A vaginal pack can be placed at the discretion of the surgeon (Fig. 10.30).

ABDOMINAL PROCEDURES FOR ANATOMIC STRESS INCONTINENCE

The patient is positioned in the low lithotomy position. With a few modifications, the supine position can be used. The vagina and lower abdomen are prepped and draped. A Foley catheter is placed per urethram and 10 mL of water is used to inflate the balloon.

A Pfannenstiel incision is made 2 cm above the pubic symphysis. The retropubic space is entered and the bladder dissected free from the posterior surface of the symphysis (Fig. 10.31). The Foley balloon is palpated with the catheter on traction to identify the bladder neck. The vagina adjacent to the bladder neck is exposed by blunt dissection with a tonsil clamp or sharp scissor dissection. If a

cystocele is present, the vagina underlying the bladder base is dissected.

Two to four #1 polypropylene sutures swedged onto or threaded through a Mayo needle are placed into the vaginal wall on each side, excluding the epithelium (Fig. 10.32A). The needle is then placed through the periosteum (modified Marshall-Marchetti-Krantz procedure) (Fig. 10.32B) or Cooper's ligament (Burch culposuspension) (Fig. 10.32C). Periurethral suture placement is avoided, but the vaginal sutures may extend as far proximal as necessary to correct a cystocele. A sponge stick placed in the vagina by the surgical assistant helps to elevate and support the vagina, facilitating dissection and suture placement.

A cystoscopy is performed to ensure adequate support of the bladder neck with traction on the sutures, to confirm ureteral efflux and to check for intravesical suture placement. If the patient is supine, the bladder dome can be opened for inspection in lieu of cystoscopy. A vaginal examination is performed to rule out perforation of the

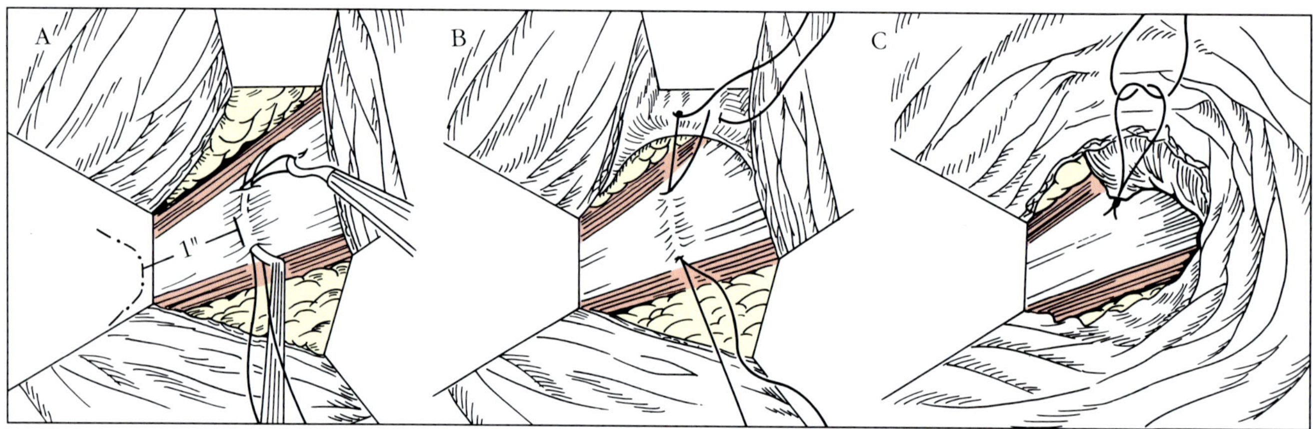

Figure 10.29 Sacrospinalis fixation. **A** Initial suture placement into ligament 2 cm medial to the right ischial spine. **B** Final suture placement into vaginal wall. **C** Vagina secured to sacrospinal ligament.

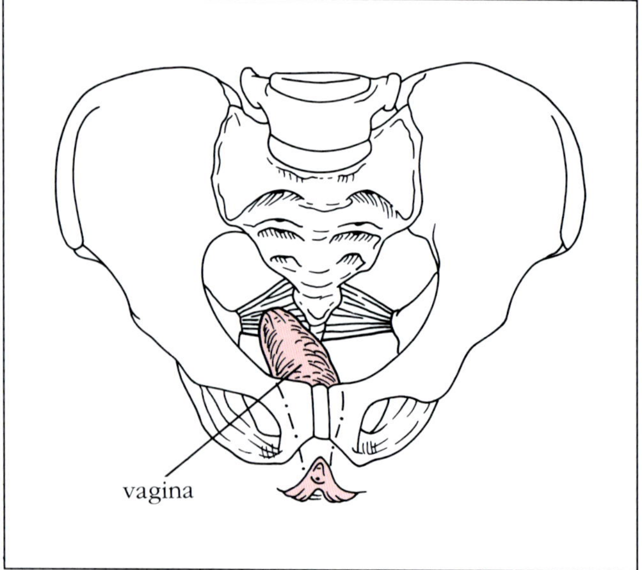

Figure 10.30 Sacrospinalis fixation. Completed repair. The vaginal wall deviates to the right, unnoticed by the patient.

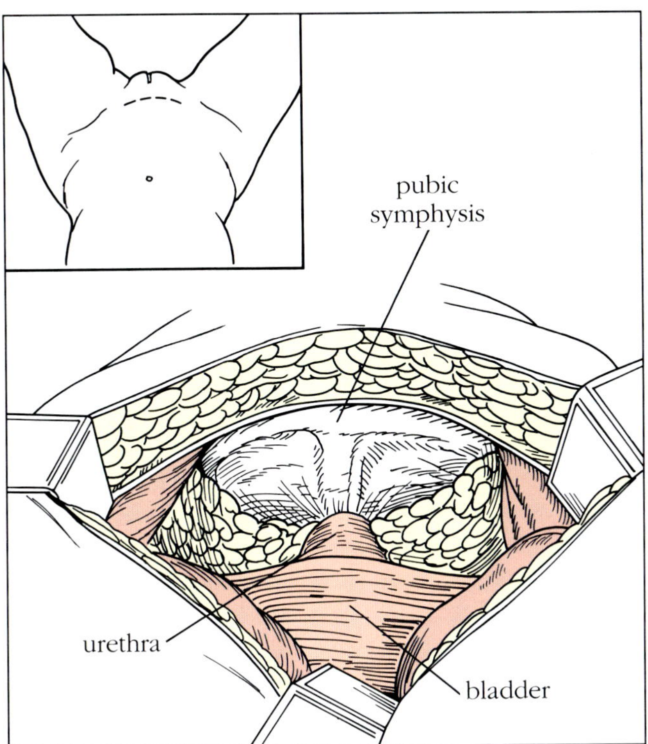

Figure 10.31 Abdominal vesical neck suspension. Entry into retropubic space with identification of bladder neck. Inset: Pfannenstiel incision.

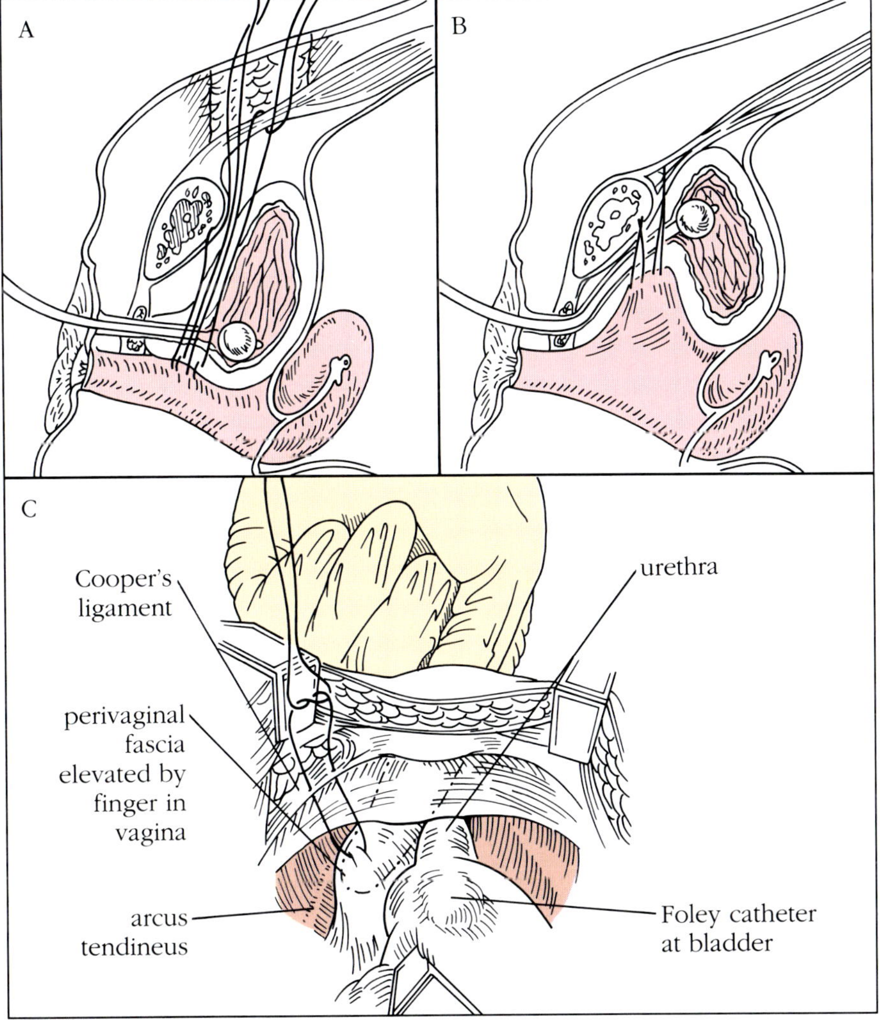

Figure 10.32 Abdominal vesical neck suspension. **A** Placement of sutures into vaginal wall at level of bladder neck. **B** Modified Marshall-Marchetti-Kranz procedure. **C** Burch suspension with correction of mild cystocele.

vaginal epithelium. The normal axis of the vagina points posteriorly towards the sacrum. If the patient has had a prior hysterectomy, anterior suspension of the vaginal wall towards the symphysis or Cooper's ligament may promote enterocele formation. To avoid this complication, the cul-de-sac can be obliterated by placing several rows of pursestring sutures between the sigmoid colon and the peritoneum anterior to the cul-de-sac (Fig. 10.33). The abdomen is closed.

Surgery for Intrinsic Sphincter Dysfunction

For the patient with severe postural incontinence and an open bladder neck at rest as seen on fluoroscopy, bladder neck suspension procedures are seldom effective in achieving continence. Proximal urethral compression or coaptation is required. This may be accomplished with sling procedures, injection of bulk-forming agents into the proximal urethra or bladder neck, or implantation of an artificial urinary sphincter. The urologist skilled in vaginal surgery will find that a vaginal approach is preferable for dissection of the urethra before most sling procedures as well as for placement of the artificial urinary sphincter, although an abdominal approach is acceptable.

SLING PROCEDURES FOR INTRINSIC URETHRAL DYSFUNCTION (TYPE III STRESS INCONTINENCE)
Pubovaginal Sling

A pubovaginal sling compresses the proximal urethra during filling of the bladder and prevents urinary stress incontinence. This is usually accomplished by harvesting a transverse graft of the anterior rectus and external oblique fascia and passing it around the urethra. The ends of the graft are sutured to the anterior rectus sheath. Urodynamic studies are helpful in the preoperative evaluation of patients with suspected type III urinary stress incontinence (ISD). Many patients with ISD have had prior surgical procedures that resulted in scarring of the periurethral and bladder neck tissues. Dissection may be difficult but is almost always possible. The pubic bone serves as a good landmark and subperiosteal dissection can be performed in difficult cases. Urinary retention and/or detrusor instability may result from an obstructing pubovaginal sling. Although it is not usually necessary, the patient should be willing to accept life-long intermittent catheterization before consenting to a sling procedure.

The patient is placed in a low lithotomy position and the lower abdomen, vagina, and perineum are prepped and draped in a sterile field. A 16 Fr Foley catheter with 10 mL of water in the balloon is used to identify the urethra and bladder neck. A Pfannenstiel incision is made and a 1.5 × 10-cm graft is harvested transversely across the anterior rectus sheath and external oblique apononeurosis. Before the graft is released, a 2-0 double-armed polypropylene suture is run up and down three times on either end of the graft. The graft, with suture and needles, is then removed and placed in a basin containing antibiotic irrigant solution. The defect is closed as the surgeon chooses, undermining the fascial edges as necessary to provide a tension-free closure.

An inverted U vaginal incision is made with the apex 0.5 cm from the urethral meatus and the lateral margins

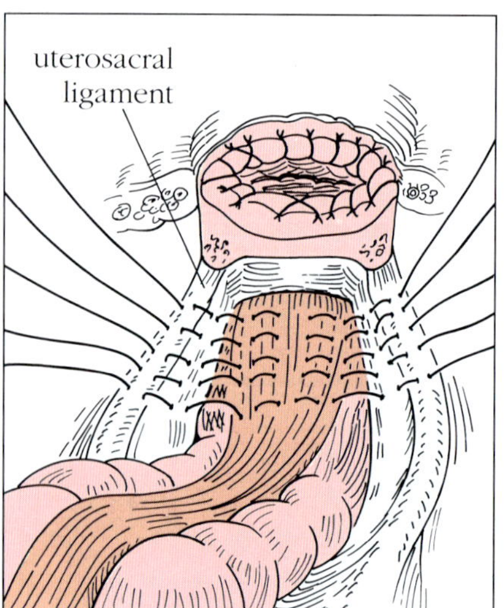

Figure 10.33 Abdominal vesical neck suspension. Obliteration of the cul-de-sac to prevent enterocele following transabdominal bladder neck suspension.

at the bladder neck. The vaginal flap is then dissected from the underlying periurethral fascia to the level of the bladder neck. Scissors are used to perforate the endopelvic fascia and enter the retropubic space bilaterally as in a Raz bladder neck suspension. The posterior surface of the anterior pubic ramus must be freed from adhesions.

A long Kelly clamp is then passed through the insertion of the rectus muscle on the right, hugging the periosteum to seat directly upon the surgeon's finger placed behind the ramus (Fig. 10.34A). The clamp is then guided through the vaginal incision. The graft is brought to the table in a kidney basin. The polypropylene sutures on the left side of the graft are grasped with the Kelly clamp and transferred suprapubically (Fig. 10.34B). The identical pro-

cedure is repeated on the right side. It is now possible to pull on each suture and compress the proximal urethra with the graft (Fig. 10.34C).

Cystoscopy is performed to evaluate urethral coaptation, which should occur with minimal tension. Indigo carmine is given intravenously and efflux from ureteral orifices is monitored. The bladder is carefully inspected for perforation. A suprapubic tube is then placed percutaneously or with a curved Lowsley tractor.

The graft is secured on one side to the anterior rectus sheath from the graft using the 2-0 double-armed polypropylene suture. The anterior vaginal flap is then replaced, using two running simple sutures of 3-0 chromic catgut. The cystoscope with 0° lens is reinserted and the bladder neck is visualized while tension is applied to the unse-

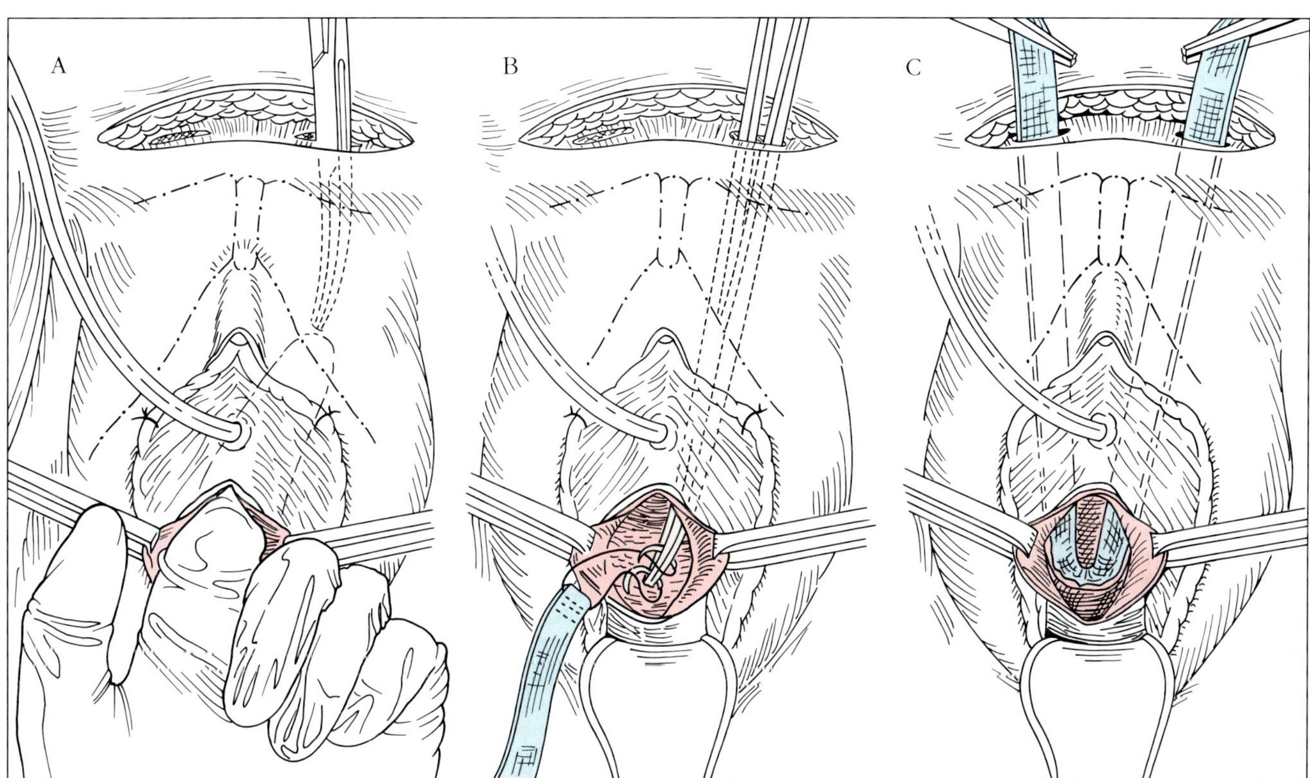

Figure 10.34 Pubovaginal sling. **A** Following dissection of a vaginal flap overlying the urethra, a finger is inserted into the retropubic space contacting the posterior rectus muscle. A Kelly clamp is passed through the rectus fascia and muscle to the surgeon's finger. **B** Graft is transferred suprapubically. **C** Graft positioned. Minimal traction on graft results in coaptation of the bladder neck and proximal urethra as seen cystoscopically.

cured suture. When the proximal urethra and bladder neck are seen just to coapt, the suture is tied. Excessive tension should be avoided (Fig. 10.35).

A Foley catheter is placed. A vaginal pack may be placed at the discretion of the surgeon.

Sling Patch

The procedure for placement of a sling patch is identical to that for a pubovaginal sling, with the following exceptions. A 2 × 4-cm patch of anterior rectus sheath is harvested. Sutures are placed into each corner of the patch, which is secured proximally to the tendinous arc (Fig. 10.36A). The sutures are transferred suprapubically with a ligature carrier (Fig. 10.36B). The sutures are tied over the anterior rectus sheath rather than affixed to it.

Vaginal Wall Sling

The patient is placed in the dorsal lithotomy position and a suprapubic tube and urethral catheter are placed.

A wide U incision is made from the urethral meatus to the bladder base (Fig. 10.37A). The urethropelvic ligament is dissected bilaterally and the retropubic space entered by perforation of the endopelvic fascia (see Fig. 10.9). A transverse incision is optionally made through the anterior vaginal wall at the level of the bladder neck, creating a rectangular island of vagina attached to the urethra in the midline (Fig. 10.37B). The vaginal wall from the bladder

neck towards the cervix or cuff may be dissected to permit advancement of the flap to the urethral meatus, covering the sling. There should be no tension on the flap if it is advanced to the meatus. Alternatively the lateral edges of the island may be freed for suture placement and the tissue overlying the bladder neck left in situ.

Two #1 Prolene sutures should be placed on each side of the sling. The proximal sutures should be placed at the level of the bladder neck and should include the pubocervical fascia and tendinous arc, as in a Raz bladder neck suspension.

A small suprapubic incision is made and the Raz needle passed on each side, transferring the sutures through the suprapubic wound. The cystoscope is used to rule out intravesical suture placement and to confirm clear efflux from both ureteral orifices. The proximal urethra should coapt with minimal tension on the suprapubic sutures. Next, the vaginal flap is advanced, using two running 2-0 or 3-0 absorbable sutures. Finally, the vaginal pack is placed and the suprapubic sutures are tied without tension. The suprapubic wound is closed.

ARTIFICIAL URINARY SPHINCTER
Transvaginal Placement

With the patient in the dorsal lithotomy position, a midline incision in the anterior vaginal wall is made from the midurethra to the bladder neck. Alternatively, the peri-

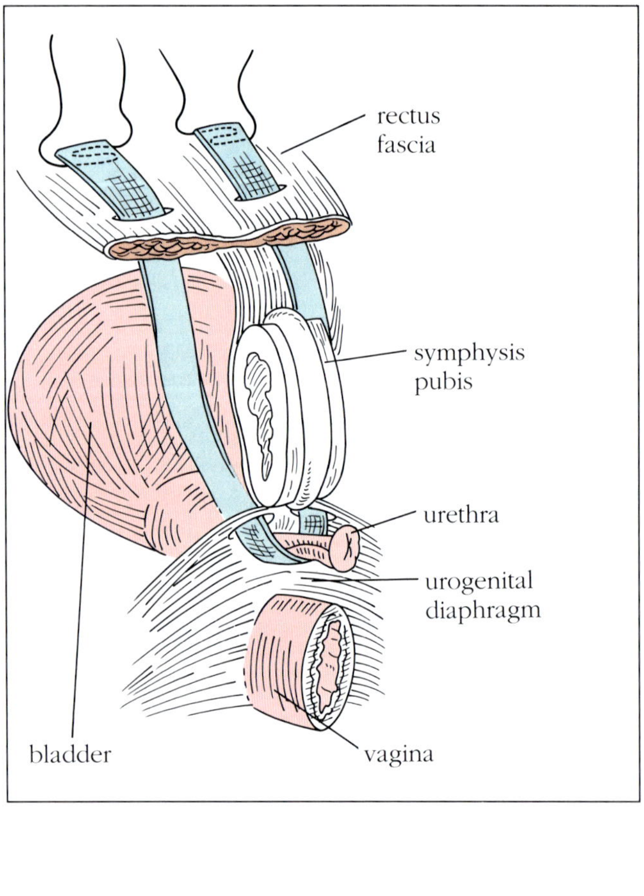

Figure 10.35 Pubovaginal sling. Graft sutured to rectus sheath.

urethral fascia is exposed through an inverted U incision. The sphincter is usually placed outside the periurethral fascia to minimize the chance of perforation and erosion.

The AS800 artificial sphincter consists of a pump, a pressure-regulating balloon, and an inflatable cuff. Within the pump are a refill/delay resistor and a valve, with a deactivation button located on the outside. Compression of the pump transfers fluid from the cuff into the balloon, which begins automatic repressurization that is delayed by the resistor in the pump. The time allowed for urination is 3 to 5 minutes. The pump then refills, followed by filling of the cuff.

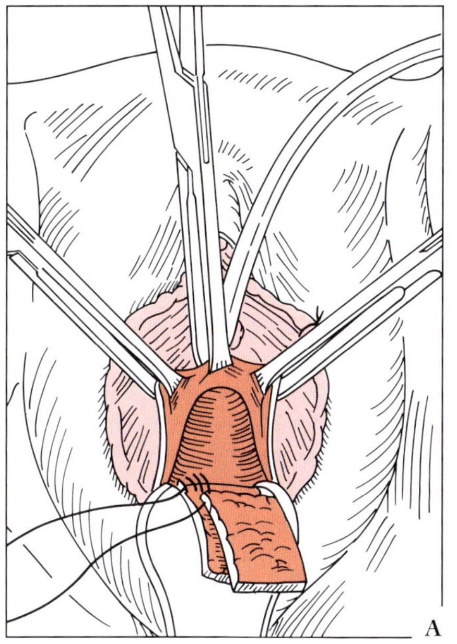
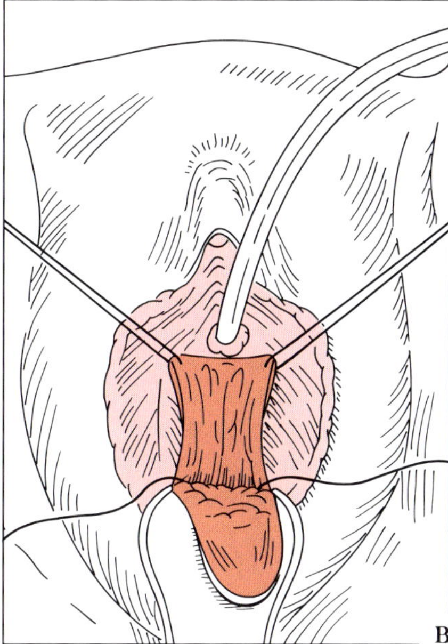

Figure 10.36 Sling patch. **A** Patch graft secured to right tendinous arc at the level of the vesical neck. **B** Sutures ready for suprapubic transfer via double-pronged (Raz) ligature carrier.

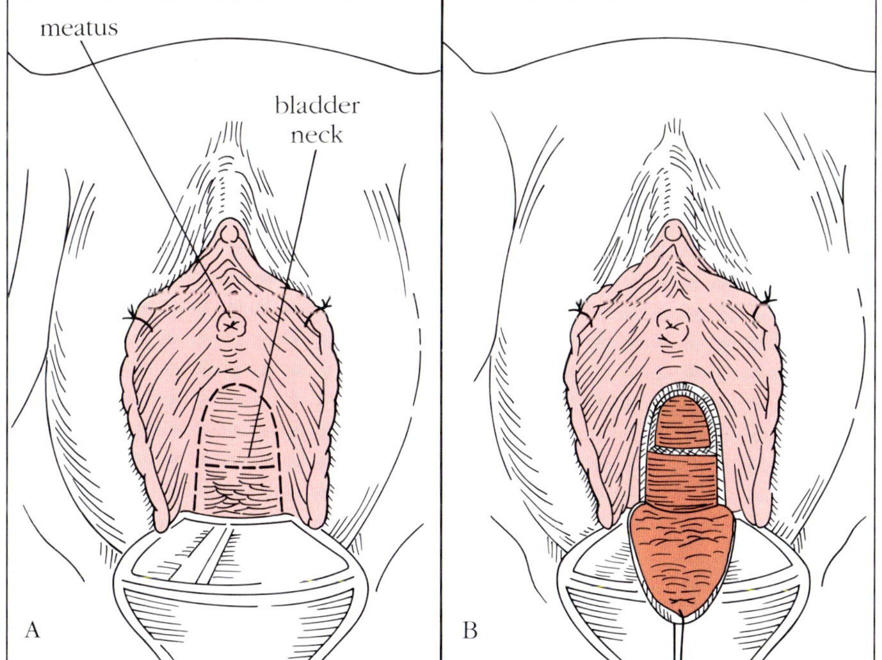

Figure 10.37 Vaginal wall sling. **A** Vaginal island flap forms sling which compresses the proximal urethra. **B** If the island flap is isolated from the vaginal wall at the bladder neck, the remaining vaginal wall may be advanced over the flap to the meatus.

A right-angle clamp is used to dissect around each side of the urethra and free the anterior urethra from the symphysis (Fig. 10.38A). A clamp is placed around the dissected urethra and a 0.25-inch Penrose drain is passed through the defect. A right-angle clamp is then used to enlarge the dissected area 2 cm anterior to the urethra (the cuff width is 2 cm) (Fig. 10.38B).

Using the right-angle clamp or a Satinsky, the flange of the cuff is grasped and guided around the urethra above the Penrose drain (Fig. 10.38C). If the pump and pressure-regulating balloon are to be located on the left side, the right-angle clamp is passed counterclockwise around the urethra, and clockwise passage places the tubing in the proper position for right-sided connections to the pressure-regulating balloon and pump. The Penrose drain is removed and the cuff snapped. The cuff tip is then excised and the snap rotated to an anterior position.

The retropubic space on the selected side is entered through a small suprapubic incision. The pressure-regulating balloon is filled with 20 mL of water and then deflated and clamped with a rubber-shod clamp. It is placed in a retropubic position above the endopelvic fascia, filled, and reclamped. A tonsil clamp is used to dissect a small subcutaneous space from the suprapubic wound to the labia majora for the pump. The tubing is trimmed and connected securely.

The device is tested by inflating and deflating the device after filling the bladder. The pump is deactivated by depressing the pump and pushing the deactivation button when it partially fills. Activation is performed 6 weeks later by vigorously compressing the pump, which opens the valve and allows the pump to refill completely. A 14 Fr Foley catheter is placed for 24 hours.

Transabdominal Placement

In the transabdominal approach, the cuff of the artificial sphincter is placed around the bladder neck and proximal urethra in the male or female patient. Through a Pfannenstiel incision, the retropubic space is developed and the endopelvic fascia is identified. Using Metzenbaum scissors or a #12 scalpel blade, the endopelvic fascia is opened on both sides. The balloon of the urethral Foley is placed on traction to identify the bladder neck.

To place the cuff, a right-angle or Satinsky clamp is used to dissect a 2-cm-wide space around the urethra at the level of the bladder neck. (If injury to the urethra or bladder neck occurs, the procedure is aborted. To identify injury, indigo-carmine-tinted saline can be injected through the urethra or the pelvis can be filled with irrigant and air injected through the urethra.) The tape sizer is passed through the defect and secured without tension to measure the circumference of the proximal urethra. Cuffs placed around the bladder neck are usually 8 to 10 cm in length. The deflated cuff is then snapped anteriorly and the tubing is passed through the anterior abdominal fascia on the side selected for the pump. A rubber-shod clamp is secured to the tubing.

The pressure-regulating balloon (usually 61 to 70 cm) is placed in a separate retropubic pocket away from the cuff. The balloon tubing is exited through the abdominal fascia a short distance away from the cuff tubing. The balloon is filled with isotonic contrast and secured with a rubber-shod clamp.

For placement of the pump, a subcutaneous tunnel from the groin to the scrotum or labia majora is created with a clamp, placing the pump as superficial as possible. A long nasal speculum aids insertion of the pump. The tubing is trimmed and connected to the balloon and cuff. The device is then cycled to ensure proper function. With the bladder filled, there should be no loss of urine through the urethra on bladder compression. The device is usually deactivated for 6 weeks.

Bulbous Urethral Cuff Placement

In the male patient, the bulbous urethra may be selected for cuff implantation. The patient is placed in the dorsal lithotomy position and a 16 Fr Foley catheter is placed. A midline perineal incision is used and the bulbocavernous muscle is divided.

For placement of the cuff, a right-angle clamp is used

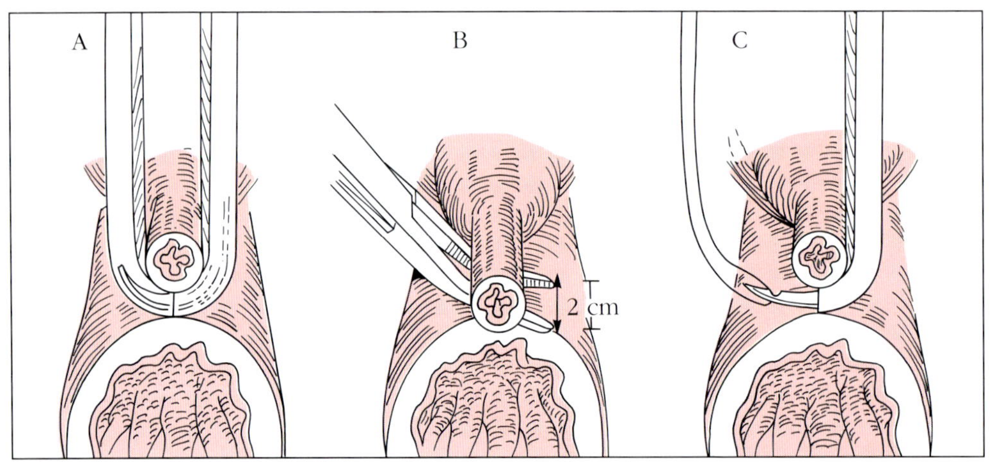

Figure 10.38 Artificial sphincter—abdominal approach. **A** Dissection of posterior urethra from vaginal wall. **B** Two-centimeter defect behind urethra allows placement of cuff without excessive mobility. **C** Cuff placement.

to dissect a space 2 cm wide around the bulbous urethra. A 4.5-cm cuff is passed around the urethra and snapped anteriorly. (If desired, the bulbous urethra can be measured with the cuff sizer before cuff selection.) Alternatively, the cuff can be placed outside the bulbocavernous muscle.

To place the deflated balloon, a small inguinal incision is made through the inguinal ring into the retropubic space. Finger dissection is used to create a pocket with adequate room for the filled balloon behind the pubis. The balloon is then inflated and a rubber-shod clamp is placed on the tubing. A tubing passer is used to advance the cuff tubing through the subcutaneous tissue and out through the groin incision.

For placement of the pump, a blunt clamp is used to create a tunnel from the inguinal incision to the scrotum. A small pocket for the pump is dissected in the dependent portion of the scrotum. A nasal speculum can be placed through the tunnel to assist with pump placement. The tubing is connected and the security is checked by vigorously pulling the tubing. The device is then cycled, tested, and deactivated for 6 weeks. The perineal wound is closed in two layers.

Complications

Infection, erosion, hydronephrosis, and persistent or recurrent incontinence may eventually follow placement of the artificial urethral sphincter. Infectious complications are minimized by administration of prophylactic antibiotics, attention to surgical technique, avoidance of urethral injury at the time of prosthesis placement, and careful patient selection. Erosion usually presents with infection, urinary retention, fistula, or urethral bleeding. Hydronephrosis can be avoided by complete assessment of filling and voiding bladder dynamics before sphincter implantation. The sphincter should not be used to control incontinence in patients with high detrusor pressure unless surgical augmentation or pharmacologic therapy provides low-pressure reservoir function of the bladder. Atrophy of the corpus spongiosum may lead to recurrent incontinence. This requires placement of a smaller cuff or increasing the balloon pressure. Persistent postoperative incontinence due to urethral dysfunction can be caused by improper cuff size or urethral scarring with decreased compressibility. In the former case the cuff is replaced with a smaller size, and in the latter a higher-pressure balloon is inserted. Bladder filling pressures should be determined (urodynamics) to rule out detrusor causes for recurrent or persistent incontinence.

PERIURETHRAL INJECTION OF BULKING AGENTS

Bulking agents, such as Teflon, fat, or collagen, may be injected periurethrally at the bladder neck in the incontinent man or woman. In female patients, three or four circumferential injections are made through a needle passed alongside or through the urethra to the bladder neck. Cystoscopy confirms occlusion of the bladder neck. In male patients, direct-vision transurethral injection through a cystoscope port with a needle designed for this purpose is simpler. Continuing improvements in the media available for injection will likely render this form of treatment more safe and effective and more often utilized in the future. The simplicity of the procedure, which is amenable to local anesthesia, appears to be the primary advantage. When the ideal agent is developed, the indications, success rate, and complications will likely be further defined along with cost and reinjection requirements.

References

Abrams P, Blaivas JG, Stanton SL, Andersen JT. Standardization of terminology of lower urinary tract function. *Neurourol Urodyn.* 1988;7:403–427.

Appel RA. Techniques and results in the implantation of the artificial urinary sphincter in women with type !II stress urinary incontinence by vaginal approach. *Neurourol Urodyn.* 1988;7:613–619.

Burns PA, Pranikoff K, Nochajski T, Desotelle P, Harwood MK. Treatment of stress incontinence with pelvic floor exercises and biofeedback. *J Am Geriatr Soc.* 1990;38:341–344.

Caine M, Raz S. The role of female hormones in stress incontinence. Presented at the 16th Congress of the Société Internationale d'Urologie; Amsterdam; 1973.

Ferguson KL, McKey PL, Bishop KR, Kloen P, Verheul JB, Dougherty MC. Stress urinary incontinence: effect of pelvic muscle exercise. *Obstet Gynecol* 1990;75:671–675.

Gittes RF, Laughlin KR. No incision pubovaginal suspension for stress incontinence. *J Urol.* 1987;138:568–570.

Hilton P, Tweddell AL, Mayne C. Oral and intravaginal estrogens alone and in combination with alpha-adrenergic stimulation in genuine stress incontinence. *Int Urogynecol J.* 1990;1:80–86.

Hodgkinson CP, Drukker BH. Infravesical nerve resection for detrusor dyssynergia: the Ingelman-Sundberg operation. *Acta Obstet Gynecol Scand.* 56:401–408.

Hodgson BJ, Dumas S, Bolling DR, Heesch CM. Effect of estrogen on sensitivity of rabbit bladder and urethra to phenylephrine. *Invest Urol.* 1978;16:67.

International Continence Society Committee for the Standardization of Terminology of the Lower Urinary Tract Function. *Br J Obstet Gynaecol.* 1990;suppl. 6:1–16.

International Continence Society. Fourth report on standardization of terminology of lower urinary tract dysfunction. *Br J Urol.* 1981;53:333.

Kaufman M, Lockhart JL, Silverstein MJ, Politano VA. Transurethral polytetrafluoroethylene injection for post-prostatectomy urinary incontinence. *J Urol.* 1984;132:463–464.

Levin RM, Jacobowitz D, Wein AJ. Autonomic innervation of the rabbit urinary bladder following estrogen administration. *Urology.* 1981;17:449.

Levin RM, Shofer FS, Wein AJ. Estrogen induced alteration in the autonomic responses of the rabbit urinary bladder. *J Pharmacol Exp Ther.* 1980;215:614.

Lewis RI, Lockhart JL, Politano VA. Periurethral polytetrafluoroethylene injections in incontinent female subjects with neurogenic bladder disease. *J Urol.* 1984;131:459–462.

Lockhart JL, Bejany D, Politano VA. Augmentation cystoplasty in the management of neurogenic bladder disease and urinary incontinence. *J Urol.* 1986;135:969–971.

McGuire E. Bladder instability and stress incontinence. *Neurourol Urodyn.* 1988;7:563–567.

Raz S, Klutke CG, Golomb J. Four-corner bladder and urethral suspension for moderate cystocele. *J Urol.* 1989;142:712–715.

Raz S, Little NA, Juma S, Sussman EM. Repair of severe anterior vaginal wall prolapse (grade IV cystourethrocele). *J Urol.* 1991;146:988–992.

Raz S, Siegel A, Short J, Snyder J. Vaginal wall sling. *J Urol.* 1989;141:43–46.

Raz S. Female urology. *Urol Clin North Am.* 1985.

Raz S. Modified bladder neck suspension for female stress incontinence. *Urology.* 1981;17:82–82.

Schmidt RA. Applications of neurostimulation. *Neurourol Urodyn.* 1988;7:585.

Stamey TA. Endoscopic suspension of the vesical neck for urinary incontinence in females: report on 203 consecutive patients. *Br J Obstet Gynaecol.* 1980;79:666–669.

Urinary Incontinence Guideline Panel. Urinary incontinence in adults: clinical practice guideline. Rockville, Md: Agency for Health Care Policy and Research, Public Health Service; March, 1992. US Department of Health and Human Services. AHCPR Pub. No. 92-0038.

Wheeless CR. *Atlas of Pelvic Surgery.* Philadelphia, Pa: Lea & Febiger; 1988.

Woodside JR, Crawford ED. Urodynamic features of pelvic plexus injury. *J Urol.* 1980;124:657.

CHAPTER 11

Impotence

Gregory A. Broderick

Analysis of male sexual function should be divided into three categories: interest, performance, and satisfaction (Fig. 11.1). Similarly, male sexual dysfunction encompasses disinterest, dysfunction, and dissatisfaction (Fig. 11.2). This chapter has been constructed to provide for the practicing urologist a review of the anatomy, physiology, and pharmacology of male sexual dysfunction. The behavioral categories of male interest/disinterest, performance/dysfunction, and satisfaction/dissatisfaction are addressed secondarily by examining what is currently known about the central nervous system as a regulator of libido and penile erection.

Impotence is a broad term often used by the patient and general medical community to express a problem with libido, penile erection, ejaculation, or orgasm. The Latin origin of the term is certainly more precise: *impotentia coeundi* refers to the inability of the male to perform the sexual act, *impotentia erigendi* refers to the inability to have a penile erection, and *impotentia generandi* refers to the inability to reproduce. The appropriate contemporary diagnostic term is *erectile dysfunction.*

The normal mechanisms of erectile function and pathophysiology of erectile dysfunction have been extensively and enthusiastically investigated in the last decade, fueled by the individual reports from Virag in 1982[1] and Brindley in 1983[2] that intracavernous injection of a vasoactive substance could produce erection without benefit of psychic or tactile stimuli. Although this review focuses on the mechanisms of penile erection, normal male sexual function involves not only initiating, maintaining, and terminating erection but also emission, ejaculation, and orgasm, events addressed during review of drug-induced sexual dysfunction. The variety, technique, and complications of penile revascularization and penile prosthetics are not discussed herein, and the reader is advised to consult other sources.[3–5]

Anatomy of Male Sexual Function

ARTERIAL ANATOMY

The arterial supply of the penis consists of the paired hypogastric–cavernous arterial beds. The vessels of penile inflow, from proximal to distal, are the internal iliac, internal pudendal, common penile, dorsal, bulbourethral, and cavernous arteries. The internal pudendal arteries cross the deep pelvis and perineum through the lesser sciatic foramen and Alcock's canal. The paired pudendal arteries are the principal supply to the common penile arteries. Recent angiographic and cadaver studies have shown that accessory supply to the penis can arise from the external iliac, obturator, or internal epigastric arteries.[6,7] After the perineal artery branches off, the internal pudendal artery becomes the common penile artery. The common penile artery is of variable but short length, composing the segment of vessel that trifurcates into the dorsal, cavernous, and bulbourethral arteries (Fig. 11.3). The paired dorsal arteries run on the surface of the tunica albuginea below Buck's fascia from the suspensory ligament to the glans. The paired cavernous arteries (arteriae profundae) enter the corporal bodies as the crura merge. At the base of the penis proximal to the suspensory ligament the cavernous arteries lie close to the septum, assuming a more central location as they run through the pendulous shaft. The paired bulbourethral arteries assume the 3 and 9 o'clock positions in relationship to the urethra and run through the corpora spongiosa to anastomose widely with dorsal branches within the glans.

In the flaccid state the cavernous artery's normal diameter is 0.5 to 0.6 mm; the cavernous arteries assume their greatest diameter—1.0 to 1.2 mm—during the tumescent phase of erection (see below).[8] Cavernous arterial diameter is controlled directly by the tone of smooth muscle composing the media of the vessel wall and indirectly by intracorporal pressure.[9] Multiple and variable anastomotic channels, first described in 1939, connect the three penile vessels.[10] Their impact on the hemodynamics of erection was not postulated until much later.[11] Observations from recent penile pharmacoarteriographic and duplex color Doppler studies have confirmed these variations in the penile arterial system. An accessory pudendal artery is the primary supply to the common penile artery in 6% to 10% of patients. Dorsal-to-cavernous and cavernous-to-cavernous arterial collaterals have been noted in one third of cases.[12–16]

VENOUS ANATOMY

Principal drainage of the corporal bodies is via the cavernous, deep dorsal, circumflex, and crural veins. Penile venous drainage is complex, with multiple levels of anastomoses (Fig. 11.4). Newman and Northrup[17] found ven-

---

FIGURE 11.1 *Sexual Function*

Interest/libido
Performance
    Erection/detumescence
    Emission
    Ejaculation
Satisfaction/orgasm

FIGURE 11.2 *Sexual Dysfunction*

Disinterest
Dysfunction
    Erection/priapism
    Emission
    Ejaculation
Dissatisfaction

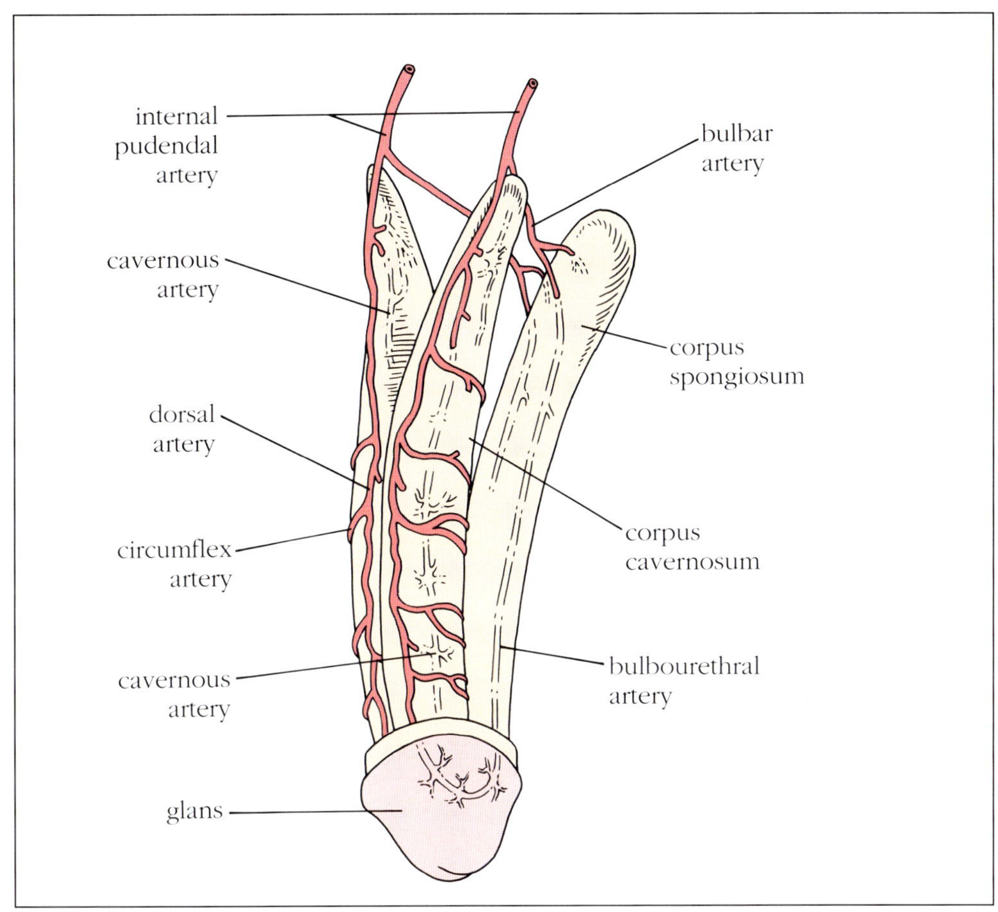

Figure 11.3 Penile arterial anatomy. (Modified with permission from Lue TF, Tanagho EA, 1988)

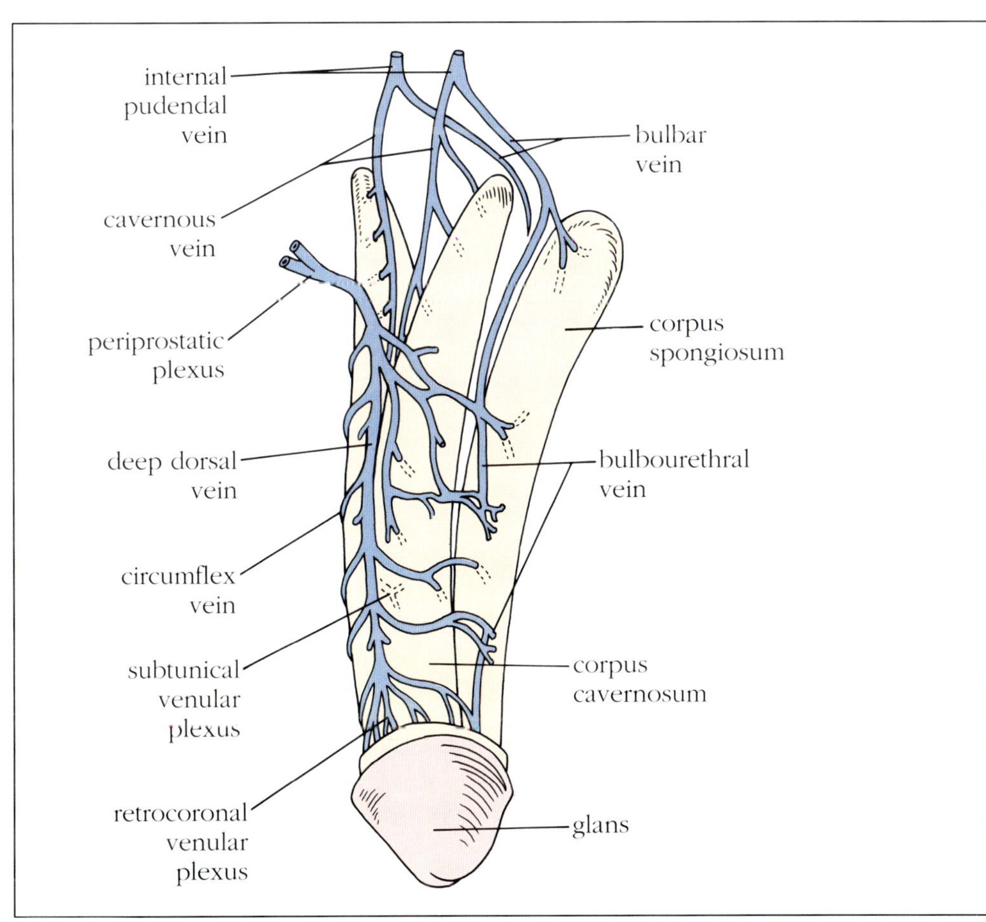

Figure 11.4 Penile venous anatomy. (Modified with permission from Lue TF, Tanagho EA, 1988)

ous drainage of the penis to be organized on three different levels: superficial, intermediate, and deep. Their observations have been confirmed in both cadaveric studies and cavernosography of potent volunteers.[6,18]

Superficial veins run between Colles' and Buck's fasciae, often coalescing into a superficial dorsal vein. Superficial veins of the penis are joined by veins from the scrotum and spermatic cord to enter either the right or left saphenous vein.

The intermediate system is composed of the deep dorsal and circumflex veins. Small venules emerge from the substance of the glans to coalesce into a retrocoronal plexus and enter the deep dorsal vein. Along its course in the groove between the corpora cavernosa, the deep dorsal vein receives circumflex veins, which arise from the undersurface of the corpus spongiosum and course laterally around the tunica albuginea. Emissary veins emerge perpendicularly or obliquely through the tunica albuginea to empty into the circumflex or deep dorsal vein. The deep dorsal vein enters the pelvis under the arch of the pubic rami, between the suspensory ligament. One to three deep dorsal veins receive three to 10 circumflex veins. Bicuspid valves are found within the deep dorsal veins.

The deep drainage system is composed of the cavernous and crural veins of the proximal third of the penis. Emissary veins arising from the dorsomedial surface of the diverging cavernous bodies unite to form one or two cavernous veins located deep and medial to the entry of the paired cavernous arteries and dorsal nerves. The cavernous veins drain into the internal pudendal veins. Just within the pelvis there are connections between the cavernous and periprostatic veins. Small crural veins emerge from the dorsal surface of each crus and drain into the internal pudendal vein.

NEUROANATOMY

Neurogenic erectile dysfunction results from surgical or traumatic severing of autonomic or somatic penile innervation or as a consequence of microscopic neuropathology with failure of cholinergic, adrenergic, or noncholinergic, nonadrenergic neurotransmission. The course and relationship of the nerves of erection to the other pelvic organs has only recently been described. Familiarity with these anatomic relationships is essential in the performance of "nerve-sparing surgery."[19–21] The cavernous nerves containing the autonomic efferents of erection lie posterolateral to the apex of the prostate at 5 and 7 o'clock; at the level of the membranous urethra they run at 3 and 9 o'clock; at the level of the proximal bulb the nerves rest at 1 and 11 o'clock in relation to the urethra, where they enter the hilum of the penis.[20]

The penis receives sympathetic, parasympathetic, and somatic innervation. Pelvic sympathetic nerves arise from the preganglionic neurons of the intermediolateral gray matter of the thoracic and lumbar spinal cord (T10–L2). Sympathetic preganglionic fibers exit the ventral roots as the white rami to the paravertebral ganglia, making synaptic connection with the postganglionic fibers of the preaortic plexus (Fig. 11.5). The hypogastric nerves contain postganglionic sympathetic fibers as well as preganglionic nerves, which descend in the pelvis to enter the pelvic nerve. The pelvic nerve is an important site of autonomic integration of erectile effectors as both pre- and postganglionic fibers of the sympathetic chain and sacral parasympathetic fibers intermingle.[9,22,23] Parasympathetic preganglionic fibers originate in the sacral cord segments (S2–S4); sacral preganglionic efferents known as nervi erigentes or pelvic nerves enter the pelvic plexus. Sympathetic preganglionic nerves also descend to the sacral ganglia with postganglionic sympathetics (gray rami) and leave within the pelvic nerves. Autonomic nerves leaving the pelvic plexus are protected (and hidden from surgical visualization) by the parietal pelvic fascia and run on the surface of the piriform muscles. Half of the pelvic plexus lies close to the anterolateral wall of the lower rectum; the other half rests on the posterior and lateral aspect of the bladder and prostate. Autonomic fibers from the pelvic plexus to the penis are known as the cavernous nerves. These fibers are beneath the pelvic fascia and associate with the posterolateral vascular bundle of the prostate.

The dorsal nerve of the penis is the somatosensory afferent of glans, prepuce, and pendulous shaft; the paired fibers pass beneath the suspensory ligament and under the pubic arch to enter the urogenital diaphragm. The pudendal nerve arising from sacral segments (S2–S4) provides somatic efferents to the external sphincter, bulbocavernous, and ischiocavernous muscles, and somatic afferents to the dorsal and perineal nerves.

PENILE ULTRASTRUCTURE

The penis consists of the paired corpora cavernosa, a perforated septum, and the single ventral corpus spongiosum. The spongiosum contains the urethra and enlarges distally to form the glans. The corpora cavernosa extend beyond the corona and into the glans. The three penile bodies are surrounded by Buck's fascia, which fuses with the suspensory ligament dorsally and Colles' fascia posteriorly. More superficial is the dartos fascia or Colles' fascia, which fuses anteriorly with the Scarpa's fascia of the abdomen. The corpora cavernosa are anchored to the inferior pubic rami by the crura, which are the divergent proximal segments.[7] The crura are covered by the ischiocavernous muscles: contraction of these muscles, which may be initiated by the bulbocavernous reflex, may transiently restrict venous outflow from the crura and augment erectile rigidity during pelvic thrusting.

Each corporal body is composed of corporal smooth muscle, fibrous tissue matrix, and endothelium-lined vascular spaces surrounded by a fibrous cover, the tunica albuginea. Recent electron microscopic investigations at the University of California, San Francisco, reveal that the tunica is bilayered, with multiple sublayers.[24] Elastic fibers provide an irregular lattice network on which collagen fibers rest. The inner layer of collagen is oriented circularly adjacent to the cavernous tissue. From this inner layer fibers radiate inward to insert on the septum. The outer layer is oriented longitudinally and inserts on the inferior pubic rami. Emissary veins run through the two layers in an oblique direction, whereas arterial perforators from the dorsal artery to the cavernous artery and, presumably, the cavernous artery to the bulbourethral artery, run perpendicularly. The structure and composition of the tunica albuginea provide the framework for erection and play a role in venous occlusion of the emissary vessels. On the other hand, the tunica of the corpus spongiosum has only one principal layer—it lacks the outer longitudinal fibers.

Morphologic changes in erectile tissue have been shown in specific conditions: Peyronie's disease, trauma, diabetes, tumor, scleroderma, priapism, and malignant infiltration.[9] In patients with diabetes mellitus, electron microscopic studies of the corpora demonstrate changes in the ultrastructure of cavernous nerves with diffuse thickening of Schwann cells and perineural basement membranes.[25] Controversy abounds as to whether the ultrastructural changes outlined by contemporary electron microscopic studies can be correlated with the degree of clinical erectile dysfunction. Persson et al.[26] noted that among patients classified as having moderate arterial insufficiency (based on assessment with intracavernous vasoactive agent and duplex Doppler ultrasound) the trabecular architecture, number, and distribution of smooth muscle cells are similar to normal patients. They found differences, though, in the abundance of mitochondria and mitochondrial morphology. They also noted cytoplasmic vacuolization and endothelial cell alterations. Changes in smooth muscle cells are apparent in patients with severe arterial disease, with smooth muscle cells showing irregular contour, fragmentation, and loss of basement lamina.[27] The cytoplasm of smooth muscles from a severe arterial disease group shows deficits of contractile myofilaments.

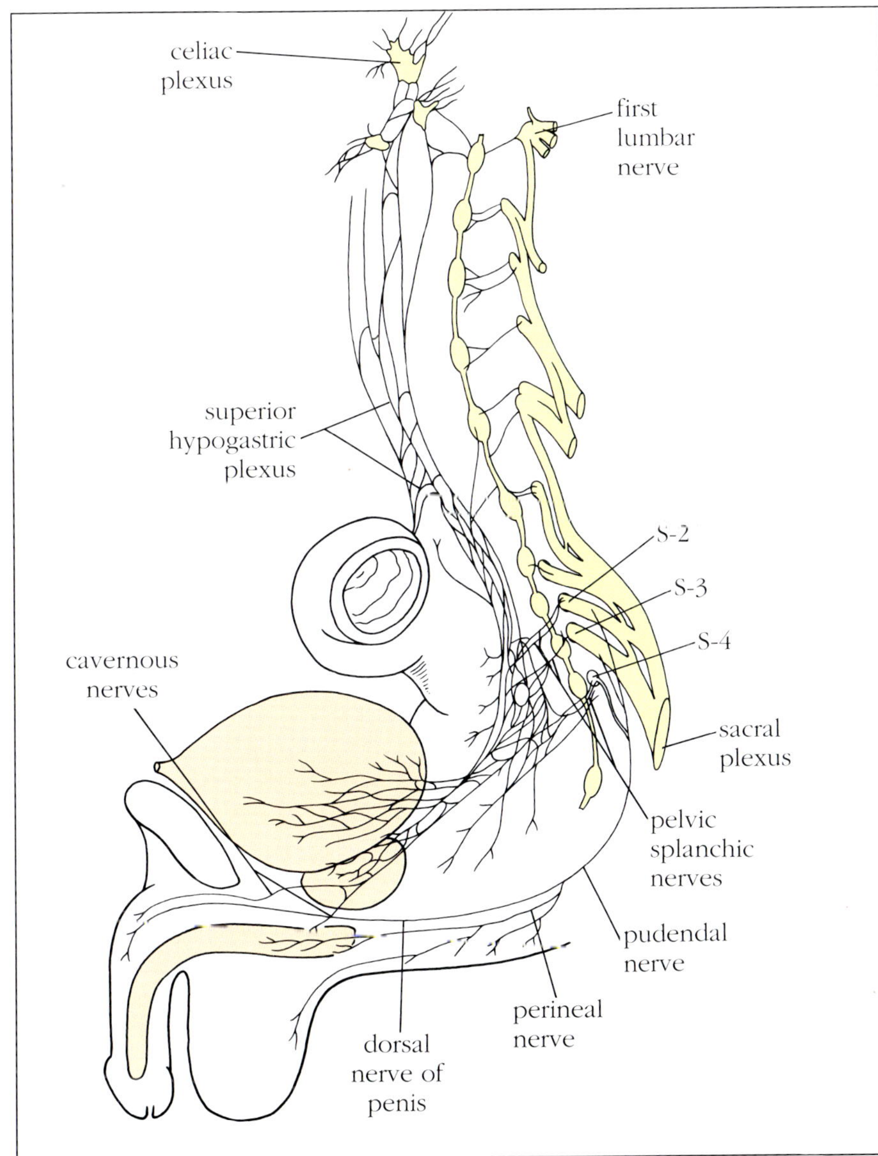

Figure 11.5 Thoracolumbar sympathetic outflow arises from the T9–L2 spinal cord segments and travels by lumbar splanchnic nerves to the prevertebral ganglia and eventually to the hypogastric chain ganglia and by the pelvic nerve to the pelvic plexus. Parasympathetic input to the cavernous tissues arises from the sacral (S2–S4) spinal cord segments and travels in the pelvic nerve to the pelvic plexus. Somatic motoneurons also originate in the S2–S4 cord segments and are conveyed by the pudendal nerve, whose terminal branches are the dorsal nerve of the penis and perineal nerve. (Modified with permission from Steers WD. Innervation of the cavernous tissue. In: Jonas U, Thon WF, Stief CG, eds. *Erectile Dysfunction.* Berlin: Springer-Verlag; 1991: 16–33)

Wespes has advocated corporal biopsies as an adjunctive technique in the diagnosis of vascular impotence, employing light microscopy and computerized morphometric analysis.[28,29] He noted that the corporal smooth muscle content of cadavers ranged from 27% to 41%; the cadaver donors had unknown potency status and a wide age range. Among patients receiving penile implants and among cadaver specimens, Wespes has observed an age-related decrease in smooth muscle content within the corpora cavernosa.[29,30] Apparently the amount of cavernous smooth muscle does not significantly vary with the site of biopsy in the same individual, contradicting earlier reports, which found varying degrees of histopathologic change in the right and left corpora among 17% of patients receiving prostheses.[31] Comparing young patients with penile curvature but hemodynamically adequate erection and elderly patients with erectile dysfunction, computerized morphometry showed that young patients (with penile curvature) had corpora cavernosa composed of 40% to 52% smooth muscle, patients with corporal veno-occlusive dysfunction had 19% to 36% smooth muscle, and patients with arterial impotence had 10% to 25% smooth muscle, with collagen contents increased accordingly.[28] Quite to the contrary, Vickers[32] examined the ultrastructure of cavernous smooth muscle and endothelium in patients with erectile dysfunction secondary to neural, arterial, venous, or fibrotic processes and found no pathognomonic changes.

Changes in the extracellular matrix have similarly been disputed. Luangkhot et al.[33] found that the collagen distribution, quantity, and types within the corpus cavernosum did not vary with age or history of erectile dysfunction. These investigators found the mean collagen content in all patients to be 47%. Collagen types I and IV predominate in the corpus proper, with lesser amounts of type III. The tunica albuginea was noted to have equal proportions of types I and III. They, and other investigators, have suggested that collagen type IV is a secretory product of the basement membrane of blood vessels, originating within the corpus from the endothelial cell linings of the sinusoids.[34] Others have noted qualitative and quantitative differences in the collagenous architecture within the corpora of impotent patients receiving prostheses.[35-38] Normal corporal collagen content has been reported to range from 40% to 65%.

It is clear that electron microscopic ultrastructural differences in smooth muscle of the corpus cavernosum are found among patients with severe erectile dysfunction; however, no single etiology of dysfunction has been associated with uniform changes in corporal tissue with the exception of diabetes, in which consistent alteration of neural architecture is seen within the cavernous bodies as in other organ systems.[39-41] Based on these morphometric studies and physiologic investigations, which will be reviewed below, it seems justified to assert that future classifications of vasculogenic erectile dysfunction must take into account pathology in the smooth muscle/endothelial cells in prepenile arteries, intrapenile arteries, and sinusoids of the corpora. At present corporal biopsies, whether processed by electron microscopy or light microscopy with computerized morphometric analysis, remain investigational techniques that require matched characterization of patients by specific etiology of impotence and/or correlation of outcomes from intervention with the response to either intracavernous agents or vascular operation (Fig. 11.6).

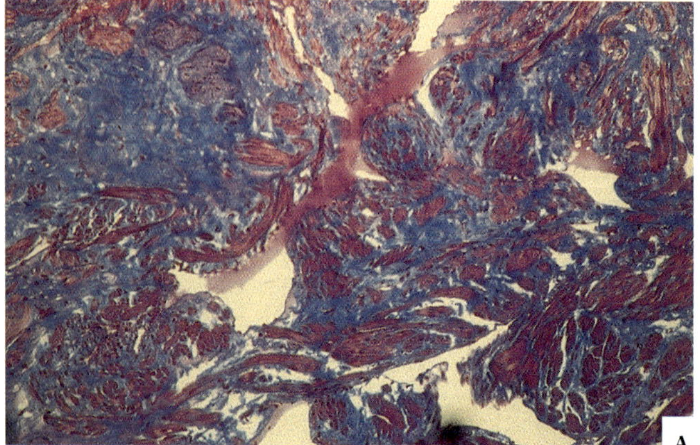 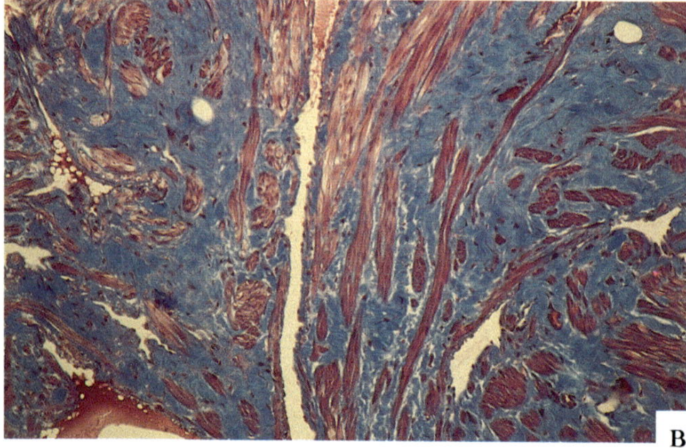

Figure 11.6 Photomicrographs of corporal biopsies taken at time of operation for correction of penile curvature **A** and placement of prosthesis for arteriogenic erectile dysfunction **B**. Accurate morphometric analysis depends on sampling and comparing several corporal areas to determine the ratio of smooth muscle to connective tissue. Trichrome staining turns smooth muscle cells red and interstitium blue. The ratio of smooth muscle to connective tissue is decreased in the patient with vasculogenic erectile dysfunction but not in the patient with curvature and normal penile hemodynamics. (Courtesy of Dr. E. Wespes, Université Libre de Bruxelles)

Hemodynamics of Erection

Erection is a complex hemodynamic event regulated by the tone of the smooth muscle of the cavernous arterioles and sinusoids.[42] A variety of theories on the mechanism of penile erection were proposed by early investigators, whose observations were limited to gross anatomic dissections and the two dimensions of the light microscope: arterial polsters,[43,44] sluice theory,[10] arterial/venous polsters,[45] and arteriovenous shunting.[17] Current appreciation of the vascular dynamics of erection is based on three-dimensional investigations of corporal microvascular architecture using corrosion casting and scanning electron microscopy.[30,46–58] The most widely acknowledged theory on the hemodynamics of erection is that attributed to the investigations of T.F. Lue (Fig. 11.7). Selecting the canine penis for corrosion casting proved to be advantageous since the internal pudendal artery could be perfused to fix one corporal body at various phases of erection. Since the septum is not perforated like the human's, the contralateral corpus in the dog served as a matched control.[50]

In the flaccid penis the smooth muscle of the cavernous arterioles and corporal sinusoids is contracted. The arterioles empty into sinusoidal spaces, i.e., smooth muscle compartments lined by endothelial cells. Although vascular resistance to inflow is elevated in the flaccid state, venular outflow is unrestricted. Regulation of venous outflow from the penis appears to be a passive phenomenon. Venules draining the sinusoidal spaces coalesce into a peripheral plexus below the outer fibroelastic tunica of the corporal

bodies. Egress from the subtunical venular plexus is via emissary veins exiting obliquely through the bilayered tunica albuginea into the deep dorsal vein or more directly via the short cavernous and crural veins at the base to the corporal bodies. Tumescence follows a decrease in corporal smooth muscle tone and vascular resistance; arterial inflow increases and the corporal sinusoids distend with oxygenated blood. The expanding sinusoids compress the subtunical plexus and restrict venous outflow.

There may actually be two circulatory trees within the corpus, with arterioles terminating in capillaries peripherally or in cavernous sinuses centrally.[30] These latter arteries are commonly referred to as helicine arterioles. The terminal portions of these helicine vessels are sharply angulated and spiral into the cavernous sinusoids. The cavernous sinuses located most centrally are larger (0.5 to 1.0 mm) and arranged parallel to the long axis of the penis; those located more peripherally are smaller and have no specific orientation. All the sinuses have anastomoses and are drained by postcavernous venules, which anastomose with the postcapillary venules in the subtunical venular plexus. Venous outflow during erection is limited dynamically by distention of the sinusoids, compressing the subtunical venular plexus against the inner layer of the tunica albuginea, and structurally by the differential stretching of the two primary layers of the tunica across which the emissary veins exit.

Observations of pudendal and cavernous arterial inflows and intracorporal pressures in the animal model reveal that erection can be divided into phases. Electro-

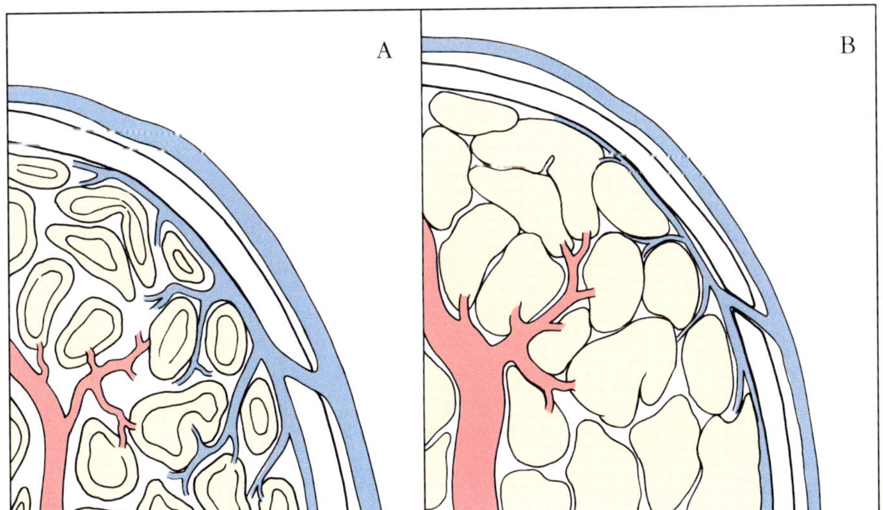

Figure 11.7 **A** In the flaccid state the arteries, arterioles, and sinusoids are contracted and the subtunical venular plexus is open, with free flow through the emissary veins perforating the tunica albuginea. **B** In erection the smooth muscle of the arteries, arterioles, and sinusoids relaxes. Maximum cavernous inflow distends the cavernous sinusoids. Intracorporal pressure rises and compresses the subtunical venous plexus, restricting venous outflow. (Reprinted with permission from Lue TF. Male sexual dysfunction. In: Tanagho EA, McAninch JW, eds. *General Urology.* 12th ed. Norwalk, Conn: Appleton & Lange; 1988:663–678)

stimulation of cavernous nerve in the animal model results in progressive erection with distinct hemodynamic phases (Fig. 11.8):

1. Latent: high flow enters the corpora throughout both diastolic and systolic cardiac cycles.

2, 3. Tumescence: the penis rapidly expands, but as rising intracorporal pressure exceeds the pressure of diastole, further inflow proceeds only during systole.

4. Full Erection: intracorporal pressure may reach 85% of systolic blood pressure.

5. Rigid Erection: stimulation of the pudendal nerve results in contraction of the ischiocavernous muscles, raising intracavernous pressure above systolic pressure.

6. Detumescence.

Cavernous nerve stimulation produces erection. Intracorporal pressure reaches 100 mm Hg during full erection and transiently exceeds 100 mm Hg during the rigid phase when pudendal nerve stimulation is added, which is analogous to contraction of the ischiocavernous and bulbocavernous muscles.[50]

Pharmacologic Regulation of Male Sexual Function and Drug-Induced Dysfunction

Normal sexual function in males involves initiating and maintaining erection, emission, ejaculation, and orgasm. Sexual response in the male can be divided into behavioral, erectile, and ejaculatory phases, each of which forms a segment of a response cascade. Responses of this cascade depend upon coordinated interaction among regulatory sites in the diencephalon, brain stem, spinal cord, and the end organs of the vascular tree of the penis, the smooth muscle of the corpora cavernosa, the skeletal muscle of the pelvis, and the accessory sex glands.[51-54]

Iatrogenic sexual dysfunction occurs when therapeutic interventions, either pharmacologic or operative, diminish the capacity of the central or peripheral neuropathways to elicit responses or that of the end organs to respond. It is important for the physician to be aware of how commonly prescribed or illicit drugs may impair the male sexual response. The incidence and type of sexual side effects elicited by pharmacotherapies depend on pharmacologic and patient-response variables. The pharmacologic variables include the biologic effects of the drug and the potency and efficacy of the drug to elicit these responses. The therapeutic variables include dosage and duration of therapy. The patient variables include the pharmacologic sensitivity of the patient and the predisposition of the patient to sexual response disorders.[54-58] The list of sexual side effects in this review represents a summary of these observations. Figure 11.9 summarizes the reported effects of commonly prescribed oral drugs on male sexual behavior.

DRUG-INDUCED CHANGES IN SEXUAL BEHAVIOR

The behavioral phase consists of the neural integration of sensory data with cognition, emotion, and desire, leading to the initiation and maintenance of sexual activity. Drug therapies can alter behavioral responses by affecting the

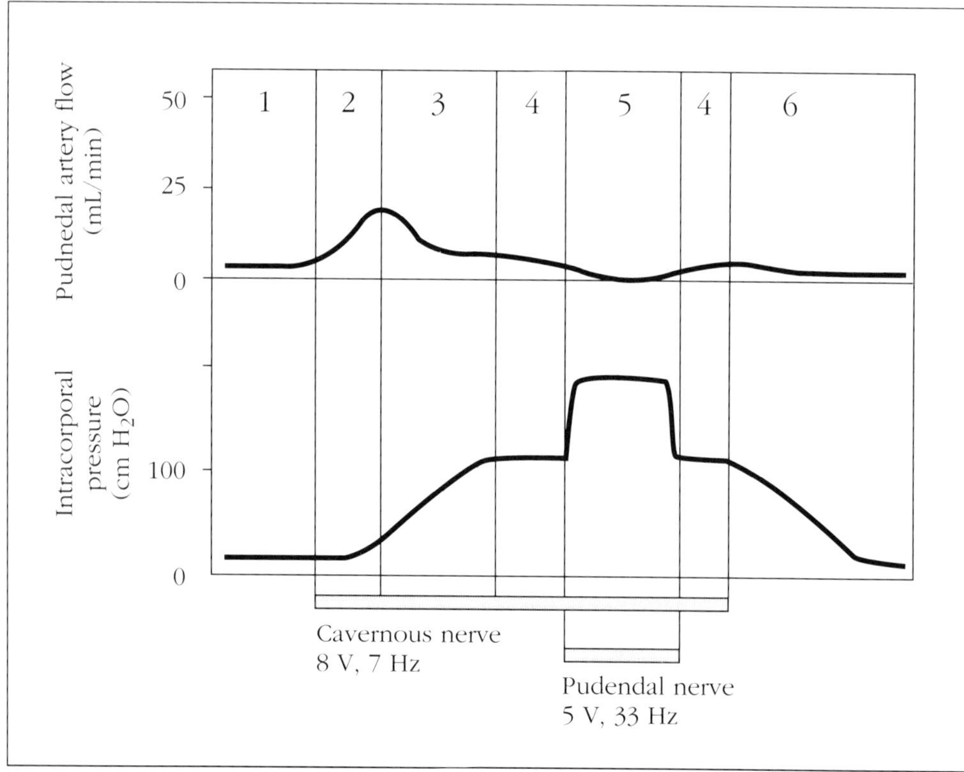

Figure 11.8 Six phases of erection. Electrical stimulation of the cavernous and pudendal nerves in simian and canine models of erection. (Reprinted with permission from Lue TF, 1988)

general mood or activity of a patient, or by directly affecting activity within the neural pathways that regulate the expression of sexual behavior.[53,58] Drugs that depress behavior include the prescription drugs with sedative side effects, which have been given various classifications, such as hypnotics, sedatives, minor tranquilizers, and major tranquilizers.[58,59] In addition to the primarily suppressive effects on sexual response, it has been claimed that low doses of notorious central nervous system depressants, such as alcohol, barbiturates, and methaqualone, increase sexual drive by suppressing social anxieties.[54,60] Oncolytic agents can affect sexual behavior through direct toxic effects on the hormonal axis or indirectly through toxic effects on multiple organ systems.

Drugs can also have selective effects on sexual behavior through brain areas that are responsible for regulating sexual drive.[51,61] One of these regions is the medial preoptic area (MPOA) of the ventral diencephalon, which functions as a sexual drive control center in a variety of mammalian species. Neurons within the MPOA receive synaptic terminals from peptidergic, dopaminergic, adrenergic, and serotonergic neurons and contain receptors for reproductive hormones.[51,52,54,60,62]

Observations of increased libido in parkinsonian, psychiatric, and impotent patients receiving the catecholamine precursor L-dopa stimulated research on the pharmacologic control of sexual behavior.[63–67] In laboratory animals and patient populations, increased sexual behavior can be induced by altering catecholamine metabolism through increasing synthesis with L-dopa or decreasing degradation with a monoamine oxidase B inhibitor, deprenyl.[68,69] Amphetamine, a catecholamine-releasing agent, and cocaine, a catecholamine uptake inhibitor, increase sexual behavior in rats and libido in men after acute administration.[69–72] Reserpine and α-methyldopa, which deplete functional pools of catecholamines in neurons, suppress sexual behavior in animals and libido in patients.[59,61,68,71]

In contrast to dopaminergic agonists, dopaminergic antagonists (e.g., antipsychotics) suppress sexual drive in patients and animals. Significant decreases in sexual drive and interest were noted in evaluations of thioridazine, fluphenazine, haloperidol, and chlorpromazine for the treatment of "deviant" sexual behavior.[52,54,60] In addition to the effects on MPOA neuronal function, dopamine antagonists can also suppress sexual response through the hyperprolactinemia and secondary hypogonadism induced by these agents with chronic dosing.

Since L-dopa, cocaine, amphetamine, and deprenyl affect the activity of all catecholaminergic neurons, it is possible that these effects on sexual drive may be mediated in part by increased adrenergic receptor activity.[51,68] Yohimbine, an α₂-adrenergic antagonist, increases sexual behavior by blocking presynaptic autoreceptors and increasing adrenergic receptor activity. The only effects of systemically or intracranially administered yohimbine on sexual response that have been consistently documented in laboratory studies are the behavioral drive-enhancing effects.[73,74]

Serotonin has been proposed to be an inhibitory transmitter in the control of sexual drive.[51,61,68] Direct or indirect augmentation of 5-HT activity by the administration of the precursor, 5-hydroxytryptophan, 5-HT uptake inhibitors, 5-HT releasing agents, or a variety of postsynaptic agonists results in suppression of sexual behavior in male rats.[75,76]

HORMONAL EFFECTS ON SEXUAL BEHAVIOR

Androgens are essential for male sexual development. Steroidogenesis begins in the Leydig cells of the testes by the sixth week of embryonic life.[77] Sexual dimorphism of the central nervous system in mammals is regulated by fetal and neonatal levels of circulating androgens and estrogens. In laboratory animals adult sexual behavior can be altered by changes in the medial preoptic area (MPOA) induced by supplementation or denial of sex steroids.[77–83]

Testosterone is synthesized within the Leydig cells under the control of luteinizing hormone (LH), a glycoprotein secreted by the anterior lobe of the pituitary gland. Normally, within the circulation 44% of testosterone is transported bound to sex-hormone-binding globulin, 54% is bound to albumin, and 2% is free.[84] Within target tissues testosterone is enzymatically converted by aromatization to estradiol or reduced to dihydrotestosterone (DHT). Aromatization to estradiol occurs within the central nervous system and reduction to DHT in the peripheral tissues: prostate, penis, hair follicles, sebaceous glands, and seminal vesicles.[77]

Hypogonadal patients receiving testosterone supplements show increases in tumescence and rigidity, the number of nocturnal erectile events, and total sleep erection time.[85] On the other hand, prepubertal boys and castrate men have reflexogenic and psychogenic erections. The concept of "andropause" remains poorly defined and controversial, but bound and free levels of testosterone decrease progressively with age.[84,86,87] Although hypogonadism has been found in one third of elderly impotent patients, impotence and hypogonadism in men over 50 years of age have been found statistically independent in recent geriatric studies.[88–90]

LH has a short half-life and its secretion is episodic; the circadian release of testosterone is regulated by the pulses in LH secretion. To overcome sampling errors most investigators recommend that a random low level of testosterone be re-assayed on two or three mornings or that serum be sampled sequentially on the same morning three times, 15 minutes apart, with pooling of the blood for assay.[84,91] Simple determination of plasma testosterone levels permits diagnosis of hypogonadism; measuring LH levels further permits differentiation between primary (hypergonadotropic, LH high) and secondary (hypogonadotropic, LH low) hypogonadism. In the majority of hyperprolactinemic patients sexual dysfunction is accom-

FIGURE 11.9 *Reported Side Effects of Oral Drugs*

DRUG	LIBIDO	ERECTION	EJACULATION
Sympatholytics			
Reserpine	−	−	−
α-Methyldopa	−	−	−
Guanethidine	−	−	−
Guanadrel	−	−	−
Bethanidine		−	−
Debrisoquine		−	
α-Adrenergic Agonists			
α1-Agonists			
Phenylpropanolamine			+
Pseudoephedrine			+
Ephedrine			+
α2-Agonists			
Clonidine		−	
α-Adrenergic Antagonists	−		
α1-Antagonists			
Prazosin		−/P	−
Phentolamine			−
Phenoxybenzamine			−
α2-Antagonists			
Yohimbine	+	+	
β-Adrenergic Antagonists			
Propranolol	−	−	−
Pindolol		−	
Labetolol		−/P	−
Atenolol		−	
Oxprenolol	−		
Metoprolol	−	−	
Timolol	−	−	
Diuretics			
Spironolactone	−	−	
Chlorthalidone	−	−	
Bendroflumethiazide		−	
Hydrochlorothiazide		−	
Acetazolamide	−	−	
Amiloride	−	−	
Dichlorphenamide	−	−	
Methazolamide	−	−	
Anticholinergics			
Anisotropine		−	
Dicyclomine		−	
Glycopyrrolate		−	
Homatropine		−	
Oxybutinin		−	
Tridihexethyl		−	
Clidinium		−	
Hexocyclium		−	
Propantheline		−	
Mepenzolate		−	
Methantheline		−	
Antipsychotics			
Chlorpromazine	−	−/P	−
Thioridiazine	−	−/P	−
Mesoridazine	−	−/P	−

DRUG	LIBIDO	ERECTION	EJACULATION
Antipsychotics			
Pimozide	−	−/P	−
Perphenazine			−
Trifluoperazine			−
Fluphenazine	−	−	−
Butaperazine			−
Thiothixene		−/P	+
Chlorprothixene			−
Haloperidol		−	
Molidone		P	
Benperidol		−	
Sulpiride		−	
Antidepressants			
Tricyclic Antidepressants			
Imipramine	−	−	−
Amitriptyline	−	−	−
Desipramine		−	
Maprotiline	−	−	
Nortriptyline	−	−	
Protriptyline	−	−	−
Clomipramine	−	−	−
Amoxapine	−	−	−
MAO Inhibitors			
Phenelzine		−	−
Pargyline		−	−
Mebanazine			−
Iproniazid			−
Isocarboxazid		−	−
Transcypromine	+	−	
Trazodone	+	P	
5-HT Uptake Inhibitors			
Sertraline			−
Fluoxetine			−
NE Uptake Inhibitors			
Viloxazine		+	
DA Uptake Inhibitors			
Nomifensine	+		
Bupropion	+		
Lithium	−	−	
Anxiolytics			
Chlordiazepoxide			−
Lorazepam			−
Alprazolam			−
Diazepam	+/−		−
Fluazepam	+		
Buspirone	+	+	+
Parkinsonian Drugs			
L-Dopa	+	+	+
Apomorphine	+	+	
Bromocriptine	+	+	
Pergolide	+	+	+
Deprenyl	+		
Opioid Agents			
Agonists			
Methadone	−	−	−
Antagonists			
Naltrexone		+	

− = reduced function; + = improved function; P = priapism (Created in collaboration with Mark Foreman, PhD) panied by low normal or abnormally low levels of testosterone. Routine measurement of serum prolactin without concomitant complaint of impaired libido or evidence of hypogonadism is of low diagnostic yield in the urologic practice.[84] The principal etiologies of hyperprolactinemia are prolactinoma of the pituitary, uremia (chronic renal insufficiency), and drugs (sedatives, neuroleptics, antiemetics, and reserpine).

The hypothalamus integrates a broad spectrum of neuronal information, routing physical or emotional stress and metabolic health into a single signal—increasing or decreasing the corticotropins.[77] LH-RH (luteinizing-hormone-releasing hormone) secretion and sexual behavior can be affected by endogenous endorphins and enkephalins. As a result of a single but substantial physical stress (e.g., marathon running), heavy exercise for twenty or more days, or psychologic stress, the endogenous opioid system is activated, suppressing LH-RH and LH release and dropping testosterone to hypogonadal levels.[86,92–94] In animals corticotropin-releasing factor (CRF) inhibits the ability of LH-RH to stimulate release of LH from the pituitary; chronic increase in corticotropins can decrease testosterone levels by this central mechanism. Elevated CRF has been found in the cerebrospinal fluid of depressed patients.[95,96]

Drugs that decrease dopaminergic receptor activity, such as antipsychotics or catecholamine depleting agents, eventually suppress sexual function through the induction of hyperprolactinemia and secondary hypogonadism. Drugs with antiandrogenic activity, such as cyproterone acetate, flutamide, finasteride, and cimetidine, can induce decreased libido and erectile dysfunction.[52,54,72] These dysfunctions are also associated with the antihypertensive agent spironolactone, which has antiandrogenic activity and suppresses the synthesis of androgens. Cyproterone acetate has actually been used to treat "deviant" sexual behavior.[52] Other agents that depress libido by decreasing testosterone levels include estrogens, gonadotropin-releasing hormone agonists and antagonists (leuprolide), corticosteroids, ketoconazole, and progestins.[53] Digoxin has a structural similarity to estrogen; it has been associated with impotence, development of gynecomastia, and increase in plasma estrogen levels.[97]

Currently, the only pharmacologic agents approved for treating behavioral sexual dysfunction (disinterest) in the United States are testosterone for hypogonadism and bromocriptine for hyperprolactinemia. Methylated androgens that can be taken orally (methyltestosterone, fluoxymesterone, methandrostenolone, and stanozolol) should be avoided due to unpredictable hepatotoxic effects.[77] Transdermal delivery systems are in clinical phase trials. Intramuscular administration of testosterone esters is the most widely used therapy: testosterone enanthate, cypionate, and cyclohexanecarboxylate.[89]

In a review of patients attending a general medical clinic, Slag[98] noted an incidence of 5% hypothyroidism and 1% hyperthyroidism among 188 patients complaining of impotence. Excess thyroid hormones increase the production of sex-hormone-binding globulin, thus binding more testosterone. Negative feedback increases the pituitary release of LH, stimulating testosterone production by Leydig cells; correction of the hyperthyroid state lowers

FIGURE 11.9 (continued) *Reported Side Effects of Oral Drugs*

DRUG	LIBIDO	ERECTION	EJACULATION
Endocrine Therapies			
Estrogen			
Ethinyl estradiol	–		
Androgen			
Methandrostenolone	–		
Norethandrolone	–	–	
Progestin			
Medroxyprogesterone	–		
Medrogesterone	–		
Hydroxyprogesterone		–	
Progesterone	–	–	
Antiandrogen			
Cyproterone acetate	–		

DRUG	LIBIDO	ERECTION	EJACULATION
Others			
Metoclopramide	–	–	
Fenfluramine	–	–	
Baclofen		–	–
Amphetamine	+	+/–	–
Disulfiram		–	
Barbiturates	+/–	–	–
Ethosuximide	–		
Carbamazepine		–	
Digoxin	–	–	
Disopyramide		–	
Phenytoin	–	–	
Hydralazine		–/P	
Verapamil		–	
Clofibrate	–	–	
Heparin		P/–	
Cimetidine	–	–	
Primidone	–	–	
Naproxen			–

– = reduced function; + = improved function; P = priapism (Created in collaboration with Mark Foreman, PhD)

testosterone to normal levels. The association between hypothyroidism and inhibition of sexual behavior is less clear.[99] Hormonal sexual dysfunction accounts for only a small percentage of patients seeking the urologist's consultation, but supplementation of deficits in testosterone is highly successful, and recognition of endocrine disturbances (hyperprolactinemia, hypothyroidism, hyperthyroidism) can have a significant impact on the patient's health.

DOPAMINERGIC EFFECTS ON ERECTION

The only agents that have been evaluated in detail in both clinical and laboratory settings have been those that affect dopamine, serotonin, and opiate receptors. In addition to the effects on libido, dopaminergic agents also affect erectile response in men and laboratory animals without changing sexual behavior. Spontaneous erections were first noted as side effects in patients treated with L-dopa or dopaminergic agonists.[63,100] More recently, subcutaneously administered apomorphine has been shown reproducibly to induce penile erections in normal and impotent patients.[65,101–103] This acute response is not accompanied by increases in libido and is dose-related, mediated by D_2-dopaminergic receptors. Only centrally acting antagonists block the response.[102,104]

SEROTONINERGIC EFFECTS ON ERECTION

Serotonin appears to have different effects on the central and peripheral components of the sexual response in animals. Amplification of serotoninergic activity through the administration of serotonin-releasing agents or agonists also induces spontaneous erections in rats and rhesus monkeys.[105,106] The erectogenic effects of serotonin have been proposed to be mediated by the 5-HT_{1c} receptor subtype. These effects may contribute to the induction of priapism in patients treated with the antidepressant trazodone and the increase in erectile activity during rapid eye movement sleep.[107,108] The trazodone metabolite metachlorophenylpiperazine (mCPP) is a serotoninergic agonist that induces erections in rats and rhesus monkeys and selectively increases the firing rate of the penile nerve and cavernosal blood pressure in rats.[105,106,109]

OPIOID EFFECTS ON ERECTION

The loss of the ability to achieve or maintain erection has been a noted side effect in heroin or methadone addicts.[110–112] Decreased sexual desire is also noted in many of these patients, which suggests a CNS depressant effect. Spontaneous erections are reported side effects during treatment with the opiate antagonists naloxone and naltrexone in heroin or methadone addiction.[113,114]

ADRENERGIC EFFECTS ON ERECTION

The maintenance of the penis in a flaccid state depends on the continuous stimulation of α_1-adrenergic receptors on cavernosal smooth muscle through the tonic release of norepinephrine from sympathetic terminals. Drug regimens that increase peripheral adrenergic tone have been reported to cause erectile failure, whereas those that decrease postsynaptic α_1-adrenergic receptor activity are associated with reports of priapism.[53,72] Chronic treatments with amphetamine and cocaine, which indirectly increase α_1-adrenergic receptor activity, have been associated with erectile failure.[52–54,110,111] In contrast, a variety of drugs with α_1-adrenergic antagonist activity, such as some antihypertensives and antipsychotics, have been reported to cause priapism. An alternative mechanism for trazodone-induced priapism is through its α_1-adrenergic antagonist activity.

CHOLINERGIC EFFECTS ON ERECTION

The cholinergic innervation of the penis is currently thought to facilitate relaxation of cavernosal smooth muscle through the release of endothelial-cell-derived relaxation factors (EDRF). The blockade of this parasympathetic function may be partly responsible for the reported erectile failure associated with drugs with anticholinergic activity, such as imipramine and other tricyclic antidepressants.

DRUG-INDUCED CHANGES IN EJACULATORY RESPONSE

Ejaculatory events include the induction of seminal emission, ejaculation, and perceptual stimuli associated with orgasm.[115] The predominant drug-induced disorders of this phase include delayed or absent ejaculation, retrograde ejaculation, and suppressed seminal emission.[59,105] These side effects are associated with agents that alter the central or peripheral components of the seminal emission–ejaculation reflex. As in the case of the behavioral and erectile phases, drugs that affect dopaminergic or serotonergic receptor activity are thought to modulate the central component of the ejaculatory reflex. The peripheral component of the ejaculatory reflex primarily involves the sympathetic control of smooth muscle contraction within the vas deferens, ejaculatory ducts, seminal vesicles, prostate, external urethral sphincter, and bladder neck for the antegrade emission of sperm and seminal fluid and the increase of pressure within the vasal ampulla for ejaculation. The somatic innervation of the striated bulbocavernosal, ischiocavernosal, and pelvic floor muscles regulates the clonic contractions that cause expulsion of the fluid during ejaculation. Orgasm is a cognitive process triggered by pressure changes in the proximal urethra and the contractions of the periurethral striated muscles.[53]

Evaluation of Erectile Dysfunction

As described above, erection is a complex neurophysiologic event mediated by corporal smooth muscle (CSM) tone. Detumescence and flaccidity are initiated and maintained by corporal smooth muscle contraction; tumescence is initiated by relaxation of vascular tone and a drop in resistance to arterial flow that bathes the cavernous tissues in highly oxygenated arterial blood. Erection involves the coordinated activity of at least five neuropharmacologic events:[22,25,42,116]

1. Decrease in α-adrenergic neurotransmission in association with possible local inhibition of α-adrenergic activity

2. Nerve-mediated release of nitric oxide, resulting in a rapid and profound relaxation of CSM

3. Activation of endothelial cells by acetylcholine neurotransmission (muscarinic), stimulating the release of nitric oxide

4. Activation of other nonadrenergic, noncholinergic (NANC) neuroeffectors (possibly ATP, substance P, or VIP)

5. β-Adrenergic neurotransmission, which, at least in vitro, is a small constituent of CSM relaxation.

Detumescence and flaccidity are mediated principally by α-adrenergic stimulation and possibly cessation of release or inhibition of relaxing neuroeffectors and stimulation by the contractile vascular mediator endothelin.

PHARMACOTESTING

The intracavernous injection of vasoactive substances for pharmacotesting and the nonprosthetic management of erectile dysfunction is an accepted and effective technique (Fig. 11.10). The ability of papaverine to induce erection was first described by Virag in 1982[1,117]; he made the observation that accidental intracavernous injection of papaverine (typically applied extraluminally to dilate vessels during a revascularization procedure) initiated an erection. Subsequently, numerous studies have reported similar therapeutic effects with α-blockers, vasoactive intestinal polypeptide, calcium channel blockers, prostaglandin E_1, and most recently, nitrosovasodilators (donors of nitric oxide). For the past decade three agents have principally been used for clinical pharmacotesting: papaverine, papaverine/phentolamine, and prostaglandin E_1. The mechanisms of action of these intracavernous vasodilators have been described well.[118–120]

Papaverine has a direct myotonlytic effect on smooth muscle by nonselective inhibition of cyclic nucleotide phosphodiesterases, which results in accumulation of intracellular cyclic adenosine 3′,5′-monophosphate (cAMP). Recent investigations suggest that a second mechanism of smooth muscle relaxation may be increasing efflux of intracellular calcium stores.[121] The adverse effects

of papaverine pharmacoerection are both systemic and local: peripheral vascular dilation, hypotension, reflex tachycardia, elevation of liver function assays (8%), corporal smooth muscle fibrosis, and priapism (2% to 10%).

Phentolamine methylate is an α-adrenoreceptor antagonist for both α_1 and α_2 receptors. When injected alone it increases corporal blood flow but does not significantly raise intracorporal pressure. It is hypothesized that by blocking prejunctional α_2 receptors phentolamine inadvertently increases intracorporal norepinephrine release, preventing complete sinusoidal relaxation. Response rates to pharmacotesting with combination papaverine/phentolamine (65%) are better than with papaverine alone (36%).[118,122]

Prostaglandin E_1 (PGE_1) is a naturally occurring substance found in high concentrations in the seminal vesicles and seminal plasma. The effects of prostaglandins are species-specific, and some congeners actually contract smooth muscle ($PGF_{2\alpha}$). PGE_1 is a potent smooth muscle relaxant and vasodilator in humans; it prevents platelet aggregation and stimulates intestinal motility. In numerous self-injection programs it has been lauded as safer than and equally efficacious to the combination of papaverine and phentolamine.[123] PGE_1 is a profound relaxant of corporal smooth muscle and has an α_2-antiadrenergic action. Its α-blocking effect may offset the sympathetic tone believed responsible for psychogenic impotence. Prostanoids are synthesized and degraded within the human corpora[124]; 80% of an administered PGE_1 dosage is inactivated during first passage through the lungs. PGE_1 use is not associated with systemic side effects and has been associated with a reduced incidence of priapism. The single consistent complaint of patients taking PGE_1 (20% of cases) is of a dull penile ache, which persists until complete detumescence.

Following experimental studies demonstrating endothelium-mediated and neuronally mediated corporal smooth muscle relaxation in vitro by nitric oxide (NO), much attention is currently being directed towards intracavernous trials of NO releasors. Nitrosovasodilators activate the arginine cyclic guanosine monophosphate pathway (Arg-cGMP). Nitric oxide (NO) is the putative nonadrenergic, noncholinergic transmitter of erection. One such NO donor is linsidomine chlorhydrate (SIN-1), a

FIGURE 11.10 *Intracavernous Agents Causing Erection*

Smooth muscle relaxants	Papaverine
α-Blockers	Phentolamine; phenoxybenzamine; moxisylyte
Calcium channel blockers	Verapamil
Peptides	Vasoactive intestinal polypeptide
Purines	ATP, adenosine
Prostaglandins	PGE_1
Nitrosovasodilators	Nitroglycerin; nitroprusside; linsidomine

metabolite of the antianginal drug *N*-ethoxycarbonyl-3-morpholino-sydnonimine. Intracorporal SIN-1 produced dose-dependent erectile responses in 63 patients, according to Stief.[125]

INVESTIGATING PENILE BLOOD FLOW

In 1971 Gaskell[126] introduced a noninvasive test of penile arterial inflow, a photometer to quantify the absorption of light by the pigment oxyhemoglobin in the glans penis. An occlusive cuff at the base of the penis was slowly loosened, and the pressure at which oxyhemoglobin became measurable in the glans was assumed to indicate penile systolic pressure. Efforts to simplify clinical measurement of penile blood flow were advanced by Abelson,[127] who in 1975 used the Doppler stethoscope to measure penile blood pressure in the flaccid penis and compared this value to systolic brachial pressure to yield the penile–brachial index (PBI, maximal systolic penile pressure divided by systolic brachial artery pressure). Michal[128] and Goldstein[129] further refined the PBI by adding lower extremity and pelvic musculature exercises and doing Doppler stethoscope auscultation before and after exercise. A decrease in the ratio of penile systolic pressure of more than 0.15 indicates pelvic steal or significant penile inflow disease.

Although inexpensive, noninvasive, and easily performed in the office, PBI has technical flaws that limit its utility: penile pressure cuff fit and occlusion is not uniform, the continuous-wave Doppler receives a mixture of signals that cannot anatomically differentiate central cavernous arteries from dorsal or bulbospongiosal arteries, pressure values often reflect the dorsal artery and lead to overestimation of systolic penile occlusion pressure, and all measurements are made in the flaccid shaft. No evaluation of the flaccid penis reflects corporal dynamics—the ability of the cavernous arteries to dilate and increase cavernous inflow. Reviews comparing the PBI to pharmacopenile arteriography have found that PBI values from normal patients overlap those from impotent patients and that penile–brachial index correlates poorly with penile arteriography.[130,131]

Goldstein has demonstrated that an accurate assessment of cavernous artery perfusion pressure requires dynamic testing, pharmacologic stimulation of cavernous artery relaxation, dilation, and penile perfusion.[8,132] He advocates use of the continuous-wave Doppler ultrasound probe with recording from the 3 o'clock or 9 o'clock position on the penile shaft to avoid auscultation of the dorsal arteries. Pulsatile infusion using heparinized saline with simultaneous corporal pressure monitoring requires indwelling needles. Infusion is increased until Doppler pulsations from the cavernous artery disappear; cessation of infusion results in cavernous pressure decline. The pressure at which arterial Doppler signal returns is the cavernous artery systolic occlusion pressure (CASOP), which is the maximal intracorporal pressure likely generated during the patient's own erection. A difference of less than 35 mm Hg between the patient's brachial systolic pressure and CASOP is considered normal. Despite a high sensitivity when compared to pharmacopenile arteriography, the test is invasive and routinely performed in concert with cavernosometry and cavernosography.[42]

Pudendal Arteriography

Arteriography remains the standard for vascular investigations. It provides the best anatomic information about the origin of the common penile arteries, although the data have been difficult to correlate with impaired function of the end organ.[133] The vessels of the flaccid shaft are not only in a low flow state but are also contracted and tortuous. It is well accepted that the specificity of penile angiographic imaging is increased by intracavernous injection of vasodilators (pharmacopenile angiography) (Fig. 11.11). Penile angiography performed in the absence of intracavernous vasoactive stimulation is of little diagnostic value. High-osmolality contrast agents are painful and require intravenous sedative or anesthesia. Many centers routinely use epidural or spinal anesthesia, which has the additional benefit of reducing vasospasm.[13,134] Low-osmolality contrast agents reduce

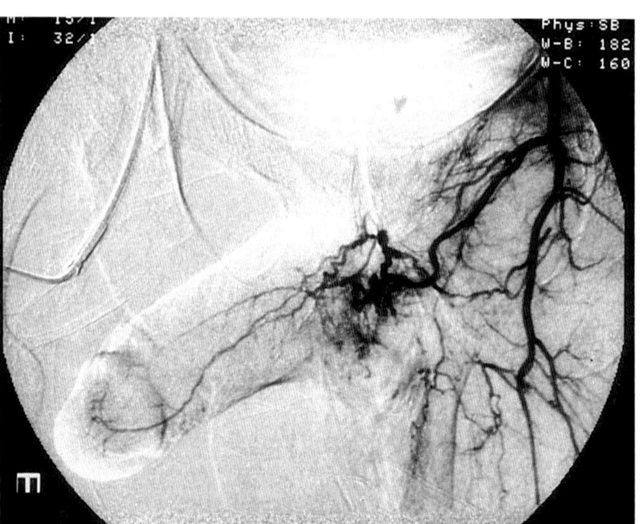

Figure 11.11 Pharmacopenile arteriography with digital subtraction technique shows the left pudendal artery, common penile artery, bulbourethral artery, and left dorsal and left cavernous arteries. The right cavernous artery arises from a branch of the left cavernous artery in this patient who had inflow disease at the level of the right pudendal artery.

angiographic morbidity but increase expense.

A technical problem is the level at which to begin vascular interrogation because, as discussed above, the common penile artery may arise from the terminus of the internal pudendal artery or from an accessory pudendal artery. Performing selective internal pudendal arteriography has an inherent false-positive rate for diagnosing penile inflow disease,[134] which affects the duration of the study, the patient's exposure to x-rays, and the amount of contrast agent used. More importantly, deviations from paired penile supply (two dorsal and two cavernous arteries) have been documented in 50% of normally potent male volunteers, and unilateral absence or hypoplasia of a dorsal artery has been shown in up to 30% of potent volunteers.[15,16] Anatomic variation of intrapenile arterial anatomy appears to be the rule rather than the exception (Fig. 11.12)—unilateral or bilateral origin of the cavernous arteries, distal shaft communications between the dorsal and central cavernous arteries, and anastomoses between the corpus spongiosum and cavernous body.[135] The essential problem is how to distinguish congenital variations in penile arterial anatomy from acquired variations and how to correlate these findings with the complaint of impotence.

The role of penile angiography cannot be dismissed, especially with ongoing developments in the interventional tools of transluminal angioplasty. Posttraumatic erectile dysfunction is clearly associated with injury to the common penile arteries in their course through the urogenital diaphragm, and bypass is indicated in the young patient who does not have concomitant neurologic injury.[136] However, patients undergoing arteriography experience the discomfort of the intraarterial contrast, exposure to ionizing radiation, the risk of minor or severe dye reaction, and disruption of an atheroma into the hypogastric-penile vascular bed. As a method of screening, penile arteriography is too invasive and nonspecific.

Color Duplex Doppler Penile Ultrasonography (CDDU)

Lue and Hricak[137] introduced the technique of high-resolution sonography and quantitative Doppler spectral analysis to evaluate vasculogenic impotence. Penile injections of papaverine, phentolamine, and PGE_1 revolutionized the diagnosis and management of impotence.[1,2,138] An excellent clinical response to the intracavernous vasoactive agent in a neurologically normal patient confirms the diagnosis of psychogenic impotence. All too often, however, the clinical response to initial intracavernous agent is suboptimal. Duplex Doppler provided the first objective evaluation of a suboptimal response using cavernous peak systolic velocity (PSV) to infer the integrity of penile circulation.[139,140] To refine the diagnosis of cavernous inflow disease and provide a noninvasive means of diagnosing cavernous veno-occlusive disease (CVOD), Doppler parameters were expanded[141–144] (i.e., end-diastolic arterial velocity (EDV), cavernous artery acceleration, percent increase in penile volume, percent increase in cross-sectional area, and resistive index [RI = PSV–EDV/PSV]). The accuracy of the penile blood-flow study has been tested through comparison to visual rating of erection following penile injection, cavernosometry/cavernosography, and phalloarteriography.[14,145–147] All parameters and real-

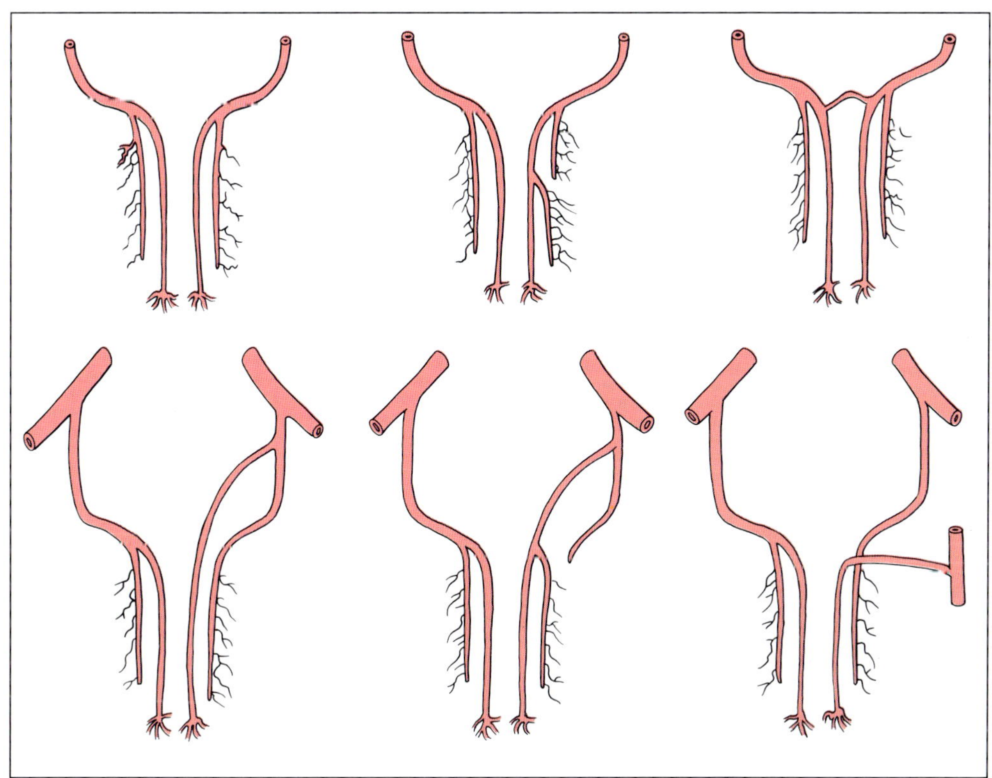

Figure 11.12 Congenital variations in the origins of the dorsal and cavernous arteries. (Adapted with permission from Bähren W, 1991)

time observations are typically made after intracavernous injection. Recent studies have assessed the additional benefits of visual sexual stimulation, sequential duplex Doppler penile measurements for up to one hour, and simultaneous assessment with a penile tumescence and rigidity device (Rigiscan, Dacomed).[144,148–150]

Real-time ultrasound imaging was originally used to measure internal cavernous arterial diameters, look for cavernous artery pulsations after stimulation, and examine the corporal tissue for fibrosis. Color Doppler (CDDU) permits real-time assessment of the cavernous arteries, vessels of the dorsal bundle, corpora spongiosa, and collaterals. With color flow these small vessels, including veins, are rapidly acquired and Doppler flow is measured accurately.[14] CDDU is specifically useful in evaluating penile pathologies (trauma, Peyronie's disease, and corporal fibrosis) and is becoming the test of first choice for evaluating a patient's failure to respond to in-office challenge with a vasoactive agent.

The corporal bodies should be scanned from base to tip to demonstrate that the echotexture is homogeneous; a fibrotic process is relatively hyperechoic (Fig. 11.13). Flow velocities are assessed in the sagittal plane. Timing is important, as arterial diameter and peak systolic velocity (PSV) maximize before full erection. Rising intracavernous pressure will dampen, then obstruct inflow during full erection and rigid erection. If the penis has not assumed an erect posture, it is held upright by the glans; this is the anatomic position of erection and serves to straighten the course of the cavernous and dorsal arteries. When there is asymmetry of cavernous peak systolic velocities greater than 10 cm/sec or when significant collateral flows are noted, examination of the crura should be made to determine if proximal inflow disease exists or intracorporal stenosis has resulted in decreased unilateral CDDU signal

(Fig. 11.14). This is easily performed by having the patient frog-leg and lift the scrotum. Scanning the perineum sagittally reveals the origin of each cavernous artery.

CDDU and Adequacy of Arterial Inflow

Flow velocites should be measured 5 minutes after injection: delay in response is typical in the chronic hypertensive patient and the anxious patient. A comfortable, warm, private setting is essential for reducing anxiety and thus sympathetic cavernous smooth muscle tone,[151] and self-stimulation enhances the penile response. CDDU assessment can be repeated immediately after self-stimulation, specifically noting erectile quality and whether the response weakens in the subsequent 5 minutes. Donatucci and Lue[152] found that among 90 patients performing self-stimulation after PGE$_1$ challenge, 74% improved; among those whose responses weakened within 5 minutes of stimulation, 84% were noted to have moderate venous leakage on follow-up cavernosography. Visual rating of erectile quality should correlate with the parameters of erectile diagnostic testing[14,118,147]:

E5: well-sustained rigidity of at least 20 minutes
E4: full erection, partial rigidity, adequate for penetration
E3: full tumescence, easily bendable
E2: moderate tumescence
E1: elongation of the shaft only
E0: no response

For purposes of statistical comparison with duplex parameters or other diagnostic testing, three categories can be assigned: E0–E3, inadequate for intromission; E4, adequate for intromission (Fig. 11.15); and E5, consistent with sustained intromission (Fig. 11.16).

Detection of flow before corporal injection is highly dependent on the patient's level of sympathetic tone, and its predictive value is uncertain.[31] The principal source of

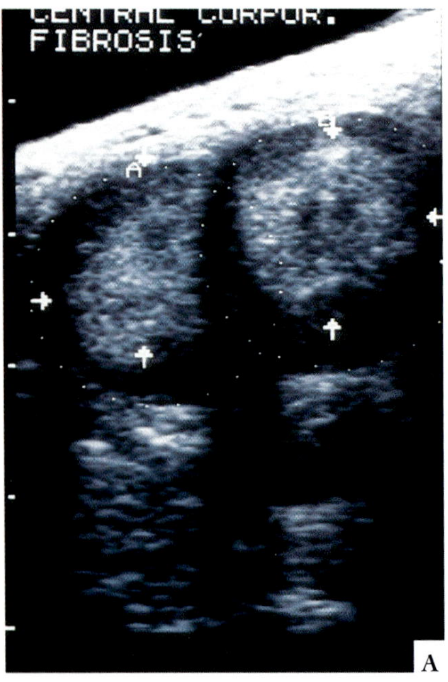

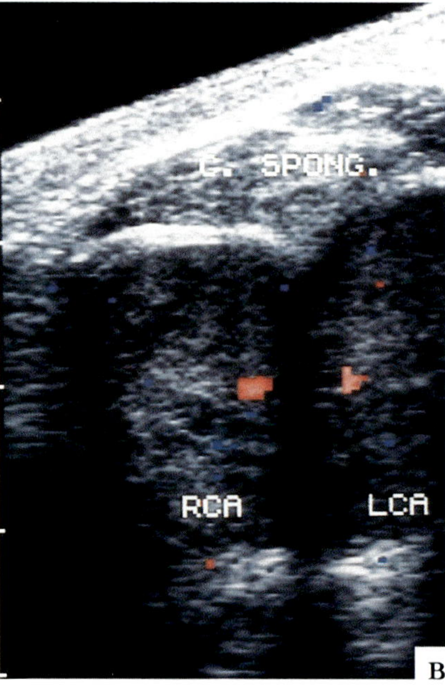

Figure 11.13 Real-time color Doppler images. **A** Distal, transverse, dorsal image of the paired cavernous bodies. Dotted lines at the level of the tunica albuginea calculate the square surface of each corpus. Central corporal fibrosis is hyperechoic (arrows) in the patient with sickle cell anemia and recurrent priapism. **B** Proximal, transverse, ventral image at the level of the perineum. The ultrasound beam travels first through compressed corpus spongiosum (C. Spong.), revealing isoechoic proximal corporal bodies with patent cavernous arteries.

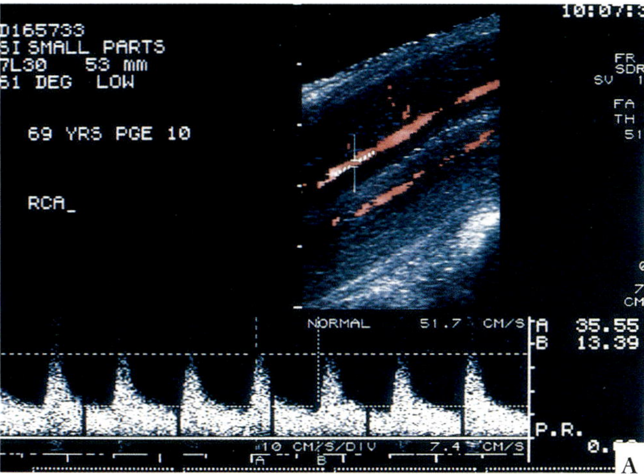

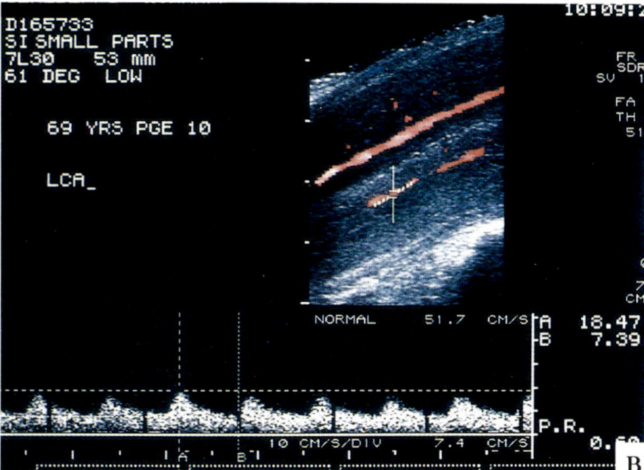

Figure 11.14 Color duplex Doppler sagittal images of the paired cavernous arteries. A 69-year-old patient with history of hypertension and coronary artery disease received prostaglandin E_1, 10 µg. **A** Right cavernous arterial (RCA) velocity is 35 cm/sec peak systolic and 13 cm/sec end-diastolic and the resistive index is 0.62. **B** Left cavernous arterial (LCA) velocity is 18 cm/sec peak systolic and 7 cm/sec end-diastolic. Diagnosis: asymmetry of cavernous arterial flow, but venous leakage cannot be ruled out. If the flow of cavernous arteries is equal at the base of the penis, the arterial disease is intrapenile, not prepenile.

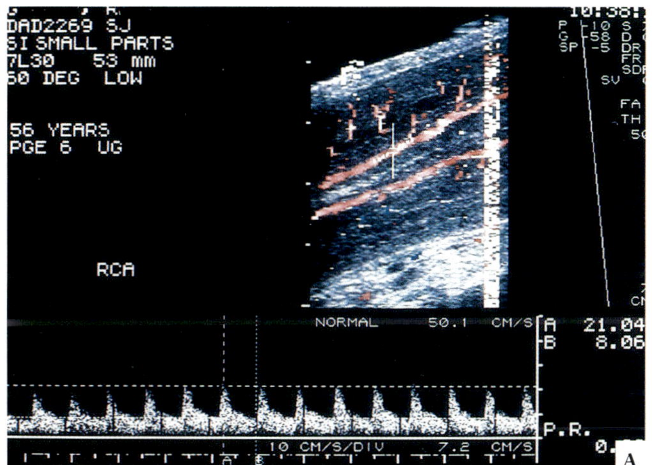

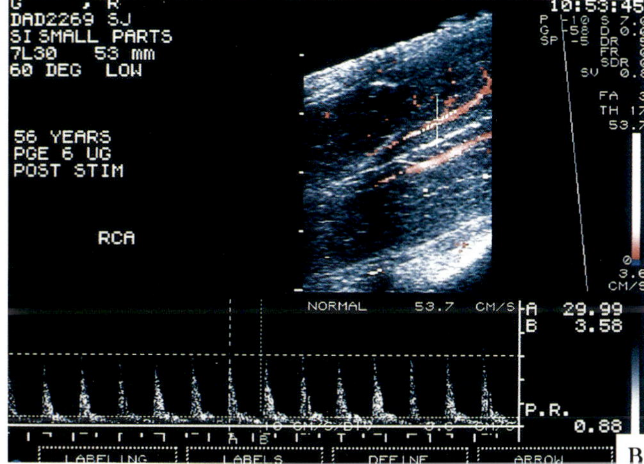

Figure 11.15 Color duplex Doppler sagittal images of the paired cavernous arteries. **A** Ten minutes following a prostaglandin E_1 injection, the right cavernous artery (RCA) velocites are 21 cm/sec peak systolic and 8 cm/sec end-diastolic and the resistive index is 0.62. Erectile quality is E3. **B** Following privacy and self-stimulation erectile quality improved (E4). RCA velocities are 29 cm/sec peak systolic and 3 cm/sec end-diastolic and the resistive index is 0.88.

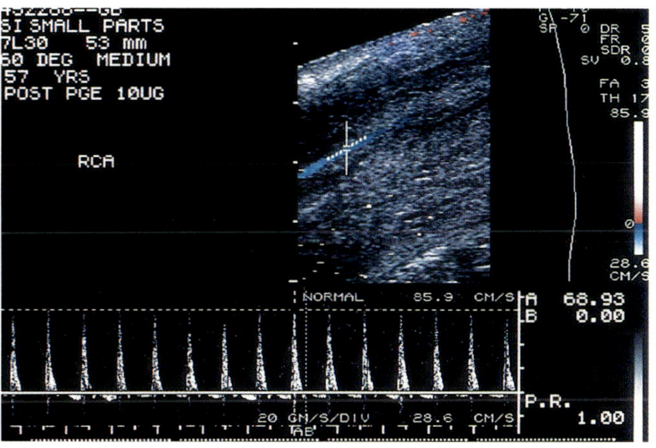

Figure 11.16 Color duplex Doppler sagittal image of the right cavernous artery (RCA). Prostaglandin E_1 (10 µg) produced a rigid erection (E5) without self-stimulation. Peak systolic velocity is 68 cm/sec with sharp waveform and reversed diastolic flow and resistive index is 1.0. Note that the cavernous artery is blue (reversed flow) and the dorsal artery antegrade flow is red. Diagnosis: adequate arterial inflow and adequate cavernous venous occlusion.

error in flow velocity determinations is an incorrectly assigned Doppler angle. Doppler flow velocity is inversely proportional to the cosine of the angle between the beam and the axis of blood flow.[147,153–155] Holding the shaft upright permits consistent measurements in line with the cavernous and dorsal vessels, with the internal Doppler angle set at 60°.

Lue has proposed that an adequate response requires an arterial diameter greater than 0.07 cm after injection, and PSV greater than 25 cm/sec. In the University of California, San Francisco, series normal subjects had mean PSV of 34.8 cm/sec and mean arterial diameter of 0.89 mm.[50,152] In a study from Baylor University normal volunteers had mean PSV of 40 cm/sec and mean arterial diameter of 1.0 mm.[156] Normal volunteers in the Harvard Medical School study had mean PSV of 47 cm/sec.[157] This study confirmed that a peak systolic velocity below 25 cm/sec correlated with severe arterial insufficiency on arteriography. The investigators cautioned against the use of mean PSV when comparing impotent patients, because asymmetry greater than 10 cm/sec was noted among 65% of patients considered to have mild to moderate arterial insufficiency. They also noted that patients with flow velocities between 25 to 30 cm/sec were effectively treated by home intracavernous therapy. The Mayo Clinic found that mean PSV less than 25 cm/sec had a sensitivity of 100% and specificity of 95% when compared to findings of pudendal arteriography.[158] Schwartz[159] correlated

progressive changes in Doppler spectral waveform patterns with increasing intracorporal pressure in potent volunteers following papaverine/phentolamine challenge. Rigid erection was associated with intracorporal pressures ranging from 83 to 106 mm Hg. During tumescence both PSV and EDV increased, with corporal pressure ranging from 11 to 25 mm Hg. With rigidity EDV approached 0, and diastolic flow reversed when intracorporal pressures reached 63 to 83 mm Hg. These progressive changes in the Doppler spectral waveform have been described by other investigators as well.[144] Contraction of the bulbocavernous and ischiocavernous muscles by direct pudendal or dorsal nerve stimulation in the animal model raises intracorporal pressures transiently and results in cessation of systolic inflow. Theoretically, supplemental compression of venous outflow increases penile rigidity during pelvic thrusting. The bulbocavernosus reflex can be stimulated during the CDDU exam with compression of the glans penis (Fig. 11.17).

CDDU and Cavernous Venous Occlusive Adequacy

The suspicion of venous leakage is raised when the patient has an excellent arterial response to injected vasodilator (PSV > 30 cm/sec), with well maintained EDV. This is accompanied by transient rigidity after self-stimulation (Fig. 11.18). Quam[158] found EDVs ranging between 0 and 24 cm/sec after intracavernous papaverine (60 mg).

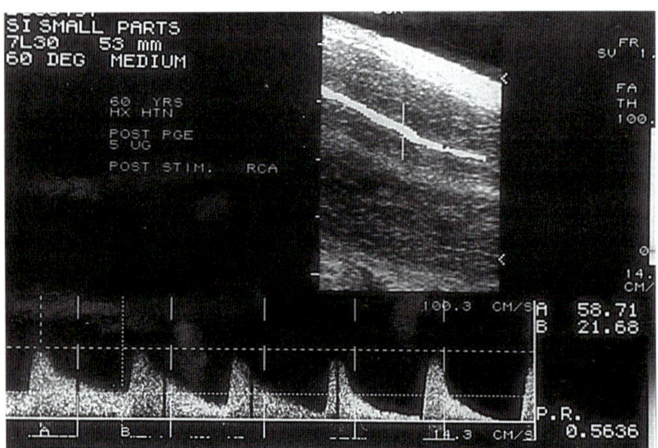

Figure 11.17 Following 5 μg of prostaglandin E$_1$ a 60-year-old man with history of hypertension achieved partial erection. He had an excellent peak systolic velocity of 58 cm/sec but a well-maintained end-diastolic velocity of 21 cm/sec and a resistive index of 0.56. The bulbocavernous reflex (BCR) is triggered by brisk squeezing of the glans penis, the contractile response of the bulbocavernous and ischiocavernous muscles transiently reduces venous outflow and the end-diastolic flow decreases. During sexual intercourse pelvic thrusting produces increased rigidity and intermittent suprasystolic intracorporal pressure by stimulating the BCR.

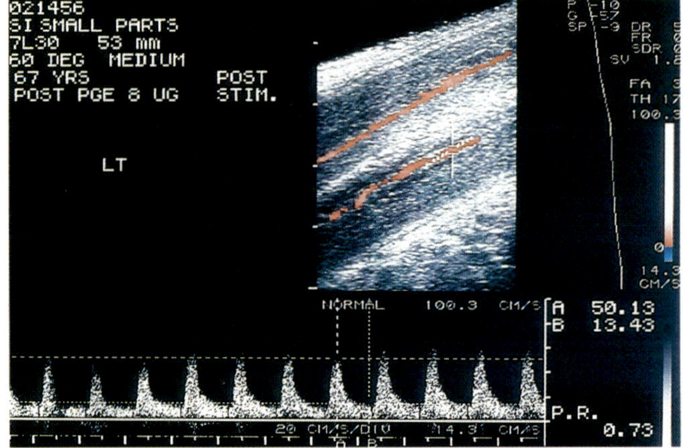

Figure 11.18 Color duplex Doppler sagittal images of the paired cavernous arteries. Prostaglandin E$_1$ 8 μg has been given, but despite privacy and self-stimulation rigidity is poor (E3). Left cavernous arterial velocities are 50 cm/sec peak systolic velocity and 13 cm/sec end-diastolic velocity and the resistive index is 0.73. Diagnosis: adequate arterial inflow and cavernous venous occlusive disease.

Among patients with peak systolic velocity greater than 25 cm/sec, venous leakage on cavernosometry was predicted with a sensitivity of 90% and specificity of 56% when end-diastolic flow was greater than 5 cm/sec. Fitzgerald,[144] using criteria of cavernous arterial adequacy (PSV > 25 cm/sec) and venous leakage (EDV > 5 cm/sec), noted that only three fourths of patients achieved maximal responses to papaverine (60 mg) at 5 minutes. Data acquistion for a total of 30 minutes yielded a sensitivity of 95% and specificity of 83% for prediction of venous leakage. Merckx[160] injected patients with PGE_1 (20 µg) and followed with Doppler analysis at 5 minute intervals. No statistical differences in Doppler parameters between 26 psychogenically impotent men and 8 potent volunteers were noted: at 5 minutes maximum PSV was 49 cm/sec, maximum EDV was 11 cm/sec, and maximum acceleration was 12.6 m/sec²; at 10 minutes PSV was 38.8 cm/sec, EDV was 3.7 cm/sec, and resistive index (RI) was 0.91. Venous leakage was diagnosed in patients with inadequate erection following PGE_1 despite high PSVs; the following Doppler parameters of the venous leak patients were noted: at 10 minutes PSV was 35 cm/sec, EDV was 7 cm/sec, restrictive index (RI) was 0.77. The RI was the only parameter that statistically differentiated the venous-incompetent group. Using this 5 and 10 minute scanning protocol, a 93% correlation between CDDU and cavernosometry was noted.

There is indeed waveform progression through the various phases of erection, with consistent increases in PSV from tumescence (E3) to partial rigidity (E4). At full erection there is peaking of the systolic waveform and actual decreases in PSV, which may fall below 25 cm/sec.[14] At maximal intracorporal pressure (E5, rigidity), Doppler analysis consistently reveals suppression of diastolic inflow associated with a resistive index approaching 1.0. The dorsal arteries are not subjected to the intracorporal pressure changes with each phase of erection; therefore, even in well sustained rigidity, antegrade diastolic flow persists.

CDDU easily detects arterial collaterals: dorsal to cavernous, cavernous to cavernous, and cavernous to spongiosal (Fig. 11.19). Anastomosis between the dorsal artery and central cavernous artery has been noted in 7 of 10

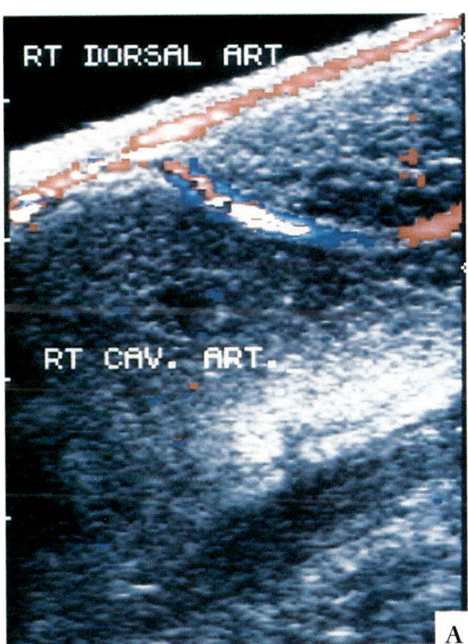

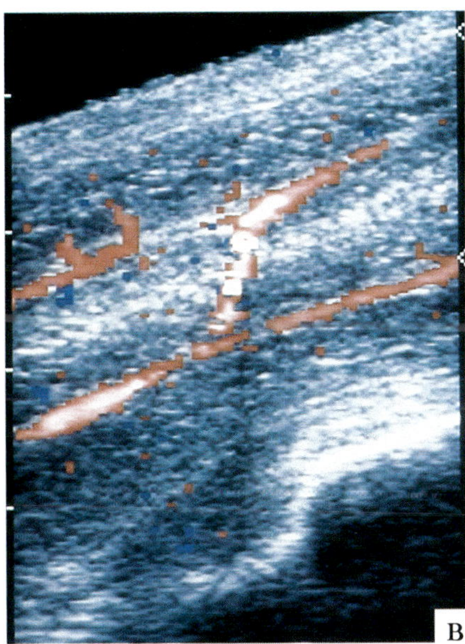

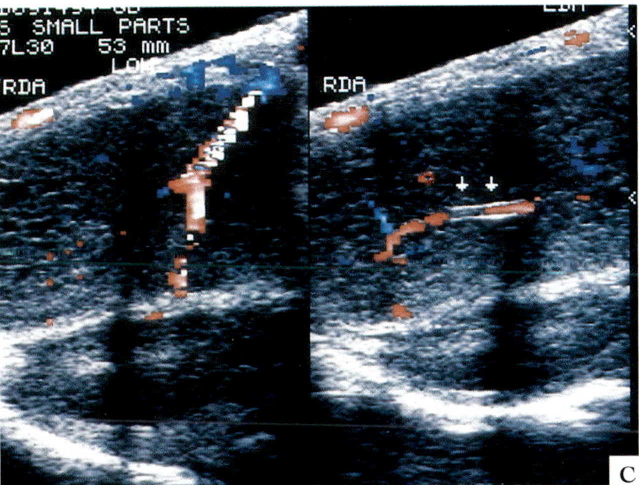

Figure 11.19 **A** Real-time color Doppler sagittal image of collateral from right dorsal artery to right cavernous artery. **B** Real-time color Doppler sagittal image of collateral from left cavernous artery to right cavernous artery. **C** Real-time color Doppler image transverse views of dorsal-to-cavernous collateral and cavernous-to-cavernous collateral (arrows).

cadaver specimens by Garibyan.[135] Most importantly, CDDU assesses the dynamics of collateral inflow; high-flow collaterals typically supplement unilateral cavernous insufficiency.[14] Measurement of the deep dorsal vein is possible without compression of venous flow (Fig. 11.20).

Peyronie's disease is a benign but nonetheless incapacitating condition resulting from inelastic focal scar of the tunica albuginea. Recent clinical investigations suggest that Peyronie's disease may alter penile hemodynamics as adversely as penile structure.[161] Traditionally, diagnosis has been based on history, patient photographs, and physical examination. Objective imaging of plaques has been attempted with plain x-rays and xeroradiography, but only lesions with overt calcifications are readily identifiable. Ultrasonography, cavernosography, computed tomography, and magnetic resonance imaging have been used to assess Peyronie's disease.[162,163]

Real-time ultrasound images of Peyronie's disease are highly informative. The tunica albuginea is normally hyperechoic compared to the corpora proper. As the corporal bodies distend with blood, the cavernous sinusoids become more hypoechoic, increasing the contrast between the tunica and corpora (Fig. 11.21). Penile plaques are hyperechoic thickenings of the tunica albuginea. The typical dorsal plaque displaces or encases the dorsal vasculature. Denser plaques cast an acoustical shadow well visualized in either transverse or sagittal planes.

Dynamic Cavernosometry and Cavernosography

Insufficient corporal veno-occlusion is implicated in 14% to 54% of patients who complain of impotence and submit to vascular diagnostic testing.[164,165] Several specific pathologies have been implicated in penile ouflow disease.[166,167]

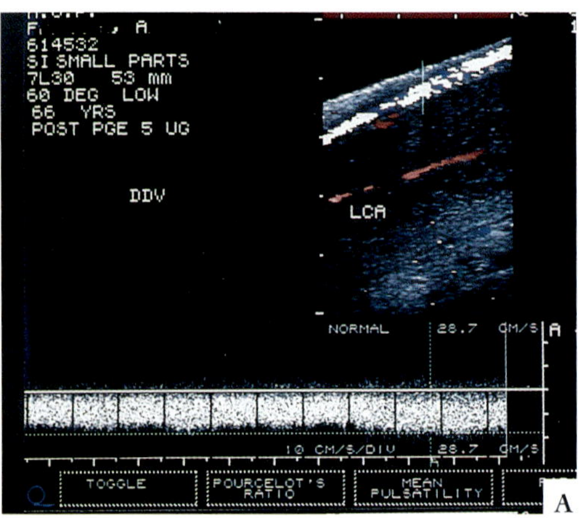

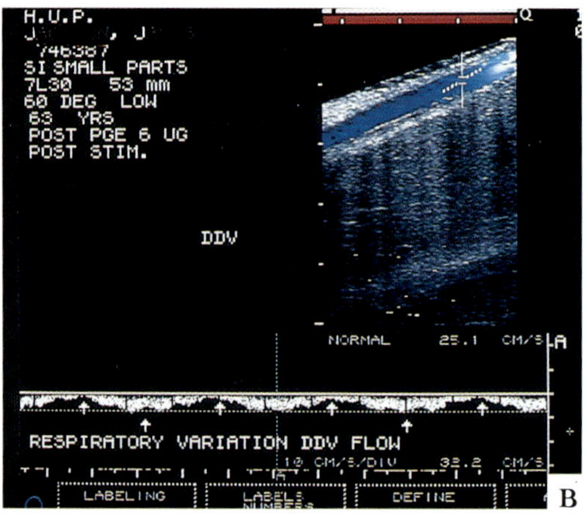

Figure 11.20 Color duplex Doppler sagittal images of the deep dorsal vein (DDV). A Nonpulsatile Doppler venous flow is 18 cm/sec. B Respiratory variation in deep dorsal vein flow(arrows).

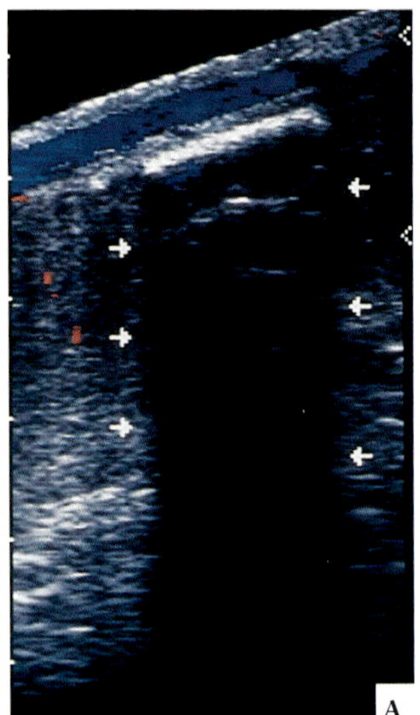

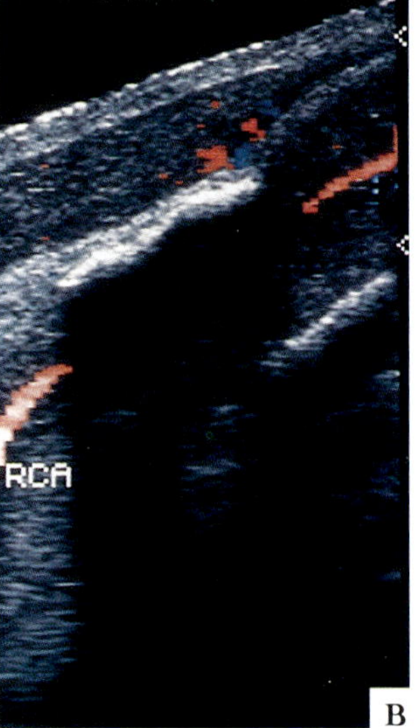

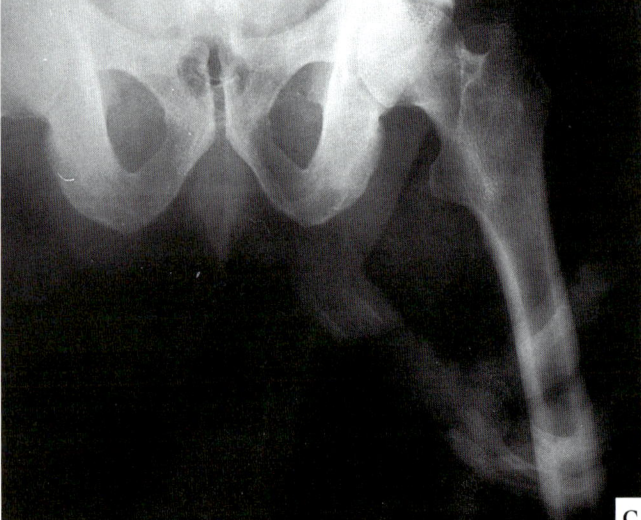

Figure 11.21 A Real-time color Doppler image, sagittal dorsal view showing hyperechoic Peyronie's plaque under the deep dorsal vein. The plaque is so dense it casts an acoustical shadow (arrows). B Real-time color Doppler image, sagittal ventral view, with hyperechoic Peyronie's plaque between the corpus spongiosum and the cavernous body. An acoustic shadow blocks the Doppler signal from the right cavernous artery (RCA). C Plain radiograph of the same patient holding his penis. Note the calcification of Peyronie's plaque. Color Doppler images reveal that the plaque is circumferential.

1. An excessive number of cavernous/crural veins or large emissary veins exiting directly from the corpora rather than obliquely through the bilayered tunica albuginea. This pathology is commonly ascribed to the young patient with primary erectile dysfunction—poorly sustained erection since the age of sexual maturity.

2. Incompetent venous channels due to weakening of the tunica albuginea as a consequence of aging or Peyronie's disease.

3. Failure to occlude subtunical venous plexus as a consequence of insufficient arterial inflow and intracorporal pressure.

4. A deficiency of stimulatory neurotransmitters or vascular mediators of smooth muscle relaxation or excessive adrenergic tone due to anxiety, psychosis, or drug effects. Nicotine, known for its arteriolar vasospastic effects, has been shown to impair directly corporal smooth muscle relaxation.

5. Impaired sinusoidal smooth muscle compliance or frank corporal fibrosis.

6. Abnormal communication between the corpora cavernosa and glans penis following shunting for priapism or a posttraumatic arteriosinusoidal fistula that bypasses the principal circulatory route within the corpora cavernosa.

The diagnosis of venous leakage requires invasive testing and is predicated on demonstrating the adequacy of arterial inflow. Partial erection after intracavernous vasoactive injection does not enable the urologist to distinguish between arterial or venous disease, and failure to achieve rigidity following a single diagnostic injection does not definitely prove vascular erectile dysfunction. Cavernosometry and cavernosography have been criticized as being "too invasive," generating patient anxiety and pain, thus predisposing the physician to make a false-positive diagnosis of veno-occlusive disease. The reader must appreciate that despite advances in ultrasound and Doppler technology, only penile pressure monitoring and penile filling characteristics done in the presence of full pharmacologic corporal smooth muscle relaxation can succinctly describe corporal hemodynamics, and only venography can provide an adequate road map for vascular reconstructive surgery (Fig. 11.22).

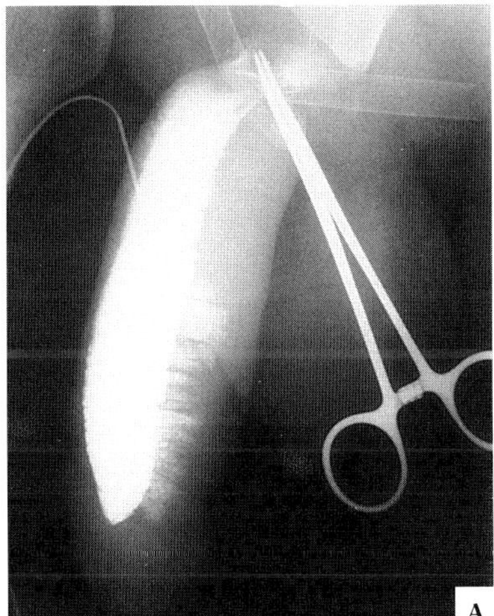
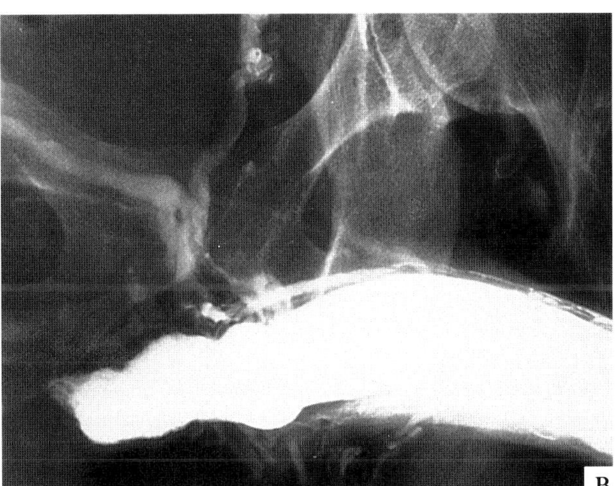
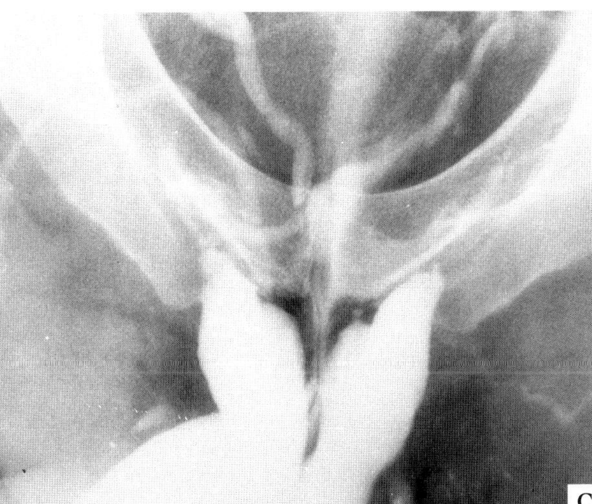
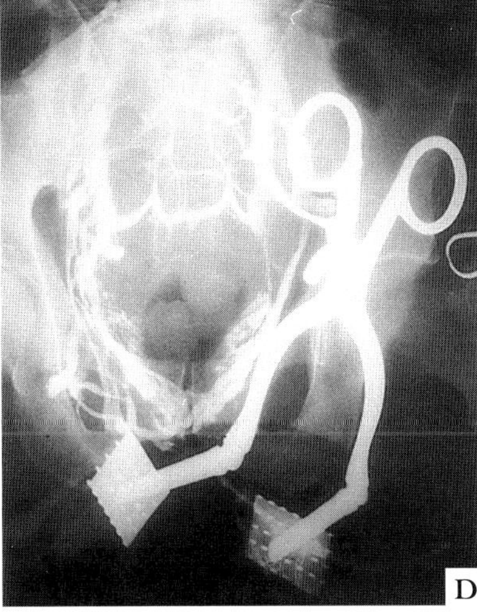

Figure 11.22 Pharmacocavernosography in a young patient with partial rigidity following 20 µg of prostaglandin E_1, despite excellent cavernous arterial inflow. **A** Low osmolar isoionic contrast is infused. There is a tourniquet at the penoscrotal junction. Initial film shows the cavernous septum is perforated; contrast is beginning to cross. **B** Short cavernous veins and deep dorsal vein drainage to preprostatic and internal pudendal veins. **C** Pelvic inlet view reveals venous leak from crural tips. **D** Intraoperative venography during penile vein ligation. Contrast infusion of a right cavernous vein and a deep dorsal vein reveals extensive pelvic venous collaterals draining the corpora cavernosa.

Kolliker first described the creation of artificial erection by penile infusion in 1892[168]; methods of dynamic infusion of contrast to permit quantification of erectile maintenence flows and visualization of leaks have only recently been developed.[117,138,169] Surgical attempts to improve sexual performance by vein ligation long antedate current understanding of the hemodynamics of erection.[170] Animal models suggest a linear relationship between intracavernous pressure and flow to maintain erection only when complete corporal smooth muscle relaxation occurs. Goldstein[91] has advocated pharmacocavernosometry/cavernosography following injection of papaverine hydrochloride (45 mg) and phentolamine mesylate (2.5 mg); he reported that the flow needed to maintain various intracavernous pressures is 3 mL/min or less, and the fall from suprasystolic cavernous pressure of 150 mm Hg over 30 seconds is less than 45 mm Hg. Lewis, in two systematic reviews of the literature on dynamic cavernosometry without and with pharmacostimulation, has noted a wide range of parameters for initiation and maintenance infusion rates.[122,171] In his own clinical studies he has found that tumescence occurs at approximately 50 mm Hg and rigid erection at 90 to 100 mm Hg, which coincides with Lue's observation that if after 60 mg of papaverine or 45 mg of papaverine with 1 mg of phentolamine intracorporal pressure rises to 80 mm Hg, both arterial and venous penile mechanisms are intact.[50] Lewis and others have dismissed initiation rates as dependent on penile size and the rate of response to smooth muscle relaxant, although a maintenance flow rate greater than 50 mL/min indicates significant veno-occlusive dysfunction.

NOCTURNAL PENILE TUMESCENCE TESTING
Maintained nocturnal erections despite a complaint of erectile dysfunction have traditionally been accepted as pathognomonic of psychogenic impotence. Some authors suggest that nocturnal penile tumescence (NPT) reflects the integrity of the corticospinal efferents of erection.[172,173] The relationship between rapid eye movement sleep and erections has long been appreciated but is of such complexity that the NPT must be correlated with other aspects of the impotent patient's evaluation. To have three to five erections per night is normal. NPT has age-specific characteristics.[148,174] Total tumescence time during sleep peaks at the age of puberty—as much of 20% of total sleep time

may be spent with an erection. In the second decade of life, the average duration of a nocturnal erection is 38 minutes. For adult males the average duration is 27 minutes. Quality of nocturnal erectile events lessens with age. Hormonal status clearly influences NPT; in hypogonadal patients there is a decrease in nocturnal erectile activity. Similarly, disturbances of sleep architecture and sleep apnea will adversely alter NPT. To further confound the diagnostic dilemma, Thase[175] has described decreased nocturnal erections among patients with anxiety, depression, and poor libido. In the sleep laboratory, at considerable expense and discomfort, NPT can be correlated with a variety of parameters: respirations, EKG, electroencephalography, jaw muscle electromyography, electrooculography, and bulbocavernous muscle activity.

Simple, inexpensive screening for the presence or absence of nocturnal erections can be accomplished with Snap Gauges (Dacomed). These are self-fastening rings with three plastic bands that break in succession under increasing force. Failure to break any bands indicates absence of nocturnal penile tumescence. More specific home testing can be accomplished with the Rigiscan (Dacomed), which records the duration of erectile events, proximal and distal tumescence, and rigidity (Fig. 11.23).

NEUROPHYSIOLOGIC TESTING
As described above, the sacral reflex arc of erection consists in somatosensory afferents via the dorsal and pudendal nerves and autonomic efferents via the pelvic and cavernous nerves. The afferent components have traditionally been measured by somatosenory evoked potentials (SSEP) and bulbocavernosus reflex (BCR) latency. The BCR is tested by electrical stimulation of the dorsal penile skin with a needle recording of the bulbocavernous muscle. The time from stimulation to contraction is sacral latency; normal latency is approximately 40 msec. Similarly, conduction velocities along the dorsal nerve can be measured. The SSEP evaluates both peripheral and central afferent pudendal pathways. The SSEP is recorded by stimulation of the penile skin and recording from the scalp with adhesive or needle electrodes. These tests are far from routine, but together BC conduction velocity, BCR latency, and SSEP can localize somatosensory afferent dysfunction (peripheral, sacral, and suprasacral).[172,173]

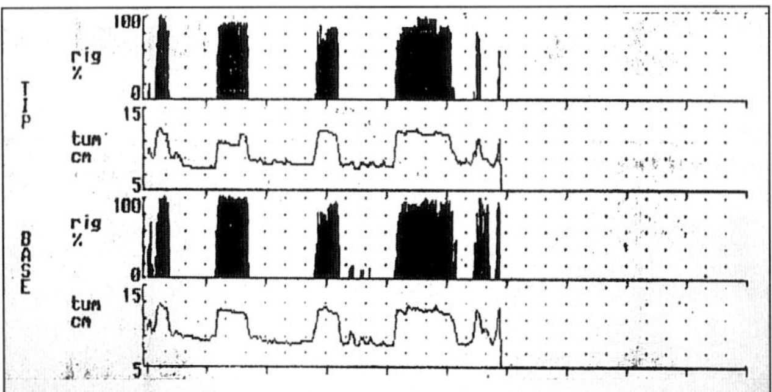

Figure 11.23 Nocturnal penile tumescence and rigidity testing (NPTR) with Rigiscan (Dacomed). Six hours of recording during sleep shows five distinct erectile events. Tumescence increases at the base and the tip, exceeding 3 to 4 cm. Proximal and distal rigidity is well sustained at 100%. Normal NPTR.

In-office testing of the dorsal nerve somatic afferents is accomplished simply and inexpensively with the penile biothesiometer, a hand-held vibrator with a fixed frequency but a variable amplitude setting. Vibratory penile perception thresholds have been determined for men of various ages.[132,172] The BCR is clinically detectable in 70% of men, according to Bors[176]; according to Blavias[177] the BCR is clinically evident in 98% of normal males with brisk compression of the glans and simultaneous visualization and palpation of the anal sphincter. The presence of the BCR is an indication of the integrity of the somatic afferents and the efferent limbs of the sacral reflex arc. The BCR is absent clinically and with urodynamic testing in all patients who have complete lower motor neuron lesions.

Tests of autonomic erectile integrity have typically been both tedious and indirect. They are based on the observation that autonomic failure results in abnormal baroreceptor responses, which are most commonly found among diabetics. The test that reflects mainly parasympathetic dysfunction is heart rate variation during quiet breathing, during deep breathing, and in response to standing upright. The test that reflects mainly sympathetic efferent dysfunction is blood pressure in response to standing upright.[178]

Gerstenberg and Wagner were the first to record electrical activity by intracavernous needle electrodes.[179–183] Subsequent authors have used both needle and skin electrodes for penile EMG, claiming to record etiology-specific penile potentials and to be able to correlate cavernous smooth muscle electrical activity with other tests of venoocclusive dysfunction.[184–187] The acronym SPACE (single potential analysis of cavernous electrical activity) is alluring but misleading, as percutaneous needle placement cannot maintain contact with a single smooth muscle cell, especially during cavernous motion from flaccidity to tumescence to erection. These recordings and those at the level of penile skin at best reflect summation of penile potentials. The value of the testing lies in the hope that the potentials originate in the cavernous tissues. Stief maintains that visual sexual stimulation of normal volunteers results in an increase in the frequency of potentials with simultaneous decrease in amplitude and polyphasity as the penis progresses from flaccidity through tumescence to full erection. In contrast electrical silence follows rigid erection induced by intracavernous injection of papaverine/phentolamine or prostaglandin E_1. He proposes that upper motor neuron and lower motor neuron lesions can be differentiated by the waveforms of cavernous electrical activity—duration, amplitude, and polyphasity. This technology is new and investigational. At the Fifth World Congress on Impotence held in Milan, September 1992, nine papers on cavernous electromyography were presented. The consensus was that electromyographic activity from the penis could be recorded but it was unclear whether cutaneous or needle electrodes were necessary, whether electrical silence invariably accompanies pharmacologic erection, and whether distinct cavernous EMG patterns can be correlated with upper or lower motor neuron lesions.[181–183,187–192]

Etiology of Erectile Dysfunction

Fifty percent to 80% of men seeking care have organic erectile dysfunction.[122,193] Not surprisingly, the ratio of organic to psychologic male sexual dyfunction is directly proportional to age, with 70% of men under 35 years of age having a psychogenic etiology and 85% of men over 50 years of age having organic impotence.[194,195] Seventy-five percent of men in their seventh decade report coital activity once monthly; weekly coitus is reported among 37% of patients 61 to 65 years old and 28% of patients 66 to 71 years old. The medical community has long appreciated the risk factors for organic erectile dysfunction: advancing age, coronary artery disease, peripheral vascular disease, diabetes mellitus, hypertension, smoking, hyperlipidemia, chronic renal insufficiency. Normative data on the prevalence of impotence have only recently become available.[196] The Massachusetts Male Aging Study assessed the prevalance of impotence complaints among 1290 men ranging in age from 40 to 70 years. During home interviews men were asked to rate their potency on a four-point scale: not impotent, minimally impotent, moderately impotent, and completely impotent. A complaint of impotence was offered by 51% of men—16% minimally, 25% moderately, and 10% completely. Diabetes under treatment was associated with a threefold increase in the probability of complete impotence, coronary disease under treatment was associated with a 78% incidence—94% among men who smoked and had heart disease. Heart disease, hypertension, diabetes, and low serum HDL cholesterol were significantly related to complaints of impotence.

The hemodynamics of erection has been reviewed above; inflow disease may reside in the prepenile hypogastric-pudendal-common penile vessels or the intrapenile cavernous arteries. Inadequacy of penile inflow is generally regarded as a symptom of the generalized para-aging process of atherosclerosis; impotence has been associated with the age and onset of coronary artery disease.[197] Virag[138] noted that men with impotence are more likely to have other clinical evidence of atherosclerotic disease than age-matched potent men. Kaiser[88,198] studied the penile–brachial index (PBI) of impotent men having stress tests and dipyridamole thallium scans and found a low PBI more often among those with abnormal cardiac tests.

The onset of impotence in diabetes is insidious and may initially be intermittent, varying with glycemic control. In a 5-year prospective study of 275 diabetic males, McCulloch[199] found the initial prevalence of impotence to be 35%; over 5 years, 28% of initially potent diabetics developed impotence, and only 9% of the impotent diabetics regained sexual function. In diabetes mellitus autonomic erectile dysfunction has its origin at the neurotransmitter level. (Clinical investigations of autonomic erectile function are discussed above.) Diabetes impairs neurogenic and endothelium-mediated relaxation of corporal smooth muscle. The corporal tissue of diabetic men and impotent nondiabetic men relaxes equally well in response to direct applications of papaverine or nitrosovasodilators, suggesting either that nonadrenergic, noncholinergic neurotransmission is impaired or that the synthesis of nitric oxide is deficient in diabetic corpora.[40,200,201]

RENAL TRANSPLANTATION

Chronic uremia and hemodialysis result in sexual dysfunction in 50% to 90% of patients.[201,202] Several metabolic culprits have been identified: uremic toxins, zinc deficiency, hyperparathyroidism, and decreased levels of free testosterone and dihydrotestosterone. Testicular morphology following chronic hemodialysis reveals maturational arrest and germ cell aplasia; the hypogonadism is believed to originate at the level of luteinizing hormone (LH) regulation. Hyperprolactinemia, a well-known central inhibitor of gonadotropin secretion, is evident in 50% of dialysis patients.[203] Erythropoietin reportedly improves erectile function and libido among patients with chronic renal insufficiency.

The majority of men with long-term function of a renal allograft are reported to regain potency. Similarly, improvements in fertility secondary to increased testosterone and sperm density have been described. The risk of vasculogenic erectile failure following anastomosis of renal graft to the internal iliac artery is 10%, but following a failed initial transplant and second transplant into the left pelvis the incidence climbs to 65%.[204]

COLORECTAL OPERATION

Abdominoperineal resection and protocolectomy can result in damage or ligation of the nerves and vessels necessary for erection. Early reports documented high impotence rates (95%) following both abdominoperineal resection for malignancy and proctocolectomy for benign disease.[205] Contemporary reviews cite significant reductions in the incidence of erectile failure following rectal excision for benign disease (0% to 20%) but no improvement following abdominoperineal resection for cancer, with the incidence of iatrogenic impotence ranging from 33% to 100%.[206,207] Improvements in postoperative potency reflect both patient age at operation and refinements in surgical technique.[208] The pelvic autonomic plexus runs anterolateral to the rectal ampulla below the lateral pelvic fascia; if dissection is extended to the walls of the pelvis for removal of lymph nodes, parasympathetic nerve damage and neurogenic erectile compromise is inevitable.

Isolated sympathetic nerve damage that spares erectile function but alters fertility status through failure of emission or retrograde ejaculation is possible. The postganglionic sympathetic nerves may be damaged during separation of the rectum from the sacrum, in the preaortic tissues below the inferior mesenteric artery near the aortoiliac bifurcation, and where they enter the seminal vesi-

cles. Potency and fertility following colorectal surgery are functions of the age of the patient and how low and wide the resection is carried: thus, sexual dysfunction is likely after abdominoperineal resection for cancer in 100% of elderly patients.

A rarely addressed factor of comorbidity in sexual dysfunction is alteration of body image following cancer procedures. Abdominal stomas for the collection of urine or feces can have a substantial impact on the sexually active patient. The psychosexual profile of the male cancer patient with an abdominal stoma suggests that even if erectile ability is maintained, sexual self-esteem is reduced.[209] Patients with urinary ileostomies undergoing reoperation for continent urinary diversion (no postoperative abdominal appliance) show improved self-image and levels of sexual activity.[210–212]

AORTOILIAC OPERATION

Leriche's syndrome, described in 1923, is characterized by fatigue and claudication in the lower extremities with exercise, absent pulsations in the femoral arteries, and impotence.[213] The incidence of iatrogenic erectile dysfunction following aortoiliac revascularization ranges from 21% to 88%, but preoperative sexual dysfunction is equally high in this group of patients, ranging from 25% to 60%. A more contemporary series (1969) shows a 21% incidence of impotence following aortic aneurysmectomy and a 34% incidence following revascularization for thrombo-occlusive disease with associated incidences of ejaculatory dysfunction being 63% and 49% respectively.[207,214]

Modifications that spare sexual function include omitting lumbar sympathectomy; opening the aorta on its right lateral surface, reflecting the overlying tissue to the left but not incising the preaortic tissue; tunneling aortofemoral bypass grafts directly anterior to the native common and external iliac vessels deep to the ureters and pelvic plexus; dissecting in the longitudinal plane over the proximal external iliac arteries; preserving internal iliac blood flow; and not resecting aortic aneurysm sacs, controlling back bleeding from the inferior mesenteric artery from within the sac.[215–217] In a collected series of non-nerve-sparing operations, 25% of patients were impotent postoperatively and 43% developed ejaculatory dysfunction. At least one subsequent series of nerve-sparing techniques, excluding patients with emergency aneurysmectomies, reported a 67% preoperative potency rate with no postoperative erectile complaints and only a 3% incidence of ejaculatory dysfunction.[216]

RADICAL PROSTATECTOMY AND CYSTOPROSTATECTOMY

Following the elegant anatomic dissections of Walsh and Donker[19] and Lepor et al.,[21] a resurgence of enthusiasm for the management of prostate cancer by radical prostatectomy occurred. The Johns Hopkins group has demonstrated the anatomic relationships of the cavernous nerves to the pelvic plexus, lateral pelvic fascia, Denonvilliers' fascia, prostatovesicular vessels, prostate, urethra, and rectum. Fibers of the autonomic pelvic plexus are microscopic and travel laterally and posteriorly to the seminal vesicles, coalescing along the posterolateral surface of the prostate from a group of fibers 11 mm wide to 5 mm at the apex of the prostate. Surgically, the nerves are only identifiable by their relationship to the capsular vessels of the prostate.[218,219] Injury and consequent impotence commonly occur during apical dissection and transection of the urethra from the prostate, separation of the prostate from the rectum, and division of the lateral pelvic fascial attachments. Refinements in surgical technique not only improve postoperative potency rates but significantly lower morbidity secondary to intraoperative bleeding.

Postoperative potency is a function of the patient's age and the progression of the disease. Patients with B1 disease (confinement to one prostate lobe) in their fifth decade of life have an 83% recovery of sexual function 12 months after surgery; similarly, men 60 to 69 years have a recovery rate of 60%, and men 70 to 79 years have a recovery rate of 50%. More extensive disease—B2 (involvement of both prostate lobes)—is often associated with a desmoplastic–fibrotic response surrounding the neurovascular bundles and postoperative potency for men in their sixth decade falls dramatically to 38%. Recovery of sexual function after resection of one neurovascular bundle occurs at rates similar to the younger patient.

Walsh's anatomic nerve-sparing modifications have been applied to radical cystectomy with consequent improvement in postoperative potency, albeit less dramatic improvements. Removal of the bladder and prostate en masse requires wider mobilization and dissection. Recent cadaver dissections reveal that in 70% the unilateral accessory pudendal artery arose from the obturator or the inferior or superior vesical arteries. In 50% of dissections this accessory pudendal artery was also found to be the major inflow to the common penile artery on that side and would be ligated during cystectomy.[6]

Assessments of postradiation impotence share the same flaw as most surgical series: no pretherapy diagnostic testing. The general incidence of postradiation impotence has been reported to range from 30% to 65% for external beam therapy and 25% for interstitial therapy.[220,221]

TRANSURETHRAL OPERATIONS

As described above, the neural bundles of erection lie posterolateral to the prostate and contain the postganglionic autonomic nerves; for the transurethral resectionist this means that potential nerve trauma could result from capsular penetration or the spread of current during electrocautery of bleeding vessels within the posterior urethra from the 3 to 5 o'clock or 7 to 9 o'clock positions. Urologists have traditionally denied a causal relationship between TURP and impotence, citing patient age and concurrent medical risk factors.

Clearly the incidence of retrograde ejaculation is 50% to 60% and will often be the basis for the patient's complaint.[206,222–224] Older series reported erectile dysfunction following TURP in 4% to 40% of patients. A cooperative study of thirteen institutions found the incidence of impotence following transurethral resection to be 4% among 3885 patients.[225]

Optical internal urethrotomy (OIU) permits direct and precise incision of urethral strictures, usually without electrocautery. In 1981 McDermott[226] reported four cases of temporary or permanent erectile dysfunction among 179 patients receiving OIU. In 1990 Graversen[227] reported a 10% incidence of partial or total erectile dysfunction following OIU. Assessments were made by interviews and dynamic testing using Doppler ultrasonography and cavernosography. These authors postulated that shunting of the normally sequestered corpus cavernosum blood during erection was occurring via communication with the corpus spongiosum, a communication established by the urethrotomy. This theory is not substantiated by their investigations. Incision for OIU is typically performed at the 12 o'clock position, where the urethra is surrounded by the least spongiosum—in cross-section the urethra resides within the corpus spongiosum like a displaced doughnut hole. If post-OIU impotence were actually due to inadvertent surgical communication between the spongiosum and corporal bodies, this long-term complication should be associated with the immediate complication of excessive bleeding through the urethra; however, no such association has been described. Moreover, the majority of OIUs are performed for stricture in the bulbar or pendulous urethra, sites distal to where the cavernous nerves enter the corporal bodies. Corporal venous drainage and spongiosal drainage communicate normally through the circumflex veins and through the corporal perforators to the glans perforators (Fig. 11.24). Perhaps it is significant, however, in the complex issue of postoperative potency, that a common origin of urethral stricture is post-TURP (endoscope) scar formation.

PRIAPISM: OVERFUNCTION OF A NORMALLY REVERSIBLE MECHANISM

Priapism is a persistent erection that fails to subside after climax and is accompanied by penile pain and tenderness; it is the overfunction of a normal mechanism.[228] Traditionally priapism has been categorized as primary (spontaneous, idiopathic) or secondary to numerous specific pathologies (sickle cell disease, leukemia, fat emboli, malignant infiltration, neurologic injury, alcohol, and psychotropic drugs).[229] With the increasing popularity of pharmacologic erection programs, iatrogenic or therapeutically induced prolonged erection is likely to be the most common etiology of priapism. Priapism is a notable complication of pharmacologic erection programs; the reported incidence is from 6% to 40%, with the greatest incidence among young men with spinal cord injuries.[230–232] Contemporary appreciation of penile hemodynamics has led to functional classification of the prolonged erection as either ischemic (veno-occlusive) or high-flow (arterial).

Of the various causes of priapism, only one—trauma—has been attributed to "dysregulation" of arterial inflow.[233,234] With the exception of malignant infiltration of the penis, the remaining clinical scenarios involve veno-occlusive priapism.

Priapism is an obvious failure of the detumescence mechanism, which may result from secondary inhibition of the intrinsic intracellular mediators of corporal smooth muscle contraction or primary inhibition of the sympathetic α-adrenergic neurotransmission normally terminating erection. Beyond a certain, as yet undefined, time the cavernous smooth muscle becomes refractory to recoiling, perhaps as a result of anoxic, hypercarbic acidotic alteration of the corporal environment.[235,236] This urologic emergency is well recognized clinically.

Early histologic investigations revealed that after 24 hours of ischemic priapism the corporal tissues became thickened and edematous.[228] The natural history of untreated priapism is impotence, with perhaps some erectile ability spared in the proximal crura. Despite surgical intervention potency rates remain no better than 55%.[237] Electron microscopic work by Spycher et al.[238] demonstrated trabecular interstitial edema after 12 hours followed by the destruction of sinusoidal endothelium, exposure of the basement membrane, and thrombocyte adherence by 24 hours. By 48 hours actual thrombus formation occurs in the sinusoidal spaces and the smooth muscle undergoes fibroblast-like cell transformation.

Permanent impotence can be avoided following pharmacologic priapism by prompt intervention.[239] Prolonged erection of 4 to 6 hours will respond to exogenously administered α-adrenergics—epinephrine (10 to 20 µg), phenylephrine (100 to 200 µg), ephedrine (10 to 50 mg), or norepinephrine (10 to 20 µg), which are directly injected every 5 to 10 minutes until detumescence. They may also be mixed into normal saline for corporal irrigation. It has been my experience that prolonged erection (2 to 4 hours) and true priapism of 6 to 12 hours (excluding posttraumatic, sickle cell, and malignant infiltrations) respond if initial or repeated penile aspiration results in freshly oxygenated bright red blood entering the corpora cavernosa before judicious injection of an α-adrenergic compound: phenylephrine 100 to 200 µg, ephedrine 10 to 50 mg, norepinephrine 10 to 20 µg, or epinephrine 10 to 20 µg. Occluding the base of the pendulous shaft after aspiration, then injecting adrenergic and waiting 10 to 30 seconds before releasing penile compression minimizes washout and the risk of systemic hypertension. Failure of administered adrenergic to detumesce the erection requires formal corporal shunting or arteriography and unilateral embolization in the case of high-flow priapism.

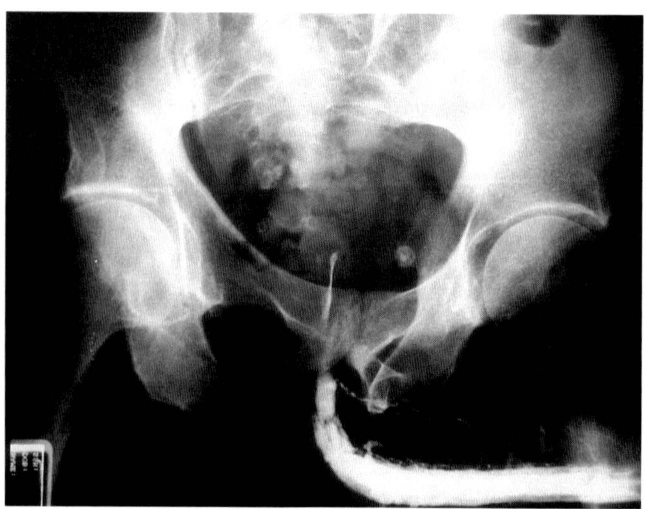

Figure 11.24 Overzealous infusion of retrograde urethral contrast produces intravasation into the corpus spongiosum in this patient who has gonorrheal strictures and multiple OIUs. Contrast leaves the spongiosum via circumflex veins to the superficial and deep dorsal veins. A jet of contrast crosses the bladder neck.

References

1. Virag R. Intracavernous injection of papaverine for erectile failure. *Lancet.* 1982;2:938. Letter.
2. Brindley GS. Cavernosal alpha-blockade: a new technique for investigating and treating erectile impotence. *Br J Psychiatry.* 1983;143:332.
3. Hinman F Jr. *Atlas of Urologic Surgery.* Philadelphia, Pa: WB Saunders Co; 1989.
4. Mulcahy JJ. The management of complications of penile implants. *Probl Urol.* 1991;5:608–627.
5. Goldstein I. Penile revascularization. *Urol Clin N Am.* 1987;14:805–813.
6. Breza J, Aboseif SR, Orivs BR, Lue TF, Tanagho EA. Detailed anatomy of penile neurovascular structures: surgical significance. *J Urol.* 1989;141:437–443.
7. Wein AJ, Van Arsdalen K, Hanno PM, Levin RM. Anatomy of male sexual dysfunction. In: Jonas U, Thon WF, Stief CG, eds. *Erectile Dysfunction.* Berlin: Springer-Verlag; 1991:3–15.
8. Goldstein AMB, Padma-Nathan H. The microarchitecture of the intracavernosal smooth muscle and the cavernosal fibrous skeleton. *J Urol.* 1990;1144–1146.
9. Lue TF. Physiology of erection and pathophysiology of impotence. In: Walsh PC, et al, eds. *Campbell's Urology.* 6th ed. Philadelphia, Pa: WB Saunders Co; 1992:709–728.
10. Deysach IJ. Comparative morphology of erectile tissue of the penis with especial emphasis on the probable mechanism of erection. *Am J Anat.* 1939;64:111.
11. Wagner G, Bro-Rasmussen F, Willis EA, Nielsen MH. New theory on the mechanism of erection involving hitherto undescribed vessels. *Lancet.* 1982;1:416.
12. Ginestie JF, Romieu A. L'éxploration radiologique de l'impuissance. Paris: Maonie; 1976:2–24.
13. Huguet JF, Clerissi J, Juhan C. Radiologic anatomy of pudendal artery. *Eur J Radiol.* 1981;1:278–284.
14. Broderick GA, Arger P. Duplex doppler ultrasonography: noninvasive assessment of penile anatomy and function. *Semin Roentgenol.* 1993;43–56.
15. Bähren W, Gall H, Scherb W, Stief C, Thon W. Arterial anatomy and arteriographic diagnosis of arteriogenic impotence. *Cardiovasc Intervent Radiol.* 1988;11:195.
16. Bähren W, Gall H, Scherb W, Holzki G, Sparwasser C. Pharmacoarteriography in chronic erectile dysfunction. In: Jonas U, Thon WF, Stief CG, eds. *Erectile Dysfunction.* Berlin: Springer-Verlag; 1991:137–161
17. Newman HF, Northrup JD. Mechanism of human penile erection: an overview. *Urology.* 1981;17:399–408.
18. Fuchs AM, Mehringer CM, Rajfer J. Anatomy of penile venous drainage in potent and impotent men during cavernosography. *J Urol.* 1989;1353–1356.
19. Walsh PC, Donker P. Impotence following radical prostatectomy: insight into etiology and prevention. *J Urol.* 1982;128:492–497.
20. Lue TF, Zeineh SJ, Schmidt RA, Tanagho EA. Neuroanatomy of penile erection: its relevance to iatrogenic impotence. *J Urol.* 1984;131:273–280.
21. Lepor H, Gregerman M, Crosby R, Mostofi FK, Walsh PC. Precise localization of the autonomic nerves from the pelvic plexus to the corpora cavernosa: a detailed anatomical study of the adult male pelvis. *J Urol.* 1985;133:207–212.
22. de Groat WC, Steers WD. Neuroanatomy and neurophysiology of penile erection. In: Tanagho EA, Lue TF, McClure RD. *Contemporary Management of Impotence and Infertility.* Baltimore, Md: Williams & Wilkins; 1988:3–27.
23. Steers WD. Neural control of penile erection. *Semin Urol.* 1990;8:66–79.
24. Hsu GL, Brock G, Martinez-Pineor L, von Heyden B, Lue TF, Tanagho EA. The three-dimensional structure of the human tunica albuginea: anatomical and ultrastructural levels. *Int J Impotence Res.* 1992;4(suppl 2):41.
25. Saenz de Tejada I, Blanco R, Goldstein I, et al. Cholinergic neurotransmission in human corpus cavernosum: responses of isolated tissue. *Am J Physiol.* 1988;254:H459–H467.
26. Persson C, Diederichs W, Lue TF, et al. Correlation of altered penile ultrastructure with clinical arterial evaluation. *J Urol.* 1989;142:1462.
27. Khawand N, Vidic B, Jevtich MJ. Clinical application of electron microscopy of the corpora cavernosa in normal and impotent men. *J Urol.* 1987;137(pt 2):233A. Abstract 519.
28. Wespes E, deGoes PM, Schiffmann S, Depierreux M, Vanderhaeghen JJ, Schulman CC. Computerized analysis of smooth muscle fibers in potent and impotent patients. *J Urol.* 1991;1015–1017.
29. Wespes E, deGoes PM, Schulman C. Vascular impotence: focal or diffuse penile disease. *J Urol.* 1992;1435–1436.
30. Banya Y, Ushiki T, Takagane H, et al. Two circulatory routes within the human corpus cavernosum penis: a scanning electron microscopic study of corrosion casts. *J Urol.* 1989;879–883.
31. Meuleman EJH, Bemelmans BLH, Van Asten WNJC, Doesburg WH, Skotnicki SH, Debruyne FMJ. The value of combined papaverine testing and duplex scanning in men with erectile dysfunction. *Int J Impotence Res.* 1990;2:87–98.
32. Vickers MA Jr, Seiler M, Weidner N. Corpora cavernosa ultrastructure in vascular erectile dysfunction. *J Urol.* 1990;1131–1134.
33. Luangkhot R, Rutchik S, Agarwal V, Puglia K, Bhargava G, Melman A. Collagen alterations in the corpus cavernosum of men with sexual dysfunction. *J Urol.* 1992;467–470.
34. Fawcett DW. Connective tissue proper. In: Fawcett DW, ed. *Bloom & Fawcett: A Textbook of Histology.* Philadelphia, Pa: WB Saunders Co; 1986:139–142.
35. Padma-Nathan H, Cheung D, Perelman N, Boyd SD, Nimni ME. The effects of aging, diabetes and vascular ischemia on the biochemical composition of collagen found in the corpora and tunica of potent and impotent men. *Int J Impotence Res.* 1990;2:75.
36. Jevtich MJ, Kass M, Khawand N. Changes in the corpora cavernosa of impotent diabetics: comparing histological with clinical findings. *J Urol (Paris).* 1985;91:287.
37. Bornman MS, du Plessis DJ, Ligthelm AJ, van Tonder HJ. Histological changes in the penis of the chacma baboon: a model to study aging penile vascular impotence. *J Med Primatol.* 1985;14:13.
38. Cohen MS, Sharpe W, Warner RS, Zorgniotti A. Morphology of corporal cavernosa arterial bed in impotence. *Urology.* 1980;25:382.
39. Mersdorf A, Goldsmith PC, Wolfgang D, et al. Ultrastructural changes in impotent penile tissue: a comparison of 65 patients. *J Urol.* 1991;749–758.
40. Saenz de Tejada I, Goldstein I, Azadzoi KM, Krane RJ, Cohen RA. Impaired neurogenic and endothelium-mediated relaxation of penile smooth muscle from diabetic men with impotence. *N Engl J Med.* 1989;320:1025.
41. Staubesand J, Wetterauer U, Kulvelis F. Ultrastructural findings in patients with erectile dysfunction. In: Jonas U, Thon WF, Stief CG, eds. *Erectile Dysfunction.* Berlin: Springer-Verlag; 1991:34–43.
42. Broderick G, Hypolite J, Levin RM. In-vitro contractile response of the rabbit corpus cavernosa to field stimulation and autonomic agonists and antagonists: a qualitative study. *Neurourol Urodynam.* 1991;10:507–515.
43. von Ebner V. Über klappenartige Vorrichtungen in den Arterien der Schwellkorger. *Anat Anz.* 1990;18:79.
44. Kiss F. Anatomisch-histologische Untersuchungen über die Erektion. *Z Anat.* 1921;61:455–521.
45. Conti G. L'erection du penis humain et ses bases morphologicovasculaires. *Acta Anat.* 1952;14:217–262.

46. Lierse W. Blood vessels and nerves of the human penis. *Urol Int.* 1982;37:145.

47. Fournier GR Jr, Jünemann KP, Lue TF, Tanagho EA. Mechanisms of venous occlusion during canine penile erection: an anatomic demonstration. *J Urol.* 1987;137:163.

48. Lue TF, Muller SC, Jünemann KP, Fournier GR Jr, Tanagho EA. Hämodynamische Veränderungen während der Erektion und funktionelle klinische Diagnostik der penilen Gefässe mittels Ultraschall und gepulstem Doppler. *Akt Urol.* 1987;18:115.

49. Aboseif SR, Lue TF. Hemodynamics of penile erection. *Urol Clin North Am.* 1988;15:1.

50. Lue TF, Tanagho EA. Hemodynamics of erection. In: Tanagho EA, Lue TF, McClure RD. *Contemporary Management of Impotence and Infertility.* Baltimore, Md: Williams & Wilkins; 1988:28–38.

51. Foreman MM, Wernicke JF. Approaches for the development of oral drug therapies for erectile dysfunction. *Semin Urol.* 1990;8:107–112.

52. Bancroft J, ed. *Human Sexuality and Its Problems.* 2nd ed. Edinburgh: Churchill Livingstone; 1989.

53. Wein AJ, Van Arsdalen KN. Drug-induced male sexual dysfunction. *Urol Clin North Am.* 1988;15:23–31.

54. Rosen RC. Alcohol and drug effects on sexual response: human experimental and clinical studies. *Annu Rev Sex Res.* 1991;2:119–179.

55. Kaplan HS, ed. *Disorders of Sexual Desire.* New York, NY: Brunner Mazel; 1979.

56. Bansal S. Sexual dysfunction in hypertensive men: a critical review of the literature. *Hypertension.* 1988;12:1–10.

57. Harrison WM, Rabkin JG, Ehrhardt AA, et al. Effects of antidepressant medication on sexual function: a controlled study. *J Clin Psychopharmacol.* 1986;6:144–149.

58. Howell JR, Reynolds CF, Thase ME, et al. Assessment of sexual function, interest and activity in depressed men. *J Affective Disord.* 1987;13:61–66.

59. Segraves RT. Effects of psychotropic drugs on human erection and ejaculation. *Arch Gen Psychiatry.* 1989;46:275–284.

60. Segraves RT. Drugs and desire. In: Leiblum SR, Rosen RC, eds. *Sexual Desire Disorders.* New York, NY: Guilford Press; 1988:313–347.

61. Sachs BD, Meisel RL. The physiology of male sexual behavior. In: Knobil E, Neill JD, Ewing LL, eds. *The Physiology of Reproduction.* New York: Karger; 1988;2:1393–1423.

62. Grant LD, Stumpf WE. Hormone uptake sites in relation to CNS biogenic amine systems. In: Stumpf WE, Grant LD, eds. *Anatomical Neuroendocrinology.* Basel: Karger; 1975:445–463.

63. Barbeau A. L-Dopa therapy in Parkinson's disease: a critical review of nine years' experience. *Can Med Assoc J.* 1969;101:59–69.

64. Angrist B, Gershon S. Clinical effects of amphetamine and L-dopa on sexuality and aggression. *Compr Psychiatry.* 1976;17:715–722.

65. Del Bene E, Fanciullacci M, Poggioni M, Principe L, Sicuteri F. Apomorphine and other dopamine modifiers of human sexual and nociceptive tonus. In: Segal M, ed. *Psychopharmacology of Sexual Disorders.* London: John Libbey; 1985:145–153.

66. Uitti RJ, Tanner CM, Rajput AH, et al. Hypersexuality with antiparkinsonian therapy. *Clin Neuropharmacol.* 1989;5:375–383.

67. Yaryura-Tobias J, Diamond B, Merlis S. The action of L-dopa on schizophrenic patients (a preliminary report). *Curr Ther Res.* 1970;12:528–531.

68. Bitran D, Hull EM. Pharmacological analysis of male rat sexual behavior. *Neurosci Biobehav Rev.* 1987;11:365–389.

69. Dallo J, Lekka N, Knoll J. The ejaculatory behavior of sexually sluggish male rats treated with (−)deprenyl, apomorphine, bromocriptine and amphetamine. *Pol J Pharmacol Pharm.* 1986;38:251–255.

70. Malmnas CO. The significance of dopamine, versus other catecholamines, for the L-dopa induced facilitation of sexual behavior in the castrated male rat. *Pharmacol Biochem Behav.* 1976;4:521–526.

71. Buffum J. Pharmacosexology: the effects of drugs on sexual function. *J Psychoactive Drugs.* 1982;14:5–44.

72. Abramowicz M. Drugs that cause sexual dysfunction. *Med Lett Drugs Ther.* 1987;29:65–70.

73. Smith ER, Lee RL, Schnur SL, Davidson JM. Alpha-2-adrenoceptor antagonists and male sexual behavior. *Physiol Behav.* 1987;41:7–14.

74. Sala M, Braida D, Leone MP, et al. Central effect of yohimbine on sexual behavior in the rat. *Physiol Behav.* 1990;47:165–173.

75. Foreman MM, Hall JL, Love RL. Effects of fenfluramine and parachloroamphetamine on sexual behavior of male rats. *Psychopharmacology.* 1992 (in press).

76. Pinder RM, Brogen RN, Sawyer PR, et al. Fenfluramine: a review of its pharmacological properties and efficacy in obesity. *Drugs.* 1975;10:241–323.

77. Schurmeyer TH, Hesch RD. Endocrinology of impotence. In: Jonas U, Thon WF, Stief CG, eds. *Erectile Dysfunction.* Berlin: Springer-Verlag; 1991:78–90.

78. Baum MJ. Effects of testosterone propionate administered perinatally on sexual behavior of female ferrets. *J Comp Physiol Psychol.* 1976;90:399–410.

79. Carter CS, Clemens LG, Hoekema DJ. Neonatal androgen and adult sexual behavior in the golden hamster. *Physiol Behav.* 1972;9:89–95.

80. Clarke IJ, Scaramuzzi RJ, Short RV. Sexual differentiation of the brain: endocrine and behavioural responses of androgenized ewes to oestrogen. *J Endocrinol.* 1976;71:175–176.

81. Edwards DA, Burge KG. Early androgen treatment and male and female sexual behavior in mice. *Horm Behav.* 1971;2:49–58.

82. Ford JJ. Differentiation of sexual behavior in swine. *Biol Reprod.* 1981;24(suppl 1):95A.

83. Pardridge WM, Gorski RA, Lippe BA, Green R. Androgens and sexual behavior. *Ann Intern Med.* 1982;96:488–501.

84. McClure RD. Endocrine evaluation and therapy of erectile dysfunction. In: Krane RH, ed. *Urol Clin North Am.* 1988:53–64.

85. Cunningham GR, Hirschkowitz M, Korenman SG, Karacan I. Testosterone replacement therapy and sleep-related erections in hypogonadal men. *J Clin Endocrinol Metab.* 1990;70:792–797.

86. Baker ER. Menstrual dysfunction and hormonal status in athletic women: a review. *Fertil Steril.* 1981;36:691.

87. Vermeulen A, Rubens R, Verdonck L. Testosterone secretion and metabolism in male senescence. *J Clin Endocrinol Metab.* 1972;34:730.

88. Kaiser FE, Udhoji V, Viosca SP, Morley JE, Mooradian AD, et al. Cardiovascular stress tests in patients with vascular impotence. *Clin Res.* 1989;37:89A.

89. Korenman SG, Morley JE, Mooradian AD, et al. Secondary hypogonadism in older men: its relationship to impotence. *J Clin Endocrinol Metab.* 1990;963–969.

90. Morley JE, Kaiser FE. Impotence in elderly men. Drugs Aging. 1992;2:330–344.

91. Goldstein I, Krane RJ. Diagnosis and therapy of erectile dysfunction. In: Walsh PC, et al, eds. *Campbell's Urology.* 6th ed. Philadelphia, Pa: WB Saunders Co; 1992:3033–3072.

92. Boyden TW, Pamenter RW, Grosso D, Stanforth P, Rotkis T, Wilmore JH. Prolactin responses, menstrual cycles, and body composition of women runners. *J Clin Endocrinol Metab.* 1982;54:711–714.

93. Brisson GR, Volle MA, DeCarufel D, Desharnais M, Tanaka M. Exercise-induced dissociation of the blood prolactin response in young women according to their sports habits. *Horm Metab Res.* 1980;12:201–205.

94. Kreuz LE, Rose RM, Jennings JR. Suppression of plasma testosterone levels and psychological stress. *Arch Gen Psychiatry.* 1972;26:479–482.

95. Yesavage JA, Davidson J, Widrow L, Berger PA. Plasma

testosterone levels, depression, sexuality and age. *Biol Psychiatry.* 1985;20:199–228.

96. Nemeroff CB, Widerlov E, Bissett G, et al. Elevated concentrations of CSF corticotropin-releasing-factor-like immunoreactivity in depressed patients. *Science.* 1984;226:1342–1233.

97. Neri A, Aygen M, Zuckerman Z. Subjective assessment of sexual dysfunction of patients on long term administration of digoxin. *Arch Sex Behav.* 1980;9:343–349.

98. Slag MF, Morley JE, Elson MK, et al. Impotence in medical clinic outpatients. *JAMA.* 1983;249:1736–1740.

99. Pogach LM, Vaitukaitis JL. Endocrine disorders associated with erectile dysfunction. In: Krane RJ, Siroky MB, Goldstein I, eds. *Male Sexual Dysfunction.* Boston, Mass: Little, Brown & Co; 1983:63.

100. Jeanty P, van den Kerchove M, Lowenthal A, DeBruyne H. Pergolide therapy in Parkinson's disease. *J Neurol.* 1984;231: 148–152.

101. Lal S. Apomorphine in the evaluation of dopaminergic function in man. *Prog Neuropsychopharmacol Biol Psychiatry.* 1988;12:117–164.

102. Lal S, Tesfaye Y, Thavundayil J, et al. Apomorphine: clinical studies on erectile impotence and yawning. *Prog Neuropsychopharmacol Biol Psychiatry.* 1989;13:329–339.

103. Segraves RT, Bari M, Segraves K, Spirnak P. Effect of apomorphine on penile tumescence in men with psychogenic impotence. *J Urol.* 1991;145:1174–1175.

104. Danjou P, Alexandre L, Warot D, et al. Assessment of erectogenic properties of apomorphine and yohimbine. *Br J Clin Pharmacol.* 1986;26:733–739.

105. Berendsen HHG, Jenck F, Broekkamp CLE. Involvement of 5-HT1c receptors in drug-induced penile erections in rats. *Psychopharmacology.* 1990;101:57–61.

106. Szele FG, Murphy DL, Garrick NA. Fenfluramine, m-chlorophenyl-piperazine and other serotonin re-uptake agonists and antagonists on penile erections in non-human primates. *Life Sci.* 1988;43:1297–1303.

107. Lal S, Rios O, Thavundayil JX. Treatment of impotence with trazodone: a case report. *J Urol.* 1990;143:819–820.

108. Saenz de Tejada I, Ware CJ, Blanco R, et al. Pathophysiology of prolonged penile erection associated with trazodone use. *J Urol.* 1991;145:60–64.

109. Steers WD, de Groat WC. Effects of m-chlorophenylpiperazine on penile and bladder function in rats. *Am J Physiol.* 1989;257:R1441–1449.

110. Segraves RT. Pharmacological agents causing sexual dysfunction. *J Sex Marital Ther.* 1977;3.157 176.

111. Segraves RT, Madsen R, Carter CS, Davis JM. Erectile dysfunction associated with pharmacological agents. In: Segraves RT, Schoenberg HW, eds. *Diagnosis and Treatment of Erectile Disturbances: A Guide for Clinicians.* New York, NY: Plenum Medical Book Co; 1985:23–64.

112. Pfaus JG, Gorzalka B. Opioids and sexual behavior. *Neurosci Biobehav Rev.* 1987;11:1–34.

113. Goldstein JA. Erectile function and naltrexone. *Ann Intern Med.* 1986;105:799.

114. Charney DS, Heninger GR. Alpha-2-adrenergic and opiate receptor blockade: synergistic effects on anxiety in healthy subjects. *Arch Gen Psychiatry.* 1986;43:1037–1041.

115. Murphy JB, Lipshultz LI. Abnormalities of ejaculation. *Urol Clin North Am.* 1987;14:583–596.

116. Andersson KE, Holmquist F. Mechanisms for contraction and relaxation of human penile smooth muscle. *Int J Impotence Res.* 1990;2:209–225.

117. Virag R, Legman M, Zwang G, Dermange H. L'utilisation de l'erection passive dans l'exploraton de l'impuissance d'origine vasculaire. *Contraception Fertilité Sexualité.* 1979;7:707.

118. Jünemann KP. Pharmacotesting in erectile dysfunction. In: Jonas U, Thon WF, Stief CG, eds. *Erectile Dysfunction.* Berlin: Springer-Verlag; 1991:104–114.

119. Andersson KE, Holmquist F, Wagner G. Pharmacology of drugs used for treatment of erectile dysfunction and priapism. *Int J Impotence Res.* 1991;3:155–172.

120. Lewis RW. The pharmacologic erection. In: Paulson DF, Lewis RW, Barrett DM, eds. *Problems in Urology: The Impotent Man.* Philadelphia, Pa: JB Lippincott Co; 1991;5:541–558.

121. Wang Q, Large WA. Modulation of noradrenaline-induced membrane currents by papaverine in rabbit vascular smooth muscle cells. *J Physiol (Lond).* 1991;439:501–512.

122. Jünemann KP, Personn-Jünemann C, Alken P. Pathophysiology of erectile dysfunction. *Semin Urol.* 1990;8:80–93.

123. Earle CM, Keogh EL, Wisniewski ZS, et al. Prostaglandin E_1 therapy for impotence: comparison with papaverine. *J Urol.* 1990;143:323–325.

124. Roy AC, Adaikan PG, Sen DK, Ratnam SS. Prostaglandin 15-hydroxydehydrogenase activity in human penile corpora cavernosa and its significance in prostaglandin-mediated penile erection. *Br J Urol.* 1989;64:180–182.

125. Stief CG, Holmquist F, Kjamilian M, Krah H, Andersson KE, Jonas U. Preliminary results with the nitric oxide donor linsidomine chlorhydrate in the treatment of human erectile dysfunction. *J Urol.* 1992;148:1437–1440.

126. Gaskell P. The importance of penile blood pressure in cases of impotence. *Can Med Assoc J.* 1971;105:104.

127. Abelson D. Diagnostic value of the penile pulse and blood pressure: a Doppler study of impotence in diabetics. *J Urol.* 1975;113:636.

128. Michal V, Kramer R, Pospichal J. External iliac "steal syndrome." *J Cardiovasc Surg.* 1978;19:355.

129. Goldstein I, Siroky MB, North RI, et al. Vasculogenic impotence: role of the pelvic steal test. *J Urol.* 1982;128:300.

130. Schwartz AN, Lowe MA, Ireton R, Berger RE, Richardson MI, Graney DO. A comparison of penile brachial index and angiography: evaluation of corpora cavernosa arterial inflow. *J Urol.* 1990;143:510.

131. Padma-Nathan H, Klavans S, Goldstein I, Krane RJ. The screening efficacy of PBI versus duplex ultrasound versus cavernosal artery systolic occlusion pressure. In: *Proceedings of the Sixth Biennial International Symposium for Corpus Cavernosum Revascularization and Third Biennial World Meeting on Impotence;* October 6–9, 1988; Boston, Mass. 32.

132. Goldstein I, Krane RJ, Greenfield AJ, Padma-Nathan H. Vascular diseases of the penis: impotence and priapism. In: Pollack H, ed. *Clinical Urography.* Philadelphia, Pa: WB Saunders Co; 1990:2231–2252.

133. Bookstein JJ, Lange EV. Penile magnification pharmacoarteriography: details of intrapenile arterial anatomy. *AJR.* 1987; 148:883.

134. Rajfer J, Canan V, Dorey FJ, Mehringer CM. Correlation between penile angiography and duplex scanning of cavernous arteries in impotent men. *J Urol.* 1990;143:1128–1130.

135. Garibyan H, Lue TF. Anastomotic network between the dorsal and cavernous arteries in the penis. *J Urol.* 1990;143:221A.

136. Lurie AL, Bookstein J, Kessler W. Angiography of posttraumatic impotence. *Cardiovasc Intervent Radiol.* 1988;11:232–236.

137. Lue TF, Hricak H, Marich KW, Tanagho EA. Vasculogenic impotence evaluated by high resolution ultrasonography and pulsed Doppler spectrum analysis. *Radiology.* 1985;155:777.

138. Virag R, Bouilly P, Frydman D. Is impotence an arterial disorder? *Lancet.* 1984;1:181–184.

139. Paushter DM. Role of duplex sonography in the evaluation of sexual impotence. *AJR.* 1989;153:1161.

140. Robinson LQ, Woodcock JP, Stephenson RP. Duplex scanning in suspected vasculogenic impotence: a worthwhile exercise? *Br J Urol.* 1989;63:432.

141. Forsberg L, Olsson AM. Doppler studies of the penile circulation. *Urol Radiol.* 1988;10:129.

142. Krysiewicz S, Mellinger BC. The role of imaging in the diagnostic evaluation of impotence. *AJR.* 1989;153:1133.

143. Lue TF, Nelson RP. Determination of erectile penile volume by ultrasonography. 1989;141:1123–1126.

144. Fitzgerald SW, Erickson SJ, Foley WD, Lipchik EO, Lawson TL. Color Doppler sonography in the evaluation of erectile dysfunction: patterns of temporal response to papaverine. *AJR.* 1991;157:331–336.

145. Rajfer J. Endocrine evaluation of impotence. In: Rajfer J, ed. *Infertility and Impotence*. Chicago, Ill: Year Book Medical Publishers; 1990:243–247.

146. Gall H, Bähren W, Scherb W, Stief C, Thon W. Diagnostic accuracy of Doppler ultrasound technique of the penile arteries in correlation to selective arteriography. *Cardiovasc Intervent Radiol*. 1988;11:225.

147. Broderick GA, Lue TF. The penile blood flow study: evaluation of vasculogenic impotence. In: Jonas U, Thon WF, Stief CG, eds. *Erectile Dysfunction*. Berlin: Springer-Verlag; 1991: 126–136.

148. Kessler WO. Nocturnal penile tumescence. *Urol Clin North Am*. 1988;15:81–86.

149. Mellinger BC, Vaughn ED. Penile blood flow changes in the flaccid and erect state in potent young men measured by duplex scanning. *J Urol*. 1990;144:894–896.

150. Shabsigh R, Fishman IJ, Shottland Y, Karracan I, Dunn JK. Comparison of penile duplex ultrasonography with nocturnal penile tumescence monitoring for the evaluation of erectile impotence. *J Urol*. 1990;143:924.

151. Diederichs W, Stief CG, Lue TF, Tanagho EA. Sympathetic inhibition of papaverine-induced erection. *J Urol*. 1991;146: 195–198.

152. Lue TF, Donatucci CF. The combined intracavernous injection and stimulation test: diagnostic accuracy. *J Urol*. 1992; 148:61–62.

153. Burns PN. Physical principles of Doppler ultrasound and spectral analysis. *J Clin Ultrasound*. 1987;15:567–590.

154. Merritt CR. Doppler color flow imaging. *J Clin Ultrasound*. 1987;15:591–597.

155. Foley WD, Erickson SJ. Color Doppler flow imaging. *AJR*. 1991;156:3–13.

156. Shabsigh R, Fishman IJ, Quesada ET, Seale-Hawkins CK, Dunn JK. Evaluation of vasculogenic erectile impotence using penile duplex ultrasonography. *J Urol*. 1989;142:1469–1474.

157. Benson CB, Vickers MA. Sexual impotence caused by vascular disease: diagnosis with duplex sonography. *AJR*. 1989; 153:1149.

158. Quam JP, King BF, James EM, et al. Duplex and color Doppler sonographic evaluation of vasculogenic impotence. *AJR*. 1989;153:1141.

159. Schwartz AN, Wang KY, Mack LA, et al. Evaluation of normal erectile function with color Doppler sonography. *AJR*. 1989; 153:1155.

160. Merckx LA, De Bruyne RMG, Goes E, Derde MP, Keuppens F. The value of dynamic color duplex scanning in the diagnosis of venogenic impotence. *J Urol*. 1992;148:318–320.

161. Roddy TM, Goldstein I, Devine CJ. Peyronie's disease, parts I+II. *AUA Update Series*. 1991;10:1–15.

162. Altaffer LF, Jordan GH. Sonographic demonstration of Peyronie's plaques. *Urology*. 1981;17:29.

163. Rollandi GA, Tentarelli T, Vespier M. Computed tomographic findings in Peyronie's disease. *Urol Radiol*. 1985;7:153–156.

164. Porst H, van Ahlen H, Vahlensiech W. Relevance of dynamic cavernosography to the diagnosis of venous incompetence in erectile dysfunction. *J Urol*. 1987;137:1163–1167.

165. Shabsigh R, Fishman IJ, Schum C, Dunn JF. Cigarette smoking and other vascular risk factors in vasculogenic impotence. *Urology*. 1991;38:227.

166. Lue TF. Physiology of penile erection. In: Jonas U, Thon WF, Stief CG, eds. *Erectile Dysfunction*. Berlin: Springer-Verlag; 1991:44–56.

167. Puech-Leao P, Reis JMSM, Glina S, Reichelt AC. Leakage through the crural edge of the corpora cavernosa: diagnosis and treatment. *Eur Urol*. 1987;13:163–165.

168. Kolliker A. Das anatomische und physiologische Verhalten der cavernosen Körper der Sexualorgane. *Verh Phys-Med Ges Würzburg*. 1852;2:118.

169. Ebbehoj J, Wagner G. Insufficient penile erection due to abnormal drainage of cavernous bodies. *Urology*. 1979; 13:507.

170. Lydston GF. The surgical treatment of impotency. *Am J Clin Med*. 1908;15:1571–1573.

171. Lewis RW. Venogenic impotence: diagnosis, management and results. In: Paulson DF, Lewis RW, Barrett DM, eds. *Problems in Urology: The Impotent Man*. Philadelphia, Pa: JB Lippincott Co; 1991;5:567–576.

172. Padma-Nathan H, Goldstein I. Neurologic assessment of the impotent male. In: Montague DK, ed. *Disorders of Male Sexual Functions*. Chicago, Ill: Year Book Publishers; 1987: 86–94.

173. Scherb WH. Neurophysiological evaluation of erectile dysfunction. In: Jonas U, Thon WF, Stief CG, eds. *Erectile Dysfunction*. Berlin: Springer-Verlag; 1991:178–186.

174. Karacan I. Clinical value of nocturnal erection in the prognosis and diagnosis of impotence. *Med Aspects Hum Sexuality*. 1970;4:27.

175. Thase ME, et al. Nocturnal penile tumescence is diminished in depressed men. *Biol Psychiatry*. 1988;24:33.

176. Bors E, Blinn KA. Bulbocavernosus reflex. *J Urol*. 1959; 82:128.

177. Blaivas JG, Zayed AAH, Labib KB. The bulbocavernosus reflex in urology: a prospective study of 299 patients. *J Urol*. 1981;126:197–199.

178. Abicht JH. Testing the autonomic system. In: Jonas U, Thon WF, Stief CG, eds. *Erectile Dysfunction*. Berlin: Springer-Verlag; 1991:187–193.

179. Gerstenberg TC, Nordling J, Hald H, Wagner G. Standardized evaluation of erectile dysfunction in 95 consecutive patients. *J Urol*. 1989;141:857–861.

180. Wagner G, Gerstenberg T. Human in vivo studies of electrical activity of corpus cavernosum. *J Urol*. 1988;139:327A.

181. Gerstenberg TC, Metz P, Nielsen SL. Corpus cavernosum smooth muscle relaxation and contraction correlates with xenon wash-out of the cavernous body. *Int J Impotence Res*. 1992;4(suppl 2):A18.

182. Wagner G, Gerstenberg T, Levin RJ. Electrical activity of the corpus cavernosum during flaccidity and erection of the human penis: a new diagnostic method? *J Urol*. 1989;142:723.

183. Gerstenberg TC, Nordling J. Corpus cavernosum electromyography measured by needle and surface electrodes. *Int J Impotence Res*. 1992;4(suppl 2):A21.

184. Stief CG, Djamilian M, Schaebsdam F, et al. Single potential analysis of cavernous electric activity—a possible diagnosis of autonomic impotence? *World J Urol*. 1990;8:75.

185. Stief CG, Thon WF, Djamilian M, Schaebsdam F, Jonas U. SPACE (single potential analysis of cavernous electric activity): a possible diagnosis of autonomic cavernous dysfunction and of cavernous smooth muscle degeneration. *Int J Impotence Res*. 1990;2(suppl 2):91.

186. Stief CG. Single potential analysis of cavernous electrical activity: a possible diagnosis of autonomic cavernous dysfunction and cavernous smooth muscle degeneration. In: Jonas U, Thon WF, Stief CG, eds. *Erectile Dysfunction*. Berlin: Springer-Verlag; 1991:194–203.

187. Stief CG, Hoppner C, Sauerwein D, Jonas U. Cavernous electric activity (SPACE) in spinalized patients. *Int J Impotence Res*. 1992;4(suppl 2):A23.

188. Merckx LA, Schmedding E, De Bruyne RM, Keuppens FI. Penile electromyography in the evaluation of neurogenic impotence: a critical appraisal. *Int J Impotence Res*. 1992;4 (suppl 2):A22.

189. Bemelmans BLH, Meuleman EJH, Koldewijn EL, Notermans SLH, Debruyne FMJ. Critical appraisal of penile electromyography: neurophysiological investigations of the electrical activity of cavernous smooth muscles. *Int J Impotence Res*. 1992;4(suppl 2):A25.

190. Shabsigh R, Te AE, Fisch H. Cavernous electromyography as an indicator of adequate smooth muscle relaxation during penile duplex ultrasonography. *Int J Impotence Res*. 1992;4 (suppl 2):A26.

191. Portner MR, Puech-Leao P, Glina S, Reis JMM. Inhibition of cavernous EMG activity during drug-induced penile erection. *Int J Impotence Res*. 1992;4(suppl 2):A27.

192. Buhrle CP, Schmidt P, Jünemann KP, Berle B, Alken P. Autonomic acquisition and analysis of EMG data from corpus cavernosum recordings in the dog. *Int J Impotence Res.* 1992; 4(suppl 2):A29.

193. Virag R. The screening of impotence by the use of visual sexual stimulation after intracavernous injection of a small dose of papaverine. Presented at the Second World Meeting on Impotence; June 17–20, 1986; Prague.

194. Masters WH. Sex and aging: expectations and reality. *Hosp Pract.* 1986;175–198.

195. Mellinger BC, Weiss J. Sexual dysfunction in the elderly male. *AUA Update Series.* 1992;11:146–152.

196. Feldman H, Goldstein I, Hatzichristou DG, Krane RJ, McKinley JB. Impotence and its medical and psychological correlates: results of the Massachusetts male aging study. *Int J Impotence Res.* 1992;4(suppl 2):A17.

197. Michal V, Ruzbarsky V. Histological changes in the penile arterial bed with aging and diabetes. In: *Vasculogenic Impotence: Proceedings of the First International Conference on Corpus Cavernosum Revascularization.* Springfield, Ill: Charles C Thomas Publisher; 1980:113–119.

198. Kaiser FE, Viosca SP, Mooradian AD, Morley JE, Korenman SG. Impotence and aging: alterations in hormonal secretory patterns. *Endocrine Society Abstracts.* 1988;778A.

199. McCulloch DK, et al. Natural history of impotence in diabetic men. *Diabetologia.* 1984;26:437.

200. Saenz de Tejada I, Moroukian P, Tessier J, Kim JJ, Goldstein I, Frohrib D. The trabecular smooth muscle modulates the capacitor function of the penis: studies on a rabbit model. *Am J Physiol.* 1991;260:H1590–H1595.

201. Azadzoi KM, Saenz de Tejada I. Diabetes mellitus impairs neurogenic and endothelium-dependent relaxation of rabbit corpus cavernosum smooth muscle. *J Urol.* 1992;148: 1587–1591.

202. Waltzer WC. Sexual and reproductive function in men treated with hemodialysis and renal transplantation. *J Urol.* 1981;126:713–716.

203. Salvatierra O Jr, Fortmann JL, Belzer FO. Sexual function in males before and after renal transplantation. *Urology.* 1975;5: 64–66.

204. Gittes RF, Waters WB. Sexual impotence: the overlooked complication of a second renal transplant. *J Urol.* 1979;121: 719–720.

205. Lue TF. Impotence after radical pelvic surgery: physiology and management. *Urol Int.* 1991;46:259–265.

206. Melman A. Iatrogenic causes of erectile dysfunction. In: Krane RJ, ed. *Urol Clin North Am.* 1988;15:33–40.

207. Weinstein M, Robets M. Sexual potency following surgery for rectal carcinoma. *Ann Surg.* 1977;185:295–300.

208. Yeager ES, Van Heerden JA. Sexual dysfunction following proctocolectomy and abdominoperineal resection. *Ann Surg.* 1980;191:169–170.

209. Santangelo ML, Romano G, Sassaroli C. Sexual function after resection for rectal cancer. *Am J Surg.* 1987;154:502–504.

210. Boyd SD, Feinberg SM, Skinner DG, Lieskovsky G, Baron D, Richardson J. Quality of life survey of urinary diversion patients: comparison of ileal conduits versus continent Kock ileal reservoirs. *J Urol.* 1987;138:1386.

211. Broderick GA, Stone AR, deVere-White RW. Neobladders: clinical management and considerations for patients receiving chemotherapy. *Semin Oncol.* 1990;17:598–605.

212. Goldwasser B, Webster GD. Continent urinary diversion. *J Urol.* 1985;134:227–236.

213. Leriche R. Des Obliterations arterielles hautes (obliteration de la termination de l'aorte) comme causes des insuffisances circulatoires des membres intérieurs. *Bull Mem Soc Chir.* 1923; 49:1404.

214. May AG, DeWeese JA, Rob CG. Changes in sexual function following operation on the abdominal aorta. *Surgery.* 1969;65:41–47.

215. DePalma RG, Levine SB, Feldman S. Preservation of erectile function after aortoiliac reconstruction. *Arch Surg.* 1978; 113:985.

216. Flanigan PD, Schuler JJ, Keifer T, Schwartz JA, Lim LT. Elimination of iatrogenic impotence and improvement of sexual function after aortoiliac revascularization. *Arch Surg.* 1982;117:544–550.

217. Ohshiro T, Kosaki G. Sexual function after aorto-iliac vascular reconstruction. *J Cardiovasc Surg.* 1984;25:47–50.

218. Walsh PC, Lepor H, Eggleston JC. Radical prostatectomy with preservation of sexual function: anatomical and pathological considerations. *Prostate.* 1983;4:474.

219. Walsh PC. Radical prostatectomy with preservation of sexual function: evolution of a surgical procedure. *AUA Update Series.* 1985;5:2–9.

220. Bagshaw MA, Cox RS, Ray GR. Status of radiation treatment of prostate cancer at Stanford University. *NCI Monogr.* 1988;7:47–60.

221. Shipley WU, Prout GR, Coachman NM, et al. Radiation therapy for localized prostate carcinoma: experience at the Massachusetts General Hospital (1973–1981). *NCI Monogr.* 1988;7:133–137.

222. Zohar J, Meiraz D, Maoz B, et al. Factors influencing sexual activity after prostatectomy. *J Urol.* 1976;116:332–334.

223. Finkle AL, Prien DV. Sexual potency in elderly men before and after prostatectomy. *JAMA.* 1966;139–143.

224. So EP, Ho PC, Bodesta W, et al. Erectile impotence associated with transurethral prostatectomy. *Urology.* 1982;19: 259–262.

225. Mebust WK. A review of TURP complications and the AUA nation cooperative study. *AUA Update Series.* 1989;8:186–191.

226. McDermott DW, Bates RJ, Heney NM, Althausen A. Erectile impotence as complication of direct vision cold knife urethrotomy. *Urology.* 1981;18:467–469.

227. Graversen PH, Rosenkilde P, Colstrup H. Erectile dysfunction following direct vision internal urethrotomy. *Scand J Urol Nephrol.* 1991;25:175–178.

228. Hinman F Jr. Priapism: reasons for failure of therapy. *J Urol.* 1960;83:420–428.

229. Broderick GA, Lue TF. Priapism and the physiology of erection. *AUA Update Series.* 1987;VII: lesson 29.

230. Fouda A, Hassouna M, Beddoe E, Kalogeropoulous D, Binik YM, Elhilali MM. Priapism: an avoidable complication of pharmacologically induced erection. *J Urol.* 1989;142: 995–997.

231. Girdley FM, Bruskewitz RC, Feyzi J, Graversen PH, Gasser TC. Intracavernous self injection for impotence: a long-term therapeutic option? experience in 78 patients. *J Urol.* 1988; 140:972–974.

232. Ishii N, Watanabe H, Irisawa C, et al. Intracavernous injection of prostaglandin E_1 for the treatment of erectile impotence. *J Urol.* 1989;141:323–325.

233. Bruhlmann W, Pouliadis G, Hauri D, Vollikofer CH. A new concept of priapism based on the results of arteriography and cavernosography. *Urol Radiol.* 1982;5:31–36.

234. Hauri D, Spycher M, Bruhlmann W. Erection and priapism: a new physiopathological concept. *Urol Int.* 1983;38:138–145.

235. Jünemann KP, Lue TF, Fournier GR. Blood gas analysis in drug induced penile erection. *Urol Int.* 1986;41:207–211.

236. Azadzoi KM, Vlachiotis J, Vardi Y, Sirokym B. On-line measurement of intracavernosal oxygen tension: an index of cavernosal blood flow. *Int J Impotence Res.* 1992;4(suppl 2):P23.

237. Macaluso JN, Sullivan JW. Priapism: a review of 34 cases. *Urology.* 1985;26:233–236

238. Spycher MA, Hauri D. The ultrastructure of the erectile tissue in priapism. *J Urol.* 1986;135:142–147.

239. Broderick GA, Lue TF. Treatment of priapism. In: Rajfer J, ed. *Current Problems in Infertility and Impotence.* Chicago, Ill: Year Book Medical Publications; 1990:290–299.

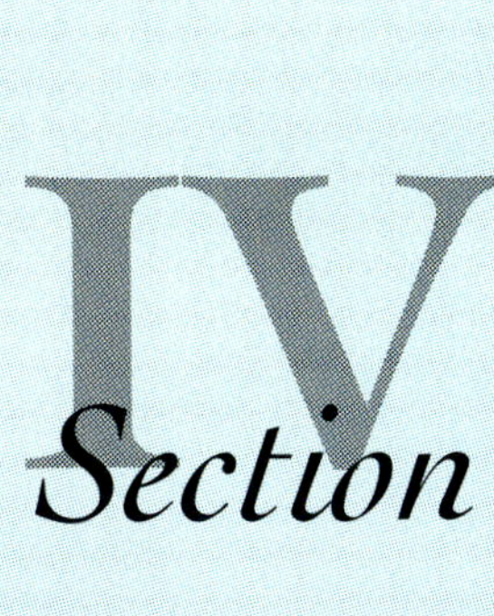

Calculus Disease

Glenn M. Preminger, editor

Metabolic Evaluation of Calculus Disease

Glenn M. Preminger

The past decade has shown unparalleled progress in the surgical treatment of nephrolithiasis. Improved endourologic devices and extracorporeal shock wave lithotripsy have revolutionized patient care, allowing efficient stone removal with a significant reduction in postoperative pain and convalescence. Indeed, the dramatic success of these innovative techniques has perhaps distracted attention from the need for proper medical evaluation and treatment of nephrolithiasis.

Equally dramatic strides have been made in the medical management of stone disease. In recent years we have witnessed the interpretation of the physicochemistry of nephrolithiasis, the diagnosis of specific abnormalities in stone-formers, and the development of selective therapies for these physiologic derangements. It is now known that the urinary environment of stone patients is conducive to the crystallization of stone-forming salts, due to increased supersaturation and/or reduced inhibitor activity. A metabolic or environmental etiology of nephrolithiasis can be found in approximately 95% of patients evaluated for their stone disease. Selective medical therapy is highly effective in preventing new stone formation, thereby reducing the need for repeated invasive procedures in patients predisposed to nephrolithiasis.

In this section on calculus disease, we will review the pathophysiology of stone disease, present the diagnostic criteria for the various conditions underlying stone formation, and discuss the selective medical management of each of these underlying conditions. Moreover, a comprehensive review of the surgical treatment of renal and ureteral stones will be presented along with certain "philosophies" for the management of symptomatic calculi.

Epidemiology

Renal calculi are abnormal concretions, occurring anywhere along the collecting system of the urinary tract, and consisting of crystalline components incorporated in organic matrix. Nephrolithiasis is a relatively common disorder affecting anywhere from 1% to 5% of the population in industrialized countries, with an annual incidence as high as 1% having been reported in middle-aged white males. Primary bladder calculi are quite uncommon in industrialized countries except when associated with bladder outlet obstruction (most commonly prostatic obstruction), neuropathic bladder disorders, or encrustation of foreign bodies.

The most common stones seen in industrialized countries contain primarily calcium oxalate occurring alone or in combination with hydroxyapatite. Calcareous calculi account for approximately 75% of renal stones. The remaining 25% of renal calculi are noncalcareous and are composed of either uric acid, struvite, or cystine.

In several unselected population surveys, the lifetime risk for stone formation in adult white males approaches 20%, while for females it is approximately 5% to 10%. In addition, the recurrence rate of nephrolithiasis has been reported to be as high as 50% within 5 years from the first stone occurrence. After 8 years, 63% of males and 18% of females were reported to form additional stones. Stone disease in black patients is one third to one fourth less common than in adult white males and blacks demonstrate a higher incidence of infection calculi.

Metabolic Classification of Nephrolithiasis

A logical method of diagnostic differentiation is to categorize nephrolithiasis on the basis of underlying physiologic-environmental abnormalities. This classification assumes that these disturbances are pathogenetically important in stone formation.

In 1972, calcium nephrolithiasis was considered to be comprised of three entities: idiopathic hypercalciuria, primary hyperparathyroidism, and normocalciuric nephrolithiasis. The cause of stone formation was not disclosed in the last category, comprising 43% of the patients. However, in 1993, dramatic progress in the diagnostic separation of nephrolithiasis paralleled by advances in analytical methodology have allowed identification of physiologic or environmental causes of stones in more than 97% of patients. Various diagnostic categories and their relative frequency are shown in Figure 12.1.

Calcareous calculi (calcium oxalate or calcium phosphate), make up approximately 75% of renal calculi. Causes of calcareous stone formation include hypercalciuria, hyperoxaluria, hyperuricosuria, hypomagnesiuria, and hypocitraturia. Hypercalciuria and hyperoxaluria contribute to stone formation by rendering urine supersaturated with respect to stone-forming calcium salts. Hyperuricosuria, in the setting of normal urinary pH (>5.5), has been associated with calcium nephrolithiasis. The pathogenetic role of hypomagnesiuria and hypocitraturia in nephrolithiasis may be ascribed to the inhibitor activity of magnesium and citrate. Citrate lowers the urinary saturation of calcium oxalate by forming a soluble complex with calcium and lowering calcium activity. Moreover, citrate may directly inhibit crystallization of calcium oxalate and calcium phosphate.

Among noncalcareous stones, the passage of unusually acid urine (pH < 5.5) would favor the formation of uric acid stones because of reduced uric acid solubility in such an environment. In gouty diathesis, uric acid lithiasis may coexist with calcium nephrolithiasis due to urate-induced crystallization of calcium salts. Patients with cystinuria may form cystine stones because of low aqueous solubility of cystine. In the presence of urinary tract infection with urea-splitting organisms, the resultant increase in ammonium ions and alkalinity may lead to struvite (magnesium ammonium phosphate) stone formation. Low urine volume contributes to formation of both calcareous and noncalcareous stones by increasing the urinary concentration of stone-forming constituents.

Physiologic Derangements of Calcium Nephrolithiasis

PATHOPHYSIOLOGY OF HYPERCALCIURIA

The association of hypercalciuria with recurrent calcium nephrolithiasis has long been recognized, although the exact cause for its relationship with nephrolithiasis continues to be debated. Hypercalciuria encountered in nephrolithiasis is heterogeneous in origin and thought to be comprised of several entities.

Absorptive Hypercalciuria

The basic abnormality in absorptive hypercalciuria is the intestinal hyperabsorption of calcium. The consequent increase in the circulating concentration of calcium enhances the renal filtered load and suppresses parathyroid function (Fig. 12.2). Hypercalciuria results from the combination of increased filtered load and reduced renal tubular reabsorption of calcium, a function of the parathyroid suppression. The excessive renal loss of calcium compensates for the high calcium absorption from the intestinal tract and helps to maintain serum calcium in the normal range. Absorptive hypercalciuria type I is considered a severe form, whereas the type II presentation is a mild or moderate form of this condition.

The exact cause for the hyperabsorption of calcium is not known. In most patients, it probably occurs by a vita-

FIGURE 12.1 *Classification of Nephrolithiasis*

	Sole Occurrence	Combined Occurrence
Absorptive hypercalciuria	30	40
Type I		
Type II		
Renal hypercalciuria	5	8
Primary hyperparathyroidism	3	8
Unclassified Ca nephrolithiasis	15	25
Hyperoxaluric Ca nephrolithiasis	2	15
Enteric hyperoxaluria		
Primary hyperoxaluria		
Dietary hyperoxaluria		
Hypocitraturic Ca nephrolithiasis	10	50
Distal renal tubular acidosis		
Chronic diarrheal syndrome		
Thiazide-induced		
Idiopathic		
Hypomagnesiuric Ca nephrolithiasis	5	10
Gouty diathesis	15	30
Cystinuria	<1	
Infection stones	1	5
Low urine volume	10	50
No disturbance and miscellaneous	<3	
	100	

The percentage for each diagnosis represents approximate estimates based on experience in Dallas, ranging from sole occurrence to combined occurrence with other abnormalities.

min-D-independent process. In some with severe absorptive hypercalciuria, enhanced renal synthesis of 1,25-(OH)$_2$ vitamin D (1,25-(OH)$_2$D), may contribute to high intestinal absorption and renal excretion of calcium.

Renal Hypercalciuria

The primary abnormality in renal hypercalciuria is believed to be an impairment in the renal tubular reabsorption of calcium. The resulting reduction in the serum calcium concentration stimulates parathyroid function (Fig. 12.3). There may be excessive mobilization of calcium from bone and an enhanced intestinal absorption of calcium because of the parathyroid hormone (PTH) excess and the ensuing stimulation of the renal synthesis of 1,25-(OH)$_2$D. These effects restore serum calcium concentration to normal. Unlike primary hyperparathyroidism,

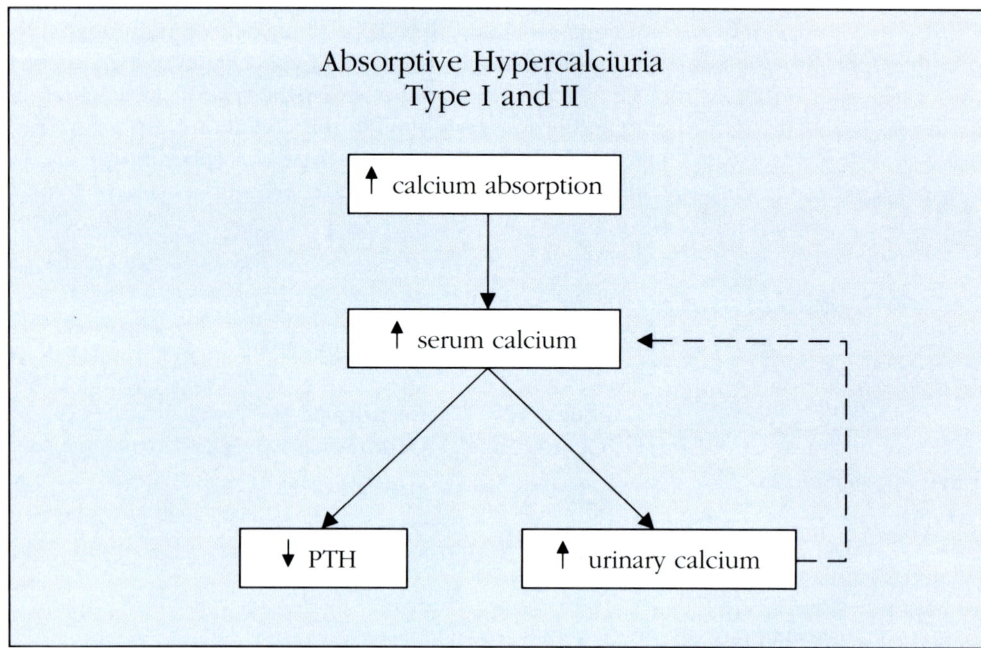

Figure 12.2 Absorptive hypercalciuria.

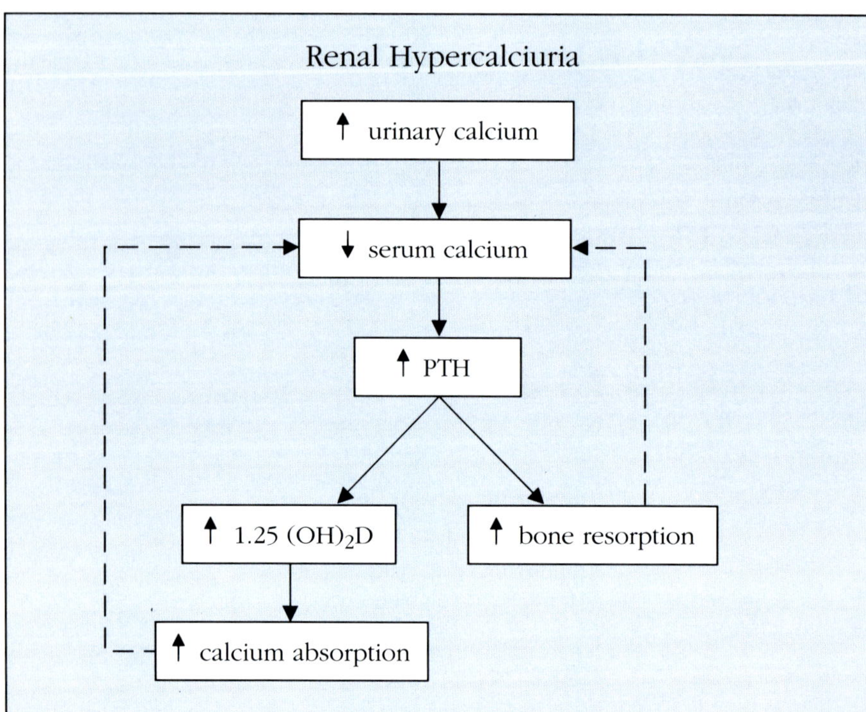

Figure 12.3 Renal hypercalciuria.

serum calcium is normal and the state of hyperparathyroidism is secondary.

Resorptive Hypercalciuria

Resorptive hypercalciuria is characterized by primary hyperparathyroidism. The initial event is the excessive resorption of bone resulting from hypersecretion of PTH (Fig. 12.4). Intestinal absorption of calcium is frequently elevated because of the PTH-dependent stimulation of the renal synthesis of 1,25-$(OH)_2D$. These effects increase the circulating concentration and the renal filtered load of calcium, often causing significant hypercalciuria.

Differential Diagnosis of Hypercalciuria

Different forms of hypercalciuria can be differentiated from their biochemical and physiologic pictures (Fig. 12.5). While the serum calcium is normal in absorptive hypercalciuria and renal hypercalciuria, patients with resorptive hypercalciuria have elevated circulating calcium levels. Serum PTH concentration is primarily elevated in resorptive hypercalciuria and secondarily elevated in renal hypercalciuria, whereas parathyroid activity is normal or suppressed in absorptive hypercalciuria. Fasting urinary calcium is normal in patients with absorptive hypercalciuria but is elevated in renal hypercalciuria and resorptive hypercalciuria. Finally, all three forms of hypercalciuria are accompanied by an intestinal hyperabsorption of calcium. However, this disturbance is a primary defect in patients with absorptive hypercalciuria and a secondary defect in renal hypercalciuria and resorptive hypercalciuria. Some patients may present with fasting hypercalciuria and normal serum PTH. While this presen-

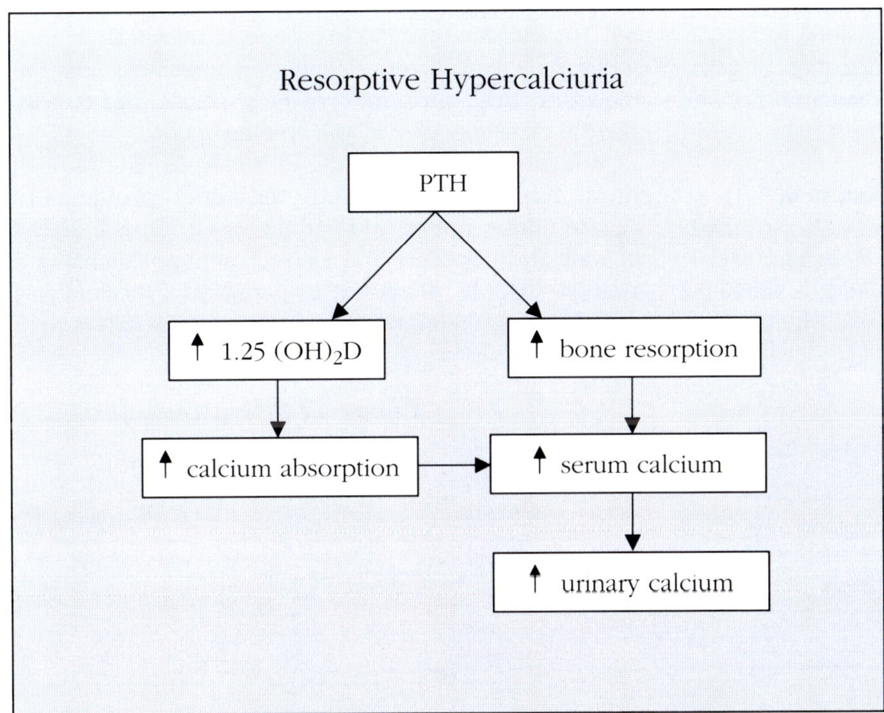

Figure 12.4 Resorptive hypercalciuria of primary hyperparathyroidism.

FIGURE 12.5 *Differential Diagnosis of Hypercalciuria*

	ABSORPTIVE	RENAL	RESORPTIVE
Serum calcium	Normal	Normal	Elevated
Parathyroid function	Suppressed	Stimulated (secondarily)	Stimulated (primarily)
Fasting urinary calcium	Normal	Elevated	Elevated
Intestinal calcium absorption	Elevated (primarily)	Elevated (secondarily)	Elevated (secondarily)

tation may be due to inadequate dietary preparation, it may represent an underlying renal phosphate leak, primary enhancement of 1,25-(OH)$_2$D production, combined renal tubular disturbances, or prostaglandin excess.

PATHOPHYSIOLOGY OF OTHER CAUSES OF CALCIUM STONES

Pathophysiology of Hyperuricosuria

Hyperuricosuria may be the only recognizable physiologic abnormality in patients with calcium nephrolithiasis (hyperuricosuric calcium oxalate nephrolithiasis). Hyperuricosuria may be due to "dietary overindulgence" of purine-rich foods or to uric acid over production (in approximately 30%).

It is believed that monosodium urate is formed in the supersaturated environment of hyperuricosuric subject (Fig. 12.6). The monosodium urate (colloidal or crystalline) may then initiate calcium oxalate stone formation by direct induction of heterogeneous nucleation of calcium oxalate or by adsorption of certain macromolecular inhibitors.

Pathophysiology of Hyperoxaluria

Urinary oxalate is derived from two major sources. Approximately 80% to 90% comes from endogenous production in the liver, whereas the remainder is obtained from dietary oxalate and/or ascorbic acid. Therefore, a primary defect of in vivo oxalate synthesis (primary hyperoxaluria), dietary overindulgence in oxalate-rich foods, or excessive vitamin C ingestion may each contribute to elevated urinary oxalate levels. While it can cause marked hyperoxaluria, primary hyperoxaluria is rare. The latter two lead to a modest rise in urinary oxalate.

The major cause of hyperoxaluria is ileal disease (enteric hyperoxaluria). A severe hyperoxaluria may result from increased intestinal absorption of oxalate. This disturbance may be encountered in patients with inflammatory bowel disease, small bowel resection, or jejunoileal bypass. Two factors probably act in concert to cause the intestinal hyperabsorption of oxalate (Fig. 12.7). Intestinal transport of oxalate may be primarily increased because of the action of bile salts and fatty acids on the permeability of intestinal mucosa to oxalate. The total amount of oxalate absorbed may also be increased because of an enlarged intraluminal pool of oxalate available for absorption. The intestinal fat malabsorption characteristic of ileal disease may exaggerate calcium-soap formation, limit the amount of "free" calcium to complex oxalate, and thereby raise the oxalate pool available for absorption.

Additional causes of stone formation in patients with enteric hyperoxaluria include the added problems of reduced urinary output due to fluid losses from the intestinal tract and hypocitraturia caused by hypokalemia and metabolic acidosis. Moreover, low urinary magnesium may result from impaired intestinal magnesium absorption.

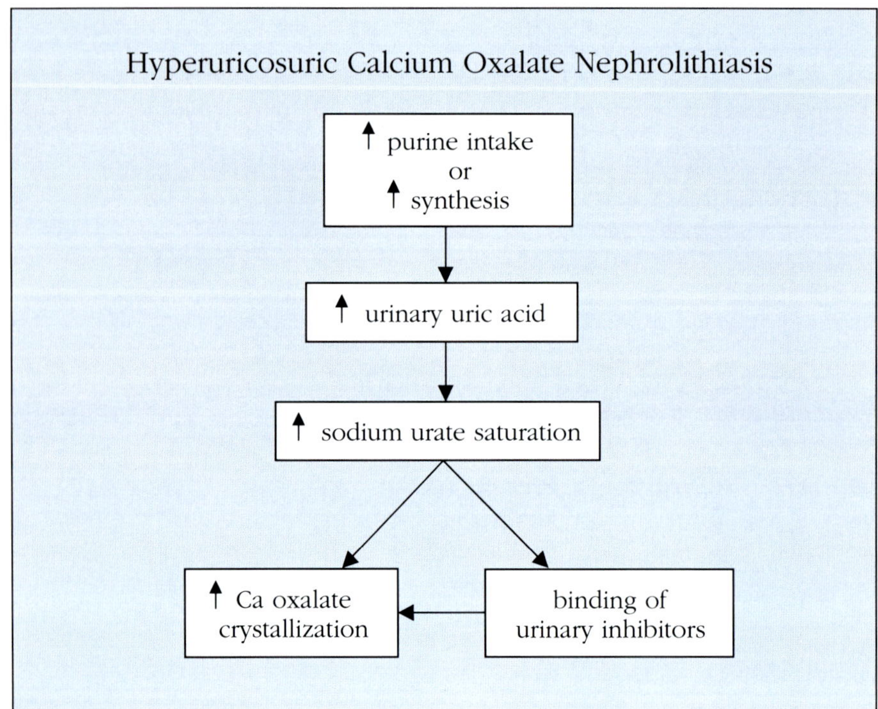

Figure 12.6 Hyperuricosuria.

Pathophysiology of Hypocitraturia

The association between urinary citrate and stone formation has long been recognized, but its major diagnositic and therapeutic implications have only recently been described. Among the factors that affect the renal handling of citrate, the acid-base status probably plays the most important role. Acidosis reduces urinary citrate both by enhancing renal tubular reabsorption and by reducing the synthesis of citrate. This mechanism accounts for the occurrence of hypocitraturia in renal tubular acidosis,

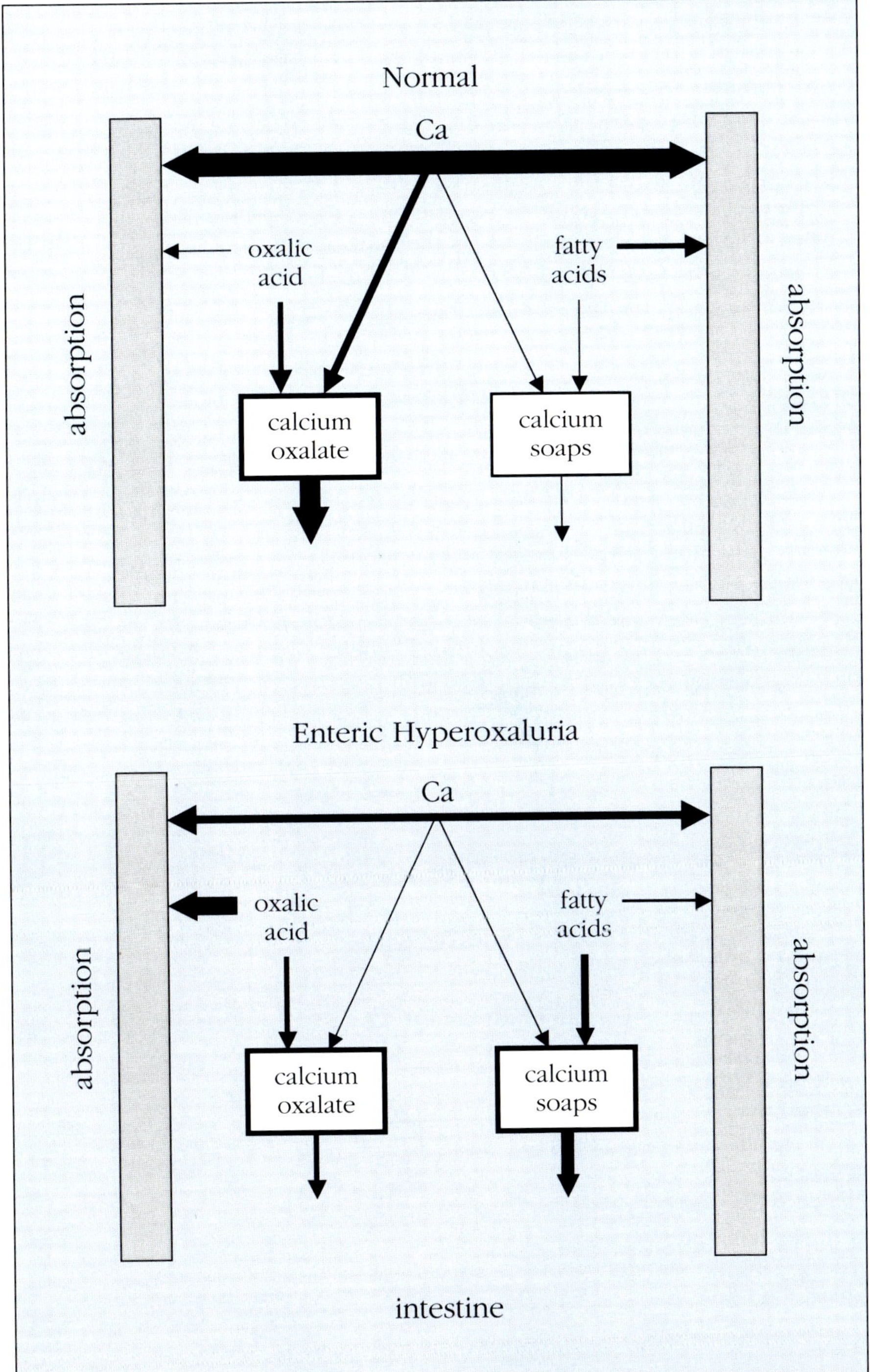

Figure 12.7 Enteric hyperoxaluria.

enteric hyperoxaluria, hypokalemia (from intracellular acidosis), and high-animal-protein diet (from elevated acid-ash content). Among patients with stones, hypocitraturia is found in all these conditions as well as with urinary tract infection (due to bacterial enzymatic action). Hypocitraturia occurs alone (10%) or with other abnormalities (50%).

Pathophysiology of Hypomagnesiuric Calcium Nephrolithiasis

Despite its infrequent occurrence, hypomagnesiuric calcium nephrolithiasis may represent a unique cause of stone formation. Besides hypomagnesiuria, this entity is characterized by hypocitraturia and low urine volume. Thus, calcium stone formation may result from the combined effects of these derangements. Although its exact pathogenetic background is not known, hypomagnesuria is probably dietary in origin.

Pathophysiology of Gouty Diathesis

Passage of acid urine (pH < 5.5) can cause both uric acid and calcium stones because the urinary pH is very close to or less than the dissociation constant of uric acid. The concentration of undissociated uric acid is high, leading to uric acid crystallization. The uric acid crystals may induce the crystallization of calcium oxalate by the same mechanism described previously for monosodium urate in patients with hyperuricosuria. In addition, uric acid has been shown to remove naturally occurring urinary macromolecular inhibitors, thereby attenuating their activity.

The term gouty diathesis has been used to describe the overall clinical entity of uric acid lithiasis. The persistent feature is the passage of unusually acid urine (pH < 5.5) in which uric acid is sparingly soluble. Some patients may present with gouty arthritis or hyperuricemia. Stone analysis will disclose uric acid alone or in combination with calcium oxalate/calcium phosphate. Some patients may display the above features except for the lack of uric acid on stone analysis. The stones may disclose only the presence of calcium oxalate and/or calcium phosphate. No specific cause has been detected for the unusually low urinary pH. Gouty diathesis may represent a phase of primary gout where the occurrence of hyperuricemia and gouty arthritis represents the full manifestation of the syndrome, whereas the picture of low urinary pH and uric acid/calcium nephrolithiasis without hyperuricemia or gouty arthritis reflects an early phase of classic gout.

PATHOPHYSIOLOGY OF NONCALCAREOUS STONES

Uric Acid Stones

Critical determinants for pure uric acid lithiasis are urinary pH less than the dissociation constant for uric acid (5.47) and/or hyperuricosuria. Uric acid stones are often formed in primary gout, which may be accompanied by low urinary pH and hyperuricosuria, but may also be found in secondary causes of purine overproduction, such as myeloproliferative states, glycogen storage disease, and malignancy (Fig. 12.8). Chronic diarrheal syndromes (ulcerative colitis, regional enteritis, jejunoileal

FIGURE 12.8 *Causes of Increased Urinary Uric Acid*

Abnormal production
  Genetic overproduction
    Enzymatic mutation (i.e., hypoxanthine-
      guanine phosphoribosyl-transferase
      [HGPRT] deficiency)
  Acquired overproduction
    Myeloproliferative disorders
    Obesity
    Alcohol ingestion
Abnormal excretion
  Diet high in purines
  Uricosuric drugs

bypass surgery) may cause uric acid lithiasis by inducing net alkali deficit and lowering urine volume (thereby reducing urinary pH and augmenting urinary concentration of uric acid respectively).

Cystine Stones

Cystinuria is an inborn error of metabolism characterized by a disturbance in renal and intestinal handling of dicarboxylic acids, including cystine. Stone formation, occurring in a minority of patients, is the result of an excessive renal excretion of cystine and its low solubility in urine. Cystine solubility is pH-dependent, with lowest solubility at low range of urinary pH, gradual increase in solubility with a rise in pH to 7.5, and rapid increase in solubility above a pH of 7.5.

The main determinant of cystine crystallization is urinary supersaturation. If the urine sample is supersaturated with respect to cystine, precipitation of cystine invariably occurs. Once the urinary saturation of cystine exceeds 250 mg/L, cystine will precipitate out of solution. If one can maintain the cystine concentration under 200 mg/L, cystine stones should not occur.

Infection (Struvite) Stones

Infection of the urinary tract with urea-splitting organisms may be associated with renal stones of struvite and of calcium carbonate-apatite. The critical determinant is the formation of ammonia in urine due to enzymatic degradation of urea by bacterial urease. The ammonia undergoes hydrolysis to form ammonium and hydroxyl ions. The resulting alkalinity of the urine augments dissociation of phosphate to form triphosphate ions and reduces the solubility of struvite. Thus, the urinary environment becomes supersaturated with respect to struvite. Although struvite stones may form de novo from infection alone, they also occur as a complication of other causes of renal calculi such as hypercalciuria.

It is most important to note that patients with infection stones have the same percentage of underlying metabolic derangements (i.e., hypercalciuria, hypocitraturia) as does the general stone-forming population. Therefore, these patients should be metabolically evaluated and prophylactic treatment offered.

Diagnosis of Nephrolithiasis

The evaluation of nephrolithiasis should identify as efficiently and economically as possible the particular physiologic defect present in a given patient with nephrolithiasis to enable selective, rational therapy of stone disease.

Such an evaluation should be able to identify specific metabolic disorders responsible for recurrent stone disease, including distal renal tubular acidosis, primary hyperparathyroidism, enteric hyperoxaluria, cystinuria, and gouty diathesis. In many of these relatively uncommon conditions, it is generally agreed that selective medical therapy is indicated not only to prevent further stone formation, but also to correct the underlying physiologic disturbance that may lead to nonrenal complications.

SELECTION OF PATIENTS FOR METABOLIC EVALUATION

There has been much debate concerning the selection of patients as to who should undergo a diagnostic evaluation. Although studies have shown that "single-stone formers" have the same incidence and severity of metabolic derangements as patients with recurrent stone disease, some patients do not form recurrent stones despite the absence of treatment. In addition, a study of single-stone formers placed on a conservative program of high fluid intake and avoidance of dietary excess revealed a low incidence of recurrent stone disease.

However, as mentioned previously, recurrent stone formation within eight years has been reported in upwards of 63% of adult males with the single stone episode. Moreover, in some patients, the initial stone episode may be a harbinger of an underlying multisystem disease such as renal tubular acidosis or renal hypercalciuria with secondary hyperparathyroidism. In such patients, diagnostic evaluation is justified solely to apply specific medical therapy in order to prevent extrarenal complications.

A final consideration is the relatively low cost of a comprehensive medical evaluation when compared to the expense of stone removal or the care of complications secondary to stone disease. Thus, a diagnostic evaluation would be cost-effective since it allows for the selection of effective prophylactic therapy for nephrolithiasis.

EVALUATION OF SINGLE-STONE FORMERS

The decision to thoroughly investigate a first-time stone former should ideally be shared by the physician and the patient. While some first-time stone formers will readily accept and follow conservative therapy, others may elect to undergo a thorough evaluation. To determine how extensive an evaluation should be, the potential or risk for new stone formation should be estimated. Patients at high risk might be middle-aged, white males with a family history of stones and those with intestinal disease (chronic diarrheal states), pathologic skeletal fractures, osteoporosis, urinary tract infection, or gout. In these patients, an extensive evaluation is recommended. Any patients with stones composed of cystine, uric acid, or struvite should undergo a complete metabolic work-up. In addition, all children should be required to undergo a complete investigation. Because stone disease is uncommon in blacks, especially in black women, one should determine the underlying etiology of nephrolithiasis in all black patients.

ABBREVIATED PROTOCOL FOR
LOW-RISK SINGLE-STONE FORMERS

In single-stone formers without increased risk, the following abbreviated protocol may be applied (Fig. 12.9). A thorough medical history should be obtained for any underlying conditions that may have contributed to the stone disease. In addition, information should be gleaned concerning the patient's dietary habits, including fluid consumption and excessive intake of certain foods, as well as a list of all medications taken. A multichannel blood screen can be helpful in identifying certain systemic problems. These include primary hyperparathyroidism (high serum calcium and low serum phosphorus), renal phosphate leak (hypophosphatemia), uric acid lithiasis (hyperuricemia), and distal renal tubular acidosis (abnormalities in serum electrolytes).

Voided urine specimens should be obtained for comprehensive urinalysis and culture. The urinalysis should include pH determination (with an electrode) since a pH greater than 7.5 is compatible with possible infection lithiasis, while a pH less than 5.5 may suggest uric acid lithiasis. The urine sediment is also examined for crystalluria since particular crystal types may give a clue to the composition of stones the patient is forming (Fig. 12.10). Urine cultures positive for urea-splitting organisms such as *Proteus, Pseudomonas,* and *Klebsiella* are suggestive of infection lithiasis. In addition, urine should be examined for the presence of cystine using a qualitative examination (nitroprusside test).

Abdominal x-rays should be obtained to document the existence of any residual stones within the urinary tract. The radiopacity of any existing stones may suggest the type of stones that are present. While magnesium ammonium phosphate and cystine stones are often radiopaque, they are not as dense as calcium oxalate or calcium phosphate stones. A plain abdominal film is also useful in identifying nephrocalcinosis (suggestive of renal tubular acidosis) and staghorn calculi (likely due to infection lithiasis). An intravenous pyelogram may be obtained to confirm the presence of radiolucent stones and also identify any anatomic abnormalities that may be responsible for stone formation.

Finally, available stones should be analyzed to determine their crystalline composition. The presence of uric acid or cystine crystals would suggest the presence of gouty diathesis or cystinuria, respectively. The finding of struvite, carbonate apatite, and magnesium ammonium phosphate would suggest infection lithiasis. A predominance of hydroxyapatite crystals suggests the presence of renal tubular acidosis or primary hyperparathyroidism. Stones composed of pure calcium oxalate or mixed calcium oxalate and hydroxyapatite are less useful diagnostically since they may occur in several entities including absorptive and renal hypercalciuria, hyperuricosuric calcium nephrolithiasis, enteric hyperoxaluria, hypocitraturic calcium nephrolithiasis, and low urine volume.

EXTENSIVE DIAGNOSIS

A more extensive evaluation, directed at the identification of underlying physiologic derangements, should be performed in patients with recurrent nephrolithiasis as well as in stone-formers at increased risk for further stone formation.

One current version of the ambulatory evaluation involves two outpatient visits, which can be completed in less than 3 weeks. Most of the required laboratory analy-

FIGURE 12.9 *Abbreviated Evaluation of Single-Stone Formers Without Risk*

HISTORY
Underlying predisposing conditions
Medications (Ca, Vit C, Vit D, acetazolamide, steroids)
Dietary excesses, inadequate fluid intake or excessive
    fluid loss

MULTICHANNEL BLOOD SCREEN
High calcium: primary hyperparathyroidism
High uric acid: gouty diathesis
Low K and CO_2, high Cl: distal renal tubular acidosis

URINE
Urinalysis
pH > 7.5: infection lithiasis
pH < 5.5: uric acid lithiasis
Sediment for crystalluria

Urine culture
Urea-splitting organisms: suggestive of infection lithiasis
Qualitative cystine

X-RAY
Radiopaque stones: calcium oxalate, calcium phosphate, magnesium ammonium phosphate (struvite), cystine.
Radiolucent stones: uric acid, xanthine, 2-hydroxyadenine, triamterene
IVP: radiolucent stones, anatomic abnormalities

STONE ANALYSIS

ses can be performed in a routine clinical laboratory with only a few of the specialized techniques being performed in a more sophisticated laboratory. The schedule of laboratory tests is outlined in Figure 12.11.

Prior to and throughout the period of evaluation, the patient is instructed to discontinue any medication known to interfere with the metabolism of calcium, uric acid, or oxalate. These medications include vitamin D, calcium supplements, antacids, acetazolamide, and vitamin C. Current medication for stone treatment (thiazide, phosphate, allopurinol, or magnesium) should be discontinued as well. Three 24-hour urine samples are collected. Two are obtained with the patient on a random diet, which is reflective of their usual dietary intake. The third 24-hour sample is collected after a week of calcium, sodium, and oxalate restricted diet. This dietary restriction is imposed to standardize the diagnostic tests, to assess better the etiology of hypercalciuria and to prepare for the "fast and calcium load" test, which is performed on the second visit. Blood samples are obtained on both visits.

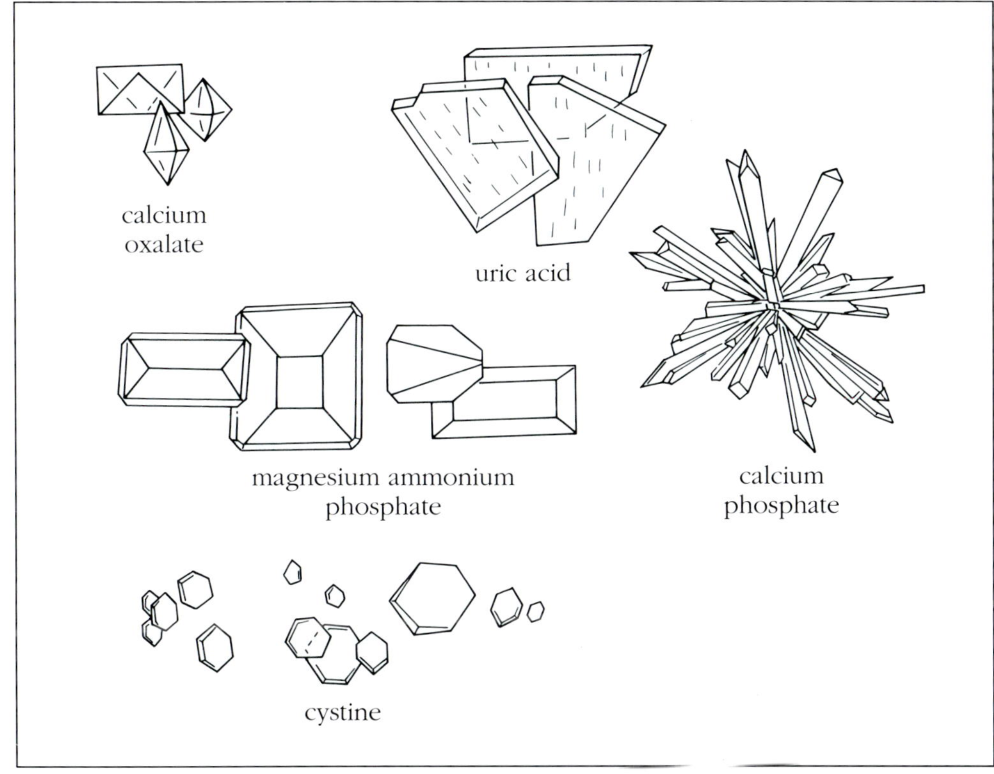

Figure 12.10 The chemical composition of renal calculi.

FIGURE 12.11 *Outline of Extensive Ambulatory Protocol*

	BLOOD			URINE								
	Complete Blood Count	SMA	PTH	Calcium	Uric Acid	Creatinine	Sodium	pH	Total Volume	Oxalate	Citrate	Qualitative Cystine
Visit 1*	X	X		X	X	X	X	X	X	X	X	X
Visit 2†		X	X	X	X	X	X	X	X	X	X	
Fast				X		X			X			
Load				X		X			X			

*History and physical examination, diet history, radiologic evaluation, two 24-hour urine samples on random diet, dietary instruction for restricted diet.

†24-hour urine sample on restricted diet (400 mg calcium and 100 mEq sodium per day), fast, load test.

Fast and Calcium Load Test

A "fast and calcium load" study is performed on the morning of the second visit. It is essential that the patient have adhered to the restricted diet for at least 7 days prior to this testing to eliminate the effects of absorbed calcium on fasting calcium excretion. To ensure adequate hydration, distilled water (300 mL each) is to be taken 12 hours and 9 hours prior to the calcium loading. Other than water ingestion at these time periods, the patients are to be fasting. Two hours prior to the scheduled calcium loading, patients empty their bladder completely, discard the urine, and drink an additional 600 mL of distilled water. Urine is to be collected as a pooled sample for the 2 hours prior to taking the calcium load (fasting urine). After the 2-hour fasting urine collection has been completed, a 1 g oral calcium load is administered using 250 mL of a liquid synthetic diet (Calcitest) as a carrier solution. This is prepared by first adding 500 mL of water to a can of Calcitest. Only 250 mL of the synthetic meal is used for each calcium load. Since 250 mL of the synthetic meal contains only 100 mg of calcium, 39 mL of Neocalglucon (900 mg of calcium) must be added to bring the total calcium up to 1 g. The final mixture should be taken slowly over a 5 to 10 minute period.

For the next 4 hours, urine is again collected as a pooled sample (postload urine). Both fasting and post-load samples are then assayed for calcium and creatinine. Fasting urinary calcium is expressed as milligrams per deciliter glomerular filtrate (GF) since this is reflective of renal function. To obtain this unit of measurement, the urinary calcium in milligrams per milligram of creatinine is multiplied by the serum creatinine in mg/dL. Normal fasting urinary calcium is <0.11 mg/dL GF. The postload urinary calcium is best expressed as milligrams per milligram of creatinine as it is a function of a fixed oral calcium load. The normal value for this measurement is <0.20 mg of calcium/mg creatinine.

CLASSIFICATION OF NEPHROLITHIASIS AND DIAGNOSTIC CRITERIA

Using this ambulatory protocol, the etiology of nephrolithiasis can be classified into thirteen categories reflecting specific physiologic derangements. In less than 3% of patients, no abnormality can be detected. These categories are listed in Figure 12.1 along with their relative frequency. The diagnostic criteria for the twelve principal presentations are compared in Figure 12.12.

SIMPLIFIED METABOLIC EVALUATION

The previously described extensive ambulatory protocol affords the physician a high diagnostic yield and is quite reliable. Unfortunately, some practicing physicians have

FIGURE 12.12 *Diagnostic Criteria*

	SERUM			URINARY							
	Ca	P	PTH	Ca fasting	Ca load	Ca restricted	UA	Ox	Cit	pH	Mg
Absorptive hypercalciuria type I	N	N	N	N	↑	↑	N	N	N	N	N
Absorptive hypercalciuria type II	N	N	N	N	↑	N	N	N	N	N	N
Renal hypercalciuria	N	N	↑	↑	↑	↑	N	N	N	N	N
Primary hyperpara-thyroidism	↑	↓	↑	↑	↑	↑	N	N	N	N	N
Unclassified hypercalciuria	N	N/−	N	↑	↑	↑	N	N	N	N	N
Hyperuricosuria	N	N	N	N	N	N	↑	N	N	N	N
Enteric hyperoxaluria	N/↑	N/↓	N/↓	↓	↓	↓	↓	↑	↓	N	N
Hypocitraturia	N	N	N	N	N	N	N	N	↓	N	N
Renal tubular acidosis	N	N	N/↑	↑	N	N/↑	N	N	↓	N/↑	N
Hypomagnesiuria	N	N	N	N	N	N	N/↓	N	↓	N	↓
Gouty diathesis	N	N	N	N	N	N	N/↑	N	N/↓	↓	N
Infection lithiasis	N	N	N	N	N	N	N	N	↓	↑	N

Fasting samples represent 2-hour collections obtained in morning following an overnight fast. Ca load samples were obtained over a 4-hour period subsequent to oral ingestion of 1 g Ca. PTH = immunoreactive parathyroid hormone; ↑ = high; ↓ = low; N = normal; UA = uric acid; Ox = oxalate; Cit = citrate; Mg = magnesium found this protocol to be time-consuming and difficult to perform due to the inability to obtain certain laboratory tests. A simplified diagnostic protocol may be performed that uses the same standard principles and procedures as a standard outpatient evaluation yet incorporates commercially available diagnostic tests, thus making it available to all physicians for evaluation of patients with recurrent stones or those with single stones at increased risk.

The cornerstone of this simplified protocol has been the development of a urine preservation method that allows collection of urine without refrigeration and submission of an aliquot to a central laboratory for the analysis of various stone-forming substances. The urinary constituents assayed include calcium, oxalate, and citrate (which may result from underlying metabolic problems) as well as total volume, sodium, and sulfate (which are influenced by environmental or dietary factors) (Fig. 12.13). From such determinations the urinary saturation with respect to stone-forming salts can be calculated. A graphic display of this information may then be generated, highlighting the increased or reduced risk for each environmental, metabolic, or physicochemical factor.

After the values of all urinary constituents and saturations have been determined, the physician receives a computerized printout that provides both a graphic and a numeric display of the test results. These results should aid the physician in formulating a metabolic/physiologic diagnosis. However, it is usually not possible to make a definitive diagnosis of a particular metabolic derangement without further testing. For example, it is desirable to confirm the presence of hypocitraturia or hyperuricosuria

by repeat measurements. In addition, while this graphic analysis will demonstrate hypercalciuria, it is not able to differentiate between the different forms of hypercalciuria. Finally, it is important to note that the "normal limits" cited on commercially available urine analysis packages, such as the StoneRisk Patient Profile, are not the same as those normal values that have been quoted previously where 24-hour urinary calcium of greater than 200 mg/d are considered abnormal. However, on the StoneRisk Patient Profile, the urinary calcium excretion is not considered abnormal until it is greater than 250 mg/d. Therefore, one should pay close attention to those patients who may fall in the "gray zone" when using a commercially available urine analysis package.

SIMPLIFIED AUTOMATED STONE RISK ANALYSIS

For repeat analysis of key urinary determinants (e.g., calcium), a simplified version of the automated stone risk analysis (StoneTrack) is available. Available tests are for calcium, uric acid, pH, citrate, oxalate, sodium, and total volume. These limited tests are also useful in assessing response to medical therapy.

Timing of the Metabolic Evaluation

As noted previously, while the innovative techniques of percutaneous nephrostolithotomy, ureteroscopy, and ESWL offer the stone patient an attractive alternative to conventional open surgery, they have no effect on the underlying metabolic or physiologic derangements that affect stone formation. Therefore, a thorough metabolic

---

FIGURE 12.13 *Summary of Risk Factors Identified by Automated Stone Risk Profile*

METABOLIC FACTORS
Calcium
Oxalate
Uric acid
Citrate
pH

PHYSICOCHEMICAL FACTORS
Calcium oxalate
Brushite
Sodium urate
Struvite
Uric acid

ENVIRONMENTAL FACTORS
Total volume
Sodium
Sulfate
Phosphorus
Magnesium

OTHER FACTORS
Creatinine
Potassium
Ammonium

evaluation accompanied by appropriately applied medical management should favorably affect the course of stone disease and significantly reduce the need for a repeat surgical procedure. The question remains, however, as to the timing of the metabolic evaluation in relation to the surgical procedure.

The exact time to schedule a diagnostic evaluation is dependent on several factors, including evidence of obstruction, infection, renal colic, and urgency for stone removal. It has been suggested that excretion of various stone-forming substances may be impaired in the presence of urinary tract obstruction by a renal or ureteral calculus. In addition, while no definitive studies exist, one might expect similar alterations of urinary function to exist after various techniques of stone removal. Open surgical procedures, endourologic stone removal, and ESWL all exert specific types of trauma on the renal parenchyma. One might therefore expect transient alterations in renal function after such procedures. In addition, stones associated with infection may also alter various transport properties of the nephron. The presence of infection may thus give misleading results during a diagnostic evaluation.

It seems advisable therefore to postpone a complete diagnostic evaluation for at least 1 month after resolution of ureteral obstruction or infection or after undergoing a stone removal procedure. This should allow recovery of normal renal function as well as reinstitution of the patient's regular dietary habits.

Along the same lines, a patient who is experiencing severe colic or recovering from a surgical procedure would not be expected to be following usual daily routine, including dietary habits and fluid intake. Therefore, a metabolic evaluation performed during an acute stone episode or with the patient still in the hospital may give misleading results (especially in relation to environmental risk factors) and not allow a proper diagnostic evaluation. On the other hand, a patient with existing stones scheduled for elective stone removal, yet able to enjoy his or her normal lifestyle, may have a simplified metabolic evaluation performed prior to undergoing stone removal.

References

GENERAL

Ljunghall S. Incidence of upper urinary tract stones. *Miner Electrolyte Metab.* 1987;13:220–227.

Pak CYC. Medical management of nephrolithiasis. *J Urol.* 1982;128:1157.

Preminger GM, Peterson R, Peters PC, Pak CY. The current role of medical treatment of nephrolithiasis: the impact of improved techniques of stone removal. *J Urol.* 1985;134:6–10.

Sarmina I, Spirnak JP, Resnick MI. Urinary lithiasis in the black population: an epidemiological study and review of the literature. *J Urol.* 1987;138:14–17.

METABOLIC EVALUATION

Hosking DH, Erickson SB, Van Den Berg CJ, et al. The stone clinic effect in patients with idiopathic calcium urolithiasis. *J Urol.* 1983;130:115–118.

Pak CYC. Should patients with single renal stone occurrence undergo diagnostic evaluation? *J Urol.* 1982;127:854–858.

Pak CY, Britton F, Peterson R, et al. Ambulatory evaluation of nephrolithiasis: classification, clinical presentation and diagnostic criteria. *Am J Med.* 1980;69:19–30.

Pak CY, Peters P, Hurt G, et al. Is selective therapy of recurrent nephrolithiasis possible? *Am J Med.* 1981;71:615–622.

Preminger GM, Pak CYC. The practical evaluation and selective medical management of nephrolithiasis. *Semin Urol.* 1985;3:170.

PATHOPHYSIOLOGY

Coe FL. Hyperuricosuric calcium oxalate nephrolithiasis. *Kidney Int.* 1978;13:418.

Coe FL, Kavalach AG. Hypercalciuria and hyperuricosuria in patients with calcium nephrolithiasis. *N Engl J Med.* 1974;291:1344–1350.

Ettinger B, Okdroyd NO, Sorgel F. Triamterene nephrolithiasis. *JAMA.* 1980;244:2443.

Nicar MJ, Skurla C, Sakhaee K, et al. Low urinary citrate excretion in nephrolithiasis. *Urology.* 1983;21:8.

Pak CYC. Physiological basis for absorptive and renal hypercalciurias. *Am J Physiol.* 1979;237:F415–F423.

Pak CYC, Ohata M, Lawrence EC, et al. The hypercalciurias: causes, parathyroid functions and diagnostic criteria. *J Clin Invest.* 1974;54:387.

Preminger GM, Baker S, Peterson R, Poindexter J, Pak CYC. Hypomagnesiuric hypocitraturia: an apparent new entity for calcium nephrolithiasis. *J Lithotripsy Stone Dis.* 1989;1:22.

Preminger GM, Pak CYC. Eventual attenuation of hypocalciuric response to hydrochlorothiazide in absorptive hypercalciuria. *J Urol.* 1987;137:1104.

Medical Management of Calculus Disease

Glenn M. Preminger

Conservative Medical Therapy

Certain conservative recommendations should be made for all patients regardless of the underlying etiology of their stone disease. These measures include increased fluids in order to maintain a urine output greater than 2000 mL/d. In addition, all patients should be placed on a diet limited in oxalate and sodium. In patients with suspected absorptive hypercalciuria, a dietary limitation of dairy products may also be enforced. A restriction of animal proteins in those with "purine gluttony" and hyperuricosuria should also be encouraged.

It is anticipated that with these conservative measures alone, a significant number of patients may be able to normalize their urinary risk factors for stone formation. Thus, only these conservative measures may be necessary to keep their stone disease under control. After 3 to 4 months on conservative management, patients should be re-evaluated using either standard laboratory assays or a less comprehensive automated urinalysis package (StoneTrack). If the patient's metabolic or environmental abnormalities have been corrected, the conservative treatment measures should be continued and the patient followed every 6 months with repeat 24-hour urine testing. It is believed that follow-up is essential not only to monitor the efficiency of treatment but also to encourage patient compliance. If, however, a metabolic defect persists, a more selective medical therapy may be instituted. For example, if significant hyperuricosuria (urinary uric acid greater than 800 mg/d) persists even after dietary restriction of meat products, medical therapy with allopurinol may be instituted.

Selective Medical Therapy of Nephrolithiasis

Improved elucidation of pathophysiology and formulation of diagnostic criteria for different causes of nephrolithiasis have made feasible the adoption of selective treatment programs. Such programs should 1) reverse the underlying physicochemical and physiologic derangements, 2) inhibit new stone formation, 3) overcome nonrenal complications of the disease process, and 4) be free of serious side effects. The rationale for the selection of certain treatment programs is the assumption that the particular physicochemical and physiologic aberrations identified with the given disorder are etiologically important in the formation of renal stones (as previously discussed), and that the correction of these disturbances would prevent stone formation. Moreover, it is assumed that such a selected treatment program would be more effective and safe than a "random" treatment. Despite a lack of conclusive experimental verification, these hypotheses appear reasonable and logical.

For many pharmacologic treatment programs recommended for nephrolithiasis, sufficient information is now available to characterize their physicochemical and physiologic actions (Fig. 13.1).

ABSORPTIVE HYPERCALCIURIA
Sodium Cellulose Phosphate

There is currently no treatment program capable of correcting the basic abnormality of absorptive hypercalciuria type I, although several drugs available have been shown to restore normal calcium excretion. When sodium cellulose phosphate is given orally, this nonabsorbable ion exchange resin binds calcium and inhibits calcium absorption. However, this inhibition is caused by limiting the amount of intraluminal calcium available for absorption, and not by correcting the basic disturbance in calcium transport.

The above mode of action accounts for the three potential complications of sodium cellulose phosphate therapy. First, it may cause a negative calcium balance and parathyroid stimulation when used in patients with normal intestinal calcium absorption or with renal or resorptive hypercalciuria. Second, the treatment may cause magnesium depletion by binding magnesium as well. Third, sodium cellulose phosphate may produce secondary hyperoxaluria, by binding divalent cations in the intestinal tract, reducing divalent cation-oxalate complexation, and making more oxalate available for absorption. These complications may be overcome by using the drug only in documented cases of absorptive hypercalciuria type I, applying oral magnesium supplementation (1.0 to 1.5 g magnesium gluconate twice a day, separately from sodium cellulose phosphate), and by imposing a moderate dietary restriction of oxalate.

When above precautions are followed, sodium cellulose phosphate at a dosage of 10 to 15 g/d (given with meals), has been shown to reduce urinary calcium and the saturation of calcium salts (calcium phosphate as well as calcium oxalate), to maintain stable bone density, and to be clinically effective.

Thiazide

Thiazide is not considered a selective therapy for absorptive hypercalciuria, since it does not decrease intestinal calcium absorption in this condition. However, this drug has been widely used to treat absorptive hypercalciuria because of its hypocalciuric action and the high cost and inconvenience of alternative therapy (sodium cellulose phosphate).

Current studies indicate that thiazide may have a limited long-term effectiveness in absorptive hypercalciuria type I. Despite an initial reduction in urinary excretion, the intestinal calcium absorption remains persistently elevated. These studies suggest that the retained calcium may be accreted in bone at least during the first few years of therapy. Bone density, determined in the distal third of the radius by photon absorptiometry, increases significantly during thiazide treatment in absorptive hypercalciuria, with an annual increment of 1.34%. With continued treatment, however, the rise in bone density stabilizes and the hypocalciuric effect of thiazide becomes attenuated. The results suggest that thiazide treatment has caused a low turnover state of bone which interferes with continued calcium accretion in the skeleton. The "rejected" calcium would then be excreted in urine. In contrast, bone density is not significantly altered in renal hypercalciuria, where thiazide has been shown to cause a decline in intestinal calcium absorption commensurate with the reduction in urinary calcium.

Guidelines for the Use of Sodium Cellulose Phosphate or Thiazide in AHI

Neither sodium cellulose phosphate nor thiazide corrects the basic underlying physiologic defect in absorptive hypercalciuria. Some guidelines are offered here until more selective therapy can be developed.

Sodium cellulose phosphate should be used in patients with severe absorptive hypercalciuria type I (urinary calcium greater than 350 mg/d) or those resistant to or intolerant of thiazide therapy. In patients with absorptive hypercalciuria type I who may be at risk for bone disease (growing children, postmenopausal women), thiazide may be the first choice. When thiazide loses its hypocalciuric action (after long-term treatment), sodium cellulose phosphate may be temporarily substituted for approximately 6 months and then thiazide therapy may be resumed.

Potassium supplementation should be employed when using thiazide therapy in order to prevent hypokalemia and a decrease in urinary citrate excretion. A typical treatment program might include trichlormethiazide (Naqua) 4 mg/d with potassium citrate 15 to 20 mEq twice a day. Amiloride in combination with thiazide (Moduretic) may be more effective than thiazide alone in reducing calcium excretion. However, it does not augment citrate excretion. Since amiloride is a potassium-sparing agent, its combined use with potassium citrate should be employed with caution.

In absorptive hypercalciuria type II, no specific drug treatment may be necessary, since the physiologic defect is not as severe as in absorptive hypercalciuria type I. In addition, many patients show disdain for drinking fluids and excreting concentrated urine. A low calcium intake (400 to 600 mg/d) and high fluid intake (sufficient to achieve a minimum urine output of greater than 2 L/d) would seem ideally indicated, since normocalciuria could be restored by dietary calcium restriction alone, and increased urine volume has been shown to reduce urinary saturation of calcium oxalate.

Orthophosphate

Orthophosphate (neutral or alkaline salt of sodium and/or potassium, 0.5 gm phosphorus three to four times per day) has been shown to inhibit 1,25-$(OH)_2$ vitamin D (1,25-$(OH)_2D$) synthesis and reduce urinary calcium excretion. Moreover, there is some preliminary evidence that this treatment restores normal intestinal calcium absorption. Orthophosphate reduces urinary calcium probably by directly impairing the renal tubular reabsorption of calcium and by binding calcium in the intestinal tract. Urinary phosphorus is markedly increased during therapy, a finding reflecting the absorbability of soluble phosphate. Physicochemically, orthophosphate reduces the urinary saturation of calcium oxalate but increases that of brushite. Moreover, the urinary inhibitor activity is increased, probably due to the stimulated renal excretion of pyrophosphate and citrate. Although contrary reports have appeared, this treatment program has been reported to cause soft tissue calcification and parathyroid stimulation.

FIGURE 13.1 *Physicochemical and Physiologic Effects of Pharmacologic Therapy*

	SODIUM CELLULOSE PHOSPHATE	ORTHO-PHOSPHATE	THIAZIDE	ALLO-PURINOL	POTASSIUM CITRATE
Urinary calcium	Marked decrease	Mild decrease	Moderate decrease	No change	Mild decrease/ no change
Urinary phosphorus	Mild increase	Marked	Mild increase/ increase	No change	No change
Urinary uric acid	No change	No change	Mild increase/ no change	Marked decrease	No change
Urinary oxalate	Mild increase	Mild increase/ no change	Mild increase/ mild decrease	No change	No change
Urinary citrate	No change	Mild increase	Mild decrease	No change	Marked increase
Calcium oxalate saturation	Mild decrease/ no change	Mild decrease	Mild decrease	Moderate decrease	No change
Brushite saturation	Moderate decrease	Mild increase	Mild decrease	No change	No change

Recently, a slow-release neutral potassium phosphate salt has been developed that signifcantly limits the gastrointestinal upset seen with earlier phosphate preparations. Orthophosphate is contraindicated in nephrolithiasis complicated by urinary tract infection.

RENAL HYPERCALCIURIA

Thiazide is ideally indicated for the treatment of renal hypercalciuria. This diuretic has been shown to correct the renal leak of calcium by augmenting calcium reabsorption in the distal tubule and by causing extracellular volume depletion and stimulating proximal tubular reabsorption of calcium. The ensuing correction of secondary hyperparathyroidism restores normal serum 1,25-(OH)$_2$D and intestinal calcium absorption. Thiazide has been shown to provide a sustained correction of hypercalciuria commensurate with a restoration of normal serum 1,25-(OH)$_2$D and intestinal calcium absorption for up to 10 years of therapy.

Physicochemically, the urinary environment becomes less saturated with respect to calcium oxalate and brushite during thiazide treatment, largely because of the reduced calcium excretion. Moreover, urinary inhibitor activity, as reflected in the limit of metastability, is increased by an unknown mechanism. These effects are shared by hydrochlorothiazide 50 mg twice a day, chlorthalidone 50 mg/d, and trichlormethiazide 4 mg/d. Potassium citrate supplementation (40 to 60 mEq/d) is advised, since it has been shown to be effective in averting hypokalemia and in increasing urinary citrate when administered to patients with calcium nephrolithiasis taking thiazide. Concurrent use of triamterene, a potassium-sparing agent, should be undertaken with caution because of recent reports of triamterene stone formation. However, amiloride may be used with thiazide since it alone has sometimes been shown to exert a hypocalciuric action, exaggerate the hypocalciuric action of thiazide, and prevent hypokalemia. Thiazide is contraindicated in primary hyperparathyroidism because of potential aggravation of hypercalcemia.

PRIMARY HYPERPARATHYROIDISM

Parathyroidectomy is the optimum treatment for nephrolithiasis of primary hyperparathyroidism. Following removal of abnormal parathyroid tissue, urinary calcium is restored to normal commensurate with a decline in serum concentration of calcium and intestinal absorption. The urinary environment becomes less saturated with respect to calcium oxalate and brushite and the limit of metastability for these calcium salts increases.

There is no established medical treatment for the nephrolithiasis of primary hyperparathyroidism. Although orthophosphates have been recommended for disease of mild to moderate severity, their safety and efficacy have not yet been proven. They should be used only when parathyroid surgery cannot be undertaken. Estrogen has been reported to be useful in reducing serum and urinary calcium in postmenopausal women with primary hyperparathyroidism.

HYPERURICOSURIC CALCIUM OXALATE NEPHROLITHIASIS

Allopurinol (300 mg/d) is the physiologically meaningful drug of choice in hyperuricosuric calcium oxalate nephrolithiasis resulting from uric acid overproduction because of its ability to reduce uric acid synthesis and lower urinary uric acid. Its use in hyperuricosuria associated with dietary purine overindulgence is also reasonable since dietary purine restriction is often impractical. Physicochemical changes ensuing from restoration of normal urinary uric acid include an increase in the urinary limit of metastability of calcium oxalate. Thus, the spontaneous nucleation of calcium oxalate is retarded by treatment, probably via inhibition of monosodium urate-induced stimulation of calcium oxalate crystallization. Because of the potential exaggeration of monosodium urate-induced calcium oxalate crystallization, a moderate sodium restriction (150 mEq/d) is also advisable.

Potassium citrate represents an alternative to allopurinol in the treatment of this condition. Treatment with potassium citrate (30 to 60 mEq/d in divided doses) may reduce the urinary saturation of calcium oxalate (by complexing calcium) and inhibit urate-induced crystallization of calcium oxalate.

Potassium citrate may be particularly useful in patients with mild to moderate hyperuricosuria (<800 mg/d) in whom hypocitraturia is also present. However, allopurinol is probably preferred in patients with more marked hyperuricosuria, especially if hyperuricemia coexists.

ENTERIC HYPEROXALURIA

Oral administration of large amounts of calcium (0.25 to 1.0 g four times a day) or magnesium has been recommended for the control of calcium nephrolithiasis of ileal disease. Although urinary oxalate may decrease (probably from binding of oxalate by divalent cations), the concurrent rise in urinary calcium may obviate the beneficial effect of this therapy, at least in some patients. Cholestyramine does not cause a sustained reduction in urinary oxalate. The replacement of dietary fat with medium-chain triglycerides may be helpful in those patients who also have malabsorption.

Patients may exhibit hypomagnesiuria due to impaired intestinal absorption of magnesium. Since magnesium has been shown to complex with oxalate, hypomagnesiuria may increase the urinary saturation of calcium oxalate. While oral magnesium supplements may correct hypomagnesiuria, they may also provoke further diarrhea. Magnesium gluconate (0.5 to 1.0 g three times a day) appears to be better tolerated than magnesium oxide or hydroxide. Treatment with potassium citrate (60 to 120 mEq/d) may correct the hypokalemia and metabolic acidosis and, in some patients, increase urinary citrate toward normal.

A high fluid intake is recommended to assure adequate urine volume. Since excessive fluid loss may be present, an antidiarrheal agent may be necessary before sufficient urine output can be achieved. Calcium citrate may theoretically have a role in management of enteric hyperoxaluria. This treatment may lower urinary oxalate by binding oxalate in the intestinal tract. Calcium citrate may also raise the urinary citrate and pH by providing an alkali load. Finally, calcium citrate may correct the malabsorption of calcium and adverse effects on skeleton by providing an efficiently absorbed calcium.

HYPOCITRATURIC CALCIUM OXALATE NEPHROLITHIASIS

In patients with hypocitraturic calcium oxalate nephrolithiasis, potassium citrate treatment is capable of restoring normal urinary citrate, lowering the urinary saturation, and inhibiting crystallization of calcium salts. Since hypocitraturia is found in a number of different conditions, each will be addressed individually.

Distal Renal Tubular Acidosis

Potassium citrate therapy is able to correct the metabolic acidosis and hypokalemia found in patients with distal renal tubular acidosis. In addition, it is capable of restoring normal urinary citrate although large doses (up to 120 mEq/d) may be required in severe acidotic states. With correction of the acidosis, urinary calcium should decline into the normal range. Since urinary pH is generally high to begin with in patients with renal tubular acidosis, the overall rise in urinary pH is small.

Potassium citrate therapy typically produces a sustained decline in the urinary saturation of calcium oxalate (from reduction in urinary calcium and in citrate complexation of calcium). The urinary saturation of calcium phosphate does not increase since the rise in phosphate dissociation is relatively small and is adequately compensated by a decline in ionic calcium concentration. In addition, the inhibitory activity against the crystallization of calcium oxalate and calcium phosphate is augmented due to the direct action of citrate.

Chronic Diarrheal States

Potassium citrate therapy is indicated for patients with hypocitraturia secondary to chronic diarrheal states. The dose of potassium citrate will be dependent on the severity of hypocitraturia in these patients. The dosages range from 60 to 120 mEq in three to four divided doses.

It is recommended that a liquid preparation of potassium citrate be used rather than the slow-release tablet preparation since the slow-release medication may be poorly absorbed due to rapid intestinal transit time. In addition, frequent dose schedules (three to four times a day) for the liquid preparation are necessary since this form of the medication has a relatively short duration of biologic action. A less frequent dose schedule (two to three times a day) is acceptable if the solid preparation is used because of its slow-release characteristic.

Thiazide-Induced Hypocitraturia

Noted previously, thiazide therapy may induce hypocitraturia due to hypokalemia with resultant intracellular acidosis. Therefore, it should be a common practice to administer potassium supplementation, preferably in the form of potassium citrate, to patients receiving thiazide for treatment of hypercalciuria. Potassium citrate has been shown to be equally effective as potassium chloride in correcting thiazide-induced hypokalemia. Moreover, the addition of potassium citrate not only prevents a fall in urinary citrate during thiazide therapy but may raise citrate excretion.

Idiopathic Hypocitraturic Calcium Oxalate Nephrolithiasis

This entity includes hypocitraturia occurring alone, as well as in conjunction with other abnormalities (e.g., hypercalciuria or hyperuricosuria). Stones formed in this condition are predominantly composed of calcium oxalate. Potassium citrate therapy may produce a sustained increase in urinary citrate and a decline in the urinary saturation of the calcium oxalate. Thus, it is apparent that potassium citrate can be used in a variety of conditions. Combined data from a recent long-term clinical trial using potassium citrate shows no significant change in serum potassium, hematocrit, bone density, or endogenous creatinine clearance during treatment. A liquid preparation of potassium citrate with a frequent dosage schedule (three to four times a day) is recommended in chronic diarrheal states. In other conditions, a solid preparation given on a twice daily schedule is generally well tolerated.

HYPOMAGNESIURIC CALCIUM NEPHROLITHIASIS

Hypomagnesiuric calcium nephrolithiasis is characterized by low urinary magnesium, hypocitraturia, and low urine volume. Therefore, management might include restoration of urinary magnesium levels with either magnesium oxide or magnesium hydroxide as well as correction of the hypocitraturia with potassium citrate. A preparation that contains both magnesium and citrate would be ideal in the treatment of this condition. A potentially useful drug, potassium-magnesium citrate, is currently undergoing clinical trials.

GOUTY DIATHESIS

The major goal in the management of gouty diathesis is to increase the urinary pH above 5.5, preferably to between 6.5 and 7.0. In the past, urine alkalinization has been accomplished with either sodium bicarbonate or various combinations of sodium and potassium alkali therapy. While sodium alkali may enhance dissociation of uric acid and inhibit uric stone acid formation by raising urinary pH, this medication may be complicated by the development of calcium-containing stones (calcium phosphate and/or calcium oxalate). Potassium citrate is advantageous because it is not only a good alkalinizing agent, but it appears to be without the complication of calcium stones. It should be given at a dose sufficient to maintain urinary pH at approximately 6.5 (30 to 60 mEq/d in two to three divided doses). Attempts at alkalinizing the urine to a pH greater than 7.0 should be avoided. At a higher pH there is a danger of increasing the risk of calcium stone formation. If the urinary uric acid excretion is elevated or hyperuricemia exists, allopurinol (300 mg/d) is recommended.

CYSTINURIA

The object of treatment for cystinuria is to reduce the urinary concentration of cystine to below its solubility limit (200 to 300 mg/L). The initial treatment program includes a high fluid intake and oral administration of soluble alkali (potassium citrate) at a dose sufficient to raise the urinary pH to 6.5 to 7.0. When this conservative program is ineffective, D-penicillamine or alpha-mercaptopropionylglycine (approximately 1 to 2 g/d in divided doses) has been used. This treatment has been shown to increase cystine solubility in urine via formation of a more soluble mixed disulfide. Penicillamine has been associated with frequent side effects including nephrotic syndrome, dermatitis, and pancytopenia. This side-effect profile appears to be less marked with alpha-mercaptopropionylglycine.

INFECTION LITHIASIS

If long-standing effective control of infection with urea-splitting organisms can be achieved, new stone formation may be averted, and some dissolution of existing stones may be achieved. Unfortunately, such control is difficult to obtain with antibiotic therapy. If there is an existing struvite stone, it is often difficult to eradicate the infection completely because the stone often harbors the organism within its interstices. For this reason, surgical removal of struvite stones is usually recommended.

Acetohydroxamic acid (AHA), a urease inhibitor, may reduce the urinary saturation of struvite and retard stone formation. When given at a dose of 250 mg three times a day, AHA has been shown to prevent recurrence of new stones and to inhibit the growth of stones in patients with chronic urea-splitting infections. In addition, in a limited number of patients, AHA has caused dissolution of existing struvite calculi. However, 30% of patients receiving chronic AHA therapy have experienced minor side effects and 15% developed deep venous thrombosis.

References

Griffith DP. Struvite stones. *Kidney Int.* 1978;13:372.

Griffith DP, Musher DM. Prevention of infected urinary stones by urease inhibition. *Invest Urol.* 1973;11:228–223.

Pak CYC, Fuller C, Sakhaee K, et al. Long-term treatment of calcium nephrolithiasis with potassium citrate. *J Urol.* 1985;134:11.

Pak CYC, Fuller C, Sakhaee K, Zerwekh JE, Adams BV. Management of cystine nephrolithiasis with alpha-mercaptopropionylglycine (Thiola). *J Urol.* 1986;136:1005.

Pak CYC, Peterson R. Successful treatment of hyperuricosuric calcium oxalate nephrolithiasis with potassium citrate. *Arch Intern Med.* 1986;146:863.

Pak CYC, Sakhaee K, Fuller C. Successful management of uric acid nephrolithiasis with potassium citrate. *Kidney Int.* 1985; 30:422–428.

Preminger GM, Harvey JA, Pak CYC. Comparative efficacy of "specific" potassium citrate therapy versus conservative management in nephrolithiasis of mild-moderate severity. *J Urol.* 1985;134:658.

Williams JJ, Rodman JS, Peterson CN. A randomized double-blind study of acetohydroxamic acid in struvite nephrolithiasis. *N Engl J Med.* 1984;311:760.

CHAPTER 14

Surgical Management of Calculus Disease

Glenn M. Preminger

Approximately 10% to 20% of all kidney stones may cause the patient enough problems to require surgical removal. Recent improvements in urologic equipment, fluoroscopic technology, and interventional radiologic techniques have given the patient and the urologist many choices when choosing the means of stone removal. When open renal and ureteral surgery are the means by which all new procedures are judged, it appears that percutaneous nephrostolithotomy, ureterorenoscopy, and extracorporeal shock wave lithotripsy offer the patient comparable success for the stone removal with significantly diminished patient morbidity and lowered patient cost.

As a consequence of the dramatic increase in the technologies available to the urologist for the treatment of stone disease there is controversy regarding their application. Thus it is difficult to formulate absolute treatment guidelines. This section is a compilation of many philosophies in surgical stone management. In an attempt to simplify this task, the text is divided into treatment philosophies for renal and ureteral calculi with discussion germane to the various options in each category.

Techniques Available for Surgical Management

EXTRACORPOREAL SHOCK WAVE LITHOTRIPSY

Since the first patient with a renal calculus was successfully treated with extracorporeal shock wave lithotripsy in 1980, rapid acceptance and widespread use have championed this form of stone therapy as the treatment of choice for the majority of renal and ureteral calculi. Worldwide clinical series have documented the efficacy of extracorporeal shock wave lithotripsy.

Shock waves are high-energy amplitudes of pressure generated in the air or water by an abrupt release of energy in a small space. They propagate according to the physical laws of acoustics and are transmitted through media with low attenuation. However, when a shock wave encounters a boundary between substances of dif-

fering acoustic impedance (density), compressive stresses are generated that may overcome the tensile strength of that object (Fig. 14.1). Shock waves travel through water and the soft tissues of the body with low attenuation because these materials have similar densities. However, when kidney stones of any composition are contacted by a shock wave of sufficient energy, a compression wave is induced along the front face of the stone. As a result, the anterior surface begins to crumble. As a shock wave crosses the posterior surface of the stone, part of the energy is reflected, creating tensile stress and fragmentation along the posterior surface. Repeated shock waves eventually reduce the stone to small fragments, ideally 2 mm or less in diameter, which may be passed spontaneously.

Extensive clinical testing has determined that the compression-tensile wave phenomenon results in an implosion rather than an explosion of the fragments and that the total kinetic energy of all fragments can be minimized by using a large number of relatively low-energy shock waves rather than fewer shocks of higher energy (Fig. 14.2). This finding explains the low incidence of adjacent tissue injury following successful stone fragmentation with high-energy shock waves.

Although the basic principles of shock wave lithotripsy remain unchanged, a myriad of technological advances and modifications in the currently available lithotripters have significantly expanded the clinical applications of lithotripsy.

Instrumentation for Extracorporeal Shock Wave Lithotripsy

All lithotripters share four main features: an energy source, a focusing device, a coupling medium, and a stone localization system (Fig. 14.3). The original Dornier HM-3 design uses a spark-plug energy generator with an elliptical reflector for focusing the shock waves. A water bath transmits the shock waves to the patient with stone localization provided by biplanar fluoroscopy. Modifications of the four basic components of this first-generation lithotripter have provided a class of second-generation lithotripters of which ten machines are currently either

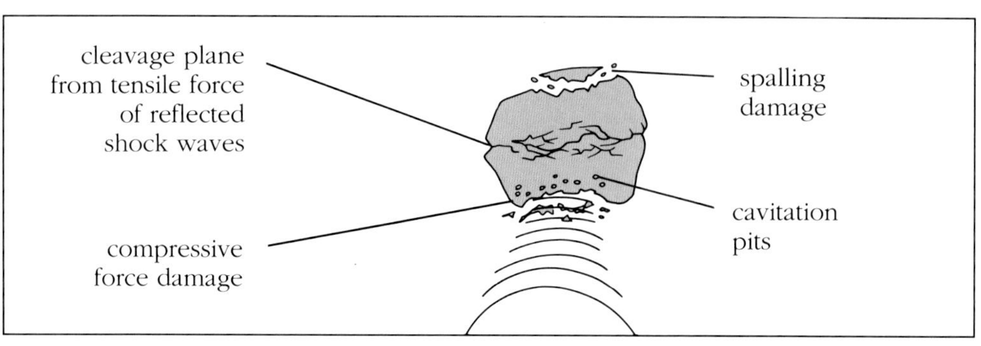

Figure 14.1 Forces generated by a focused, high-energy shock wave cause various types of damage.

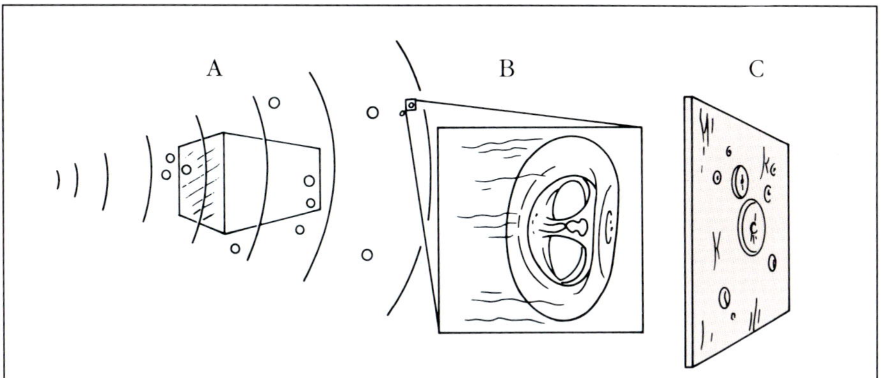

Figure 14.2 Cavitation.

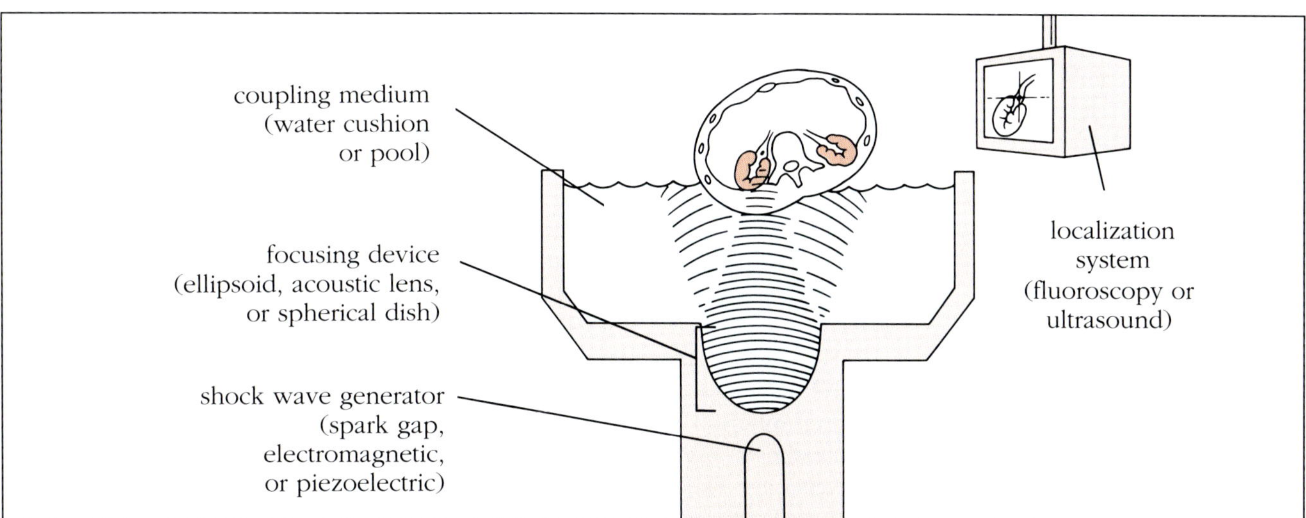

Figure 14.3 Basic lithotripsy design.

FIGURE 14.4 *Second Generation Lithotripters*

MANUFACTURER	SHOCK WAVE GENERATION	PATIENT FOCUSING	COUPLING	LOCALIZATION
Diasonics	Piezoelectric	Spherical	Membrane	Fluoroscopy/ultrasound
Direx	Spark gap	Ellipsoid	Membrane	Fluoroscopy/ultrasound*
Dornier HM-4	Spark gap	Ellipsoid	Membrane	Biplane fluoroscopy
EDAP LT-01	Piezoelectric	Spherical	Membrane	Ultrasound
Medstone	Spark gap	Ellipsoid	Membrane	Plain x-ray
Northgate	Spark gap	Ellipsoid	Membrane	Ultrasound
Siemens	Electromagnetic	Acoustic lens	Membrane	Biplane fluoroscopy
Technomed	Spark gap	Ellipsoid	Pool	Ultrasound
Wolf Piezolith 2300	Piezoelectric	Spherical	Pool	Ultrasound

*This unit does not have its own localization system. Separate ultrasound or fluoroscopy must be used.

available commercially or undergoing clinical trials (Fig. 14.4). This section on new instrumentation reviews the features of and principal differences among the second-generation lithotripters with regard to shock wave generation, focusing, patient coupling, and stone localization.

SHOCK WAVE GENERATION The two basic types of energy sources for generating shock waves are point sources and extended sources. The electrohydraulic devices (Dornier, Direx, Medstone, Northgate, and Technomed) use point sources for energy generation, whereas extended sources are incorporated in the piezoelectric (Diasonics, EDAP, and Wolf) and the electromagnetic (Siemens, Storz) devices.

The electrohydraulic shock wave generator is located at the base of a water bath and produces shock waves by an electric spark gap of 15,000 to 25,000 volts of 1 μs duration (Fig. 14.5). This high-voltage spark discharge produces rapid evaporation of water, which generates a shock wave by expanding the surrounding fluid (F_1). This electrohydraulic generator is located within an ellipsoidal reflector that concentrates the reflected shock waves at the second focal point (F_2).

Multiple, repeated electrohydraulic shock waves from a first-generation machine produce pain at the skin level and within the focal region, thus requiring general or regional anesthesia during lithotripsy. "Anesthesia-free" second-generation electrohydraulic lithotripters have been developed by widening the aperture of the ellipse and decreasing the overall energy intensity of the shock wave generator. However, some form of analgesia, sedation, or local anesthesia is usually required with the majority of second-generation electrohydraulic lithotripters (Fig. 14.6).

Piezoelectric shock waves are generated by the sudden expansion of ceramic elements excited by a high-frequency, high-voltage energy pulse (Fig. 14.7). The motion of the piezoceramic elements generates an ultrasonic wave that in turn produces a shock wave directed to the focal point. The shock wave is then propagated through a water-filled bag (EDAP, Diasonics) or basin (Wolf). The spherical focusing mechanism of the piezoelectric lithotripters provides a wide region of shock wave entry at the skin's surface, and a very small focal region (4 × 8 mm in the Wolf lithotripter). The combination of a wide aperture of the focusing sphere, a larger skin entry zone, a small focal region, and lower peak pressures generated by the piezoelectric machines have provided a truly anesthesia-free form of lithotripsy.

In the electromagnetic devices (Siemens, Storz), shock waves are generated when an electrical impulse moves a metallic membrane that is housed within a "shock tube" (Fig. 14.8). The resulting shock wave produced in the water-filled shock tube cylinder, is focused by an acoustic lens and coupled to the body surface with a water cushion. Some form of sedation and/or local anesthesia is usually required during treatment on this electromagnetic lithotripter due to the smaller aperture and moderate peak pressures generated. Recent studies have demonstrated that a transcutaneous electric nerve stimulator (TENS) will provide adequate analgesia during lithotripsy on the Siemens machine.

SHOCK WAVE FOCUSING Once shock waves are generated, they must be focused on the target calculus. The method of focusing is dictated by the type of shock wave generation. Machines that use point sources, such as the electrohydraulic lithotripters, generate shock waves that travel in an expanding circular pattern and require ellipsoidal reflectors for focusing the shock waves at the second focal point, F_2. The array of piezoceramic elements is positioned on a spherical disc that allows focusing at a very small focal region, F_1, whereas the vibrating metal

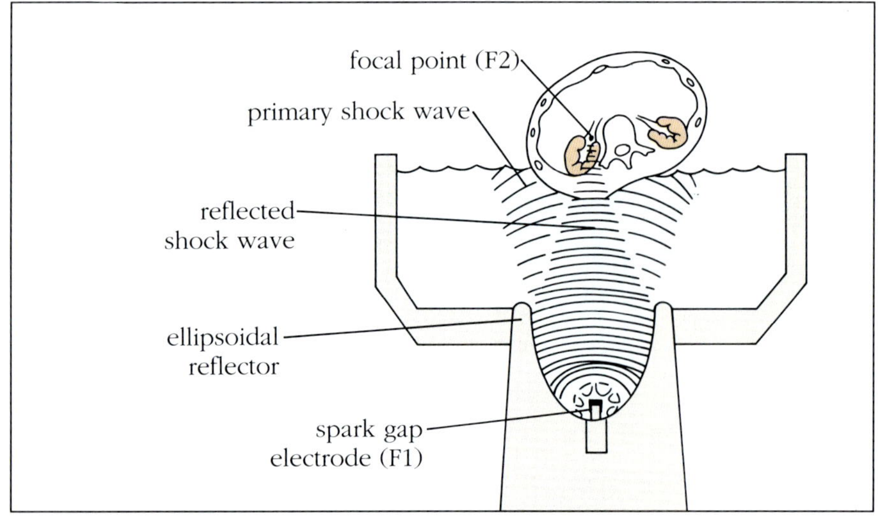

Figure 14.5 During spark gap shock wave generation, F_1 is the origin of the primary shock wave; F_2 is the concentration of reflected shock waves at a focal point such as the kidney stone.

FIGURE 14.6 *Anesthesia Requirements Versus Lithotripter Efficiency*

	DORNIER HM-3	DORNIER HM-4	TECHNOMED SONOLITH	SIEMENS LITHOSTAR	EDAP LT-01	WOLF PIEZOLITH
Aperture (mm)	156	170	205	120	N/A	300
Focal size (mm)	12 × 50	10 × 40	N/A	11 × 90	N/A	4 × 8
Maximum pressures (bar)	500	N/A	780	440	1050	1140
Anesthesia	General	75% sedation	Sedation/ general	Sedation local/tens	Sedation	None
Average number of shock waves used	1200	2100	3600	3200	N/A	3600
Secondary Rx	16%	22%	13%	18%	32%	29%

N/A = not available

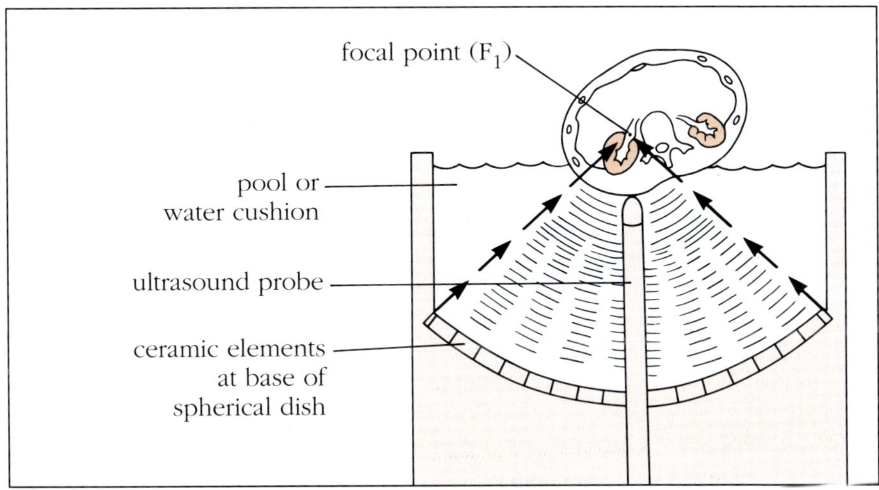

Figure 14.7 Piezoelectric shock wave generation provides a wide point of shock wave entry at the skin.

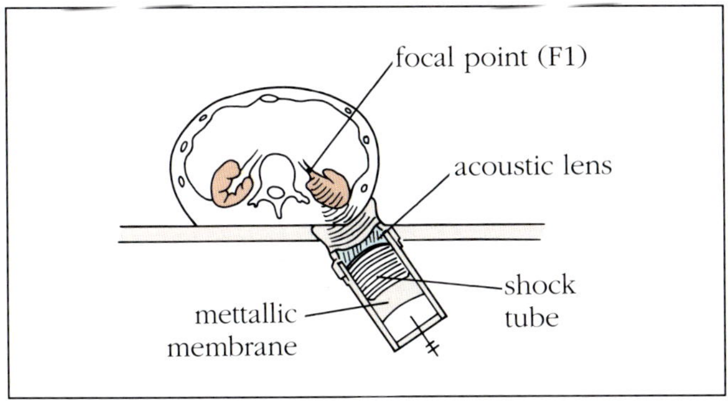

Figure 14.8 With electromagnetic shock wave generation, an acoustic lens focuses the shock waves, which are produced by an electrical impulse.

membranes of the electromechanical lithotripter produce an acoustical wave that requires a lens for focusing the shock wave at F_1.

COUPLING OF THE SHOCK WAVE The coupling media currently used by the different lithotripters ranges from a 1000 L water bath to an enclosed water cushion. The water bath requires unique positioning of the patient in the tub so that the calculus is at the second focal point. Recent modifications in the patient gantry system of the first-generation Dornier HM-3 lithotripter have allowed the treatment of children as well as distal ureteral calculi. Second-generation machines have adopted designs for coupling that minimize the space requirements as well as the physiologic and functional disadvantages of a large water bath. Current models use an enclosed water cushion, a small exposed pool of water, or a totally contained shock tube. The water-filled cushions and shock tubes contain the shock wave source, conditioned water, and a coupling membrane to allow simplified positioning and "dry" lithotripsy. However, the direct water-skin interface used by two units (Technomed and Wolf) is believed by some to offer improved shock wave coupling.

STONE LOCALIZATION Stone localization during lithotripsy is accomplished with either fluoroscopy or ultrasonography. Fluoroscopy provides the urologist with a familiar modality and has the added benefits of effective ureteral stone localization. Moreover, fluoroscopy facilitates the use of contrast material to help delineate the anatomy of the collecting system. However, fluoroscopy requires more space, carries the inherent risk of ionizing radiation to both the patient and medical staff, and is not useful in localizing radiolucent calculi.

Ultrasonography is becoming an increasingly important modality for the urologist. Sonography-based lithotripters offer the advantages of stone localization with continuous monitoring and effective identification of radiolucent stones, without radiation exposure. Additionally, ultrasound has been documented to be effective in localizing stone fragments as small as 2 to 3 mm and is as good or better than routine KUB to assess patients for residual stone fragments following lithotripsy. The ultrasound-based machines also have the important capability of gallstone localization for biliary lithotripsy (multipurpose lithotripters: Direx, EDAP, Technomed, Wolf). The major disadvantages of ultrasound stone localization include the basic mastery of ultrasonic techniques by the urologist and the difficulty in localizing ureteral stones. Current efforts are in progress to develop echogenic ureteral stents to aid in ultrasonic localization of ureteral calculi.

Third Generation Lithotripters

Currently, there are a number of third-generation lithotripters in clinical trials in an attempt to incorporate many of the characteristics of an "ideal" lithotripter. The basic design of the third-generation machines includes dual imaging capabilities as well as variable shock wave power. These machines include the Dornier MFL 5000 (HM5), Siemens Lithostar Plus, Storz Modulith SL20, and Wolf Piezolith 2500 (Fig. 14.9).

DUAL IMAGING Dual imaging capabilities entail having fluoroscopic as well as sonographic localization systems available in the same machine. Such a design has the advantage of using fluoroscopy for imaging stones within the kidney, as well as the ureter, while having the option to use sonography for the identification of radiolucent or biliary tract calculi. Moreover, sonographic capabilities allow one initially to target a stone using fluoroscopy and then to switch over to ultrasound to avoid an excessive amount of ionizing radiation. Moreover, having fluoroscopy capabilities may lessen the "learning curve" for many urologists who are unfamiliar with sonographic stone localization procedures.

FIGURE 14.9 *Third-Generation Lithotripters*

MANUFACTURER	SHOCK WAVE GENERATION	FOCUSING	PATIENT COUPLING	IN-LINE LOCALIZATION*
Dornier HM-5	Spark gap	Ellipsoid	Membrane	Fluoroscopy
Siemens Lithostar Plus	Electromagnetic	Acoustic lens	Membrane	2 fluoroscopy tubes
Storz Modulith SL 20	Electromagnetic	Parabolic reflector	Membrane	Ultrasound
Wolf Piezolith 2500	Piezoelectric	Spherical	Membrane	Ultrasound and fluoroscopy

*Describes which localization system is "in line" with the shock wave generator.

Interestingly, while the Dornier, Siemens, and Storz machines have all added ultrasound capabilities to provide dual imaging, none of these systems provides "in-line" imaging for both the fluoroscopic or sonographic localization devices. For example, with the Dornier and Siemens devices, one can use sonography to target a radiolucent or biliary tract calculus, yet the patient must be moved "blindly" to the fluoroscopy unit, which is in line with the shock wave generator. Alternatively, one can use the fluoroscopic localization system with the Storz machine, yet only the ultrasound is in line with the shock wave generator.

The Wolf Piezolith 2500 provides the only third-generation device that has both the fluoroscope and sonography in line with the piezoelectric shock wave generator. This permits rapidly changing from fluoroscopic to sonographic stone localization, without moving the patient off of the treatment dish.

VARIABLE POWER All four of the aforementioned third-generation devices have variable power shock wave generators, which allow the operator to apply the appropriate amount of shock wave energy for a particular stone. One can turn down the generator power to provide significantly reduced anesthesia/analgesia requirements with the Dornier, Siemens, and Storz machines as well as provide totally anesthesia/analgesia-free lithotripsy with the Wolf device. Moreover, the shock wave intensity can be increased with all four machines to allow adequate fragmentation of extremely hard or large calculi. However, one must understand that when using these lithotripters in the "high-power mode," various forms of anesthesia/analgesia will be necessary.

So in fact we still have not developed the "ultimate shock wave," which allows totally anesthesia-free lithotripsy with maximum efficiency. Yet, by varying the shock wave energy, one can administer a highly efficient shock wave with the need for anesthesia/analgesia when high shock wave pressures are indicated. On the other hand, with a small or soft stone, the shock wave energy can be significantly decreased to provide minimal-anesthesia lithotripsy.

Interestingly, while much of the industry has pushed for anesthesia-free capabilities over the past few years, many physicians have perhaps not been as aware and/or ignored the potential deleterious effect that may result from excessive administration of the higher-powered electrohydraulic shock waves. Now, with the availability of variable-powered lithotripters that use electrohydraulic, electromagnetic, and piezoelectric energy sources, one must continue to monitor closely the total amount of energy delivered to a particular kidney to limit the incidence of significant renal injury.

PERCUTANEOUS NEPHROSTOLITHOTOMY

The development of percutaneous endoscopic manipulation of stones in the renal collecting system is without precedent in the history of urologic surgery. Within one decade, the technique has evolved from an adventure undertaken only by a few physicians to a routine procedure performed by thousands of urologists worldwide, only to be forced into the background by an even more revolutionary procedure for stone treatment, namely extracorporeal shock wave lithotripsy.

Initially, a percutaneous nephrostomy tract needs to be established in order to gain access to the intrarenal collecting system. At our institution, this procedure is performed by a uroradiology team. The urologist, usually present during the access procedure, will have definite suggestions concerning the optimal positioning of the nephrostomy tract. The access tract should enter the kidney through a posterior calyx, which is usually facilitated by positioning the patient at 30° on the fluoroscopy table. In most cases, the lower or middle pole calyces may be accessed below the twelfth rib, but occasionally a supracostal approach is necessary to reach the targeted stone optimally (Fig. 14.10A). One should anticipate possible cephalad renal movement during nephrostomy access placement, which may alter the proposed approach.

The nephrostomy tract is then formed by dilating the skin, fascia, muscles, and renal tissues over the guide wire. Nephrostomy tract dilatation can be performed using graduated plastic dilators (Amplatz dilator) or a balloon catheter (Fig. 14.10B,C). After the nephrostomy tract has been dilated up to a 30 Fr (10 mm in diameter) size, a hollow plastic sheath is placed into the renal pelvis. A variety of endoscopic instruments may then be passed directly into the renal collecting system to perform various manipulations.

Endoscopy is begun by performing rigid or flexible nephroscopy. Although specially designed nephroscopes with a 30° side-arm viewing system are available, a traditional panendoscope of 24 Fr is equally well suited for rigid nephroscopy and allows visualization and manipulation inside the renal collecting system (Fig. 14.10D). Once the renal pelvis and the calyces accessible to a rigid nephroscope have been visualized and the surgeon is familiar with the intrarenal anatomy, flexible nephroscopy can be performed to inspect individual calyces that may not be within the reach of the rigid instrument. With the help of these flexible instruments, the entire collecting system can be visualized by taking advantage of the tip deflection and rotating the instrument inside the kidney

The diameter of the working sheath is usually 32 Fr, which equals about 1 cm. Therefore, stones up to this size can be extracted intact through the sheath. For the fragmentation of stones inside the renal collecting system (and the ureter) which are too large to be extracted (>1 cm), three modalities of "power lithotripsy" are available: ultrasonic lithotripsy (UL), electrohydraulic lithotripsy (EHL), and laser lithotripsy.

Ultrasonic Lithotripsy

Ultrasonic energy was first described to fragment kidney stones in 1979 by Alken. Commercially available units consist of a power generator and an ultrasound transducer and probe, which form the "sonotrode." A piezoceramic element in the handle of the sonotrode is stimulated to resonate. This converts electrical energy into ultrasound waves (with a frequency of 23,000 to 27,000 Hz) that are transmitted along the hollow metal probe and vibrate its tip (Fig. 14.11). When the vibrating tip is brought in contact with the surface of a stone, the calculus can be disintegrated. The probe must be rigid since sound waves cannot be transmitted without energy loss along flexible probes. The probes come in 10 and 12 Fr sizes and are passed through the straight working channel of a rigid nephroscope with a 30° or 90° offset lens (24 or 26 Fr nephroscope diameter). Suction tubing can be connected to the end of the sonotrode probe, thus converting the unit into a "vacuum cleaner" for stone fragments. Normal

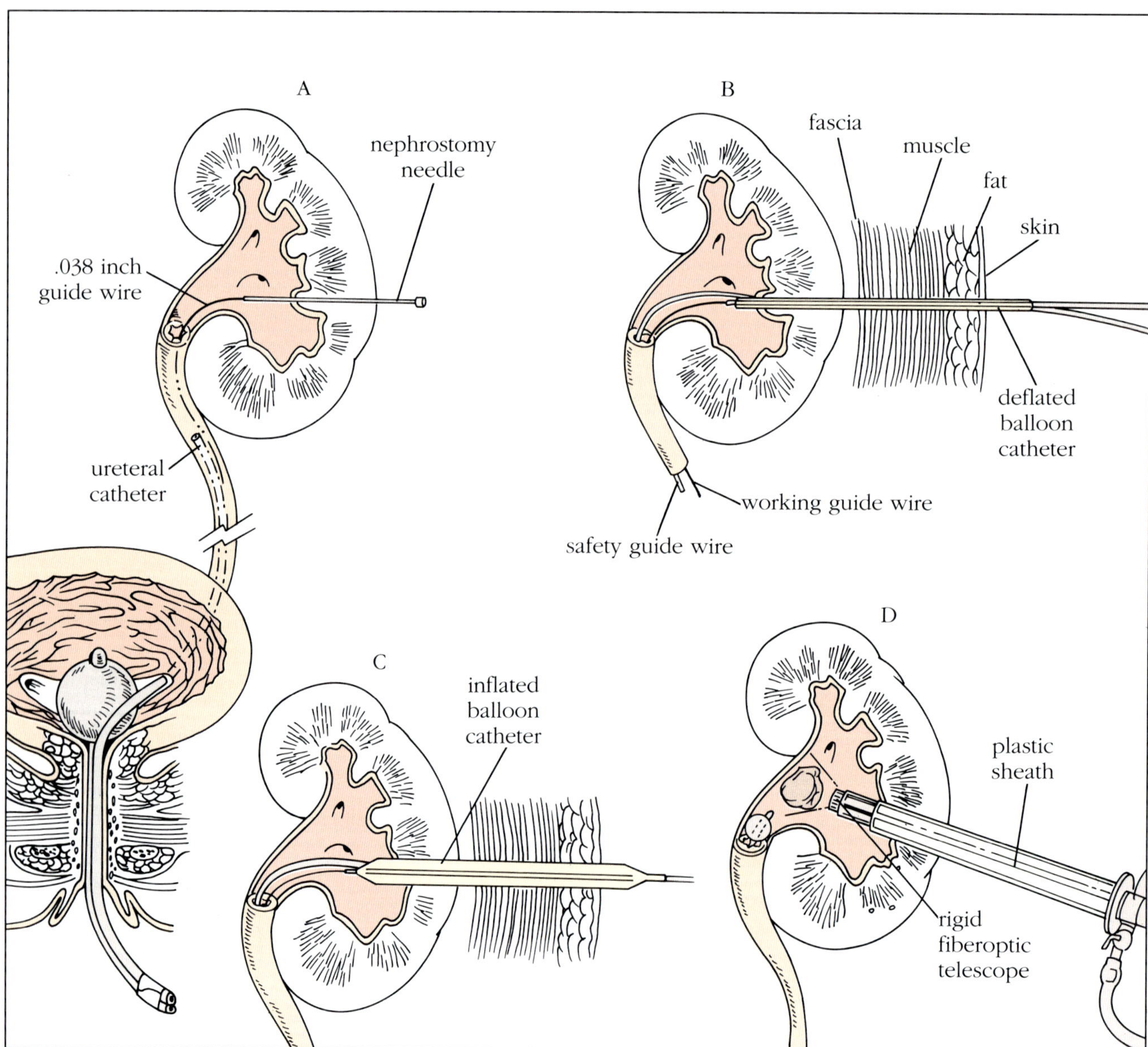

Figure 14.10 A–D Percutaneous urinary stone removal.

saline at body temperature should be used as irrigant.

Ultrasonic lithotripsy should be the procedure of choice for fragmentation of large renal stones. However, some uric acid, calcium oxalate monohydrate, or cystine stones may not break up easily, necessitating EHL. Besides the risk for perforation and extravasation of irrigant, UL is associated with noise levels of around 90 dB several inches from the transducer. For lengthy UL sessions, ear plugs are therefore recommended. Depending on the location of the stones, retained fragments are seen in 3% to 35% of all cases treated with ultrasonic lithotripsy. This cannot be considered a failure in many cases because the UL is often performed for the debulking of large stones to be followed by extracorporeal shock wave lithotripsy as a planned two-stage procedure.

Electrohydraulic Lithotripsy

The principles of electrohydraulic lithotripsy (EHL) were described and developed by a Russian engineer in 1950. This technology has been used extensively for the destruction of bladder stones, and in 1975, reports were published on its use for the fragmentation of kidney stones. The EHL unit consists of a probe, a power generator, and a foot pedal. The probe consists of a central metal core and two layers of insulation with another metal layer between them. Probes are flexible and available in Fr sizes 5, 7, and 9 to be used through rigid and flexible nephroscopes.

Commercially available EHL units are manufactured with power up to 120 volts. The electrical discharge is transmitted to the probe, where it generates a spark at the tip. The intense heat production in the immediate area surrounding the tip results in a cavitation bubble that produces a shock wave that radiates spherically in all directions. Collapse of the bubble causes a second shock wave. These shock waves, repeated at a frequency of 50 to 100 per second, result in destruction of the stone.

EHL will effectively fragment all kinds of urinary calculi, including the very hard cystine, uric acid, and calcium oxalate monohydrate stones. Since the probes are small and flexible, they can be used through flexible nephroscopes and ureteroscopes to fragment stones in calyces unaccessible for UL through a rigid instrument. The primary disadvantage of EHL is the inability to remove the stone fragments efficiently. All particles have to be either washed out during intraoperative irrigation or grasped with forceps. It is therefore advantageous to fragment the stone into the smallest number of particles allowing extraction with grasping devices (usually <1.0 cm). There is no virtue in transforming a large stone into hundreds of small particles or even sand-like material, because a significant amount of time will be required to remove the debris

Overall, EHL in the kidney should be the procedure of second choice for routine stone fragmentation but the procedure of choice in the ureter. Its main application should be for very hard stones or stones not within reach of the rigid nephroscope/UL probe.

Laser Lithotripsy

Laser lithotripsy is the newest modality available for stone fragmentation. The 250 μm quartz fiber of the pulsed dye laser is easily passed through the smallest flexible nephroscope for treatment of renal calculi. Although the indications for use of laser lithotripsy on renal calculi are similar to that of EHL, the majority of the applications for laser lithotripsy are for intraureteral fragmentation of stones and therefore will be discussed in the section on ureteroscopy.

URETEROSCOPY

The advent of ureterorenoscopy has dramatically altered the management of symptomatic ureteral calculi. Rigid ureteroscopy has been used in conjunction with ultrason-

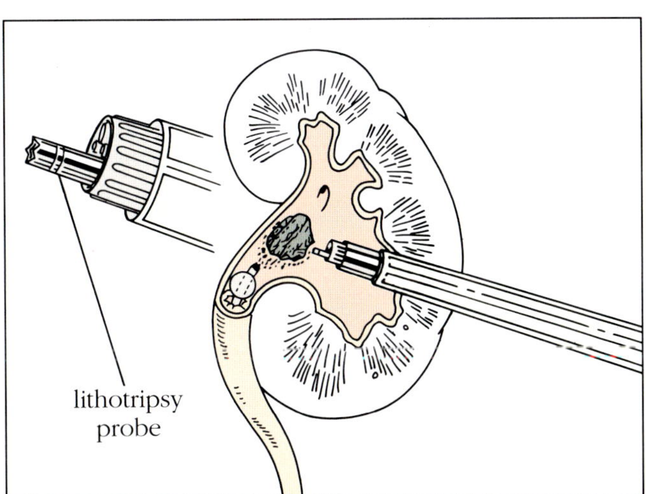

Figure 14.11 An ultrasonic lithotripsy probe through a nephroscope is used to fragment and remove a large intrarenal calculus.

ic and electrohydraulic lithotripsy and pulsed dye laser probes to fragment ureteral calculi successfully. While improvements in fiber optics and irrigation systems have fostered the use of smaller semi-rigid ureteroscopes (6.9 to 8.5 Fr), it is the introduction of flexible deflectable ureterorenoscopes that has made access to the upper ureter and intrarenal collecting system a safer and less tedious procedure.

The extremely small working channel of the semi-rigid and flexible instruments, which ranges from 2.4 to 4.0 Fr, has limited the size and usefulness of instruments that can be passed through these ureterorenoscopes and used for stone removal. Indeed, for larger stones in the proximal ureter, the 3.0 Fr basket or grasping forceps are often inadequate to accomplish successful stone extraction. This limitation of available instrumentation has prompted the use of intracorporeal lithotripsy for the management of larger upper ureteral and intrarenal calculi.

Currently the two most commonly employed methods for intracorporeal lithotripsy of ureteral stones via the flexible or semirigid ureterorenoscope are EHL and the pulsed dye laser. Ultrasonic lithotripsy is occasionally used for lower ureteral calculi, but its use has been supplanted to a large extent by EHL and laser lithotripsy. Although the choice of intracorporeal fragmentation is frequently based on the location and composition of the stone to be treated, the experience of the clinician and availability of equipment more often dictate this decision.

Electrohydraulic Lithotripsy

The first experience with electrohydraulic lithotripsy in the ureter entailed a 6 Fr EHL probe which was fluoroscopically guided to the obstructing calculus. The most common cause of failure in this early experience was secondary to the operator's inability to pass the probe to the level of the stone. Additional early experience with EHL within the ureter included the use of a 9 Fr probe, which provided excellent fragmentation of the stone, but 40% of the patients had ureteral extravasation following the lithotripsy procedure. This high complication rate was believed to be due mainly to the large probe size. The use of a smaller 5 Fr EHL probe through the rigid ureteroscope was compromised by decreased stone visualization because the probe occupied the majority of the working channel of the rigid ureteroscope. The development of a smaller 3 Fr EHL probe used through a flexible ureteroscope was reported in 1988. Recently, a 1.9 Fr EHL probe has been developed which is quite successful at fragmenting ureteral and intrarenal stones. Moreover, an additional benefit of these small caliber probes is the improved visualization through the flexible ureteroscope, as a larger portion of the working channel is available for irrigation.

Laser Lithotripsy

As noted before, laser lithotripsy is also used for the management of ureteral calculi. The significant advances in laser fibers and power generation systems have made laser lithotripsy, in many practitioners' hands, the treatment of choice for ureteral stones. The pulsed dye laser delivers short 1 μs pulsations at 5 to 10 Hz produced from a coumarin green dye. A plasma is formed at the stone surface, resulting a highly localized shock wave. The 504 nm wavelength produced by the laser is selectively absorbed by the stone and not the surrounding ureteral wall. Because the energy is delivered in short pulses, minimal heat is generated, likewise protecting the ureter. Initial experience has yielded fragmentation rates from 64% to 95%. Failures have been related to equipment malfunction (4% to 19%) or, more often, to stone composition. Moreover, use of EHL and/or basketing has been necessary as an adjunct to the laser in some cases of successful stone removal. Use of the pulsed dye laser in the ureter in all series appears to be safe, as no significant intraoperative or postoperative complications have been noted.

Continued development in laser technology has yielded larger-diameter laser fibers that are able to fragment hard calculi more effectively. Newer 300 and 320 μm laser fibers are superior to the 200 μm fibers in the fragmentation of calcium oxalate monohydrate and cystine stones. Fragmentation rates greater than 90% have been obtained with these new fibers. As the field continues to advance, new materials are being tested as sources for new laser lithotripsy units (alexandrite). Currently, cost is the most prohibitive aspect of laser lithotripsy, as most laser units command an approximate $200,000 initial investment with equally expensive yearly labor contracts.

OPEN LITHOTOMY

As percutaneous nephrostolithotomy, extracorporeal shock wave lithotripsy, and ureteroscopy have became widely embraced as the treatments of choice for the majority of renal and ureteral calculi, the indications for open lithotomy have decreased dramatically. Currently, with the available technology, only 1% to 5% of stones will require an open procedure for removal. Of 893 stone procedures performed since the introduction of extracorporeal lithotripsy at their institution, Assimos et al. found that 4.1% required open lithotomy for renal calculi. The most common indication for open lithotomy was failure of extracorporeal lithotripsy or percutaneous nephrolithotomy.

Morbidly obese patients often require open lithotomy because their body habitus precludes fluoroscopic or sonographic localization or effective treatment of renal calculi, since the shock waves become attenuated in the excess tissue. Also, the large amount of adipose tissue in the flank may prevent placement of an Amplatz sheath into the renal pelvis during percutaneous nephrostolithotomy. As percutaneous nephrostolithotomy often requires extended operative time, patients with multiple medical problems or diminished cardiac reserve may benefit from a shorter open procedure. Stones found in a collecting system with distal obstruction may require open lithotomy with concomitant pyeloplasty. In addition, obstructed or scarred calyceal infundibula may be repaired with calycorrhaphy or calycoplasty after removal of the stone. Coagulum pyelolithotomy may be helpful in patients with many small stones in multiple calyces. This procedure may also be of benefit in clearing small residual calculi in patients who have undergone anatrophic nephrolithotomy.

For branched renal calculi, surgical procedures beyond simple open pyelolithotomy may be necessary for stone removal. Pyelonephrolithotomy may be used for isolated lower pole branched calculi in a small pelvis or in a system with stenotic infundibula. Anatrophic nephrolithotomy is based on the blood supply to the kidney using the relatively avascular plane of Brodel's line for the lateral renal parenchymal incision prior to entering the collecting system. This approach permits wide exposure of the renal pelvis, enabling en bloc removal of the branched calculi with minimal residual calculi. Patients with complex stones or evidence of parenchymal loss may benefit from either partial or complete nephrectomy for stone disease.

Management of Renal Calculi

Several possibilities exist for the treatment of renal calculi. Extracorporeal shock wave lithotripsy, percutaneous nephrolithotripsy, ureterorenoscopy, and open lithotomy all provide the means to remove renal calculi effectively in given clinical situations. Other issues germane to any discussion of the treatment of renal calculi are the size of the stone being treated, stone composition (in particular cystine or calcium oxalate monohydrate), location of the stone within the kidney, and renal anatomy.

SMALL CALCULI

Although multiple treatment options exist for small renal calculi, extracorporeal shock wave lithotripsy has repeatedly been shown to be extremely effective for smaller stones. As a result, percutaneous nephrostolithotomy has been relegated to a less significant role in the management of small renal calculi, though several indications still exist for percutaneous stone removal. Failure of either of these modalities to remove the renal stone burden completely may necessitate open lithotomy or, in some cases, flexible ureterorenoscopy.

The first-generation Dornier HM-3 lithotripter represents the existing standard in terms of efficacy in stone fragmentation to which second-generation lithotripters must be compared. As the shock wave pressure (power)

and focal region of the second-generation machines have been reduced, so has the requirement for anesthesia or analgesia. However, the price paid for anesthesia-free lithotripsy is a reduction in fragmentation efficiency. For stones less than 1.5 cm in maximal dimension, the Dornier HM-3 lithotripter averages 1200 shocks per treatment, yielding a stone-free rate of approximately 85%, with a retreatment rate of 16%. For stones less than 2 cm, a 91% stone-free rate can be expected. However, as one alters the configuration of the shock wave by widening the aperture of the ellipsoid (modified Dornier HM-3 and HM-4), the average number of shock waves required increases to 2100 while maintaining a stone-free rate ranging from 56% to 82%. However, the retreatment rate has been reported to increase to a range of 22% to 37%.

Similarly, there is a compromise in efficiency with the piezoelectric lithotripters. Clinical series with piezoelectric lithotripsy (Wolf Piezolith 2300, EDAP LT-01) have reported an 84% to 90% stone-free rate at three months for stones less than 1.5 cm in diameter. However, upwards of 30% of these patients may require a secondary treatment. Moreover, the average number of shock waves increases to approximately 3500 shocks per treatment. The requirement for repeat treatments with the piezoelectric machines is somewhat offset by the fact that each treatment is performed as an "office" procedure, without anesthesia, analgesia, or significant recovery time.

Electromagnetic lithotripsy is usually performed with intravenous or oral sedation, with or without the use of local anesthesia at the skin entry site, although some centers have found that a transcutaneous nerve stimulator unit provides adequate analgesia in 90% of patients treated. The mean number of shock waves per treatment is approximately 3600, with a stone-free rate of 66% and a retreatment rate of 11%.

Currently, many variable-power third-generation lithotripters are in clinical use (Dornier HM-5, Sonolith 2000, and Wolf Piezolith 2500). Using the lower power setting, these machines have approximately a 70% stone-free rate, with a 14% to 25% retreatment rate. Therefore, in order to achieve an anesthesia-free status, one must expect the number of secondary treatments to increase and therefore the efficiency of that lithotripter to be diminished.

Though extracorporeal lithotripsy is the standard for treatment of renal calculi of less than 2 cm, some stones are recalcitrant to this mode of treatment. In these cases, percutaneous nephrostolithotomy would be the treatment of second choice. Stone-free rates greater than 90% to 95% can be expected for renal calculi less than 2 cm in size. Morbidly obese patients often require percutaneous stone removal, since imaging is hampered by the excess tissue, as is the effectiveness of the shock waves. Hard stones, composed of cystine or calcium oxalate monohydrate, are relative indications for performing percutaneous nephrostolithotomy. Although extracorporeal shock wave lithotripsy and percutaneous nephrostolithotomy are occasionally met with failure, only rarely will open lithotomy be necessary for the management of small renal calculi.

LARGE CALCULI

Though most large renal calculi may be managed like smaller renal calculi, the clinician will find a larger number of patients that require some modality other than extracorporeal shock wave lithotripsy for stone removal. As fragmentation efficiency decreases with increasing stone size, percutaneous nephrostolithotomy may become, in certain cases, the treatment of choice. As with smaller stones, open lithotomy will be required only for those stones resistant to previous treatment attempts.

As the stone's volume increases, the efficacy of all lithotripters diminishes significantly. For example, for a stone burden greater than 3 cm in a dilated collecting system, only 30% of patients will be rendered stone-free with Dornier HM-3 monotherapy. While the stone-free rate for large calculi will increase to approximately 70% for patients with normal collecting system anatomy, many clinicians prefer the use of percutaneous nephrolithotripsy as the initial form of therapy for large renal calculi. Studies have found the combination of percutaneous nephrolithotripsy and extracorporeal shock wave lithotripsy to be more effective than extracorporeal shock wave lithotripsy alone. With this type of combination therapy, stone-free rates approaching 85% to 90% have been reported for large renal calculi.

Previous studies have shown that the critical stone burden in considering extracorporeal lithotripsy monotherapy is a stone diameter of 2 cm. With stones greater than 2 cm, the number of ancillary procedures required after extracorporeal shock wave lithotripsy rises from 11% to 27% and the incidence of significant residual fragments from 3% to 10% (57% for stones greater than 3 cm in diameter). Approximately 77% of all stones greater than 3 cm required additional treatment. Therefore, for complete and incomplete staghorn calculi as well as for stones larger than 3 cm in diameter, percutaneous nephrostolithotomy should be the initial procedure, since occasionally it will be the only one required. The use of percutaneous nephrostolithotomy for stones between 2 and 3 cm depends on the preference of the physician. Percutaneous nephrostolithotomy is indicated if there is obstruction of the urinary tract between the stone location and the ureterovesical junction (e.g., infundibular stenosis, primary or secondary ureteropelvic junction obstruction, ureteral stricture, ureteral stricture, ureterovesical junction obstruction). For stones larger than 2.5 cm previous studies have shown an 83% stone-free rate after percutaneous nephrostolithotomy with a 17% auxiliary procedure rate. Although the total hospital cost is slightly higher for patients undergoing percutaneous

management of larger renal calculi, the convalescence period was significantly shorter than those patients undergoing open lithotomy.

Again, open lithotomy would not be the principal choice for large renal calculi but must always be considered in patients with existing renal anomalies or previous failures with either extracorporeal lithotripsy or percutaneous nephrostolithotomy.

STAGHORN CALCULI

One of the current controversies in stone management is the treatment of staghorn calculi. Treatment philosophies vary from single modality treatment of all staghorn calculi with extracorporeal lithotripsy to combined treatment with percutaneous nephrolithotomy and extracorporeal shock wave lithotripsy to open lithotomy. The differences in opinion are based in the inferior results obtained with the treatment of renal calculi by extracorporeal shock wave lithotripsy and the increased patient morbidity caused by the other modalities.

Initially, staghorn calculi were treated solely with open lithotomy with reasonable success rates. But with the advent of percutaneous nephrolithotomy in the early 1980s new avenues for treatment of this troublesome stone were opened. Though one could expect anatrophic nephrolithotomy to render a patient free of stones approximately 65% to 90% of the time, there was a high complication rate (up to 50%) and significant time needed for convalescence. Complete removal of staghorn calculi by percutaneous nephrolithotomy varies from 62% to 95% with a 20% to 57% complication rate. Most clinicians employ a single treatment session but sometimes require multiple tracts to access completely a branched calculus percutaneously. Often clinicians prefer to stage the percutaneous procedure, with patients returning for a secondary percutaneous nephrolithotomy.

As extracorporeal lithotripsy became widely available for the treatment of renal calculi, attempts to treat staghorn calculi with this modality were reported in the literature. Initially, the reports were dismal, as most patients underwent only a single treatment and follow-up was quite short. With multiple treatments, prolonged follow-up, and ureteral stenting, stone-free rates at 3 to 6 months have been reported from 36% to 72% with complication rates similar to percutaneous nephrostolithotomy (12% to 64%).

Recently, many centers have suggested the combined use of percutaneous nephrostolithotomy and extracorporeal lithotripsy for treatment of staghorn calculi. The initial treatment session is for stone debulking through a percutaneous tract with ultrasonic and/or electrohydraulic lithotripsy (Fig. 14.12). If retained renal calculi are noted on postprocedure radiographs, then extracorporeal lithotripsy, with or without internal ureteral stenting, is used to fragment the remaining stone burden. Also, flexible nephroscopy may be used as a final procedure to remove additional fragments. Success rates of 80% to 95% have been reported with this combined approach. Kahnowski et al. studied combination therapy with extracorporeal lithotripsy and percutaneous nephrostolithotomy and found that percutaneous nephrostolithotomy was the only procedure required to render the patient stone-free in 14 of 44 patients with complete staghorn calculi. Moreover, the incidence of urosepsis was reduced and the nephrostomy tract allowed irrigation to be performed to wash out fragments and to allow postoperative chemolysis. In a direct comparison between extracorporeal lithotripsy and percutaneous nephrostolithotomy, Winfield et al. demonstrated that the number of rehospitalizations after extracorporeal lithotripsy monotherapy was as high as 48%, while it was only 6% to 13% for primary percutaneous nephrostolithotomy therapy. Placement of a nephrostomy tube was necessary in upwards of 40% of patients after extracorporeal lithotripsy. In this study, the stone-free rate after extracorporeal lithotripsy monotherapy was only 39% at 8 months. Yet, only 14% of patients treated with percutaneous nephrostolithotomy alone had residual calculi.

A few alternative methods have been explored to treat staghorn calculi. Aso and associates have used ureterorenoscopy and electrohydraulic lithotripsy to treat patients with partial and complete staghorn calculi. They report that 88.2% were successfully treated with this method but operative time was markedly increased. Also, ureteroscopy with ultrasonic stone fragmentation has also been used to debulk staghorn calculi prior to extracorporeal lithotripsy.

As mentioned, the controversy over the appropriate modality to employ in treatment of staghorn calculi exists because no modality is clearly superior. Based on these reports, initial debulking with percutaneous nephrostolithotomy followed by extracorporeal shock wave lithotripsy, if necessary, appears to be the procedure of choice for complete and incomplete staghorn calculi. But for incomplete staghorn calculi, initial treatment could consist of either percutaneous nephrostolithotomy alone or extracorporeal lithotripsy with internal ureteral stenting, especially if the lithotripter to be used is a high-power spark gap generator or variable-power third-generation machine. Treatment of residual calculi can be repeat extracorporeal lithotripsy or staged percutaneous nephrostolithotomy with flexible nephroscopy through the established tract. For complete staghorn calculi, treatment is most efficacious with the combination of percutaneous nephrostolithotomy and extracorporeal lithotripsy.

Open pyelolithotomy or anatrophic nephrolithotomy may be considered for patients with extremely dilated collecting systems. Also, staghorn calculi with multiple calyceal extensions may best be managed with anatrophic nephrolithotomy since multiple secondary percutaneous procedures may be required to clear all affected calyces. As previously mentioned, anatomic abnormalities associated with staghorn calculi may be corrected surgically at the time of stone removal. Moreover, those patients with calyceal or ureteropelvic junction obstruction may require adjunctive postprocedure measures and are at increased risk for complications during extracorporeal shock wave lithotripsy or percutaneous nephrostolithotomy for treatment of staghorn calculi.

CALYCEAL DIVERTICULAR STONES

Treatment of calculi in calyceal diverticula have long been a source of controversy. Some question the clinical significance of these stones and their ability to cause symptoms of such severity as to mandate intervention. Experience with extracorporeal shock wave lithotripsy as monotherapy is varied, with stone-free rates ranging from 20% to 56%. Though the stone-free rate for treatment of calyceal diverticular stones is routinely poor, 75% of patients in one series reported an improvement in or resolution of their symptoms, despite a 25% stone-free rate. Recently, the success rates of extracorporeal lithotripsy, extracorporeal lithotripsy combined with percutaneous nephrostolithotomy, and percutaneous nephrostolithotomy alone were compared for the treatment of calyceal diverticular stones. In the group treated with extracorporeal shock wave lithotripsy alone, the stone-free rate was only 4% with an equally unimpressive symptom-free rate of 36%. In those patients treated with percutaneous nephrostolithotomy alone or combined with extracorporeal shock wave lithotripsy, the stone-free rate was 92%, with 100% of the patients being rendered symptom-free. Therefore, percutaneous nephrostolithotomy may be the

FIGURE 14.12 *Management of Staghorn Calculi*

	STONE-FREE RATE (%)	COMPLICATIONS (%)	HOSPITAL STAY (DAYS)
Shock wave lithotripsy	31–67	28–50	10
PNL	74–68	19–40	5–10

procedure of choice, with small residual calculi secondarily treated with extracorporeal shock wave lithotripsy. Alternatively, because extracorporeal shock wave lithotripsy is noninvasive, the physician and patient may opt for this modality as initial treatment for calyceal diverticular calculi, despite its apparent shortcomings.

LOWER POLE RENAL CALCULI

As the results of the initial clinical series using extracorporeal shock wave lithotripsy were reported, it was clear that treatment of lower pole renal calculi by extracorporeal shock wave lithotripsy was associated with a lower stone-free rate than that of calculi located in other parts of the kidney. In 1986, the U.S. Cooperative Study of Extracorporeal Shock Wave Lithotripsy found by stratifying the stone-free rate by original location of calyceal stones that the stone-free rate for lower pole calculi was 71.1% compared to 83.8% for stones treated in the renal pelvis. Of interest, only 64.1% of stones originally in the superior calyx and 75.7% of middle calyx stones were completely cleared at 3 months in this series. Also, 44.3% of all residual stone fragments were found in the lower pole calyx. A more obvious difference in the stone-free rate of dependent calyceal stones was noted in a later series. In this series, 58% of lower pole calyces were rendered stone-free by extracorporeal shock wave lithotripsy versus 84%, 78%, and 76% respectively, in the renal pelvis, upper pole calyx, and middle calyx.

One study has compared percutaneous stone extraction and extracorporeal shock wave lithotripsy treatment of solitary lower pole calculi. Of the patients treated with percutaneous nephrostolithotomy, 85% were stone-free at 13 months compared to 59% of patients treated with extracorporeal lithotripsy. However, the hospital stay and recovery time were increased in the percutaneous nephrolithotomy group, as were the complication rate and retreatment/auxiliary procedure rate. Extracorporeal lithotripsy was therefore recommended as the treatment of choice for lower pole calculi. In an attempt to overcome this apparent anatomic disadvantage, some centers employ positional techniques to improve clearance of lower pole calyceal stone debris following extracorporeal shock wave lithotripsy.

HORSESHOE KIDNEY

Stones form in approximately 20% of patients with a horseshoe kidney. The ureters arise high in the renal pelvis and pass anteriorly. It is believed that this configuration leads to the common finding of hydronephrosis in patients with horseshoe kidneys, with resultant urinary stasis, infection, and subsequent stone formation. Approximately 50% of patients with stones in horseshoe kidneys treated with extracorporeal lithotripsy monothera-

py will became stone-free. The anteromedial and inferior position of the horseshoe kidney makes stone localization with ultrasound and often fluoroscopy difficult, if not impossible, in some cases. Also, the dilated collecting system of the horseshoe may prevent fragment passage after extracorporeal lithotripsy. A recent study reported on 15 patients with calculi in horseshoe kidneys treated with percutaneous nephrostolithotomy. Approximately 78% of these patients were stone-free at follow-up and this figure improved to 88.8% when extracorporeal lithotripsy was used to treat residual fragments. Caution should be exerted when treating horseshoe kidneys, as anomalous vessels may complicate development of a percutaneous nephrostomy tract by the inexperienced radiologist or urologist.

SOLITARY KIDNEY

Treatment of stones in a solitary kidney provides a significant challenge for the urologist. Prior to the introduction of percutaneous nephrostolithotomy and extracorporeal lithotripsy, retrospective studies failed to reveal any changes in renal function after anatrophic nephrolithotomy of a solitary kidney. Experience with percutaneous nephrostolithotomy in solitary kidneys has been found to be safe and efficacious. Treatment of renal calculi by extracorporeal lithotripsy also was shown to have minimal to no effect in renal function nor was it associated with an increased incidence of complications.

Recently, a long-term comparison of renal function in patients with solitary kidneys and/or moderate renal insufficiency after treatment of renal calculi by percutaneous nephrostolithotomy or extracorporeal lithotripsy was reported. In patients with a solitary kidney and creatinine level less than 2 mg/dL, 13% of patients undergoing percutaneous stone removal and 29% of patients who underwent extracorporeal shock wave lithotripsy showed at least a 25% deterioration of renal function approximately 4 years after their procedure. In patients with a solitary kidney or two kidneys with a creatinine level of 2 to 3 mg/dL, none experienced renal deterioration. In contrast, among patients with a creatinine level greater than 3 mg/dL with either two kidneys or a solitary kidney, 80% of patients undergoing extracorporeal lithotripsy showed a decrease in renal function compared to 0% of patients who underwent percutaneous nephrostolithotomy. The investigators concluded that extracorporeal lithotripsy may be contraindicated in patients with a solitary kidney or two kidneys with a creatinine level greater than 3 mg/dL.

It appears that all modalities available for stone removal are safe and effective in a solitary kidney. Therefore, treatment philosophies for patients with stones in a solitary kidney should for the most part be based on those used in patients with paired kidneys.

Management of Ureteral Calculi

Concomitant to the development of the technologies associated with extracorporeal lithotripsy has been the remarkable advance in modalities for treatment of ureteral calculi. The development of the rigid ureteroscope and, later, the semi-rigid and flexible fiberoptic ureteroscopes has made the entire ureter and renal pelvis accessible for treatment of ureteral and renal stones. Advances in the fiberoptic lens systems of more recent ureteroscopes have decreased the size of the instrument, allowing the ureter to be traversed without prior dilation. Additionally, intracorporeal stone fragmentation has improved with recent developments in electrohydraulic lithotripsy and laser lithotripsy. While most proximal ureteral stones are currently managed by extracorporeal shock wave lithotripsy, ureterorenoscopy continues to be used by many physicians to treat mid and distal ureteral stones. Moreover, ureteroscopic and/or percutaneous access is often useful for the management of ureteral calculi when shock wave lithotripsy has failed.

PROXIMAL URETERAL CALCULI

The options for treatment of proximal ureteral calculi are numerous. Proximal ureteral stones are easily localized and treated with fluoroscopic and ultrasound imaging systems used with various first- and second-generation lithotripters. Stones in the proximal ureter may easily be approached by percutaneous antegrade techniques. Also, with flexible ureteroscopy, the upper ureter is routinely accessible and treatment of proximal stones with various modalities has been quite successful.

A large number of centers are using in situ extracorporeal shock wave lithotripsy monotherapy to treat proximal ureteral stones. First- and second-generation lithotripters that employ fluoroscopy to localize ureteral stones may be used to achieve stone-free rates between 61% to 100% when treating upper ureteral stones. Proximal ureteral calculi may also be pushed into the renal pelvis to facilitate extracorporeal visualization, targeting, and fragmentation (the so-called push-bang technique). Extracorporeal shock wave lithotripsy of proximal ureteral stones can occasionally be tedious with second-generation units that use ultrasound for localization, but fragmentation rates of up to 90% can be expected. Placement of a ureteral stent appears to aid in the fragmentation and visualization of the stone. Recently, an echogenic stent has been developed that may provide additional aid to the urologist using ultrasound to localize ureteral calculi. The renal coil of this stent provides a sonographic landmark that may then be traced through the ureteropelvic junction to the level of the stone.

Proximal ureteral calculi may be approached endoscopically with the flexible ureteroscope and fragmented with either electrohydraulic (EHL) or laser lithotripsy (Fig. 14.13). Initial success with EHL was overshadowed by a relatively high complication rate (up to 40%). With rigid ureteroscopy, 75% and 22% fragmentation rates, respectively, were reported for intracorporeal lithotripsy by EHL for mid and proximal ureteral calculi. Recent studies are more encouraging, with stone-free rates approaching 95% using either 3 Fr or 1.9 Fr EHL with flexible ureteroscopy and insignificant complication rates. Laser lithotripsy of proximal ureteral calculi has proven to be highly efficacious—

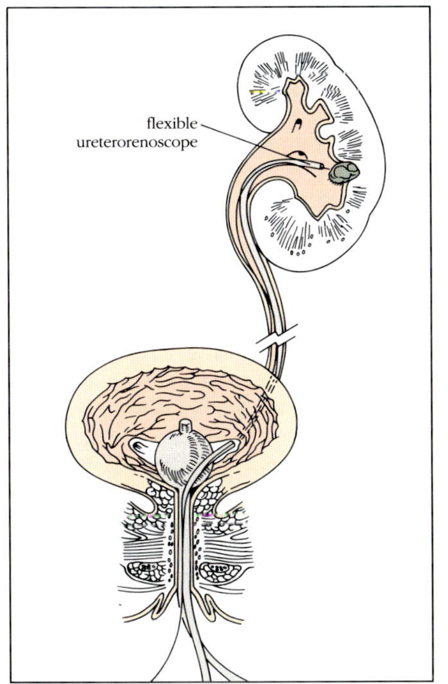

Figure 14.13 Flexible ureterorenoscope used to reach stones trapped within a calyceal diverticulum.

cious and for some investigators is the treatment of choice. Several authors have reported their experiences, with fragmentation rates ranging from 60% to 88%. Cystine and calcium oxalate monohydrate calculi were often poorly fragmented by the early laser prototypes. Fragmentation rates have been improved with larger, higher-power laser fibers and with new lasers (alexandrite).

The percutaneous antegrade approach to proximal ureteral calculi is also a viable treatment option. In one series, 35 of 37 proximal ureteral calculi and 20 of 20 midureteral calculi were successfully removed intact by flexible nephroscopy, fragmented with EHL or ultrasonic lithotripsy, or basketed under fluoroscopic guidance.

MIDURETERAL CALCULI

Treatment of calculi in the midureter has become significantly less troublesome with the advent of the ureteroscope and associated instrumentation used for in situ fragmentation. Extracorporeal lithotripsy is now being used extensively for midureteral stone fragmentation. Earlier studies have reported decreased stone-free rates for midureteral calculi using extracorporeal shock wave lithotripsy. With treatment performed in the prone position, one series reported a 94% stone-free rate with treatment on the HM-3 lithotripter. This position decreases the attenuation of shock waves that is normally encountered with traditional shock wave entry through the patient's back. Again, incorporating the prone position, 100% of patients were stone-free at 3 months after treatment with the second-generation Siemens Lithostar lithotripter. Because of the bony pelvis and sacrum as well as the lack of easily identified sonographic landmarks, extracorporeal shock wave lithotripsy of midureteral calculi using second-generation ultrasound-guided lithotripters has presented significant difficulty. Despite this, some series have shown stone-free rates in excess of 75% for in situ treatment of midureteral stones using ultrasound-guided lithotripters. As with proximal ureteral stones, midureteral calculi may be pushed into the renal pelvis for "routine" extracorporeal shock wave lithotripsy.

If a general anesthetic is required to perform extracorporeal shock wave lithotripsy, ureteroscopy may be considered for stone removal. Midureteral stones are easily accessible by both rigid and flexible ureteroscopy. New, small-diameter, semirigid fiberoptic ureteroscopes obviate the need for dilatation while providing excellent optics, enabling the urologist to treat ureteral calculi in a minimally invasive fashion, and in select cases, under sedation only (Fig. 14.14). In most series, stones in the midureter treated with ureteroscopy are removed in 80% to 95% of cases with EHL, laser lithotripsy, or ultrasonic lithotripsy, with or without basketing. If extracorporeal shock wave lithotripsy is available, it may be reasonable to make an initial attempt to fragment the midureteral stone in situ or proceed with either the "push-bang" technique or with a stent past the stone. Failures may then be approached with repeat extracorporeal lithotripsy or ureteroscopy. If the available lithotripter uses ultrasound for stone localization, or if extracorporeal shock wave lithotripsy is not available, it seems prudent to make the initial attempt at stone removal with the ureteroscope using either EHL or laser lithotripsy to fragment the stone; the stone-free rates are equivalent or superior to extracorporeal shock wave lithotripsy alone.

DISTAL URETERAL STONES

For many clinicians, ureteroscopy is the preferred treatment of distal ureteral calculi, though extracorporeal shock wave lithotripsy is used as treatment of choice by some centers. Recently, several investigators have touted the use of extracorporeal shock wave lithotripsy for the treatment of distal and prevesicular stones with the patient in a prone or modified sitting position. One study demonstrated an 87% stone-free rate with one treatment on the HM-3 lithotripter, with patients positioned in the prone position. Similar results have been noted in other series using the Dornier HM-3 lithotripter for the in situ treatment of distal ureteral stones.

Treatment of distal ureteral stones with rigid ureteroscopy has proven to be reliable and safe, and it requires less technical expertise than more proximal calculi. Lower ureteral stones can be removed by ureteroscopy in approximately 90% to 99% of cases. Although controversy exists as to which intraureteral fragmentation method is superior, it is clear that any of ultrasonic lithotripsy, EHL, or laser lithotripsy will be effective in at least 90% of distal ureteral stones treated. Therefore, the means of intracorporeal fragmentation should be based primarily on the clinician's familiarity with the method chosen and the available equipment.

In summary, some investigators think the treatment of distal ureteral stones may best be managed initially with endoscopic techniques. As excellent results have been obtained with in situ treatment of distal ureteral stones by extracorporeal shock wave lithotripsy, this may become the treatment of choice for some clinicians. Of course, failure of both treatment options may require antegrade percutaneous management or open ureterolithotomy.

Summary

The surgical management of urinary calculus disease has changed dramatically in the past decade. The development of percutaneous nephrostomy techniques has allowed new access to upper tract stones. Percutaneous removal of large calculi was made possible by the development of ultrasonic and electrohydraulic lithotripsy. All upper tract calculi can now successfully be removed in 70% to 100% of cases with minimal complications. Percutaneous techniques have reduced transfusion rates and hospital costs and have markedly shortened convalescence when compared to open surgery.

Ureteroscopy followed percutaneous stone procedures as advanced fiberoptic technology allowed the development of small-caliber instruments required for this procedure. With experience, successful stone retrieval has occurred in upwards of 90% of cases, again with minimal complications. As percutaneous nephrostolithotomy and ureteroscopy have become available, the subspecialty of endourology has emerged and significantly changed the management of urinary tract calculi.

Perhaps the most significant advance in stone therapy has been the design and implementation of extracorporeal shock wave lithotripsy. With this noninvasive technique, most renal and proximal ureteral calculi can be effectively treated with minimal morbidity and convalescence. Research in lithotripter design is ongoing, with more advanced and effective machines on the horizon. The applicability of extracorporeal shock wave lithotripsy to biliary tract calculi is currently under investigation.

Finally, one should not disparage the importance of medical therapy for recurrent nephrolithiasis. Selective medical therapy of nephrolithiasis is highly effective in preventing new stone formation. A remission rate higher than 80% and overall reduction in individual stone formation rate of more than 90% can be obtained in patients with nephrolithiasis. In patients with mild to moderate stone disease, virtually total control of stone disease can be achieved with a remission rate greater than 95% (Fig. 14.15). The need for stone removal may be dramatically reduced by an effective prophylactic program. Selective pharmacologic therapy of nephrolithiasis also encompasses the advantages of overcoming nonrenal complications as well as averting certain side effects that may be caused by nonselective medical therapy. Despite these advantages, it is clear that selective medical therapy cannot provide total control of stone disease. A satisfactory response requires continued, dedicated compliance by patients to the recommended program and a commitment by the physician to provide long-term follow-up and care.

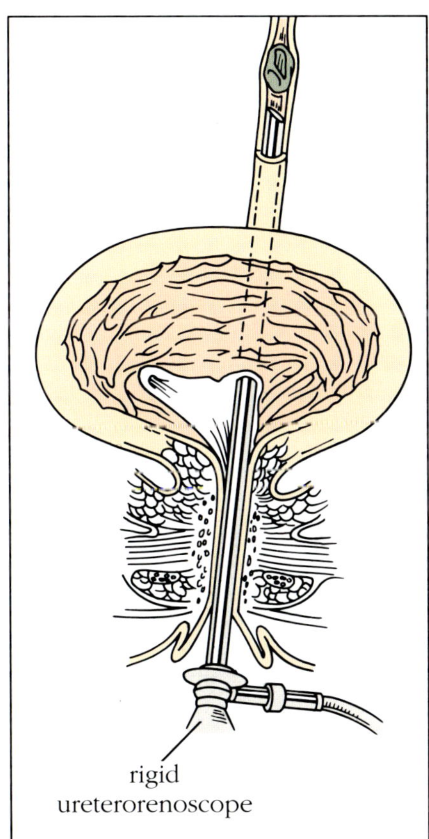

Figure 14.14 An obstructing calculus with a rigid ureterorenoscope passed to the midureter.

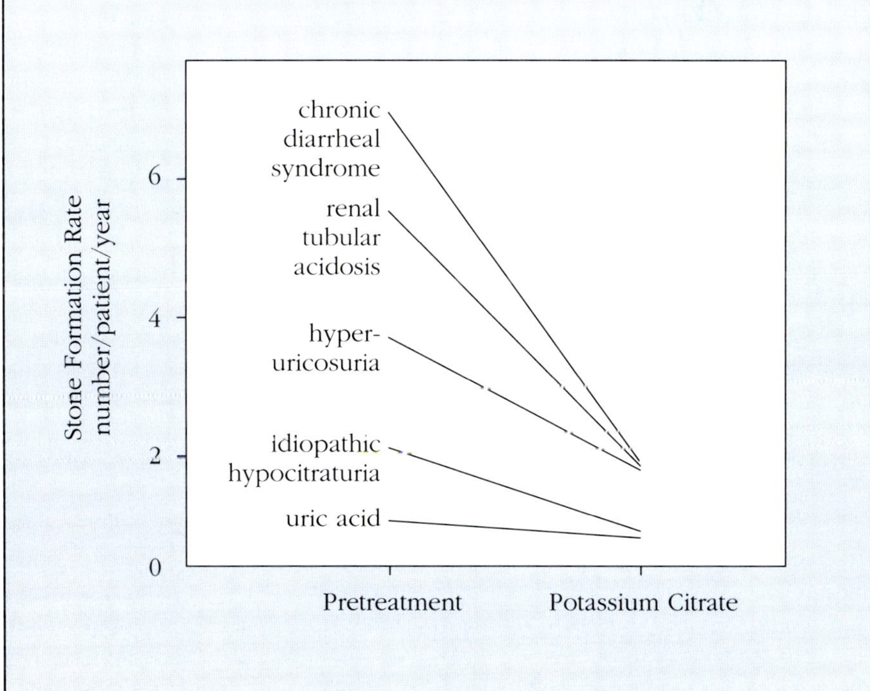

Figure 14.15 The impact of medical therapy on the rate of stone formation.

References

EXTRACORPOREAL SHOCK WAVE LITHOTRIPSY

Becht E, Moll V, Neisius D, Ziegler M. Treatment of provesical ureteral calculi by extracorporeal shock wave lithotripsy. *J Urol.* 1988;139:916–918.

Chaussy C, Schmiedt E, Jocham D, Brendel W, Forssmann B, Walther V. First clinical experience with extracorporeally induced destruction of kidney stones by shock waves. *J Urol.* 1982;127:417–420.

Constantinides C, Recker F, Jaeger P, Hauri D. Extracorporeal shock wave lithotripsy as monotherapy of staghorn renal calculi: 3 years experience. *J Urol.* 1989;142:1415–1418.

Gleeson MJ, Griffith DP. Extracorporeal lithotripsy monotherapy for large renal calculi. *Br J Urol.* 1989;64:329–332.

Graff J, Diederichs W, Schulze H. Long-term follow up in 1003 extracorporeal shockwave lithotripsy patients. *J Urol.* 1988;140:479.

Haupt G, Benkert S, Graff J, Senge T. Results of more than 1500 ESWL treatments with the MFL 5000. *J Endourol.* 1990;4:S151.

Keele LL, McNamara TC, Dorey FO, Milster RE. *De novo* extracorporeal shock wave lithotripsy for lower ureteral calculi: treatment of choice. *J Endourol.* 1990;4:71.

Lingeman JE, Newman D, Mertz JH, et al. Extracorporeal shock wave lithotripsy: the Methodist Hospital of Indiana experience. *J Urol.* 1986;135:1134–1137.

Marberger M, Turk C, Steinkogler I. Painless piezo-electric extracorporeal lithotripsy. *J Urol.* 1988;139:695.

Mazone DJ, Chiang B. Extracorporeal shock wave lithotripsy of stones in the upper, middle, and lower ureter. *J Endourol.* 1988;2:107.

Neisius D, Zwergel TH, Jung P, Ziegler M. Extracorporeal piezoelectic lithotripsy (EPL) with the new Piezolith 2500: first clinical experiences. *J Endourol.* 1990; 4:S92.

Preminger GM. Sonographic piezoelectric lithotripsy: more bang for your buck. *J Endourol.* 1989; 3:321–327.

Rassweiler J, Gumpinger R, Mayer R, et al. Extracorporeal piezoelectric lithotripsy using the Wolf-Lithotripter versus low energy lithotripsy with the modified Dornier HM-3: a cooperative study. *World J Urol.* 1987;5:218.

Rassweiler J, Kohrmann KU, Wess O, Alken P. Modulith SL20—its clinical establishment. *J Endourol.* 1990;4:S90.

Rassweiler J, Westhauser A, Bub P, Eisenberger F. Second-generation lithotripters: a comparative study. *J Endourol.* 1988;2:193–204.

Rodriques Netto N, Casterta Lemos G, Claro JFA: *In situ* extracorporeal shock wave lithotripsy for ureteral calculi. *J Urol.* 1990;144:253.

Tiselius HG, Pettersson B, Anderson A. Extracorporeal shock wave lithotripsy of stones in the mid ureter. *J Urol.* 1989;141:280.

Turk C, Steinkogler I, Krings F, Marberger M. First experience with a lithotripter with in-line ultrasonic and flouroscopic stone localization. *J Endourol.* 1990;4:S90.

Vallancien G, Aviles J, Munoz R, et al. Piezoelectric extracorporeal lithotripsy by ultrashort waves with the EDAP LT01 device. *J Urol.* 1988;139:689.

Zwergel U, Neisius D, Zwergel T, Ziegler M. Results and clinical management of extracorporeal piezoelectric lithotripsy (EPL) in 1321 consecutive treatments. *World J Urol.* 1987;5:213.

PERCUTANEOUS NEPHROSTOLITHOTOMY

Cohen ES, Schmidt JD. Extracorporeal shock wave lithotripsy for stones in solitary kidney. *Urology.* 1990;36:52.

Jones JA, Lingeman JE, Steidle CP. The roles of extracorporeal shock wave lithotripsy and percutaneous nephrostolithotomy in the management of pyelocaliceal diverticula. *J Urol.* 1991;146:724–727.

Lingeman JE, Coury TA, Newman DM, et al. Comparison of results and morbidity of percutaneous nephrostolithotomy and extracorporeal shock wave lithotripsy. *J Urol.* 1987;138:485–490.

Preminger GM, Clayman RV, Hardeman SW, Franklin J, Curry T, Peters PC. Percutaneous nephrostolithotomy versus open surgery for renal calculi: a comparative study. *JAMA.* 1985;254:1054.

Schulze H, Hertle L, Kutta A, Graff J, Senge T. Critical evaluation of treatment of staghorn calculi by percutaneous nephrolithotomy and extracorporeal shock wave lithotripsy. *J Urol.* 1989;141:822–825.

Segura JW, Patterson DE, Leroy AJ, et al. Percutaneous removal of kidney stones: review of 1,000 cases. *J Urol.* 1985;134:1077–1081.

Streem SB, Zelch MG, Risius B, Geisinger MA: Percutaneous extraction of renal calculi in patients with solitary kidneys. *Urology.* 1986;27:247–252.

Winfield HN, Clayman RV, Chaussy CG, Weyman PJ, Fuchs GJ, Lupu AN. Monotherapy of staghorn renal calculi: comparative study between percutaneous nephrolithotomy and extracorporeal shock wave lithotripsy. *J Urol.* 1988;139:895.

URETEROSCOPY

Aso Y, Ohta N, Nakano M, Ohtawara Y, Tajima A, Kawabe K. Treatment of staghorn calculi by fiberoptic transurethral nephrolithotripsy. *J Urol.* 1990;144:17–19.

Begun FP, Jacobs SC, Lawson RK. Use of a prototype 3F electrohydraulic electrode with ureteroscopy for treatment of ureteral calculous disease. *J Urol.* 1988;139:1188–1191.

Blute ML, Segura JW, Patterson DE. Ureteroscopy. *J Urol.* 1988;139:510.

Denstedt JD, Clayman RV. Electrohydraulic lithotripsy of renal and ureteral calculi. *J Urol.* 1990;143(1):13–17.

Dretler SP. Laser photofragmentation of ureteral calculi: analysis of 75 cases. *J Endourol.* 1987;1:9.

Dretler SP. An evaluation of ureteral laser lithotripsy: 225 consecutive patients. *J Urol.* 1990;143(2):267–272.

Dretler SP, Keating MA, Riley J. An algorithm for the management of ureteral calculi. *J Urol.* 1986;136: 1190–1193.

Dretler SP, Watson G, Parhish L, Murray S. Laser fragmentation of ureteral calculi: initial experience. *J Urol.* 1987;137:386.

Feagins BA, Wilson WT, Preminger GM. Intracorporeal electrohydraulic lithotripsy with flexible ureterorenoscopy. *J Endourol.* 1990;4:347–351.

Higashihara E, Horie S, Takeuchi T, et al. Laser ureterolithotripsy with combined rigid and flexible ureterorenoscopy. *J Urol.* 1990;143:273.

Huffman JL. Experience with the 8.5 French compact rigid ureteroscope. *Semin Urol.* 1989;7:3–6.

Kahn RL. Endourological treatment of ureteral calculi. *J Urol.* 1986;135:239.

Lingeman JE, Sonda LP, Kahnoski RJ, et al. Ureteral stone management: emerging concepts. *J Urol.* 1986; 135:1172.

Politis G, Griffith DP: Ureteroscopy in management of ureteral calculi. *Urology.* 1987;30:39.

Preminger GM, Roehrborn CG. Special applications of flexible deflectable ureterorenoscopy. *Semin Urol.* 1989;7:16–24.

OPEN SURGERY

Assimos DG, Boyce WH, Hamson CH, McCullough DL, Kroovand RL, Sweat KR: Role of open stone surgery since extracorporeal shock wave lithotripsy. *J Urol.* 1989;142:263.

Chang CR, Webb DR, Payne SR, Wichhara JE. Comparison of treatment of renal calculi by open surgery, percutaneous nephrolithotomy and extracorporeal shock wave lithotripsy. *Br Med J.* 1986;292:879.

COMBINATION THERAPY

Kahnoski RJ, Lingeman JE, Lowry TA, Steele RE, Mosbaugh PG. Combined percutaneous and extracorporeal shock wave lithotripsy for staghorn calculi: an alternative to anatrophic nephrolithotomy. *J Urol.* 1986;135:679.

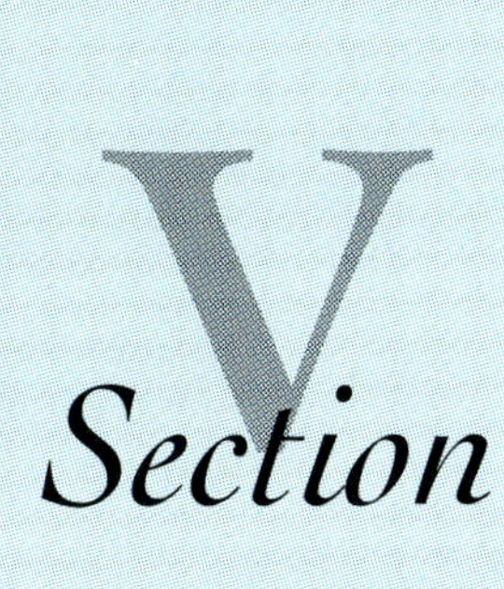

Inflammatory Disease

Robert Moldwin, editor

CHAPTER 15

Recurring Cystitis in the Sexually Active Female Patient

Robert Moldwin

Ten percent to 20% of women develop a urinary tract infection (UTI) during their lifetimes. Most of these infections are confined to the bladder (cystitis) and are easily eradicated with one of a wide variety of antibiotics. In most patients cystitis never recurs or, at worst, recurs sporadically and infrequently. Unfortunately, some women acquire bacterial cystitis two or more times per year. Most of these patients are premenopausal, sexually active women who are understandably frustrated by their repeated bouts with dysuria, frequency, and urgency (Fig. 15.1).

Over the past 15 years remarkable advances have been made towards understanding the pathogenesis of recurring UTIs. This has led to useful methods of prevention and treatment, which are discussed below.

Defining the Jargon: What Is Cystitis?

"Bacterial cystitis" implies an invasive infection of the bladder resulting in an inflammatory reaction. Typical symptoms include dysuria, urinary frequency and urgency, and a feeling of suprapubic fullness. A urinalysis usually reveals many leukocytes and erythrocytes. High fever, chills, flank tenderness, and white cell casts seen on microscopic examination of the urinary sediment are more typical of pyelonephritis. Even with these differential criteria available, many patients with an infection seemingly confined to the bladder prove to have a subclinical focus of upper tract infection.[1]

The urine culture, our gold standard for the diagnosis of bacterial cystitis, has undergone changes in interpretation over the past 10 years. Originally, significant bacteriuria was defined as $>10^5$ colony-forming units (CFU)/mL. This value enabled the diagnosis of pyelonephritis to be made within 95% confidence limits[2] yet excluded 30% to 50% of women with the classic symptoms of acute bacterial cystitis. Stamm et al.[3] were instrumental in redefining the criterion for bacterial cystitis as $>10^2$ CFU/mL. Nevertheless, women with symptoms of acute cystitis who demonstrate fewer than 10^2 CFU/mL of urine account for approximately 31% of patients.[4] Moreover, cystitis can be caused by pathogens not detectable on standard cultures (e.g., *Mycobacterium tuberculosis* and the etiologic agents of nongonococcal urethritis, *Chlamydia trachomatis* and *Ureaplasma urealyticum*) (Fig. 15.2).

The presence of bacteria on microscopic examination of the urine sediment is often helpful in diagnosing a UTI. However, its sensitivity is limited when the diagnosis of cystitis is considered, as bacterial counts must be at least 30,000/mL for the organisms to be detected under the microscope.[5]

Pathogenesis

The bacteria that cause most UTIs are acquired from the large bowel. The higher overall incidence of UTIs in women is thought to be attributable to the close proximity of the urethral meatus to the fecal reservoir. The retrograde movement of bacteria into the bladder is further facilitated by the relatively short (2 to 4 cm) female urethra.

Enterobacteria appear to be more likely to colonize the vaginal introitus of women who develop recurrent UTIs than of control subjects.[6] Recent studies suggest that

FIGURE 15.1 *Types of Infection in Women with Recurring Cystitis (After Stamey[5])*

FIRST INFECTION	Uniformly symptomatic, community acquired; 80% are caused by *Escherichia coli*. Responds well to variety of antibiotics
BACTERIAL PERSISTENCE	Return of infection several days after discontinuance of antibiotics with isolation of the same organism. Such infections have been described as "complicated"[12] and may indicate an anatomic abnormality
UNRESOLVED BACTERIURIA	Continuance of infection despite antibiotic or surgical therapy. Usually indicates previous or acquired antibiotic resistance or poor bioavailability (e.g., azotemia, calculus disease with infected stone)
REINFECTION	New infection involving different organism or strain. Reinfection accounts for almost all recurring UTIs

this abnormal colonization is mediated by increased binding of uropathic bacteria to the vaginal and bladder mucosa.[7,8] Such binding seems to be related to the presence or unmasking of specific receptors on the mucosal surface that interact with bacterial pili. Schaeffer et al.[9] recently demonstrated that uropathic bacteria also adhere more readily to buccal cells from women with recurrent UTIs, suggesting a generalized phenotypic alteration in receptor expression in these patients.

PERSONAL HYGIENE

To date, there is no evidence that bathroom habits such as the direction of wiping oneself after a bowel movement, the wearing of tight clothing, and vaginal douching have any effect on the development of repeated bouts of cystitis.[10]

SEXUAL ASPECTS

For many years, clinicians had noted a dramatic rise in the incidence of cystitis with the onset of sexual activity. Indeed, many women seemed to develop cystitis within 24 to 48 hours after sexual intercourse. This "honeymoon cystitis," however, was dismissed by many investigators as coincidental.

In 1978, Buckley et al.[11] demonstrated that 23 (30%) of the 76 patients they studied had a tenfold increase in urinary bacterial counts after sexual intercourse, which was thought to "milk" bacteria (normally dwelling in the periurethral region) in a retrograde fashion into the urethra and bladder. Another supporting study revealed that nuns 18 to 35 years of age were 12.8 times less likely to develop urinary tract infections than were white working women of the same age group.[12] Finally, the dramatic

decrease in infection rates with a program of postcoital antibiotic prophylaxis spoke for the important role of sexual intercourse in recurring cystitis.[13,14]

CONTRACEPTIVE USE
Diaphragm

The diaphragm is the only method of birth control that has a confirmed role in the development of urinary tract infections. Both vaginal colonization and urinary tract infections are significantly more common in diaphragm users than in women using other forms of contraception.[15–17] Gillespie[18] suggested that the diaphragm's effect is mediated by a mild urethral obstruction, pointing out the greater time needed to achieve peak urine flow when a diaphragm is in place. However, no significant volume of postvoiding residual urine (suggestive of urine stasis) was noted in her patients.

Spermicides

Spermicidal foams and jellies may be more important in predisposing the patient to cystitis than the diaphragm itself.[16,17] Recent studies show that the active component of such products, nonoxynol-9, promotes vaginal colonization and bacteriuria with *Escherichia coli*.[16] Other investigators point out that the reduced numbers of lactobacilli in the vaginal vault in women who use spermicides may predispose them to bacterial vaginosis.[19]

An interesting side issue has been the finding that nonoxynol-9-impregnated contraceptive sponges reduce the incidence of chlamydial and gonoccocal infections.[20] In addition, recent in vitro studies suggest that nonoxynol-9 may have protective value against HIV[21] and trichomonal infections.[22] The higher prevalence of candiduria found

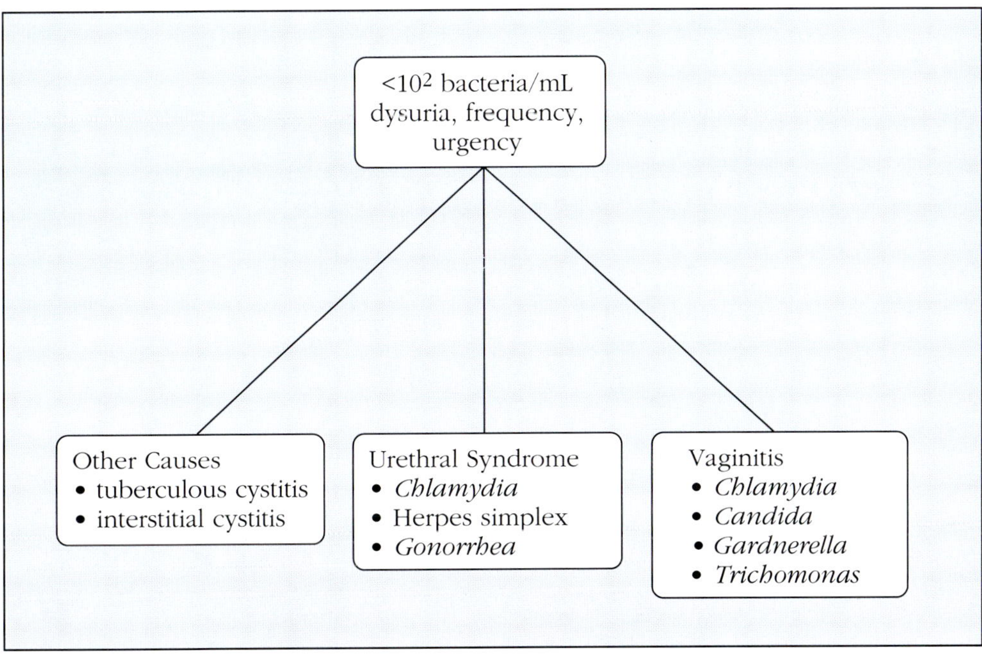

Figure 15.2 Causes of recurrent cystitis.

with these preparations is believed to be secondary to changes in the *Lactobacillus* colonization of the vaginal vault.[16,20]

Oral Contraception

Although hormonal factors appear to be involved in susceptibility to UTI, at present no data demonstrate a clear association between oral contraceptive use and recurrent cystitis.[23]

Evaluation

The initial evaluation of patients with recurring cystitis begins with a history and physical examination. In addition to eliciting the typical symptomatology of cystitis, patients should be questioned regarding the type of contraception used and the temporal relations of the symptoms to sexual intercourse. A history of gynecologic complaints such as vaginal discharge, a foul vaginal odor, and pruritus, all suggestive of vaginitis, should also be sought. A history of childhood pyelonephritis, renal stones, unusual cultured organisms, or previous urologic surgery places the patient at higher risk for complicated urinary tract infections, and a more aggressive work-up may be indicated. Surgically correctable structural abnormalities may finally declare themselves through the failure of standard antibiotic therapy.

We usually base our initial diagnosis of bacterial cystitis on the clinical presentation, a microscopic examination of the urinary sediment, and the esterase dipstick test, which is specific for the presence of leukocytes and has a sensitivity of 80%. This test, combined with microscopic analysis, brings the overall confidence limits of a diagnosis of infection to 85% to 90%. The final diagnosis of cystitis is achieved with a cultured clean-catch midstream urine specimen.

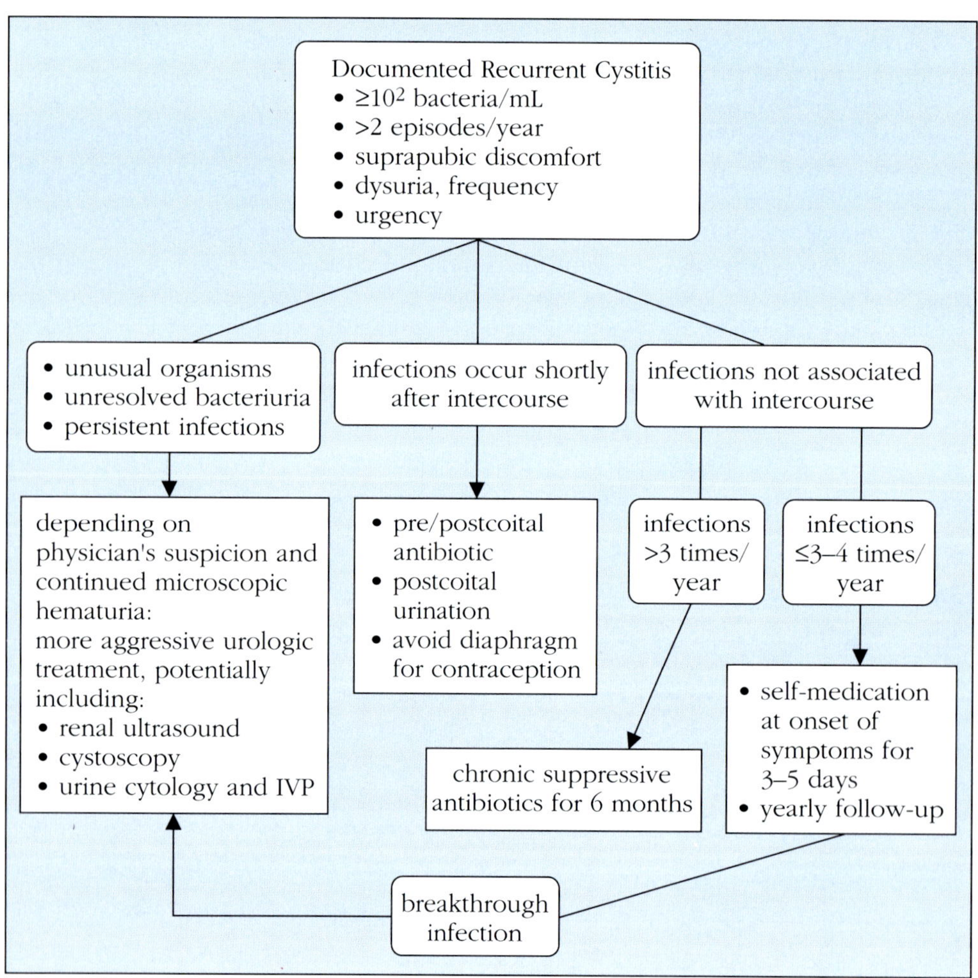

Figure 15.3 Algorithm for treatment of recurrent cystitis.

Routine intravenous urography and cystoscopy, once commonly performed on patients with recurrent UTIs, are used much less frequently today because the yield of significant findings is so low. The screening renal ultrasound scan, a relatively low-cost and noninvasive procedure, has, for the most part, become standard for identification of the 5% of patients who develop repeated UTIs secondary to a structural abnormality. As previously mentioned, a more aggressive work-up may be necessary based on the physician's index of suspicion.

Treatment

Our algorithm for the treatment of recurrent cystitis (Fig. 15.3) is based on the infection's temporal relation to sexual intercourse. If the infections occur immediately (within 24 to 48 hours) after intercourse, we recommend precoital or postcoital antibiotic prophylaxis. Drug resistance and alterations in the vaginal flora (with subsequent yeast vaginitis) are uncommon with such measures because of the short course of therapy. Agents with good success rates include nitrofurantoin macrocrystals, trimethoprim with or without sulfamethoxazole, cephalosporins, penicillins, and fluoroquinolones. We also recommend postcoital urination to wash out any bacteria that were introduced into the bladder. If the patient uses a diaphragm, we suggest changing to an alternative method of contraception.

If the development of cystitis does not appear to be related to sexual intercourse, two other methods of treatment are available.

CHRONIC PROPHYLAXIS

Long-term therapy involves one suppressive dose of an antibiotic each night or every other night. It is believed that the resulting constant presence of antibiotics in the urine decreases bacterial adherence to the urothelial surface.[24] The choice of drug is more important in these situations than in postcoital prophylaxis. The ideal drug has few side effects, achieves high urine concentrations, is unlikely to be associated with the development of drug resistance, and has little effect on the vaginal flora. Parsons[25] has reviewed the medications available and suggests nitrofurantoin macrocrystals as first-line therapy. The frequency of gastrointestinal upset seems to be this medication's chief disadvantage. Other appropriate medications are listed in Figure 15.4. Recurrent breakthrough infections during chronic prophylaxis suggest the need to reevaluate the patient for evidence of structural abnormalities or subclinical pyelonephritis.

SELF-THERAPY

Once the diagnosis of recurring cystitis has been established, we usually have the patients self-medicate. They are instructed to begin full-course therapy for 3 to 5 days at the onset of symptoms. This is a particularly helpful technique for those patients who experience less than three infections per year. We have found that such early treatment decreases the patient's symptomatic interval, gives her a sense of control over the problem, and enhances her overall satisfaction with medical care.

Although single-dose therapy has a high success rate, we do not use it routinely. Our concern is with the occasional patient who does not respond favorably to this regimen and misinterprets this outcome as the result of undertreatment. Also, many patients remain symptomatic for 24 to 48 hours after the onset of therapy and feel more comfortable if they take antibiotics during this time.

Patients are followed on a yearly basis or at shorter intervals if breakthrough infections arise. They are instructed to keep a diary of any infections to help guide future care.

Conclusion

Recurring cystitis is commonly seen in the sexually active woman. Coliform bacteria tend to colonize the vaginal vault and periurethral region of frequently infected women much more readily than in normal subjects. In many patients, sexual intercourse appears to potentiate the passage of these bacteria into the urethra and bladder.

The practitioner must be cautious when initially evaluating these patients to exclude complicating conditions (i.e., pyelonephritis, structural abnormalities) and other entities with similar symptomatology (i.e., vaginitis, urethritis). With an accurate diagnosis established, effective therapy can be achieved by pre/postcoital prophylaxis, chronic prophylaxis, or self-medication. The drug should be chosen on the basis of cost-effectiveness, lack of side effects, and a low propensity for microbial resistance and yeast vaginitis. Also helpful in preventing repeated episodes of cystitis may be a change in contraception from the diaphragm to alternative methods.

FIGURE 15.4 *Commonly Used Antibiotics in the Treatment of Cystitis*

ANTIBIOTIC	USUAL DOSAGE FOR ACUTE INFECTION (3 to 5 days)	PROPHYLACTIC DOSE (q.h.s. or pre-/postcoital)	DRUG RESISTANCE	RISK OF YEAST INFECTION
Nitrofurantoin macrocrystals	50 mg q.i.d.	50 mg	Low	Low
Trimethoprim-sulfamethox-azole	2 tablets, 80 mg TMP 400 mg SMX, b.i.d.	1/2–1 tablet	Moderate	Moderate
Trimethoprim	100 mg b.i.d.	50 mg	Low with suppression; high with full course	Moderate
Cephalexin	250–500 mg q.i.d., t.i.d.	250 mg	Low with suppression; high with full course	Moderate
Fluoroquinolones				
Norfloxacin	400 mg b.i.d.	400 mg	Low	Moderate
Ofloxacin	200 mg b.i.d.	200 mg	Low	Moderate
Ciprofloxacin	500 mg b.i.d.	250 mg	Low	Moderate
Enoxacin	200 mg b.i.d.	200 mg	Low	Moderate
Amoxicillin	250 mg t.i.d.	250 mg	High	Very high (25%)

ANTIBIOTIC	MAJOR ADVERSE EFFECTS	USE IN PREGNANCY	COST	COMMENTS
Nitrofurantoin macrocrystals	GI upset, pulmonary fibrosis, peripheral neuropathy	Associated with hemolytic anemia in G6PD deficiency	Low	Nausea less with macrocrystalline form; should be taken with meals; pulmonary fibrosis with long-term use; best overall first-line antibiotic
Trimethoprim-sulfamethox-azole	Blood dycrasias at term and during lactation	May cause kernicterus if administered at term or first 2 months post-partum	High	—
Trimethoprim	Blood dyscrasias, rash	—	Moderate	Not recommended for full-course therapy owing to development of resistant organisms
Cephalexin	—	—	High	Recommended only for pre-/postcoital and suppressive therapy
Fluoroquinolones				
Norfloxacin	Nausea, diarrhea, headache	Contraindicated during pregnancy and lactation	Very high	These drugs cover a wide range of Gram-negative bacteria; not recommended as first-line therapy owing to high cost and potential development of resistance
Ofloxacin			Very high	
Ciprofloxacin			Very high	
Enoxacin			Very high	
Amoxicillin	—	—	Moderate	Good for pre-/postcoital prophylaxis; limited role in full-course or chronic suppressive therapy owing to profound effect on vaginal flora

References

1. Johnson JR, Stamm WE. Urinary tract infections in women: diagnosis and treatment. *Ann Intern Med.* 1989;111:906–917.

2. Kass EH, Savage W, Santamarina BA. The sigificance of bacteriuria in preventive medicine. In: Kass EH, ed. *Progress in Pyelonephritis.* Philadelphia, Pa: FA Davis; 1965:3–10.

3. Stamm WE, et al. Diagnosis of coliform infections in acutely dysuric women. *N Engl J Med.* 1982;307:463–468.

4. Pfau AS, Sacks TG. An evaluation of midstream urine cultures in the diagnosis of urinary tract infections in women. *Urol Int.* 1970;25:326–341.

5. Shortliffe LM, Stamey TA. Infections of the urinary tract: introduction and general principles. In: Walsh PC, Perlmutter AD, et al, eds. *Campbell's Urology.* 5th ed. Philadelphia, Pa: WB Saunders; 1985:738–784.

6. Pfau A, Sacks T. The bacterial flora of the vaginal vestibule, urethra and vagina in premenopausal women with recurrent urinary tract infections. *J Urol.* 1981;126:630–634.

7. Fowler JE, Stamey TA. Studies of introital colonization in women with recurrent urinary infections, VII: the role of bacterial adherence. *J Urol.* 1977;117:472–476.

8. Stamey T. Recurrent urinary tract infections in female patients: an overview of management and treatment. *Rev Infect Dis.* 1987;9(suppl 2):S195–S211.

9. Schaeffer A, Jones JM, Dunn JK. Association of *in vitro Escherichia coli* adherence to vaginal and buccal epithelial cells with susceptibility of women to recurrent urinary-tract infections. *N Engl J Med.* 1981;304:1062–1066.

10. Strom BL, Collins M, West SL, Kreisberg J, Weller S. Sexual activity, contraceptive use, and other risk factors for symptomatic and asymptomatic bacteriuria. *Ann Intern Med.* 1987;107:816–823.

11. Buckley RM, McGuckin M, MacGregor RR. Urine bacterial counts after sexual intercourse. *N Engl J Med.* 1978; 298:321–324.

12. Kunin CM, McCormack RG. An epidemiologic study of bacteriuria and blood pressure among nuns and working women. *N Engl J Med.* 1968;278:635–642.

13. Stapleton A, Latham RH, Johnson C, Stamm WE. Postcoital antimicrobial prophylaxis for recurrent urinary tract infection: a randomized, double-blind, placebo-controlled trial. *JAMA.* 1990;264:703–706.

14. Pfau A, Sacks T, Engelstein D. Recurrent urinary tract infections in premenopausal women: prophylaxis based on an understanding of the pathogenesis. *J Urol.* 1983;129: 1153–1157.

15. Fihn SD, Latham RH, Roberts P, Running K, Stamm WE. Association between diaphragm use and urinary tract infection. *JAMA.* 254:240–245.

16. Hooton TM, Hillier S, Johnson C, Roberts PL, Stamm WE. *Escherichia coli* bacteriuria and contraceptive method. *JAMA.* 1991;265:64–69.

17. Fihn SD, Johnson C, Pinkstaff C, Stamm WE. Diaphragm use and urinary tract infections: analysis of urodynamic and microbiological factors. *J Urol.* 1986;136:853–856.

18. Gillespie L. The diaphragm: an accomplice in recurrent urinary tract infections. *Urology.* 1984;24:25–30.

19. Hooton TM, Fihn SD, Johnson C, Roberts PL, Stamm WE. Association between bacterial vaginosis and acute cystitis in women using diaphragms. *Arch Intern Med.* 1989;149: 1932–1936.

20. Rosenberg MJ, Rojanapithayakorn W, Feldblum PJ, Higgins JE. Effect of the contraceptive sponge on chlamydial infection, gonorrhea, and candidiasis. *JAMA.* 1987;257:2308–2312.

21. Hicks DR, Martin LS, Getchell JP, et al. Inactivation of HTLV-III/LAV-infected cultures of normal human lymphocytes by nonoxynol-9 in vitro. *Lancet.* 1985;2:1422–1423.

22. Stone KM, Grimes DA, Magder LS. Personal protection against sexually transmitted diseases. *Am J Obstet Gynecol.* 1986;155:180–188.

23. Evans DA, Hennekens CH, Miao L, et al. Oral contraceptive use and bacteriuria in a community based study. *N Engl J Med.* 1978;299:536–537.

24. Beachey EH. Adhesin-receptor interactions mediating the attachment of bacteria to mucosal surfaces. *J Infect Dis.* 1987;143:325–345.

25. Parsons CL. Protocol for treatment of typical urinary tract infection: criteria for antimicrobial selection. *Urology.* 1988;32:22–25.

CHAPTER 16

Epididymitis

Robert Moldwin

Acute epididymitis can occur in men and boys of all ages but is more common after the onset of sexual activity. Although relatively rare in children, epididymitis is frequently associated with structural or neurologic anomalies and usually coexists with bacteriuria. Coliforms are the most common pathogens seen in this group of patients.

Epididymitis caused by sexually transmitted pathogens is usually seen in heterosexual men under the age of 35. The pathogens involved are usually *Neisseria gonorrhoeae* and/or *Chlamydia trachomatis,* organisms that are commonly associated with urethritis. Homosexual males who practice anal intercourse are more likely to develop a coliform infection. These findings support the retrograde inoculation of the epididymitis in most cases.

In men over the age of 35, coliforms again become the leading cause of epididymitis. As in the male child, epididymitis is often precipitated by bacteriuria. The bacteriuria is usually associated with structural and/or neurologic pathology. Iatrogenic sources of infection (i.e., cystoscopy, indwelling Foley catheters) are also common in this group of patients.[1]

Evaluation

Diagnosing acute epididymitis is often difficult. Other intrascrotal pathologies that can mimic the signs and symptoms of acute epididymitis include testicular torsion, tumors, trauma, incarcerated hernia, and thrombosis of the pampiniform plexus. Torsion is more common in patients under 20 years of age, whereas testicular tumors are more common in patients over 20 years of age.

The patient with acute epididymitis usually presents with a several-day history of gradually worsening testicular pain, although occasionally the pain is of sudden onset and associated with straining. When bacteriuria is present the patient may also complain of urinary frequency, urgency, and dysuria. Fever and leukocytosis are common and can be associated with pyelonephritis. A rectal examination to rule out acute prostatitis is extremely important in these patients. Epididymitis caused by sexually transmitted pathogens is often accompanied by concomitant urethritis and an associated discharge.[2]

The findings at physical examination may change as the disease progresses (Fig. 16.1). Inflammation usually involves the tail of the epididymis first, then gradually progresses to the head and ultimately to the testicle. In the interim, landmarks such as the epididymal–testicular sulcus may become obscured. An anesthetic block of the spermatic cord is often helpful to relieve severe pain temporarily for the examination. Finally, a "reactive" hydrocele may form, which makes an accurate examination impossible. In these instances the fluid can be aspirated or an ultrasound study of the region obtained.

The epididymis is usually exquisitely tender and indurated to palpation. This finding is not necessarily diagnostic, since approximately 15% of testicular torsions present in this manner as a consequence of venous engorgement.[3] Tenderness solely in the upper pole of the epididymis should raise the question of torsion of the appendix testes. Unlike testicular torsion, foreshortening of the spermatic cord is not seen until the later stages of acute epididymitis. Because of contiguous infection, the spermatic cord is usually tender early in patients with epididymitis but only during the later stages of testicular torsion.

Sexually active men should have a Gram stain of a urethral smear performed for evaluation of *N gonorrhoeae*

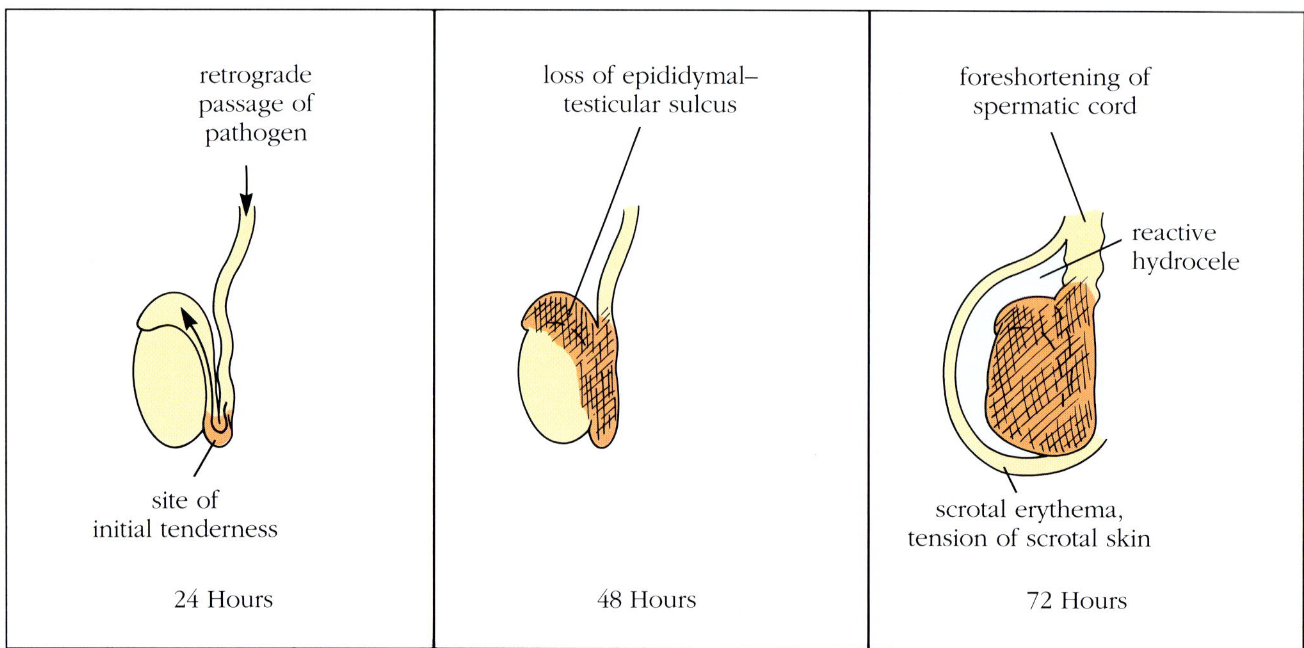

Figure 16.1 Stages of epididymitis.

(intracellular Gram-negative diplococci). The presence of leukocytes alone on urethral smear suggests infection with *C trachomatis,* which also can be assumed to be present in approximately 30% of patients who harbor gonococcal organisms.[2] Only after material is obtained for a urethral smear should midstream urine be obtained for analysis and culture, as the urine stream may wash many leukocytes and organisms from the urethra and result in a false-negative evaluation.

It is extremely important to pair laboratory and clinical findings. For example, pyuria is occasionally present in patients with testicular torsion and may lead to an incorrect diagnosis if not interpreted with other clinical data.[4] In the case of an equivocal diagnosis, a testicular nuclear scan is usually diagnostic. However, I tend to reserve this testing for patients with a very low suspicion of torsion, since delays in performing scrotal exploration may be associated with loss of the testicle.

A relatively new modality to distinguish epididymitis from acute testicular torsion is color-flow Doppler. The main advantages of this technique are that it is noninvasive and provides a *rapid,* acurate diagnosis.

Treatment

Three general measures should be instituted in all cases of epididymitis: bed rest, scrotal support/elevation, and nonsteroidal antiinflammatory agents (Fig. 16.2). The patient with bacteriuria in the midstream urine collection should receive initial broad-spectrum antibiotic coverage. Hospital admission for administration of parenteral antibiotics should be dictated by the clinical situation such as signs of sepsis, abscess formation, or significant pain. All patients in this category should undergo a thorough urologic evaluation to rule out structural anomalies. If bladder dysfunction is suspected, urodynamic evaluation is indicated. Bacteriuria also suggests an underlying prostate infection. Therefore, I tend to treat these patients for long periods of time (6 to 8 weeks) to prevent the development of chronic bacterial prostatitis. The choice of antimicrobials is discussed below.

Patients who present without bacteriuria are more common in clinical practice. If the evaluation suggests *N gonorrhoeae,* the patient should be treated with one dose of ceftriaxone, 250 mg IM and doxycycline, 100 mg P.O.

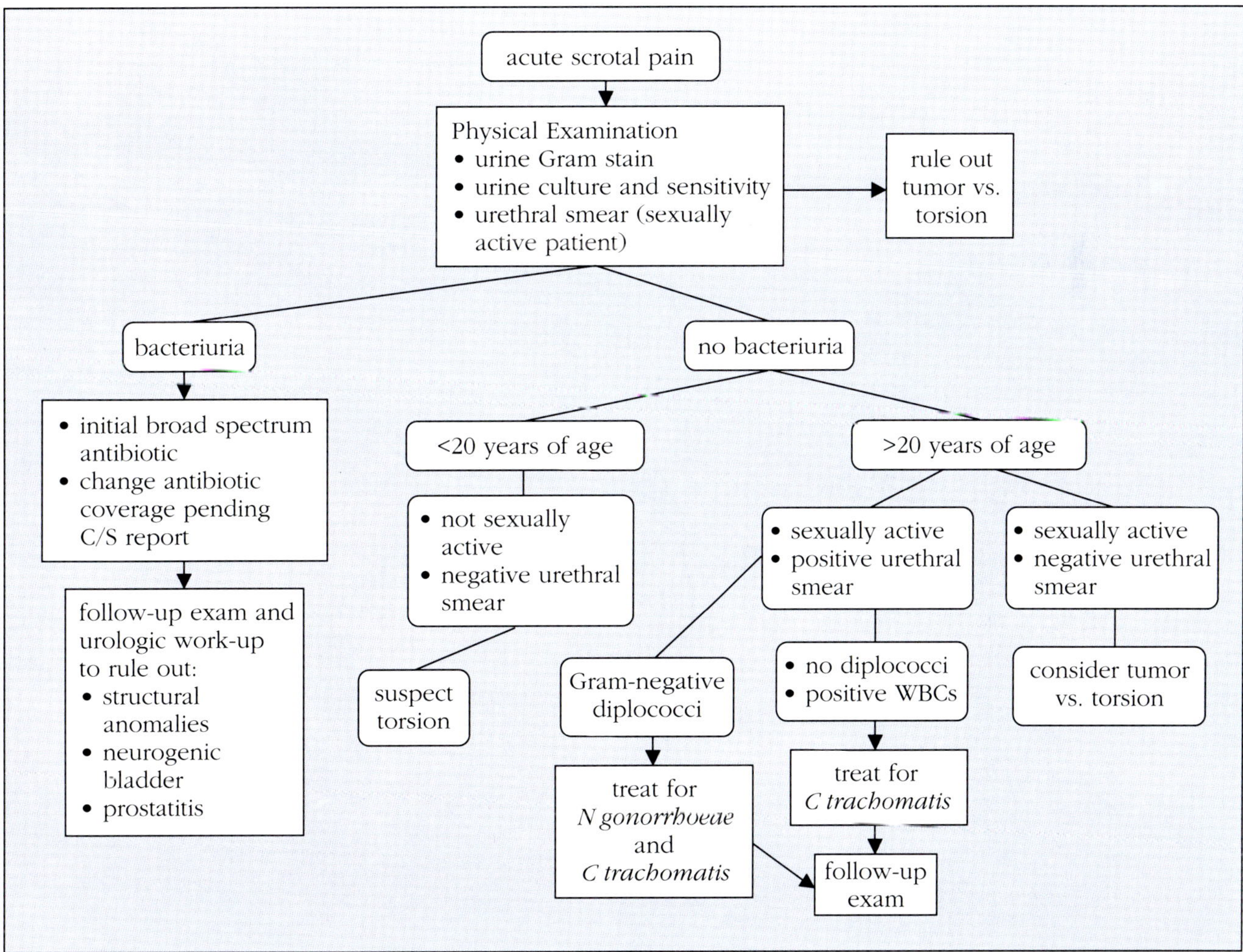

Figure 16.2 Algorithm for treatment of epididymitis.

for 10 days for empiric management of chlamydial infection. Doxycycline is also appropriate when many leukocytes are the only finding on urethral smear. I do not routinely obtain chlamydial cultures or enzyme assays because the false-negative rate is approximately 15% to 20% and because the organisms are exquisitely sensitive to doxycycline, making precise identification unnecessary. Sexual partners must be evaluated and treated with the same antibiotic regimen if infected.

Follow-up examination is very important for the patient with epididymitis. Generally speaking, the patient should be seen within a week after the initial evaluation. A significant decrease in pain should be noted. However, swelling may take 2 to 3 months to resolve completely.

Persistent regions of induration should alert the physician to the possibility of a testicular tumor.

Conclusion

Epididymitis is frequently seen in urologic practice. The etiology in most young adults is a sexually transmitted organism such as *N gonorrhoeae* or *C trachomatis*. In older adults, Gram-negative rods are the most common cause. The diagnosis should be based on history, physical examination, and the results of urine culture and/or urethral smear. In the absence of a clear diagnosis, the examining physician should suspect testicular tumor or torsion.

References

1. Kunin CM. The concepts of significant bacteriuria and asymptomatic bacteriuria: clinical syndromes and the epidemiology of urinary tract infections. In: *Detection, Prevention and Management of Urinary Tract Infections.* Philadelphia, Pa: Lea & Febiger; 1987:72–73.
2. Berger RE, Alexander ER, Harnisch JP, et al. Etiology, manifestations and therapy of acute epididymitis: prospective study of 50 cases. *J Urol.* 1979;121:750–754.
3. Delvillar RG, Ireland GW, Cass AS. Early exploration in acute testicular conditions. *J Urol.* 1972;108:887–890.
4. Stage KH, Schoenvogel R, Lewis S. Testicular scanning: clinical experience with 72 patients. *J Urol.* 1985;125:334–136.

CHAPTER 17

Prostatitis

Robert Moldwin

Prostatitis can be defined as an inflammation of the prostate gland characterized by the microscopic demonstration of more than 12 to 15 white blood cells/high-power field (WBC/HPF) in the prostatic secretions. Prostatitis has been subdivided into several distinct categories[1] on the basis of their unique clinical presentations and laboratory findings (Fig. 17.1). Treatments for the various forms differ, and an accurate initial diagnosis is therefore important to optimize the results of therapy.

Acute Bacterial Prostatitis

Acute bacterial infection is the easiest form of prostatitis to diagnose and treat. The patient usually presents with systemic signs of an infectious illness, most commonly fever and chills. A urologic problem is suggested by irritative and, occasionally, obstructive voiding symptoms and low back, suprapubic, and perineal pain.

EVALUATION

A thorough physical examination is mandatory because spread of infection to the kidneys or testes is common. On rectal examination the prostate is quite swollen and tender. Regions of fluctuance are consistent with an abscess and require further evaluation (Figs. 17.2, 17.3).

Urinalysis uniformly demonstrates pyuria. Urine cultures typically include Gram-negative rods, with *Escherichia coli* being the most common pathogen. Gonococcal urethritis was, in the past, a significant cause of prostatitis and prostatic abscess formation. Although this form of prostatitis is relatively rare today, the diagnosis should be strongly considered in any patient with a history of untreated urethritis.

Prostate massage and urethral manipulation are contraindicated in acute bacterial prostatitis, as both maneuvers will further potentiate bacteremia. If the patient presents in acute urinary retention, placement of a suprapubic catheter is recommended until he is able to void.[2]

TREATMENT

General treatment measures include initial broad-spectrum antibiotic coverage until sensitivity results are available, bed rest, hydration, antipyretics, and stool softeners. Barriers between the prostate and serum normally exclude many antimicrobials, but these barriers appear to be disrupted in the severe inflammation seen in acute prostatitis, thus permitting drug penetration. Therefore, the choice of antimicrobial therapy should be based on the final urine culture report. The response to treatment is usually very dramatic because of the rapid clearing of secondary cystitis. The prostate should be reinspected during the course of therapy to identify any developing regions of fluctance.

When an abscess is suspected a CT scan of the pelvis is recommended to confirm the diagnosis and further evaluate the extent of disease. Transrectal ultrasound scanning of the prostate is also helpful in making the diagnosis of prostatic abscess, but this modality will not demonstrate extracapsular extension as well as the CT scan. If an abscess is confirmed, immediate surgical drainage by transurethral resection or perineal incision is indicated. The results of both techniques are good and recurrences are rare.[3,4]

Antibiotic therapy should be continued for at least 6 to 8 weeks to prevent chronic bacterial prostatitis. The antimicrobial agent to be used after the acute inflammatory reaction has subsided is one of those appropriate for

FIGURE 17.1 *Categories of Prostatitis*

Acute bacterial
Chronic bacterial
Nonbacterial (prostatosis)
Prostatodynia (pelvic floor
   or bladder neck dysfunction)

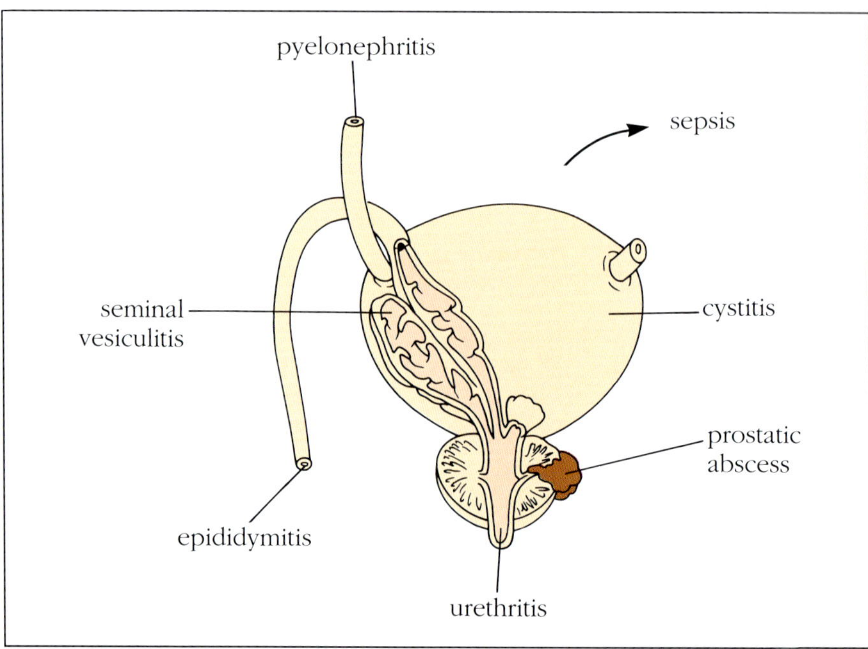

Figure 17.2 Possible sequelae of prostatitis.

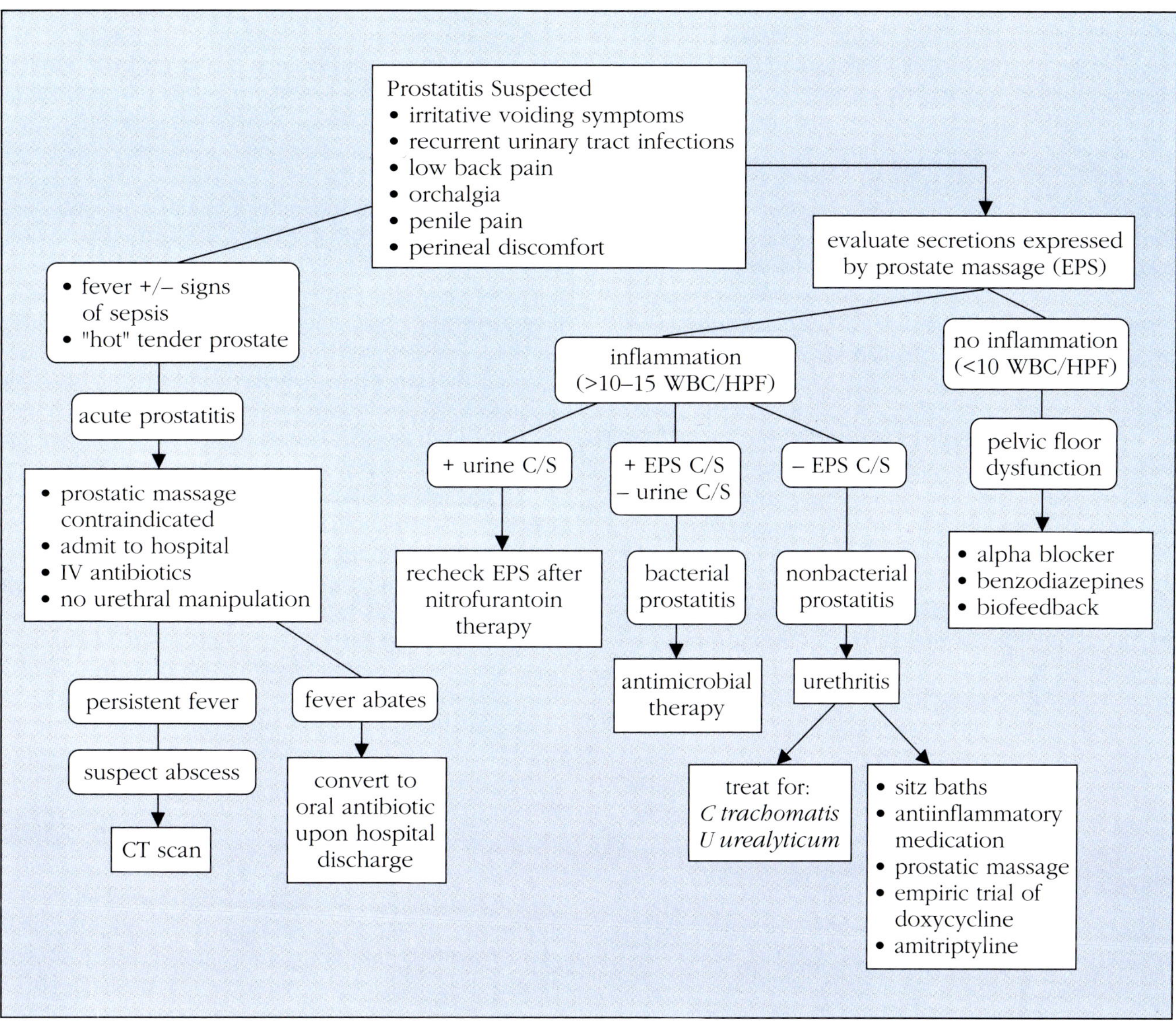

Figure 17.3 Algorithm for evaluation of prostatitis.

FIGURE 17.4 *Medications Useful in the Treatment of Bacterial Prostatitis*

MEDICATION	PROSTATE TISSUE/ PLASMA RATIO	WHOLESALE COST/WK*
Fluoroquinolones	1.5–3.0	$35–$40
Ciprofloxacin		
Ofloxacin		
Lomefloxacin		
Enoxacin		
Norfloxacin		
Trimethoprim-sulfamethoxazole	1.0–3.0	$14–$15
Generic		$3.22
Carbenicillin indanyl sodium	0.25	$89.60
Erythromycin (generic)	—	$4.20
Doxycycline (generic)	—	$1.40

*Medical Letter. 1992;34(872):60.

the treatment of chronic bacterial prostatitis (Fig. 17.4), which gain entry into the prostate tissue in the absence of significant inflammation.

Chronic Bacterial Prostatitis

Chronic bacterial prostatitis (CBP) accounts for only 5% of symptomatic individuals. Patients most often present with relapsing urinary tract infections, and the diagnosis of CBP is unlikely to be correct if the patient does not have this history. Other possible symptoms are urinary frequency, urgency, and perineal, testicular, low back, or suprapubic discomfort.

EVALUATION

Prostate examination is characteristically unrevealing. Study of the secretions expressed by prostate massage (EPS), as described by Meares and Stamey[5] (Fig. 17.5), is necessary for accurate diagnosis and choice of appropriate therapy. To evaluate the EPS adequately, several other urine cultures are necessary to confirm that the infection is localized to the prostate. First, the urethral meatus is

cleansed after the foreskin is retracted. The patient initiates a urine stream and collects the first 5 to 10 mL in a sterile container, which is designated VB1 (voided bladder specimen #1). Bacteria isolated from this sample represent urethral flora. The patient immediately collects his midstream urine (VB2).

Next, the patient undergoes prostate massage to collect the EPS. This involves digital "stripping" of the prostate in a lateral to medial direction, then in a superior to inferior direction. This is usually very uncomfortable for the patient, and slow progression with periodic rest periods is advisable. Only a few drops are obtained. The final drop can be placed on a microscope slide directly from the urethral meatus and the remainder sent for quantitative cultures. If no EPS is obtainable, the patient should void 5 to 10 mL into another sterile container (VB3).

All specimens should be sent for quantitative culture. The physician should speak with the receiving laboratory in detail about the incoming specimen: the laboratory must understand that exact bacterial colony counts are requested on small-volume specimens. Colony counts should be reported even if very low (i.e., <100 CFU/mL).

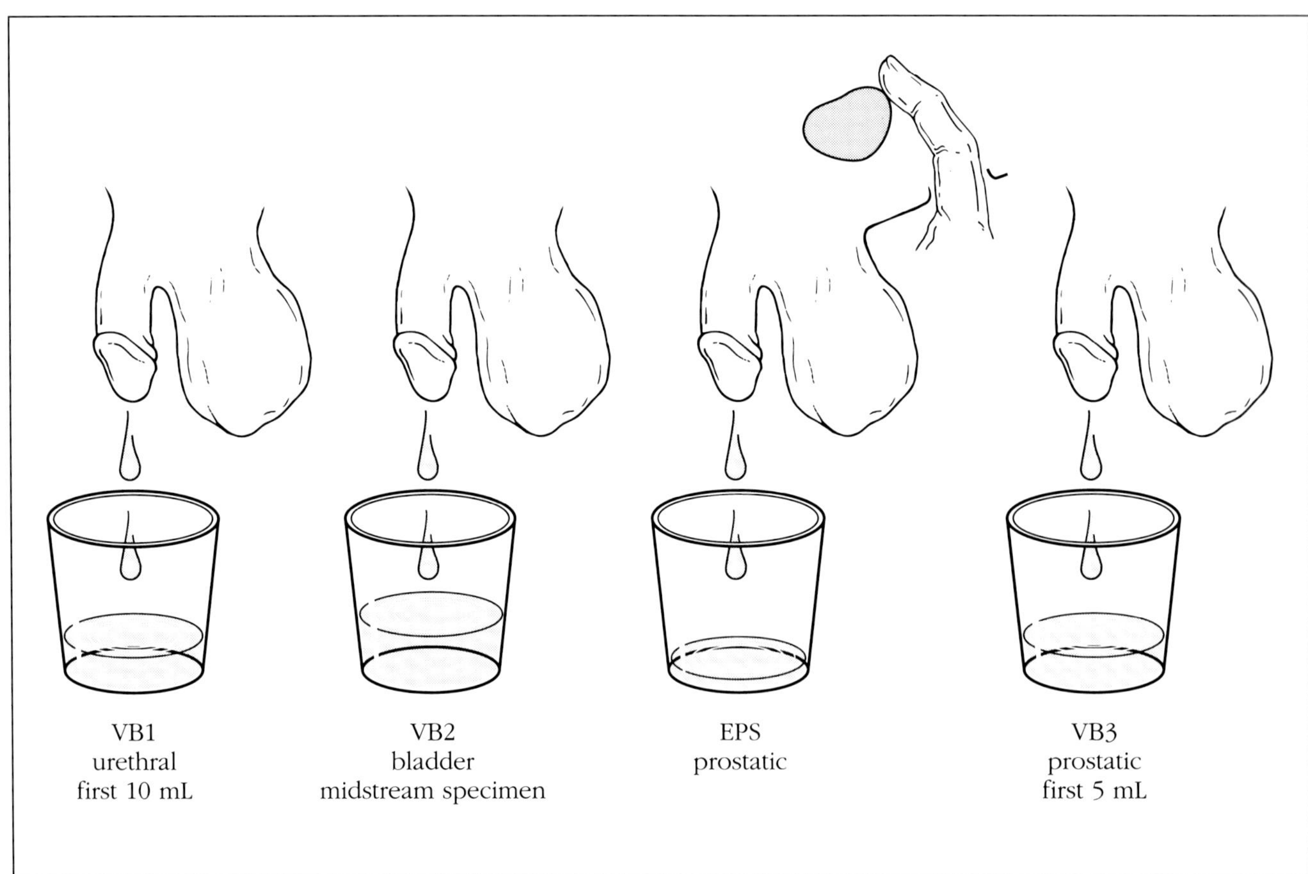

Figure 17.5 The secretions expressed by prostate massage (Meares and Stamey) must be studied to diagnose prostatitis accurately and to treat it. (Adapted from Nickel C, 1990)

The EPS is evaluated by the physician at the time of examination. Individuals with more than 15 WBC/HPF most likely have prostatitis; however, differentiation of nonbacterial prostatitis from CBP is confirmed by culture. Another characteristic finding of CBP is lipid-laden macrophages, which are exclusively prostatic in origin. Patients with less than 10 WBC/HPF are unlikely to have prostate inflammation. On microscopic examination, it is often difficult to differentiate immature sperm from leukocytes. A variety of vital stains are now available to make this distinction in the office laboratory.

The diagnosis of CBP can finally be made when cultures of the EPS are positive *and* the EPS has at least a tenfold (1 log) higher quantitative colony count than either the VB1 or the VB2 specimen. If the patient has bacterial cystitis at the time of localizing cultures, the results cannot be assessed accurately. I therefore screen the patient's VB2 specimen with a leukocyte esterase and nitrite dipstick test before proceeding further with localization studies (EPS, VB3). If the patient has cystitis it should be treated with a medication that will eradicate the organisms from the urine but will be excluded from the prostate. Examples include nitrofurantoin and ampicillin. Once the cystitis is resolved, localization studies can be repeated to establish an accurate diagnosis.

A local immunologic response to the offending bacteria occurs in patients with CBP.[6,7] The concentrations of both IgG and IgA (predominantly IgA) levels in the EPS are elevated, whereas serum concentrations are unchanged. The diagnostic utility is limited, however, as mild elevations of EPS immunoglobulins can also be seen in patients with nonbacterial prostatitis. These antibodies appear to be directed against specific bacterial antigens and can easily be measured by enzyme-linked immunoabsorbent assay (ELISA). When specific antibodies are measured, signficant differences between CBP and nonbacterial prostatitis (NBP) are usually seen. Patients with the former condition will have elevated immunoglobulins for 12 to 18 months after successful treatment, whereas immunoglobulin concentrations will remain unchanged if treatment is ineffective. Although this assay technique has been primarily experimental, it may eventually have clinical usefulness for detection of bacterial prostatitis in patients in whom localization studies are equivocal because of either poor specimen collection or previous antimicrobial therapy.

TREATMENT
Medical Therapy

One should choose an antibiotic with a low MIC for the cultured organism and good prostatic penetration. Useful agents are listed in Figure 17.4. Trimethoprim and the fluoroquinolone class of drugs are known to have the highest prostatic penetration, as much as three times the plasma concentration. These medications may therefore offer the best chance of cure, depending on the offending organism's sensitivity patterns.

Therapy is given for 6 to 12 weeks. The optimal duration of treatment has not been established for any antimicrobial agent. Short-course therapy appears to be less effective, which may reflect harboring of bacteria in prostate calculi or corpora amylacea or low antibiotic concentrations in the prostatic fluid (as opposed to prostate tissue). New evidence suggests that some bacteria encase themselves within a glycoprotein matrix or "biofilm," which protects them from antimicrobial exposure.[8] Unfortunately, many reports of antibiotic treatment successes have been flawed by inadequate control populations, poorly performed localization studies, and imprecise definitions of "cure." It is therefore not surprising that reported cure rates range from 30% to 90%. Antibiotic treatment of CBP is often frustrating, as reinfections are seen in approximately 50% of "cured" patients 6 months after therapy,[3,9,10] and bacterial persistence is common. Localization studies can be carried out after 4 weeks to assess the response to treatment. If the EPS still shows prostatic infection, the chance of cure after further antibiotic therapy is minimal.[11]

If infection recurs, another course of antibiotic therapy is recommended. In the event that infections continue to recur, chronic low-dose antibiotic suppression is advisable. In these instances, it is *not* necessary to rely on medications with good prostatic penetration, as the goal is to avoid repeated urinary tract infections and their accompanying symptoms.

Invasive Therapy

Direct injection of antibiotics has been advocated by several investigators to provide tissue concentrations not achievable by oral or parenteral administration. Plomp et al.[12] treated 29 patients with CBP refractory to trimethoprim-sulfamethoxazole by intraprostate injection of thiamphenicol. Bacteriologic cures were noted in 19 patients at 1 and 6 months after treatment. Jimenez-Cruz et al.[13] treated 51 patients with two to four courses of ultrasound-guided intraprostate injection of amikacin or tobramycin. The microbiologic cure rate was approximately 70% at 3-month follow-up. Although these results are promising, few other studies have been conducted using this technique.

Radical prostatectomy is the most reliable method to rid the patient of CBP; however, this represents an extreme approach. A near-complete prostatectomy by a transurethral route has been suggested as a less morbid solution. However, one difficulty with the transurethral approach is the potential failure to remove all infected tissue. This is of particular concern because infection commonly resides in the peripheral zone, a region that is difficult to resect completely. In addition, approximately 25% of the prostate lies distal to the verumontanum, a region not available for resection because of concerns about rendering the patient incontinent. Bacteriologic cures have nevertheless been noted in about 30% of cases when this technique was combined with antibiotic therapy. The most important advantage of radical TURP may be the removal of colonized prostatic calculi and corpora amylacea. This technique appears to be most justified in men with persistent infections and accompanying obstructive prostatic hyperplasia.

Nonbacterial Prostatitis (Abacterial Prostatitis or Prostatosis)

DIAGNOSIS AND EVALUATION

Nonbacterial prostatitis is the most common form of prostate inflammation. These patients present in the same manner as patients with CBP, except that relapsing UTIs are not seen. The diagnosis of NBP is made on the basis of prostatic inflammation as assessed by microscopic examination of the EPS; however, bacterial cultures are negative. Examination of the prostate is usually unremarkable, although occasionally tenderness of the periprostatic tissue and the levator ani muscles is demonstrated. Neurologic examination is normal. Further work-up should include urine cytology study and cystoscopy to rule out bladder pathology (i.e., carcinoma in situ) as a cause for the patient's irritative symptoms. An initial intravenous urogram is obtained to exclude referred discomfort from distal ureteral pathology. Finally, a urethral smear for Gram staining and culture should certainly be obtained if there is any indication of urethritis.

The cause of NBP is unknown, although several proposals have been offered (Fig. 17.6). Controversy exists about the roles played by *Ureaplasma urealyticum* and *Chlamydia trachomatis* in NBP. Although their involvement as causative agents in nongonococcal urethritis suggests a role in NBP, studies showing a clear cause and effect relationship are lacking. In addition, examination of the prostate fluid from patients with NBP has failed to demonstrate a local immune response to these organisms.[14]

A possible cause of NBP is intraprostatic reflux of urine. It is thought that this well-documented phenomenon is intermittent and may be responsible for bacterial inoculation of the prostate in acute and chronic prostatitis.[15] Indeed, intraprostatic urine reflux appears to be necessary for the formation of prostatic calculi. In the case of NBP, intraprostate reflux is postulated to cause a "chemical prostatitis" or to initiate an immunologic response to urine constituents.[16] Neither of these hypotheses has been substantiated.

TREATMENT

General treatment measures include warm sitz baths, anticholinergic drugs, and nonsteroidal antiinflammatory agents. Prostate massage is often helpful for patients who have infrequent sexual activity and "congested" prostates. An empirical trial of doxycycline, 100 mg b.i.d. for 2 weeks, is reasonable in cases where *Ureaplasma* or *Chlamydia* is a suspected pathogen. This treatment rarely improves the symptoms, however, and if symptoms remain unchanged no further antibiotic therapy should be administered.

If this conservative therapy fails, the patient may have an associated component of prostatodynia (see below) and should be treated accordingly. Otherwise, I have found low-dose amitriptyline to be of great value in the relief of symptoms. I usually begin therapy with 10 to 25 mg at bedtime and slowly increase the dose to 75 mg as needed. The principal side effects of this medication are related to its anticholinergic properties, constipation being the most frequently encountered. Patients with obstructive prostate hyperplasia may experience a worsening of symptoms. Another often distressing side effect is morning lethargy. This is usually self-limiting and abates during the first 4 to 6 weeks of therapy. However, simply adjusting the time of the evening dose to dinnertime is all that is usually necessary to alleviate this problem.

Prostatodynia

Ideally, prostatodynia should not be placed in the general category of prostatitis syndromes because no prostate pathology is present. The expressed prostate secretions are normal and patients typically do not give a history of urinary tract infections. Prostatodynia has nevertheless become part of the prostatitis classification because of its symptoms, which resemble with those of CBP and NBP. Discomfort may be referred to the suprapubic region, perineum, lower back, testicles, or penis. Pain may also be associated with ejaculation. Irritative voiding symptoms, urinary hesitancy, an intermittently poor urine flow, and constipation are other common complaints.

ETIOLOGY

The cause of this symptom complex is not completely understood. However, it is believed that most patients suffer from a functional obstruction of the bladder neck. This obstruction has been postulated to be secondary to

FIGURE 17.6 *Etiologies of Nonbacterial Prostatitis*

Infectious
    Gonococcus*
    *Ureaplasma**
    *Chlamydia**
    *Mycoplasma**
    Tuberculosis
    Parasites
    Mycosis
Intraprostatic reflex (chemical prostatis)*

*Not definitively proved.

improper funneling of the bladder neck during voiding by the sympathetically innervated smooth muscle of the prostatic urethra (i.e., smooth muscle dyssynergia).[17] Other evidence suggests that pelvic floor dysfunction[18] is present in some patients, causing inappropriate contraction of the striated sphincter during voiding. Schmidt and Vapnek[19] demonstrated abnormalities of external sphincter and levator ani/puborectalis function in these patients. Pelvic floor dysfunction is believed to be a learned behavior, and no neurologic abnormalities are seen. Many of these patients have stressful lifestyles, which may potentiate their symptoms. The 70% symptomatic improvement rates obtained with pelvic floor relaxation techniques (personal observations) provide indirect support for pelvic floor dysfunction as a cause of prostatodynia.

DIAGNOSIS

The diagnosis of prostatodynia is initially based on the characteristic symptoms in the absence of inflammatory cells or bacteria in the EPS. The clinician should keep in mind that this condition is often present in the face of CBP and NBP. In addition the patient's irritative voiding symptoms may reflect conditions such as interstitial cystitis or carcinoma in situ, and he should be evaluated in the same manner as for NBP. Rectal examination may demonstrate a "tight" anal sphincter with tenderness of the periprostatic tissues, in the absence of bladder outlet obstruction.

Urodynamic evaluation is often helpful to rule out associated (but uncommon) bladder dysfunction. Videourodynamic study is the definitive method to detect dysfunction of the bladder neck. A uroflow examination will usually reveal decreased mean flow rates with an associated strain pattern (in the absence of prostatic urethral obstruction). Uroflow examination is also quite useful to measure a patient's progress quantitatively during treatment as well as his symptomatic improvement.

TREATMENT

Medical therapy of prostatodynia has centered on treatment of the smooth and skeletal muscle components of the pelvic floor. Alpha-1-blocking agents such as prazosin and terazosin have been used. Both of these medications are antihypertensives and have a first-dose syncopal phenomenon associated with their use as a result of orthostatic hypotension. Their other predominant dose-limiting side effect is drowsiness. Of the two preparations, I prefer terazosin because of its once-a-day dosing. An initial dose of 1 mg can be given at bedtime (which avoids problems with syncope). After a few days the dose can be raised to 2 mg. Thereafter, the dose can be increased gradually while the patient's blood pressure is monitored; however, doses larger than 5 mg are rarely successful. Surgical correction of prostatodynia with transurethral incision of the bladder neck has been said to be successful, but these reports are anecdotal.

General treatment measures for pelvic floor dysfunction are listed in Figure 17.7. Pelvic floor relaxation is helpful in patients whose prostatodynia associated with tenderness of the pelvic floor. Patients are first instructed to identify the pelvic floor muscles. To accomplish this, they are told to begin voiding, then to stop the flow of urine midstream while identifying the muscle groups responsible for this effect. Patients then concentrate on relaxing those muscle groups while voiding or defecating. They should also be instructed not to strain while voiding, as this is likely to worsen their symptoms. Constipation, which is a common accompanying complaint, should be aggressively treated to avoid straining. Low-dose diazepam, 2 mg t.i.d., is often helpful in conjunction with pelvic floor relaxation as both an anxiolytic and a skeletal muscle relaxant. Patients should be informed that changes in their symptoms will take from 1 to 3 months. The best results with pelvic floor relaxation are achieved in the well-motivated patient. The roles of EMG biofeedback, transcutaneous electrical nerve stimulation, neurostimulation, and prostatic hyperthermia are under study, and the early results appear promising.

Significant stress and psychiatric disturbances are common in patients with prostatodynia. Whether these problems are a cause or a result of prostatodynia is unknown. Psychiatric assistance may be helpful in selected patients. Finally, and most importantly, a comprehensive discussion of the patient's problem with added reassurance is often the most helpful therapy.

Conclusion

Prostatitis is one of the problems most commonly encountered by the urologist. Unfortunately, it is also often one of the most difficult and frustrating problems for both the physician and the patient. The form of therapy chosen and its ultimate outcome are directly related to the form of prostatitis present. It is therefore mandatory to make an accurate diagnosis *early* in the patient's care.

FIGURE 17.7 *General Treatment Measures for Pelvic Floor Dysfunction*

Warm sitz baths b.i.d. or t.i.d.
Nonsteroidal antiinflammatory agents
Laxatives (if constipation is present)
Avoidance of sitting for long periods
Firm seat support
Pelvic floor relaxation

References

1. Drach GW, Meares EM Jr, Fair WR, Stamey TA. Classification of benign diseases associated with prostatic pain: prostatitis or prostatodynia? *J Urol.* 1978;120:266.
2. Meares EM Jr. Prostatitis. *Med Clin North Am.* 1989;15:405–424.
3. Meares EM Jr. Prostatitis syndromes: new perspectives about old woes. *J Urol.* 1980;123:141–147.
4. Orland SM, Hanno PM, Wein AJ. Prostatitis, prostatosis, and prostatodynia. *Urology.* 1985;25:439–459.
5. Meares EM Jr, Stamey TA. Bacteriologic localization patterns in bacterial prostatitis and urethritis. *Invest Urol.* 1968;5:492–518.
6. Shortliffe LMD, Elliott K, Sellers RG. Measurement of urinary antibodies to crude bacterial antigen in patients with chronic bacterial prostatitis. *J Urol.* 1989;141:632–636.
7. Wishnow KI, Wehner N, Stamey TA. The diagnostic value of the immunologic response in bacterial and nonbacterial prostatitis. *J Urol.* 1982;127:689–694.
8. Nikel C, Costerton JW. Bacterial localization in antibiotic-refractory chronic bacterial prostatitis. *J Urol.* 1991;145:236A(93).
9. Aagaard J, Madsen PO. Bacterial prostatitis: new methods of treatment. *Urology.* 1991;37(suppl):2–8.
10. Lipsky BA. Urinary tract infections in men; epidemiology, pathophysiology, diagnosis, and treatment. *Ann Intern Med.* 1989;110:138–150.
11. Meares EM Jr. Long-term therapy of chronic bacterial prostatitis and trimethoprim-sulfamethoxazole. *Can Med Assoc J.* 1975;112:22s–25s.
12. Plomp TA, Baert L, Maes RA. Treatment of recurrent bacterial prostatitis by local injection of thiamphenicol into prostate. *Urology.* 1980;15:542–547.
13. Jimenez-Cruz JF, Boronat Tormo F, Gallego Gomez J. Treatment of chronic prostatitis: intraprostatic antibiotic injections under echography control. *J Urol.* 1988;139:967–970.
14. Shortliffe LMD, Wehner N, Stamey TA. Measurement of chlamydial and ureaplasmal antibodies in serum and prostatic fluid of men with nonbacterial prostatitis. *J Urol.* 1985;133:276A.
15. Kirby RS, et al. Intra-prostatic urinary reflux: an aetiological factor in abacterial prostatitis. *Br J Urol.* 1982;54:729–731.
16. Meares EM Jr. Nonbacterial prostatitis. In: Drach GW, ed. *Common Problems in Infections and Stones.* St. Louis, Mo: Mosby–Year Book; 1992:95.
17. Barbalias GA, Meares EM, Sant GR. Prostatodynia: clinical and urodynamic characteristics. *J Urol.* 1983;130:514–517.
18. Segura JW, Opitz JL, Greene LF. Prostatosis, prostatitis or pelvic floor tension myalgia? *J Urol.* 1979;122:168–169.
19. Schmidt RA, Vapnek JM. Pelvic floor behavior and interstitial cystitis. *Semin Urol.* 1991;9:154–159.

CHAPTER 18

Acute Pyelonephritis in the Adult

Robert Moldwin

Acute pyelonephritis should be suspected in the patient who presents with fever, chills, flank pain, and bacteriuria. Other common clinical features include nausea, vomiting, and abdominal pain. A history of renal calculus disease, urologic surgery, or pyelonephritis in childhood, obstructive urinary symptoms, or the presence of unusual organisms on culture should raise the suspicion of an associated structural abnormality.

Evaluation

Physical examination typically demonstrates a flushed patient with costovertebral angle tenderness on the affected side. Urinalysis invariably reveals bacteriuria, often associated with hematuria. Leukocyte casts in the urinary sediment are particularly suggestive of pyelonephritis. Urine culture shows *Escherichia coli* in approximately 85% of cases.[1] Other Gram-negative rods commonly cultured include *Klebsiella pneumoniae* and *Proteus mirabilis*. Frequently seen coccal forms include enterococci and *Staphylococcus saprophyticus*. A single organism will be identified in 85% of patients.[2] Characteristic

FIGURE 18.1 *Radiographic Findings of Acute Pyelonephritis*

INTRAVENOUS UROGRAPHY
Normal in 75% of cases
Smooth renal enlargement
Delayed excretion of contrast; poor contrast enhancement of parenchyma or caliceal system secondary to diminished concentrating ability
Streaking pattern within nephrogram
Streaking pattern within renal pelvis and ureter secondary to mucosal edema

ULTRASONOGRAPHY
Most patients show no changes
Diffuse renal enlargement
Small patchy hyperechoic or hypoechoic regions
Loss of caliceal/parenchymal interface

COMPUTED TOMOGRAPHY
Most sensitive for detection of pyelonephritis
Wedge-shaped zones of decreased attenuation after contrast administration. Affected areas are approximately 30 to 80 HU; normal renal parenchyma is about 120 to 130 HU.
This finding is probably reflective of local ischemia.
Nondistinct borders of kidney, suggesting perinephric reaction

radiographic findings are listed in Figure 18.1. Blood cultures should be performed as indicated.

Approximately 20% of adult patients who experience having an episode of acute pyelonephritis develop focal cortical scars. However, progression of disease with associated renal failure is very rare. Likewise, the development of chronic pyelonephritis is unlikely unless neurologic or structural abnormalities are present.[3,4]

Treatment and Follow-up

Antibiotic administration should begin immediately after urine cultures are obtained. Patients can be treated on an outpatient basis when they are mildly or moderately symptomatic and can eat, drink, and take their prescribed medications. Treatment should continue for 2 weeks. Longer courses of therapy are unwarranted and have more associated side effects. Trimethoprim-sulfamethoxazole and the fluoroquinolones are useful agents, whereas ampicillin and oral first-generation cephalosporins have lower success rates. Final drug selection should be based on antibiotic sensitivities.

Patients should monitor their temperature and symptoms. If no improvement is noted within 48 hours, the patient must return for reevaluation, as most cases of uncomplicated acute pyelonephritis will respond within this time.

Absolute indications for hospital admission include changes in mental status, nausea and vomiting, fever greater than 102°F in a catheterized patient, and evidence of structural abnormality.[5] Broad-spectrum antibiotic coverage should be administered initially. The gentamicin/ampicillin combination has been the standard of therapy; however, *E coli* may be resistant to ampicillin in as many as 50% of cases. Replacing the ampicillin with a combination "cillin"/β-lactamase inhibitor (e.g., ampicillin plus subactam or ticarcillin plus clavulanate) may obviate this problem. Aztreonam or imipenem is useful when nephrotoxicity is of concern. Symptoms and fever should diminish significantly after 3 to 4 days of therapy. The patient can then be changed to an oral antibiotic for 2 weeks. Patients who present with bacteremia should undergo a full 10-day course of parenteral antibiotics.[5]

Failure of the infection to respond to therapy may indicate obstruction, intense focal inflammation (focal or multifocal bacterial nephritis, lobar nephronia), or perinephric abscess. Although obstruction is usually obvious on IVU, signs of lobar nephronia and perirenal abscess may be subtle. Ultrasound or CT scans of the kidneys will be helpful to differentiate these lesions further.[6] Small intrarenal abscesses and lobar nephronia can usually be treated successfully with more aggressive antimicrobial therapy. Combination parenteral antibiotics should be continued 3 to 5 days after the patient becomes afebrile before switching to oral delivery. If fever persists beyond 2 weeks of appropriate antibiotic therapy or if the patient's condition worsens (e.g., follow-up radiographic studies demonstrate enlargement of an abscess), CT-guided needle aspiration for culture and drainage should be considered before surgical exploration is undertaken.

Urine cultures should be performed during the course of antimicrobial therapy. Additional cultures should be taken 2 weeks and 8 weeks thereafter to confirm the absence of infection. Structural or urodynamic abnormalities can be evaluated if clinically indicated.

Conclusion

Acute pyelonephritis is commonly seen in both urologic and general medical practice. In the adult patient these episodes usually are easily treated and have no significant clinical sequelae. A poor response to treatment should alert the physician to the possibility of an underlying structural anomaly.

References

1. Kunin CM. The concepts of significant bacteriuria and asymptomatic bacteriuria: clinical syndromes and the epidemiology of urinary tract infections. In: *Detection, Prevention and Management of Urinary Tract Infections*. Philadelphia, Pa: Lea & Febiger; 1987:73–74.
2. Safrin S, Seigel D, Black D. Pyelonephritis in adult women: inpatient versus outpatient therapy. *Am J Med*. 1988;85:793–798.
3. Meyrier A. Long term risks of acute pyelonephritis. *Nephron*. 1990;54:197–201.
4. Huland M, Busch R, Riebel TH. Renal scarring after symptomatic and asymptomatic upper urinary tract infection: a prospective study. *J Urol*. 1982;128:682–685.
5. Smith JW. Southwestern Internal Medicine Conference: prognosis in pyelonephritis: promise or progress. *Am J Med Sci*. 1989;297:53–62.
6. Resnick MI, Hughs P. Advances in the diagnosis of renal infections. *Infect Urol*. May/June 1988:43–55.

CHAPTER 19

Perinephric Abscess

Robert Moldwin

Perinephric abscess is defined as a collection of pus between the renal capsule and Gerota's fascia. Most cases are secondary to renal disease such as obstruction or focal bacterial nephritis, extension of a renal medullary abscess, or xanthogranulomatous pyelonephritis. In these conditions, Gram-negative rods are the most commonly encountered pathogens. Hematogenous dissemination of *Staphylococcus aureus* (the most common cause of renal cortical abscess or carbuncle), which was responsible for 80% of perinephric abscesses in the preantibiotic era, still accounts for 15% of cases.[1,2] Approximately 30% of patients are diabetics.

Natural History

In most cases, an abscess will be identified and treated before significant extension can occur. If allowed to progress, the abscess may bulge anterolaterally through Petit's triangle (formed by the borders of the latissimus dorsi and external oblique muscles and the iliac crest), leading to abscess pointing and spontaneous drainage. Inferior extension between the leaves of Gerota's fascia may result in a psoas, groin, or paravesical collection. Progression of the collection superiorly may cause a subdiaphragmatic abscess. Violation of the pleural cavity will lead to empyema. Transperitoneal extension may produce peritonitis or colonic perforation (Fig. 19.1).

Evaluation

Patients usually report having had symptoms, particularly fevers, chills, and flank pain, for at least 2 weeks before seeking medical intervention. Pleuritic chest pain and hiccups may indicate diaphragmatic irritation. Inferior extension may be indicated by abdominal and unilateral back and hip pain. Flank or abdominal masses are rarely palpable.

Leukocytosis with bandemia is almost invariably present and blood cultures are positive in 10% to 40% of cases. Urine cultures are positive in as many as 80% of patients. However, in hematogenously disseminated disease the abscess will not necessarily be in continuity with the collecting system, and urinalysis or urine cultures may therefore not be diagnostic.

The findings on radiographic evaluation are listed in Figure 19.2. An IVU or ultrasound examination of the kidneys is usually abnormal, but when an abscess is suspected a CT scan should be ordered, as this study provides excellent definition of the lesion and surrounding structures. Needle aspiration of the abscess cavity is performed for microbiologic diagnosis (Gram staining and culture for aerobes, anaerobes, and acid-fast organisms). Cytology study is performed on the fluid to rule out associated neoplasm. A Cope catheter can be left to provide drainage.[3–5] The CT scan can be used to follow the response of the abscess to medical or aspirational therapy.

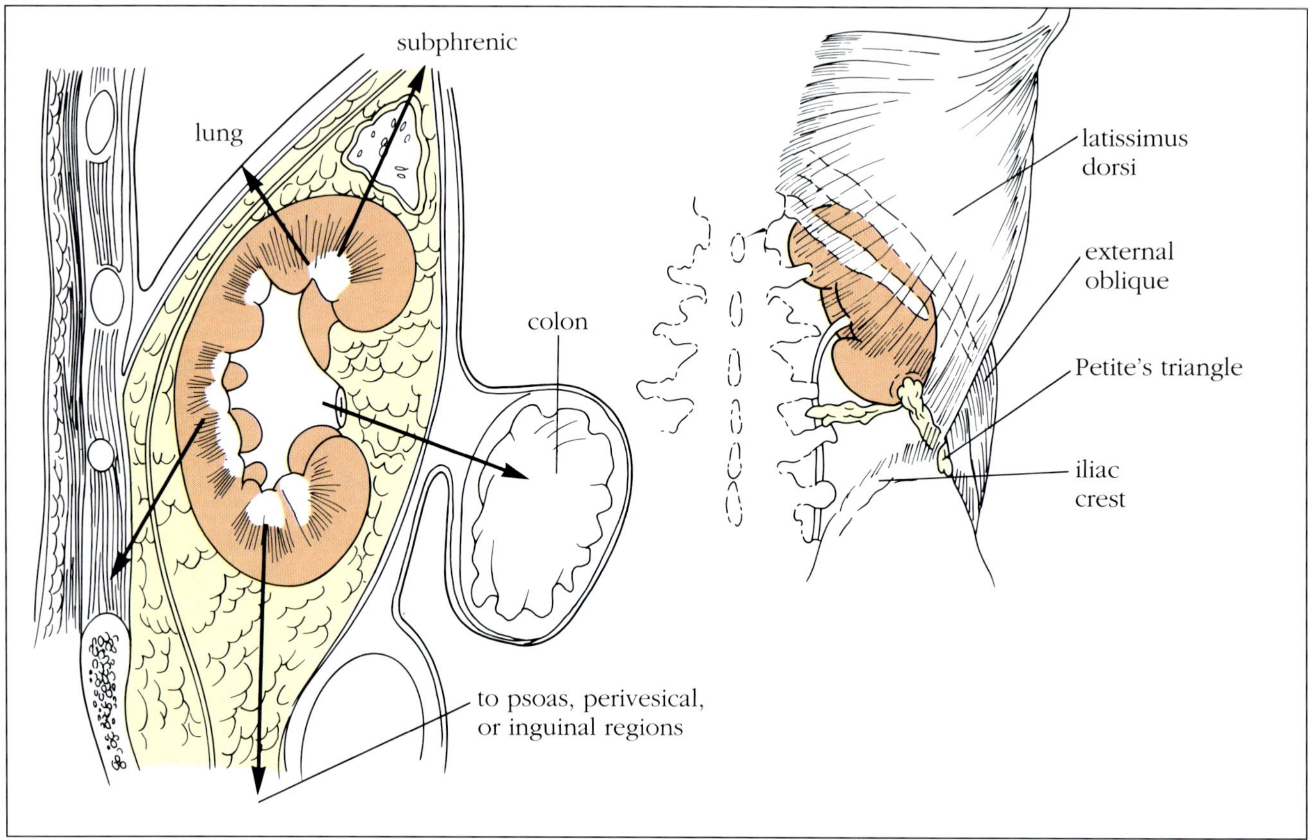

Figure 19.1 Perinephric abscess: routes of spread.

Treatment

After urine and blood cultures have been obtained for culture, the patient should be started on broad-spectrum coverage including an aminoglycoside and a ß-lactamase-resistant penicillin. Other approaches for antimicrobial management can be found in Chapter 18.

A second site of percutaneous puncture is occasionally chosen to optimize drainage. Percutaneous drainage along with appropriate antimicrobial therapy may be curative, especially for small collections with minimal loculations. The clinical improvement after percutaneous drainage is often dramatic, making eventual open surgical intervention less hazardous. Catheters should be removed only after the patient is afebrile, no leukocytosis is seen, drainage has ceased, and a repeat CT scan shows no evidence of the abscess.

Persistence of an abscess collection indicates the need for further percutanous drainage or surgical intervention. Multiloculated collections are notoriously difficult to treat percutaneously and require open surgical intervention. The choice of open surgery may be further warranted in the face of a poorly functioning kidney, which may need to be removed or significantly debrided.

When open surgery is elected, a retroperitoneal approach should be used. The kidney surface should be inspected and grossly necrotic tissue removed. Loculations must be aggressively broken down. Several wide Penrose drains are left in place. I discourage the use of Jackson-Pratt drains in these instances because of the potential for tissue ingrowth and subsequent difficulty in removal. In cases of sepsis with an associated structural abnormality, it is often wise to drain the abscess surgically, allowing the patient to improve clinically before addressing the underlying cause surgically.

Conclusion

Perirenal abscess is a uniformly deadly disease if left untreated. Its diagnosis is often confounded by its variable presentation and the occasional disparity between urine and abscess culture findings. A CT scan provides detailed information regarding the extent of the abscess and its relation to adjacent structures. This study facilitates percutaneous aspiration for microbiologic and cytologic diagnosis and the placement of drainage catheters. The mainstay of treatment is a combination of antibiotic therapy and abscess drainage. The choice of open versus percutaneous drainage is based on the patient's clinical status.

FIGURE 19.2 *Radiographic Findings of Perinephric Abcess*

CHEST FILM
Elevation and fixation of ipsilateral hemidiaphragm
Ipsilateral atelectasis or effusion
Apical scarring (in cases of tuberculosis)

INTRAVENOUS UROGRAPHY
Abnormal but nonspecific findings in 80%
   of patients
Renal displacement
Poorly visualized ipsilateral psoas shadow
Obliteration of perirenal fat shadow
Poor renal mobilization on inspiration
Changes of associated pyelonephritis

ULTRASOUND
Hypodense mass with internal echos
   (particulate matter)
Thick capsule wall
Multiple loculations are common

COMPUTED TOMOGRAPHY
Excellent detail of abscess extension and adjacent
   structures
Low attenuation of abscess (0 to 20 HU)
Enhancement of the thickened abscess wall with
   contrast administration

References

1. Rives RK, Harty JI, Amin M. Renal abscess: emerging concepts of diagnosis and treatment. *J Urol.* 1980;12:446-450.
2. Schienfeld J, Erturk E, Spararo RF, Cockett ATK. Perinephric abscess: current concepts. *J Urol.* 1987;137:191-194.
3. Resnick MI, Hughs P. Advances in the diagnosis of renal infections. *Infect Urol.* May/June 1988:43-55.
4. Gerzof SG. Percutaneous drainage of renal and perirenal abscess. *Urol Radiol.* 1981;2:171-173.
5. Godek CJ, et al. Diagnostic strategy in evaluation of renal abscess. *Urology.* 1981;18:535-541.

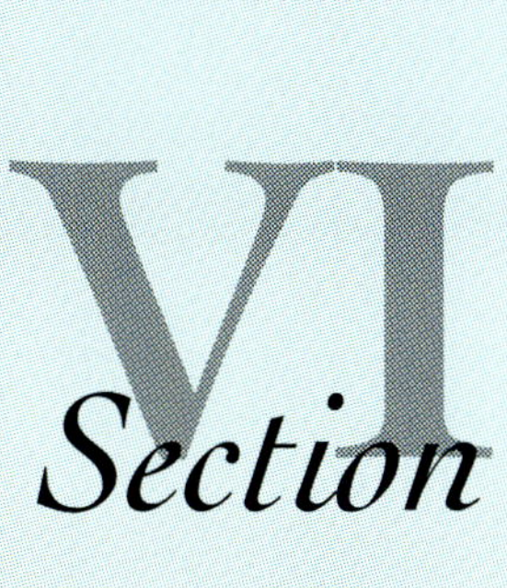

Trauma

Peter R. Carroll, editor

CHAPTER 20

Renal Trauma

Noel A. Armenakas
Jack W. McAninch
Peter R. Carroll

Pathophysiology

The kidney is the most frequently injured genitourinary organ, involved in 8% to 10% of all abdominal trauma. Renal injuries can be classified, according to their cause, as blunt or penetrating. Blunt renal injuries account for approximately 80% of all renal trauma.[1] Motor vehicle accidents are the most frequent cause, followed by assaults and falls. Penetrating renal injuries primarily result from stab and gunshot wounds.

BLUNT TRAUMA

Most blunt renal injuries are minor. The mechanism by which a kidney sustains blunt trauma and the reasons for the different patterns of such injuries remain obscure. A direct blow to the flank or abdomen can cause parenchymal injury by compressing the kidney against the vertebral bodies or back muscles. Moreover, rib or transverse process fractures can lacerate the kidney. Renal parenchymal lacerations from blunt trauma usually transect the organ in the transverse plane. In most instances, the injury begins on the border of the renal cortex and advances into the medulla and collecting system. Because larger vessels are found in the more central areas of the kidney, the deeper the parenchymal laceration, the greater the likelihood of major renal bleeding.

Arterial injury from blunt trauma appears to result from rapid deceleration.[2] The kidney is relatively mobile in the retroperitoneum and during an accident it has a different deceleration from that of the aorta. As the kidney moves relative to the aorta, the renal artery is subjected to tensile (stretching) forces. When the magnitude of these forces reaches a critical value, the intimal layer of the artery, which is relatively deficient in elastin fibers, ruptures. This initiates thrombus formation, which can cause total arterial occlusion and renal ischemia (Fig. 20.1).[3]

PENETRATING TRAUMA

Penetrating renal injuries are more likely to result in severe damage to the renal parenchyma, collecting system, and vasculature. The extent of injury cannot be judged on the basis of hematuria or the appearance of the entrance or exit wound. Because of the so-called blast effect, bullet wounds create more extensive injury than may be initially apparent.[4] Vascular pedicle injury to the kidney from gunshot and stab wounds creates major blood loss and hypovolemic shock.

Diagnosis

Renal injury is diagnosed by combining a carefully performed history and physical with laboratory and radiographic evaluation. In this way, the injury will be accurately staged (i.e., the extent and type defined) and appropriate management can be instituted.

HISTORY AND PHYSICAL

The historic details of the injury can provide significant information regarding potential renal involvement. Deceleration injuries from high-speed motor vehicle accidents or falls from heights may be associated with major vascular and/or parenchymal renal damage. With penetrating trauma, knowledge of the type and caliber of the gun is helpful when debriding injured tissue, and knowing the length of the knife may help to determine the depth of penetration.

On physical exam, flank contusions, seat-belt marks, lower rib fractures, lumbar vertebral fractures, and upper abdominal or flank tenderness are clinical indicators of blunt renal trauma and warrant further evaluation. Initial blood pressure should be noted as patients with renal vascular injuries often present in shock. Penetrating injuries to the flank or upper abdomen are indicators of possible renal trauma, although the site of injury (i.e., abdomen, flank, lumbar) does not reliably indicate the extent of renal or associated injuries.[5]

URINALYSIS

Urine should be obtained and evaluated for hematuria, by either dipstick or microscopic urinalysis. It is impor-

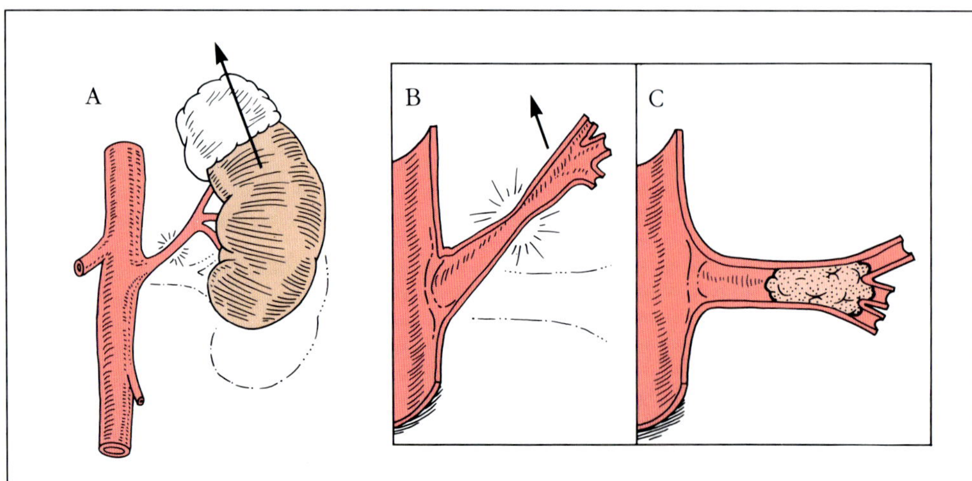

***Figure 20.1* A–C** Renal artery injury from blunt trauma: excessive stretch on the renal artery results in an intimal tear and subsequent thrombus formation.

tant to collect the first voided or catheterized specimen to avoid false-negative results from dilution after intravenous hydration.

Hematuria is the best indicator of renal injury, and more than five red blood cells per high-power field is considered abnormal. However, it is well established that the degree of hematuria does not correlate with the degree of injury[6]: patients with major deceleration injuries causing arterial thrombosis usually have microhematuria, although 28% have none[2]; conversely, patients with only minor renal injuries may have numerous red blood cells on urinalysis.

IMAGING

Radiographic imaging enables the extent of the injury to be fully defined. It is indicated in all patients with penetrating renal trauma and in those with blunt trauma who present with gross hematuria or shock and microscopic hematuria (Fig. 20.2). Also, patients with lower rib or lumbar transverse process fractures or severe deceleration injuries should be suspected of having sustained a renal injury, and thus radiographic assessment is indicated. In the adult patient with blunt trauma who is hemodynamically stable and presents only with microhematuria, a clinical diagnosis of a minor renal injury can be made without

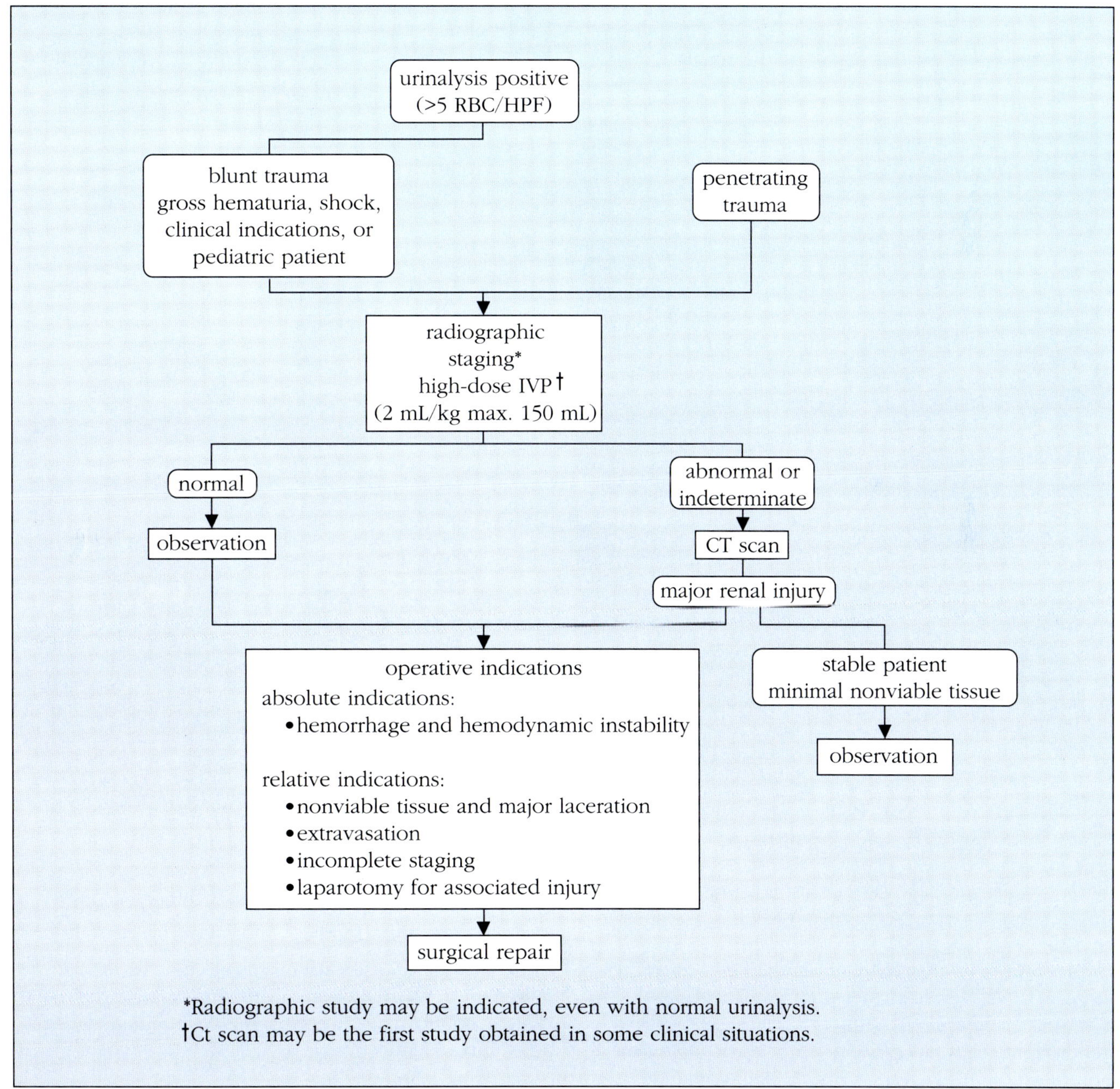

Figure 20.2 Algorithm for management of patients in whom renal injury is suspected.

radiographic renal assessment. These criteria do not pertain to the pediatric patient, in whom radiographic imaging should be performed with any degree of hematuria.

In hemodynamically stable patients, a complete excretory urogram (IVP) is obtained. This should demonstrate two normally functioning kidneys and clearly delineate the parenchymal borders, renal pelvis, collecting system, and ureters. With the addition of nephrotomography, 90% of renal injuries will be detected.[7] However, findings may be nonspecific, (i.e., decreased opacification, irregular margins) and staging incomplete.

If the results of the IVP are indeterminate and precise staging of the renal injury is not possible, computed tomography (CT) should be performed in the stable patient (Fig. 20.3). This provides excellent information regarding the depth and extent of the renal laceration, the amount of urinary extravasation, the size of any retroperitoneal hematoma, and the presence of any associated intraabdominal organ injury.[8] CT can also diagnose renal pedicle injuries; characteristic findings include an almost total lack of renal enhancement and excretion with preservation of normal size and contour.[9] The added information provided by this noninvasive imaging mode aids the selection of appropriate management.

If CT is unavailable or inconclusive, arteriography, which defines arterial injuries and renal lacerations, can be used.[10] Ultrasonography has been advocated in Europe, but its inability to differentiate blood from urine renders it less precise than CT.

In seriously injured patients, an infusion bolus of contrast medium (2.0 mL/kg) should be given and a film taken 10 minutes after contrast injection. This can be

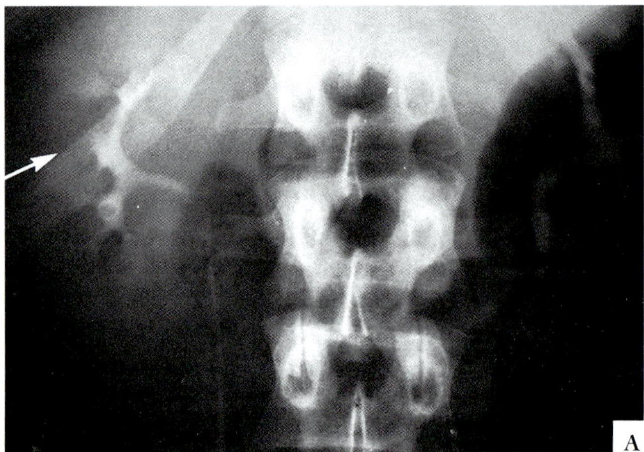

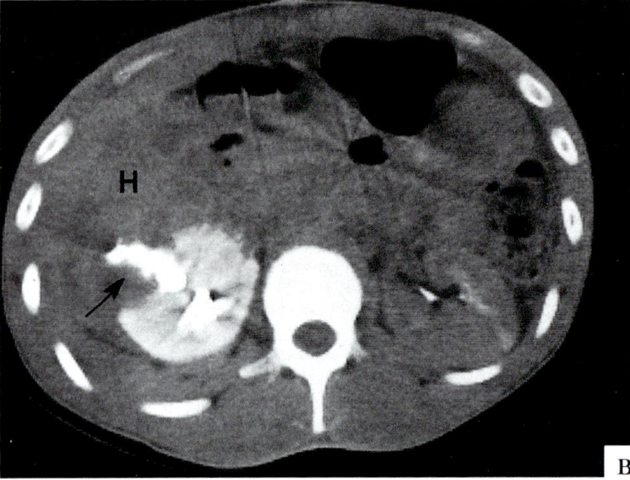

Figure 20.3 Radiographic imaging of a blunt renal injury: **A** IVP demonstrates poor visualization of the right upper pole; **B** subsequent CT scan shows a major right renal laceration with urinary extravasation (arrow) and a large perirenal hematoma (H).

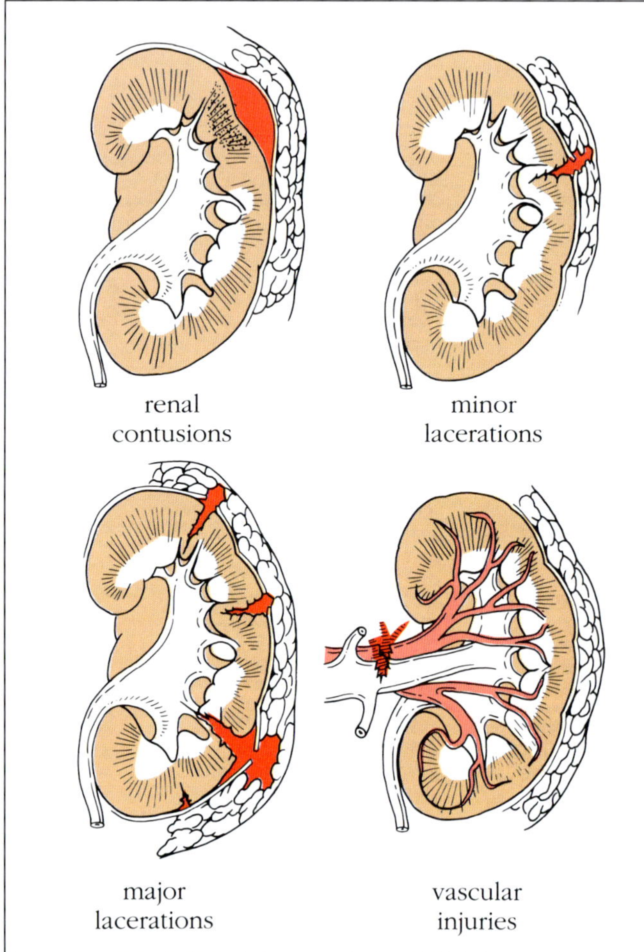

Figure 20.4 Classification of renal injuries: *(top)* minor injuries, including contusions and minor lacerations; *(bottom)* major injuries, including major lacerations and vascular injuries.

done in the resuscitation suite or operating room and will provide immediate information regarding the presence of two kidneys and their functional status.

CLASSIFICATION

Renal trauma can be classified according to severity (Fig. 20.4):

1. Minor renal injuries represent 90% of all blunt renal injuries and include contusions and superficial lacerations.[0] The latter extend only into the renal cortex. Surgical exploration is seldom necessary.

2. Major renal injuries include lacerations that extend into the deep medullary portion of the kidney and may involve the collecting system, resulting in urinary extravasation. Deep parenchymal lacerations are more prone to significant bleeding, making surgical intervention more likely.[12] Major renal injuries also include injuries to the main renal artery, vein, or segmental branches.

Management

Patients with microscopic hematuria and isolated well-staged minor injuries do not require hospitalization. Patients with gross hematuria who are shown to have contusions or minor lacerations should be hospitalized and placed at strict bed rest. If bleeding persists, repeat radiographic evaluation may be necessary. Ambulation is allowed once gross bleeding has resolved, usually in 24 to 48 hours.

Approximately 95% of blunt renal injuries can be managed nonoperatively.[13] Penetrating trauma from gunshot and stab wounds requires surgical exploration unless the renal trauma has been accurately staged and there are no other associated intraabdominal injuries requiring surgery.

Approximately 50% of renal stab wounds and 20% of renal gunshot wounds can be managed nonoperatively.

SURGICAL MANAGEMENT

Absolute indications for renal exploration include an expanding or pulsatile retroperitoneal hematoma and hemodynamic instability from renal hemorrhage. Relative indications include urinary extravasation, nonviable renal parenchyma with a major laceration, and vascular injury.[14] Patients whose injuries cannot be completely staged on the basis of clinical and radiographic criteria are also candidates.

Surgical exploration is performed by adhering to the following steps:

1. A midline transabdominal incision is made, and the transverse colon and small bowel are lifted superiorly to expose the retroperitoneum.

2. The posterior peritoneum is incised over the aorta, extending superiorly to the ligament of Treitz. If the aorta is not palpable because of a large hematoma, the incision is made medial to the inferior mesenteric vein (Fig. 20.5).

3. After exposing the anterior surface of the aorta, the dissection is carried superiorly to expose the left renal vein crossing anteriorly (Figs. 20.6, 20.7).

4. The renal arteries and right renal vein are rapidly isolated. Initially, soft vessel loops are used; vascular clamps or Rummel tourniquets may be required with heavy renal bleeding.

5. Once vascular control is achieved, the kidney can be safely explored by reflecting the colon medially and opening Gerota's fascia (Fig. 20.8).

6. The kidney is bluntly mobilized and completely exposed for thorough inspection and injury assessment.

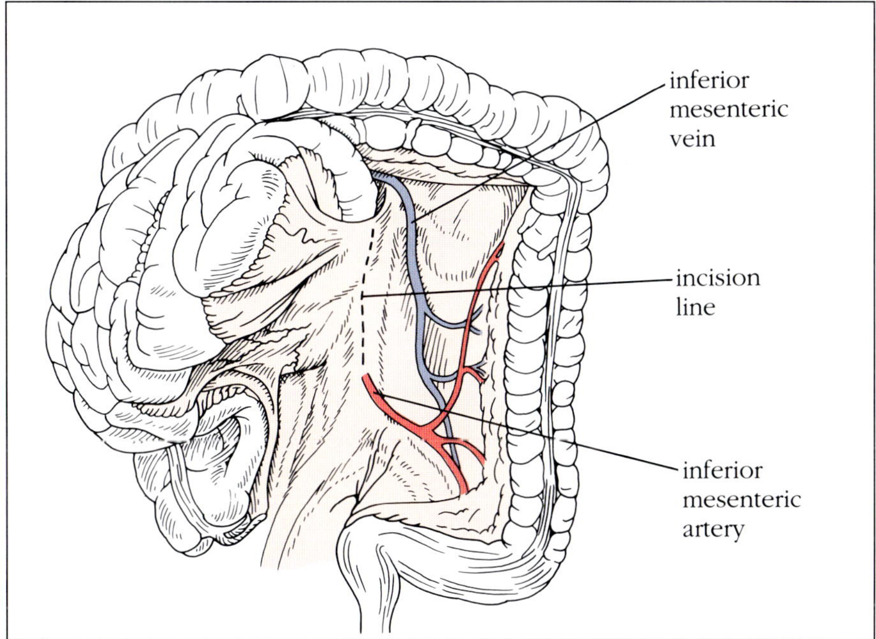

Figure 20.5 Posterior peritoneal incision over the aorta.

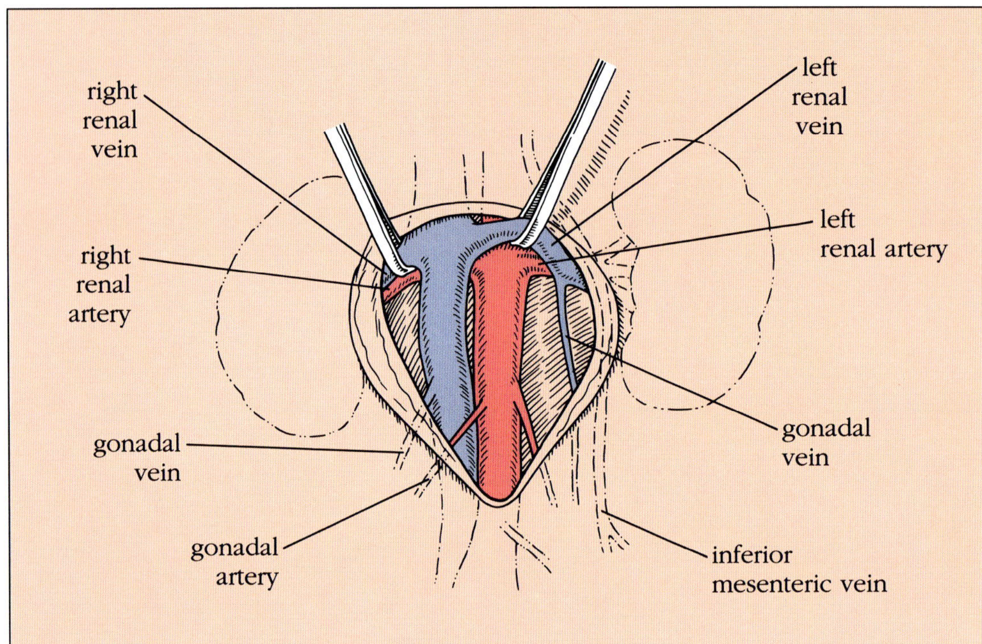

Figure 20.6 Relationship of the renal and great vessels.

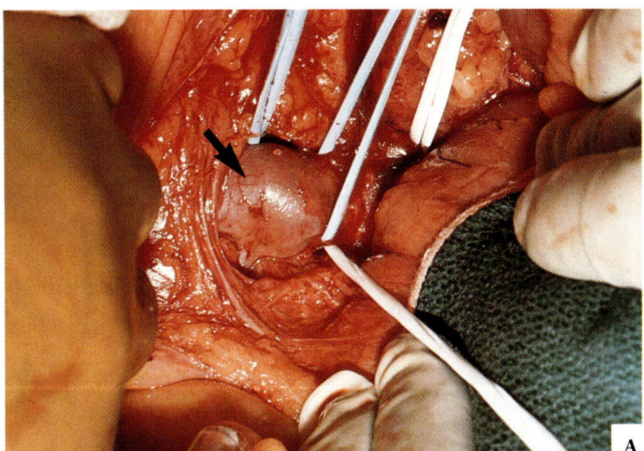

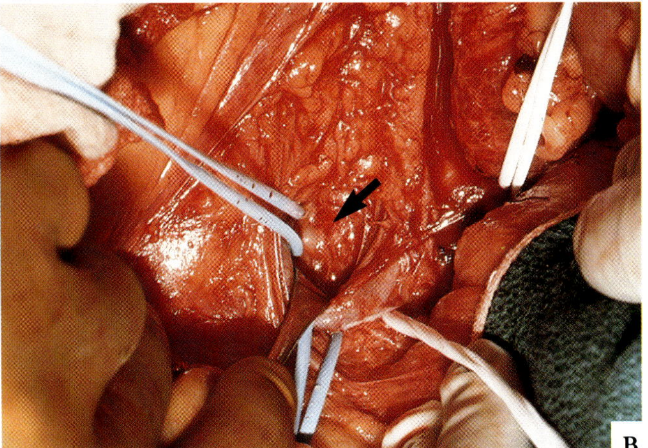

Figure 20.7 Intraoperative photographs showing the isolated left renal vein **A** and artery **B.**

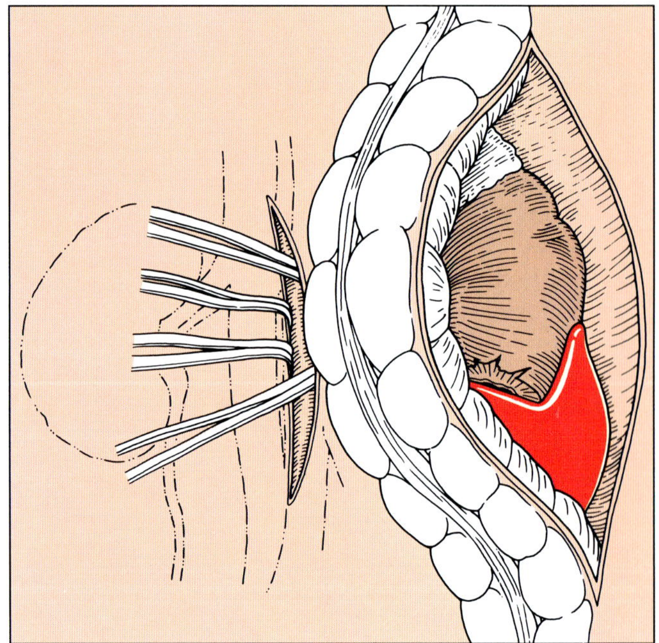

Figure 20.8 Incised Gerota's fascia exposing the injured kidney.

All nonviable tissue and any intrarenal hematoma are removed, and hemostasis is obtained with 4-0 chromic sutures placed in a figure-of-eight fashion. Lacerations extending into the collecting system are closed with fine chromic sutures (Figs. 20.9, 20.10). Partial nephrectomy can be performed in extensive polar injuries (Fig. 20.11). If the ureter or pelvis has been injured, internal stents can be used to provide improved drainage. Nephrostomy is rarely necessary. The parenchymal margins should be held in approximation by the renal capsule. If the capsule has been destroyed, the laceration margins can be covered with omentum, free peritoneum, or absorbable collagen bolsters to prevent delayed bleeding and urinary extravasation (see Fig. 20.10).

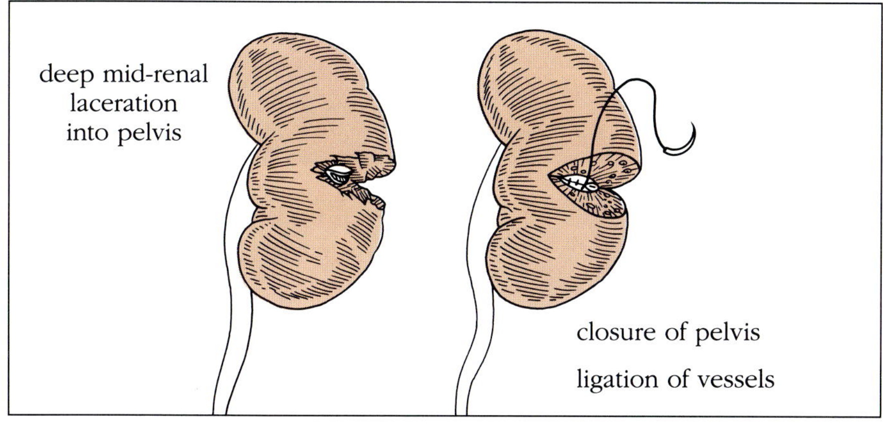

Figure 20.9 Repair of a renal injury extending into the collecting system.

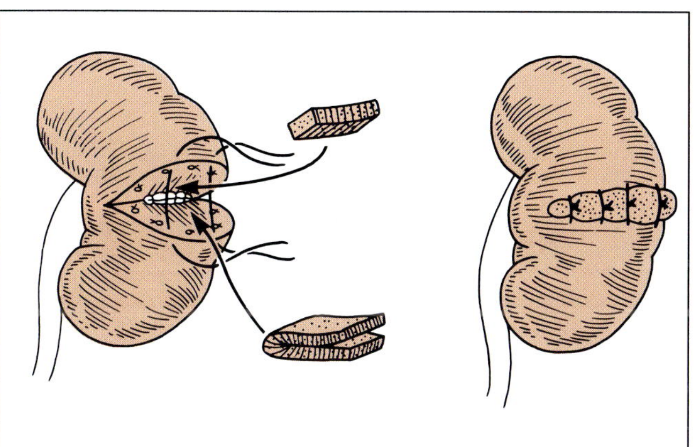

Figure 20.10 Renorrhaphy over bolsters.

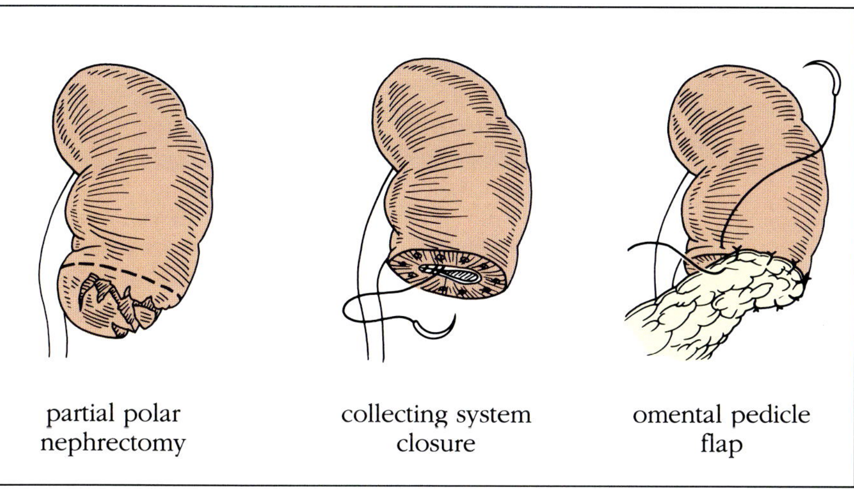

Figure 20.11 Technique for partial nephrectomy with an omental flap.

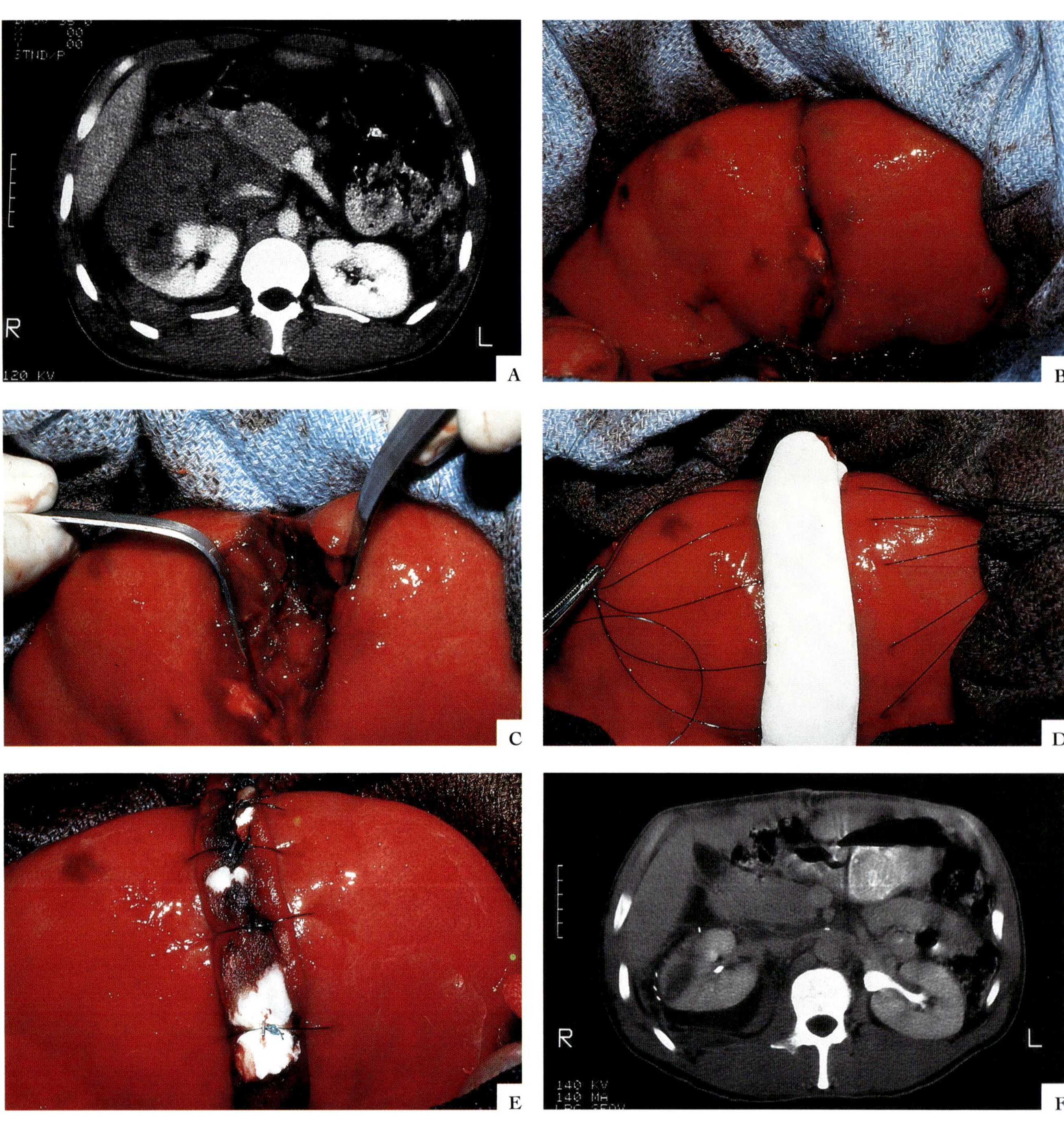

Figure 20.12 A 23-year-old man with a major right renal injury from a stab wound to the right flank. **A** CT demonstrates a deep parenchymal laceration with significant perirenal hematoma; **B** careful inspection, after complete exposure of the right kidney, reveals the laceration; **C** thorough debridement demonstrates the depth of injury; **D** renorrhaphy over a Gelfoam bolster; **E** completed renorrhaphy; **F** CT at 10 days postoperatively shows a lucent area at the level of injury corresponding to the Gelfoam bolster; **G** DMSA renal scan at 10 days also confirms symmetrical renal function. A linear area of decreased uptake can be seen on the right lateral renal border.

Management of vascular injuries is more difficult. Incomplete arterial injuries in a nonischemic kidney are amenable to repair, whereas complete arterial thrombosis with renal ischemia may be best managed by nephrectomy.[3] Injuries to the main renal vein can be repaired in the majority of cases. On the left side, the renal vein can be ligated at its origin, with adequate collateral drainage obtained by the gonadal and adrenal veins.

Reconstruction of vascular injuries, when indicated, should be performed promptly, limiting warm ischemia time.[15] Often temporary occlusion of both the renal artery and vein is required. Injuries to the main renal vessels can be repaired with fine vascular sutures. Segmental venous branches can be safely ligated because of their extensive collaterals. However, ligation of segmental arteries will result in parenchymal ischemia.

In patients with bilateral renal trauma or with injuries to a solitary renal unit, aggressive management becomes even more important. In these situations, thrombectomy with excision of the damaged artery and end-to-end anastomosis, use of a saphenous vein graft, or even autotransplantation should be attempted to preserve adequate renal function and avoid dialysis.

Outcome

Aggressive, accurate staging of renal trauma and careful attention to reconstruction are paramount in avoiding renal loss. Although most renal injuries are managed nonsurgically, renal salvage can be expected in almost 90% of cases requiring exploration (Fig. 20.12).[16]

Follow-up functional and anatomic studies, with dimercaptosuccinic acid scan (DMSA), IVP or CT, are obtained before discharge and at 6 weeks.

Hypertension is an acknowledged complication of renal trauma, occurring in approximately 5% of cases. Although it usually manifests within the first few months of injury, delayed onset (after 10 to 15 years) has been documented. Blood pressure should be measured regularly for the first year and annually thereafter. Other complications such as infection, bleeding, and continued urinary extravasation occur rarely.

References

1. Peters PC, Bright C. Blunt renal injuries. *Urol Clin North Am.* 1977;4:17.
2. Stables DP, Fouche RF, de Villiers Niekerk JP, Cremin BJ, Holt A, Peterson E. Traumatic renal artery occlusion: 21 cases. *J Urol.* 1976;115:229.
3. Carroll PR, McAninch JW, Klosterman P, Greenblatt M. Renovascular trauma: risk assessment, surgical management, and outcome. *J Trauma.* 1990;30:547.
4. Fackler M. Wound ballistics: a review of common misconceptions. *JAMA.* 1988;259:2730.
5. Carroll PR, McAninch JW. Operative indications in penetrating renal trauma. *J Trauma.* 1985;25:587.
6. Bright TC, White K, Peters PC. Significance of hematuria after trauma. *J Urol.* 1978;120:455.
7. Cass AS. Immediate radiologic and surgical management of renal injuries. *J Trauma.* 1982;22:361.
8. McAninch JW, Federle MP. Evaluation of renal injuries with computerized tomography. *J Urol.* 1982;128:456.
9. Steinberg DL, Jeffrey RF, Federle P, McAninch JW. The computerized tomography appearance of renal pedicle injury. *J Urol.* 1984;132:1163.
10. Lang K. Arteriography in the assessment of renal trauma: the impact of arteriographic diagnosis on preservation of renal function and parenchyma. *J Trauma.* 1975;15:553.
11. Nicholaisen GS, McAninch JW, Marshall G, Bluth RF, Carroll PR. Renal trauma: re-evaluation of indications for radiographic assessment. *J Urol.* 1985;133:183.
12. Cass AS, Cass BP. Immediate surgical management of severe renal injuries in multiple-injured patients. *Urology.* 1983;21:140.
13. Peterson NE. Intermediate-degree blunt renal trauma. *J Trauma.* 1977;17:425.
14. McAninch JW, Carroll PR. Renal exploration after trauma: indications and reconstructive techniques. *Urol Clin North Am.* 1989;16:203.
15. Brawley RK, Fisher RD, DeMeester TR, Elkins RC. Deliberate renal ischemia: a valuable and safe adjunct during operations upon the abdominal aorta. *Ann Thorac Surg.* 1972;13:356.
16. McAninch JW, Carroll PR, Klosterman PW, Dixon CM, Greenblatt MN. Renal reconstruction after injury. *J Urol.* 1991;145:932.

CHAPTER 21

Ureteral and Bladder Trauma

Noel A. Armenakas

Jack W. McAninch

Peter R. Carroll

Pathophysiology of Ureteral Trauma

Ureteral injuries from external trauma constitute approximately 1% of all genitourinary injuries. The low rate of injury to the ureter is due to its anatomic characteristics—its narrow diameter and retroperitoneal location between major muscle groups and the spine protect it from external forces.

Penetrating trauma is the most common cause, usually involving complete or partial ureteral transection. The heat generated by the rapid deceleration of a bullet can also cause major injury. This is usually detected after several days when urinary extravasation develops subsequent to necrosis of the ureteral wall.[1]

Ureteral injuries from blunt trauma are rare.[2] They usually occur in children and involve ureteral disruption at the level of the ureteropelvic junction because a child's vertebral column is extremely flexible and the ureteropelvic junction relatively fixed. During rapid deceleration, excessive bending of the vertebral column causes the ureter to separate (Fig. 21.1).[3] This can occur bilaterally and is usually associated with significant spinal injuries.[4,5]

The ureter is a three-layered structure (Fig. 21.2): an outer adventitial sheath, through which its blood supply courses; a medial layer made of longitudinal and circular smooth muscle fibers; and an inner mucosal lining consisting of transitional epithelium. The upper portion of the ureter receives its blood supply mainly from the renal arteries, its midportion from the aorta and iliac arteries,

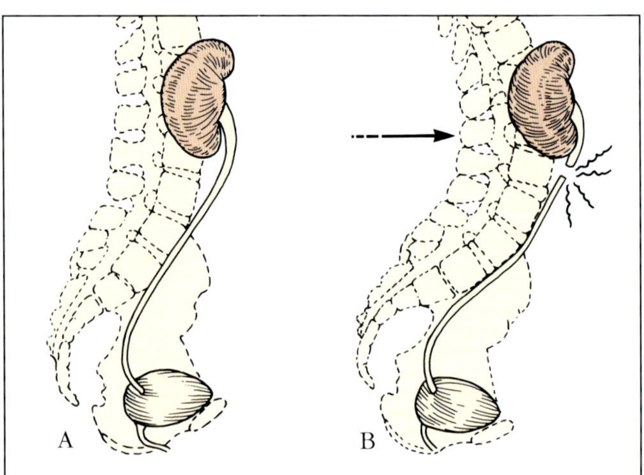

Figure 21.1 Pediatric ureteral injury. **A** Normal relationship between the urinary tract and the vertebral column. **B** Hyperextension of the lumbosacral spine with avulsion of the ureteropelvic junction.

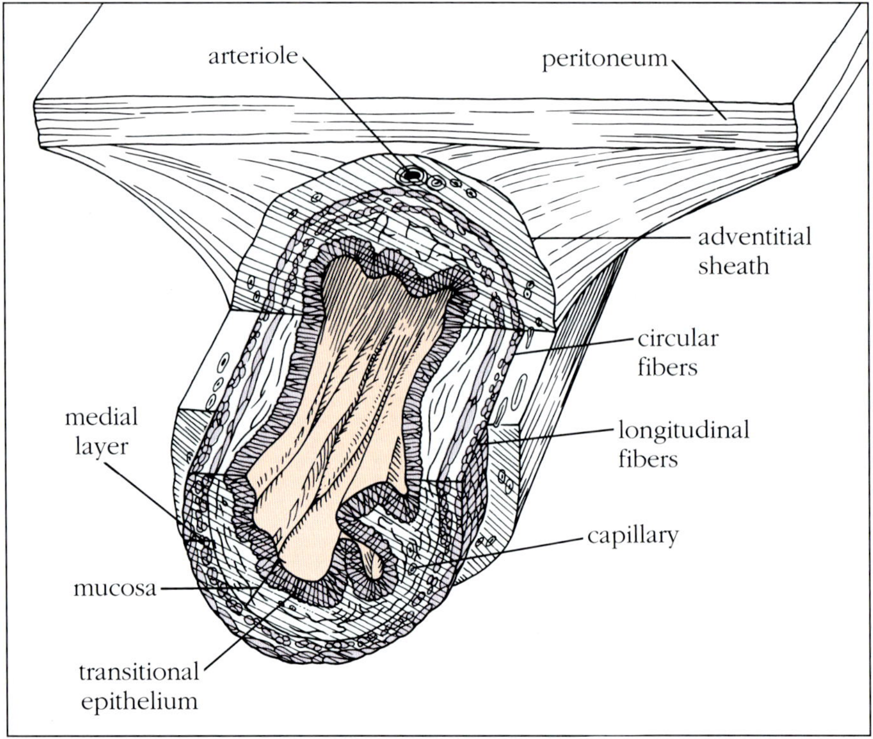

Figure 21.2 Cross-section of the ureter.

and its lower portion from the superior vesical, vaginal, middle hemorrhoidal, and uterine arteries (Fig. 21.3).[6] As these numerous sources are highly variable, ureteral dissection should be performed with great care to preserve the vasculature.

Diagnosis

A diagnosis of ureteral injury is based primarily on suspicion; there are no classic signs or symptoms. In patients with penetrating trauma, the site of injury should raise suspicion. Hematuria is an unreliable indicator and can be absent in more than 30% of cases.[7,8] Any patient with penetrating flank or abdominal trauma and a potential ureteral injury should have a renal contrast study, irrespective of the presence or absence of hematuria. Similarly, children with significant blunt abdominal trauma who cannot be adequately examined because of associated injuries should undergo radiographic evaluation, regardless of the findings on urinalysis.

RADIOGRAPHIC ASSESSMENT

Initial imaging is obtained with a complete excretory urogram (IVP). This may demonstrate extravasation of contrast, delayed function, or mild ureteral dilation proximal to the injury (Fig. 21.4). If these results are inconclusive, a retrograde ureterogram is indicated. Occasionally the diagnosis is made in the operating room during abdominal exploration. Intravenous injection of indigo carmine or methylene blue that is then excreted in the urine can be a helpful adjunct.

Management

Most patients with ureteral injury require operative exploration for management of associated abdominal injuries.[9] The most frequently involved sites are the small bowel, colon, and vascular system, and these should be repaired before ureteral exploration.[10]

The injured ureter is carefully inspected for evidence of contusion, discoloration, or lack of bleeding suggestive of ischemia. Selection of appropriate surgical management depends on the patient's condition, the site and extent of injury, and the time of diagnosis. Ureteral injuries with a significant delay in diagnosis or in an unstable patient can be managed by percutaneous nephrostomy drainage; otherwise, surgical repair should be performed.

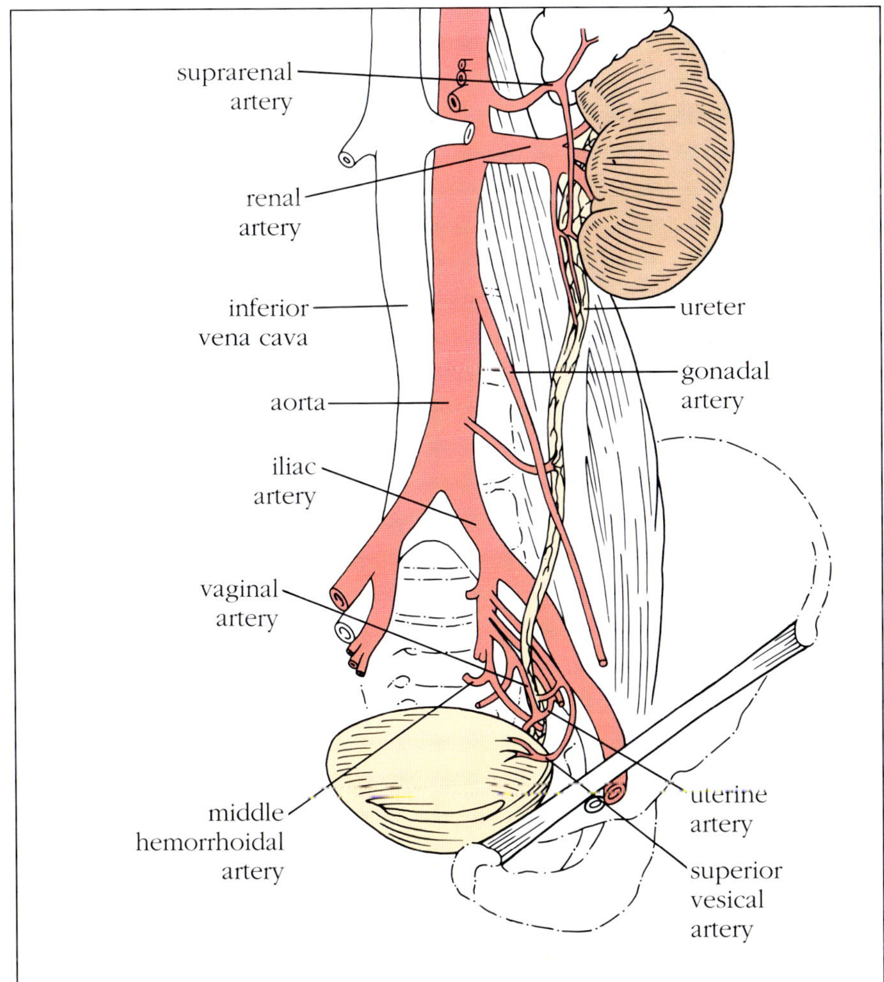

Figure 21.3 Ureteral anatomy, showing its blood supply.

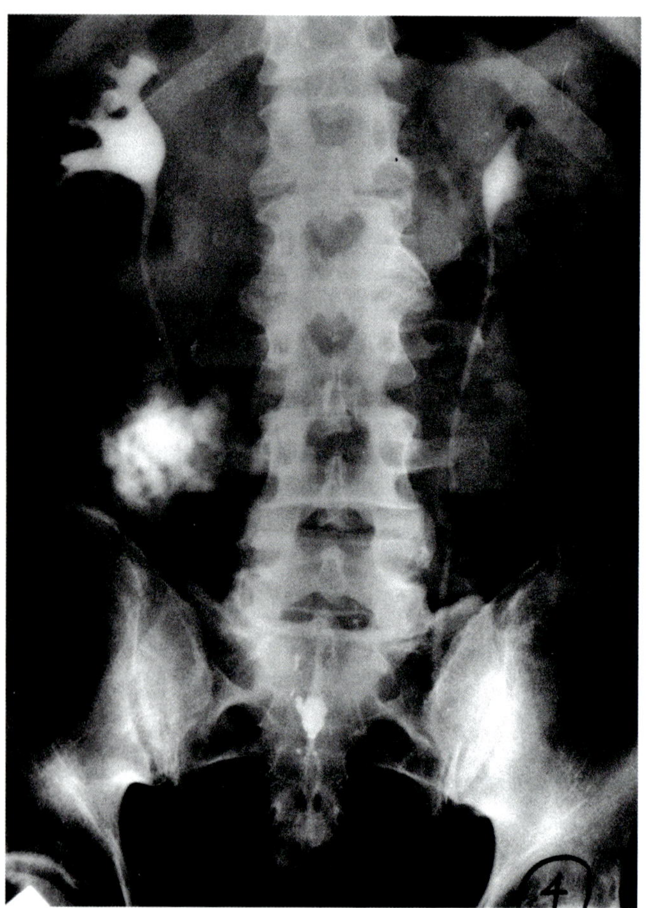

Figure 21.4 IVP showing right ureteral extravasation from a gunshot wound to the abdomen.

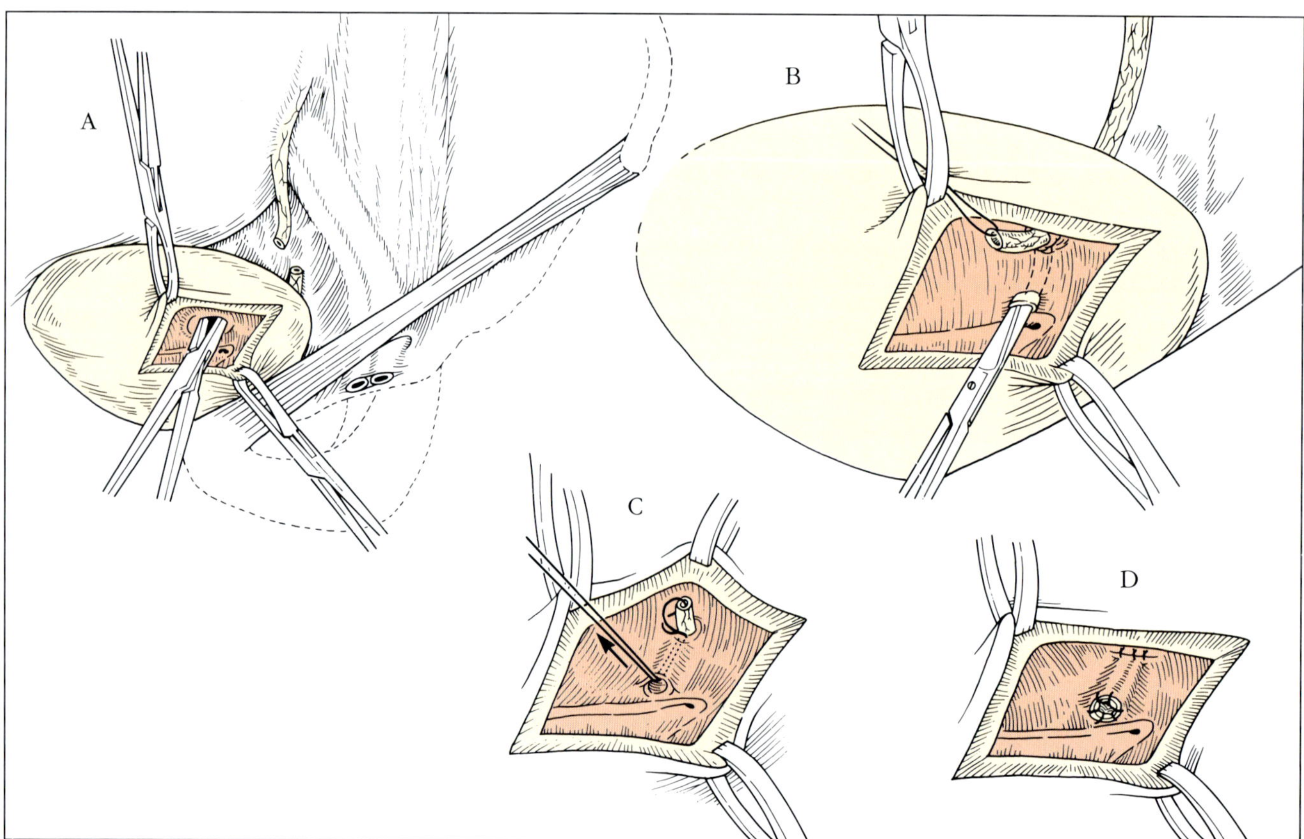

Figure 21.5 **A–D** Management of a lower ureteral injury by reimplantation.

URETERAL RECONSTRUCTION

General principles of ureteral reconstruction include careful debridement, creation of a watertight tension-free spatulated anastomosis, and adequate ureteral and retroperitoneal drainage. Various reconstructive techniques can be used, depending on the site and type of ureteral injury[11]:

1. Injuries to the lower third of the ureter are best managed by submucosal bladder reimplantation (Fig. 21.5). This can be done with a combined intra- and extravesical approach, bringing the ureter through the posterior bladder wall just medial to the original hiatus. A submucosal tunnel is created based on the standard 3:1 ratio (tunnel length:ureteral diameter). The distal ureter is then spatulated and secured to the bladder wall with interrupted 4-0 chromic sutures. The repair is stented and the bladder closed in two layers. A psoas hitch or Boari-Ockerblad flap can be used to facilitate mobilization (Fig. 21.6).

2. Injuries to the middle or upper third of the ureter are best managed by primary ureteroureterostomy (Fig. 21.7). This is performed after careful debridement and adequate dissection, allowing a tension-free anastomosis with fine absorbable sutures. With concomitant intraabdominal organ injury, the omentum can be used to exclude the ureter and protect the repair.

3. Long segmental ureteral injuries can be managed by transureteroureterostomy (Fig. 21.8). This is done by incising the posterior peritoneum and exposing both ureters. The diseased ureter is brought through a retroperitoneal window carefully to avoid any angula-

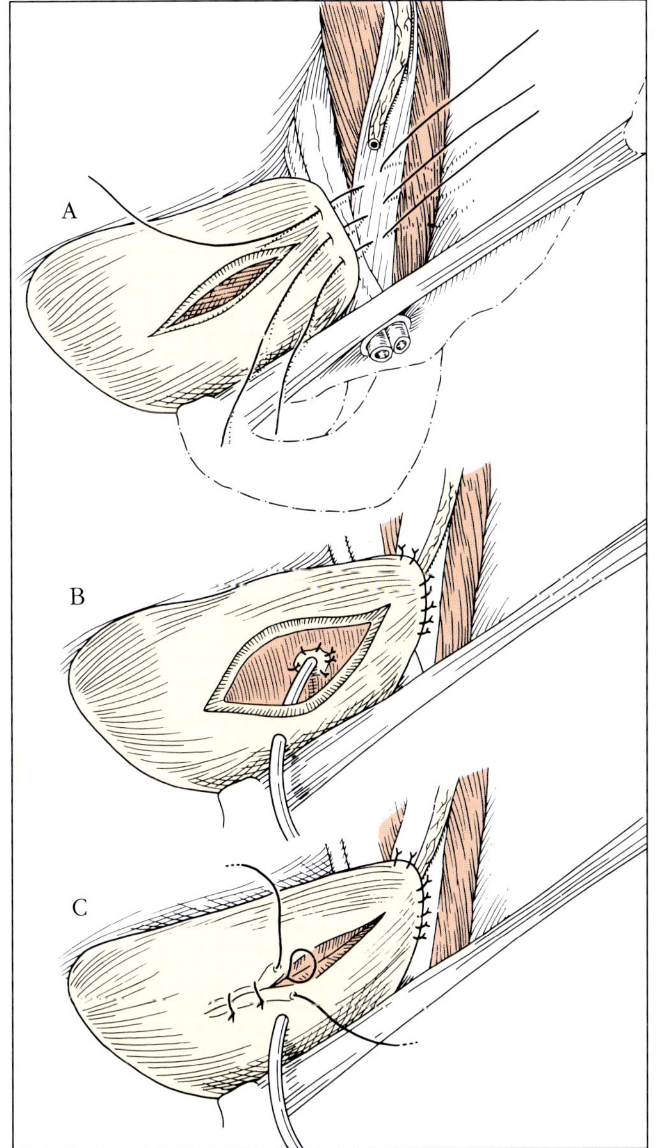

Figure 21.6 **A–C** Psoas hitch, allowing a tension-free ureterovesical anastomosis.

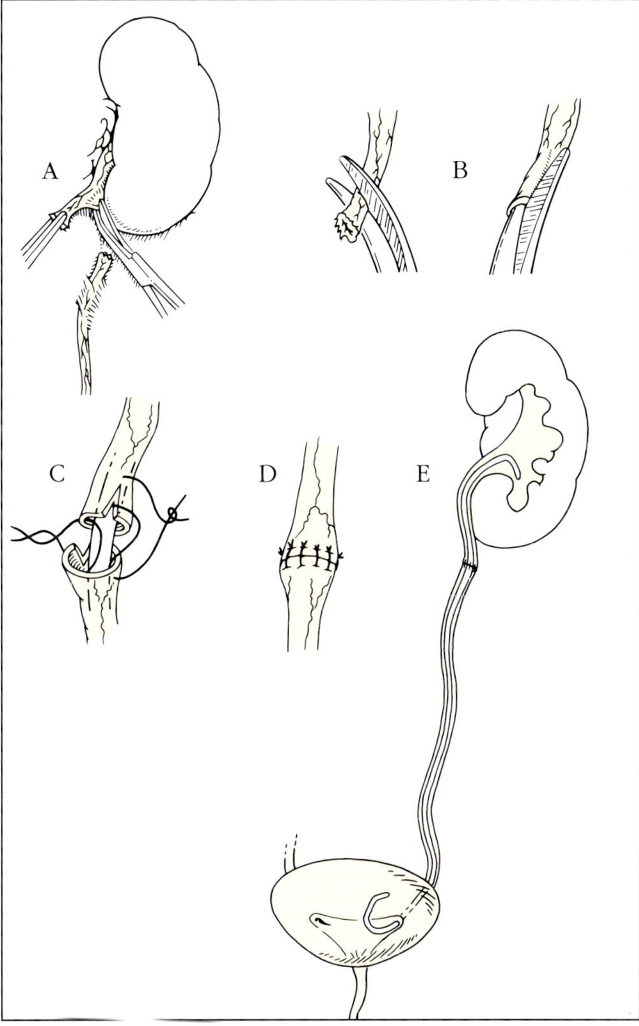

Figure 21.7 Repair of a mid-ureteral injury.
A Mobilization. **B** Debridement. **C** Spatulation.
D Completed end-to-end anastomosis. **E** Double-J stent in place.

tion. A 1.5-cm longitudinal ureterotomy is made on the medial surface of the recipient ureter, and an end-to-side tension-free anastomosis is created with running 4-0 chromic sutures.

4. In extensive ureteral injuries, autotransplantation or, rarely, ileal interposition can be used for renal salvage. Injuries that are recognized late are best managed by percutaneous nephrostomy drainage.

Outcome

Early diagnosis and careful reconstruction of ureteral injuries are important to minimize complications and preserve renal function. Complications are rare, but include fistula formation, stricture, extravasation, and infection. Radiographic evaluation with an IVP should be performed at 6 weeks and 3 months to assure proper healing.

Pathophysiology of Bladder Trauma

The bladder is second to the kidneys in frequency of injury, accounting for 22% of all genitourinary injuries. Bladder injuries are caused by either blunt or penetrating trauma to the lower abdomen, pelvis, or perineum. Blunt trauma, the more common cause, occurs from motor vehicle accidents, falls, and crush injuries and is associated with pelvic fracture in 97% of cases.[12] Most lacerations are remote from the pelvic fracture site.[13] The major mechanism of injury appears to be the shock wave gener-ated from the impact and the inertia forces in rapid deceleration. Moreover, fragments of the pubic rami may perforate the bladder, resulting in extraperitoneal rupture. Rarely, bladder rupture is seen without pelvic fracture: this occurs with a distended bladder and is invariably intraperitoneal.

The location of the bladder deep within the bony pelvis protects it from most penetrating trauma. However, the possibility of bladder trauma should be considered in lower abdominal gunshot and knife injuries.

Diagnosis

HISTORY AND PHYSICAL

Blunt bladder injury should be suspected after external abdominal trauma. The patient usually complains of abdominal tenderness and distention and is often unable to void. Associated injuries exist in almost all patients. Of these, the most frequently encountered are pelvic and long bone fractures, as well as central nervous system and chest injuries. Hemodynamic instability is common because of extensive blood loss in the pelvis and from the associated injuries.

URINALYSIS

Gross hematuria occurs in 95% of bladder ruptures from blunt injuries; the remainder will have microhematuria.[12] Urine is best obtained by urethral catheter passage. However, before catheterization the urethral meatus should be carefully inspected; blood at the meatus is indicative of a urethral injury that requires retrograde urethrography before manipulation.

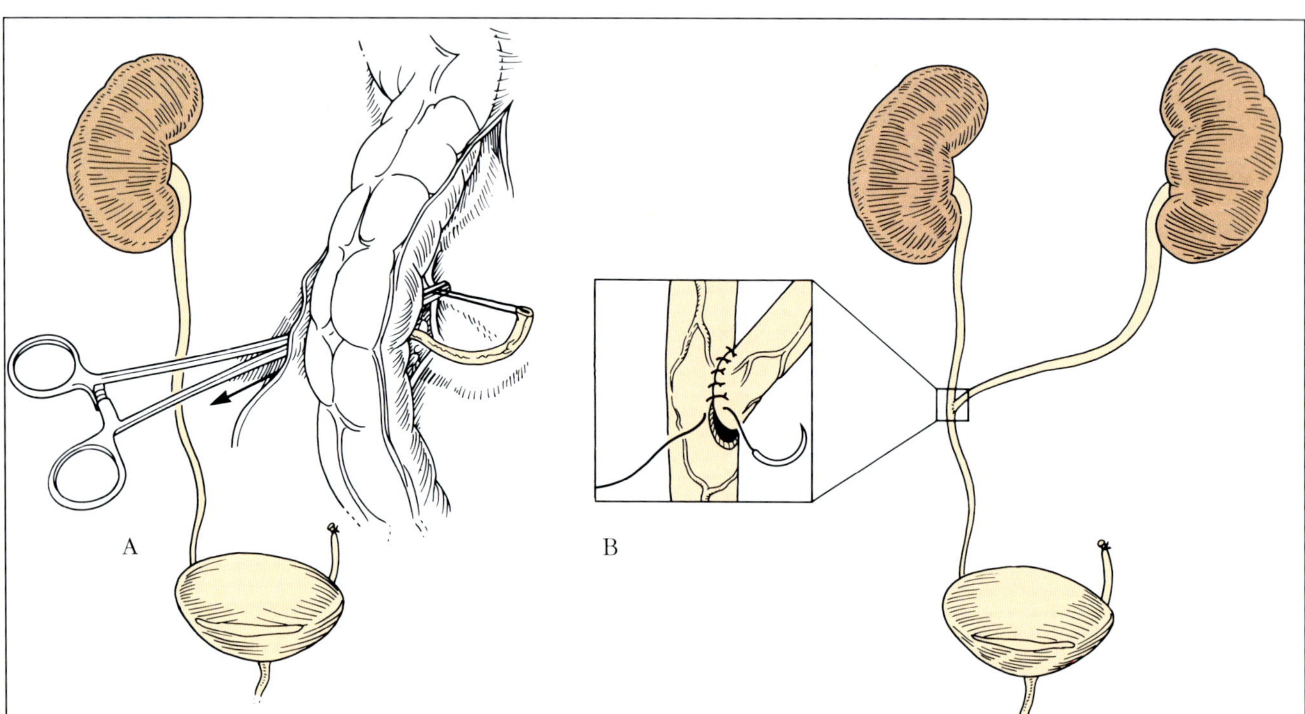

***Figure 21.8* A,B** Technique of transureteroureterostomy.

IMAGING

Cystography is the most accurate method of diagnosis.[14] A plain film of the pelvis is first obtained; 350 mL of water-soluble contrast material is infused by gravity to distend the bladder completely, and anteroposterior and drainage films are taken. The drainage film is very important because 15% of extraperitoneal ruptures are seen only on it. Extraperitoneal bladder rupture characteristically shows extravasation confined to the perivesical soft tissues (Fig. 21.9). In the presence of a large pelvic hematoma, the bladder is often compressed into a teardrop configuration (Fig. 21.10). Intraperitoneal bladder rupture shows extravasation in the peritoneal cavity, with bowel loops outlined by contrast (Fig. 21.11). Although the cystogram is accurate in diagnosing bladder injuries, the amount of contrast extravasated does not correlate with the extent of injury.

CLASSIFICATION

Bladder trauma can be classified by the type of injury:
1. Contusions, which are not associated with urinary extravasation and represent damage to the mucosa or muscularis, without resultant loss of bladder wall continuity.
2. Intraperitoneal ruptures, which most often involve the dome, this being the weakest, most mobile portion of the bladder.
3. Extraperitoneal ruptures, which represent the most common pattern of major injury and usually involve the anterior or lateral bladder walls.

Approximately 12% of bladder ruptures are both intra- and extraperitoneal.[12]

Management

The choice of management depends on the overall status of the patient, the type of bladder injury sustained, and the extent of associated injuries.

Bladder contusions can be treated by transurethral catheter drainage alone, which is maintained until hematuria completely resolves. Extravesical ruptures in patients who do not require laparotomy for repair of associated injuries can also be managed nonoperatively, provided that the urine is sterile at the time of injury.[15] In such cases, bladder drainage is maintained for 2 weeks, at which time a low-pressure cystogram can be obtained to document adequate healing.

SURGICAL MANAGEMENT

Surgical exploration is performed through a midline infraumbilical incision by adhering to the following steps:
1. Initially a small peritoneotomy is made. If free peritoneal blood is found, the peritoneotomy can be extended to allow complete inspection of abdominal viscera.
2. The space of Retzius is exposed by dissecting in the midline, avoiding any lateral pelvic hematomas.
3. An anterior cystotomy is made, allowing complete inspection of the entire bladder wall.
4. The ureteral orifices are inspected for injury. Intravenous

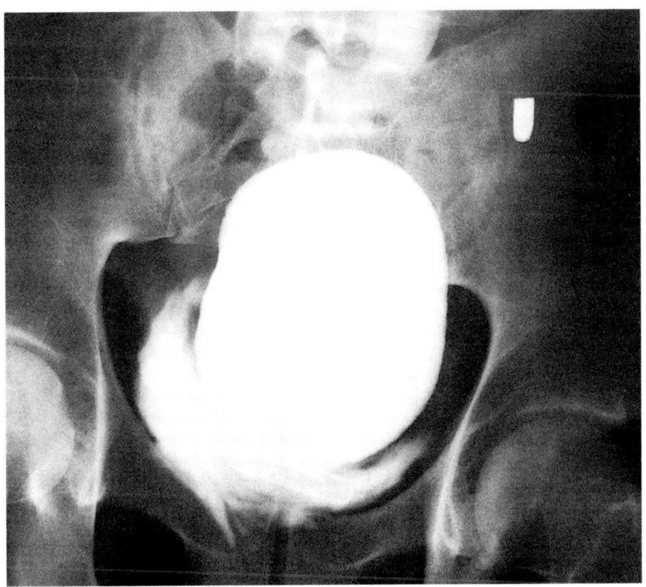

Figure 21.9 Cystogram of extraperitoneal bladder rupture.

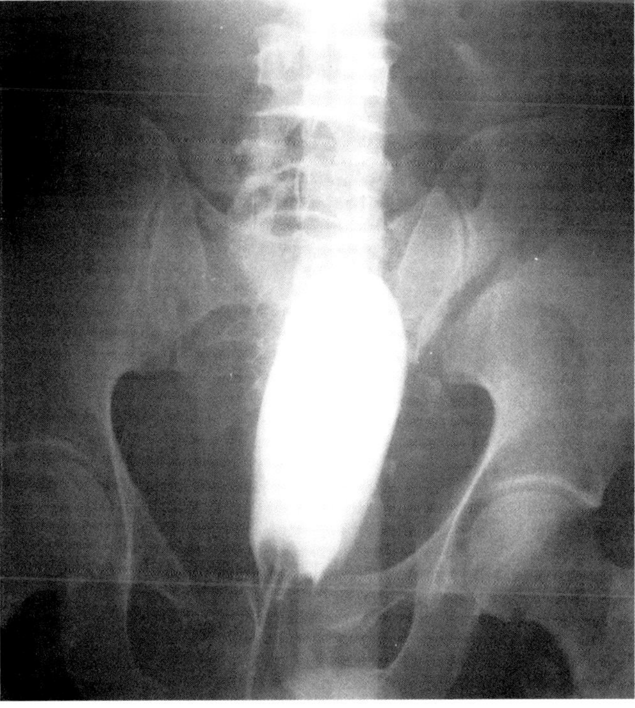

Figure 21.10 Cystogram showing characteristic "teardrop" configuration of extensive pelvic hematoma.

infusion of indigo carmine or ureteral intubation can be used to confirm integrity of the distal ureter.

5. Extraperitoneal lacerations are repaired from within the bladder lumen, in one or two layers, with interrupted or running 3-0 absorbable sutures.

6. Lacerations extending into the bladder neck are carefully repaired by reconstructing the sphincteric components with fine absorbable sutures. This decreases the likelihood of posttraumatic incontinence or contracture.

7. Intraperitoneal ruptures are closed in multiple layers, incorporating the peritoneum and bladder muscle in one layer and the bladder mucosa in another.

8. A large suprapubic tube is used to drain the bladder and the anterior cystotomy is closed in two layers. Retropubic drains should be avoided because of the risk of infection and hematoma. A urethral catheter is maintained until gross hematuria clears. The suprapubic tube is left in place for 7 to 10 days, and contrast studies are performed before its removal.

Outcome

Mortality in patients with bladder trauma is over 20%[12] and is usually related to the associated injuries rather than to the bladder rupture. Complications of the bladder injury rarely occur. Incontinence is seldom seen, and initial urinary urgency, frequency, or bladder instability usually subsides. Bladder infections resulting from prolonged catheter drainage can be managed with appropriate antibiotic therapy.

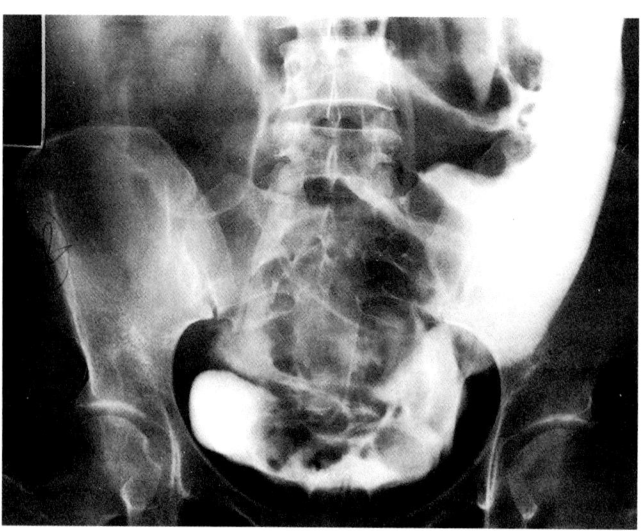

Figure 21.11 Cystogram of intraperitoneal bladder rupture demonstrating bowel loops outlined by contrast.

References

1. Cass AS. Ureteral contusion with gunshot wounds. *J Trauma.* 1984;24:59.
2. Carlton CE Jr, Scott R, Guthrie AG. The initial management of ureteral injuries: a report of 78 cases. *J Urol.* 1971;105:335.
3. Diokno AC. Avulsion of the proximal ureter secondary to blunt trauma. *J Urol.* 1974;111:412.
4. Jaffray DC, Jones HWF, Pringle RG. Renal pelviureteric injury in traumatic paraplegia. *Injury.* 1985;16:244.
5. Heath AD, May A. Bilateral avulsion of the upper ureters. *Br J Urol.* 1975;47:386.
6. Guerriero WG. Ureteral trauma. In: McAninch JW, ed. *Trauma Management: Urogenital Trauma.* New York, NY: Thieme-Stratton; 1985;2:50.
7. Presti JC Jr, Carroll PR, McAninch JW. Ureteral and renal pelvic injuries from external trauma: diagnosis and management. *J Trauma.* 1989;29:370.
8. Liroff SA, Pontes JES, Pierce JM. Gunshot wounds of the ureter: five years of experience. *J Urol.* 1977;118:551.
9. Carlton CE Jr, Guthrie AG, Scott R Jr. Surgical correction of ureteral injury. *J Trauma.* 1969;9:457.
10. Gangai MP, Agee RE, Spence CR. Surgical injury to the ureter. *Urology.* 1976;8:22.
11. Presti JC Jr, Carroll PR. Intraoperative management of the injured ureter. *Perspect Colon Rectal Surg.* 1988;1:98.
12. Carroll PR, McAninch JW. Major bladder trauma: mechanisms of injury and a unified method of diagnosis and repair. *J Urol.* 1984;132:254.
13. Corriere JN Jr, Sandler CM. Mechanisms of injury, patterns of extravasation and management of extraperitoneal bladder rupture due to blunt trauma. *J Urol.* 1988;139:43.
14. Carroll PR, McAninch JW. Major bladder trauma: the accuracy of cystography. *J Urol.* 1983;130:887.
15. Corriere JN Jr, Sandler C. Management of the ruptured bladder: seven years of experience with 111 cases. *J Trauma.* 1986;126:830.

CHAPTER 22

Urethral Trauma

Noel A. Armenakas

Peter R. Carroll

Jack W. McAninch

Anatomically, the male urethra is divided into four portions: prostatic, membranous, bulbous, and penile-pendulous. However, a more appropriate classification, when evaluating urethral trauma, is the division into posterior and anterior segments. The posterior urethra includes the prostatic and membranous portions; the anterior urethra is composed of the bulbous and pendulous urethral segments.

Pathophysiology

The major cause of urethral rupture is blunt trauma at the level of the urogenital diaphragm.[1] Most injuries are caused by motor vehicle accidents or falls, and over 95% occur in conjunction with pelvic fracture. The shearing force, generated by disruption of the pelvis, pulls the prostatic urethra and its attachments on the inferior pubis in one direction, while the membranous urethra, attached to the urogenital diaphragm, is pulled in another (Fig. 22.1).

Anterior urethral injuries are also commonly caused by blunt trauma,[2] and most are from straddle injuries. In anterior urethral injuries confined by Buck's fascia, extravasation of urine and blood is contained within the penis; disruption of Buck's fascia allows extravasation extending along the abdominal wall just below Scarpa's fascia (Fig. 22.2).

Penetrating injuries to the anterior urethra are less common. They are usually iatrogenic, occurring during urethral instrumentation.

Injuries to the female urethra are exceedingly rare. They are more common in children than in adults and are usually accompanied by pelvic fracture. These lacerating injuries often extend into the bladder neck or vagina and can disrupt the normal continence mechanism.

Diagnosis

HISTORY AND PHYSICAL

A history of perineal trauma or pelvic fracture should alert the examining physician to a potential urethral injury. Blood at the urethral meatus is the single best

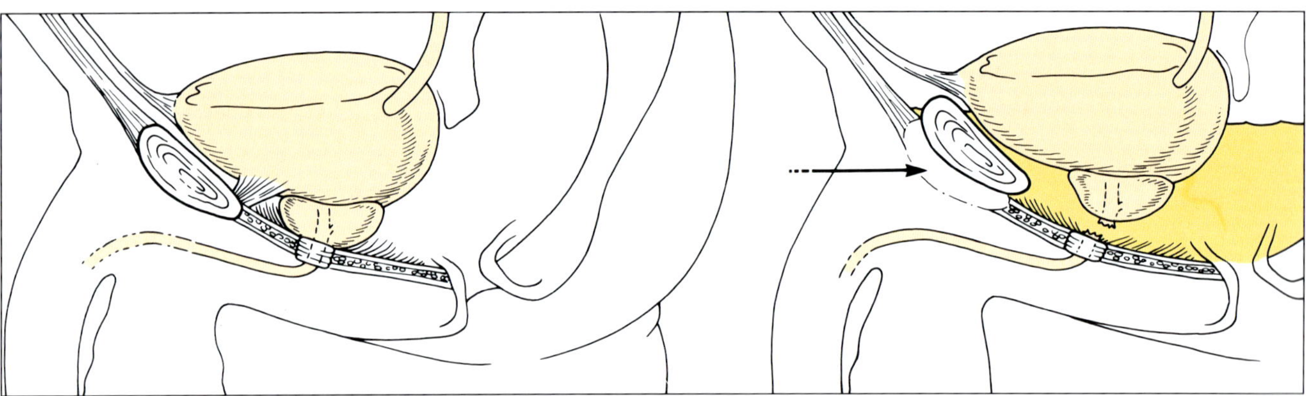

Figure 22.1 Posterior urethral rupture with superior displacement of the prostate.

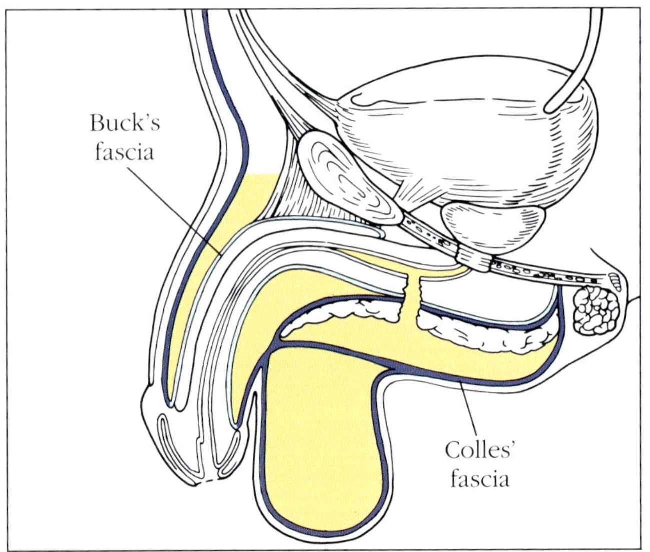

Figure 22.2 Anterior urethral rupture with disruption of Buck's fascia, allowing extravasation of urine into the scrotum and anterior abdominal wall.

indicator of urethral trauma (Fig. 22.3).[3,4] Before urethral catheter passage, the meatus should be carefully inspected. A rectal exam should be performed in all cases. With posterior urethral disruption, the prostate may be elevated or "high-riding."

Absence of blood at the meatus and an orthotopic prostate on rectal exam are sufficient evidence that safe passage of a urethral catheter is possible (Fig. 22.4).

IMAGING

Retrograde urethrography is the best method to establish the diagnosis of urethral injury.[1] A small Foley catheter is introduced in the distal pendulous urethra, and its balloon inflated to 2 mL. Approximately 20 mL of undiluted water-soluble contrast material is injected and a roentgenogram is taken. In complete urethral disruption, contrast is not visible within the urinary tract proximal to the

injury; in partial disruption, contrast material enters the bladder.[3]

Management

INITIAL MANAGEMENT

The preferred initial management of urethral injury is suprapubic cystostomy urinary diversion.[3,5] This is most often performed as an open procedure to allow identification of coexisting bladder injury, which occurs in 33% of posterior urethral injuries.[3] A percutaneously placed cystostomy tube can be used for anterior urethral injuries, although its small lumen and the passage of blood clots may impede adequate drainage.

Urethral realignment has been advocated as initial treatment of selected prostatomembranous disruptions.[4,6] It should be considered only in a hemodynamically stable

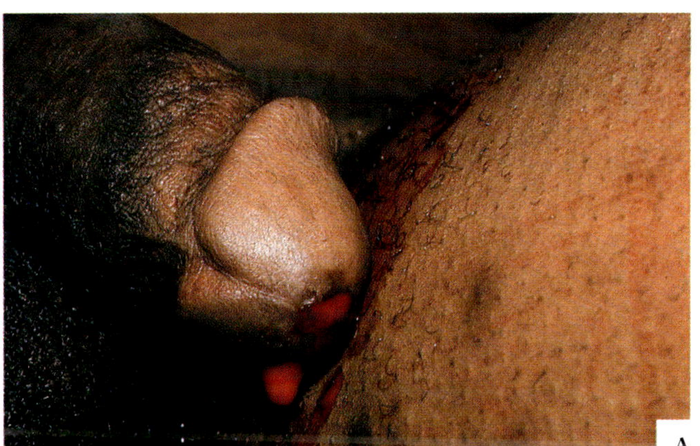
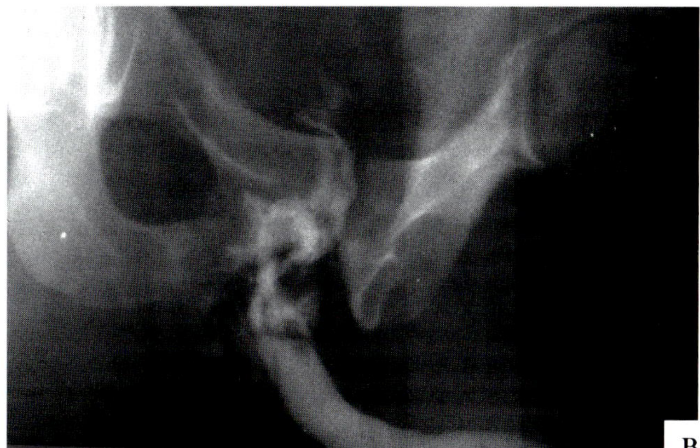

Figure 22.3 **A** Blood at the meatus after blunt pelvic trauma. **B** Retrograde urethrogram shows complete posterior urethral disruption.

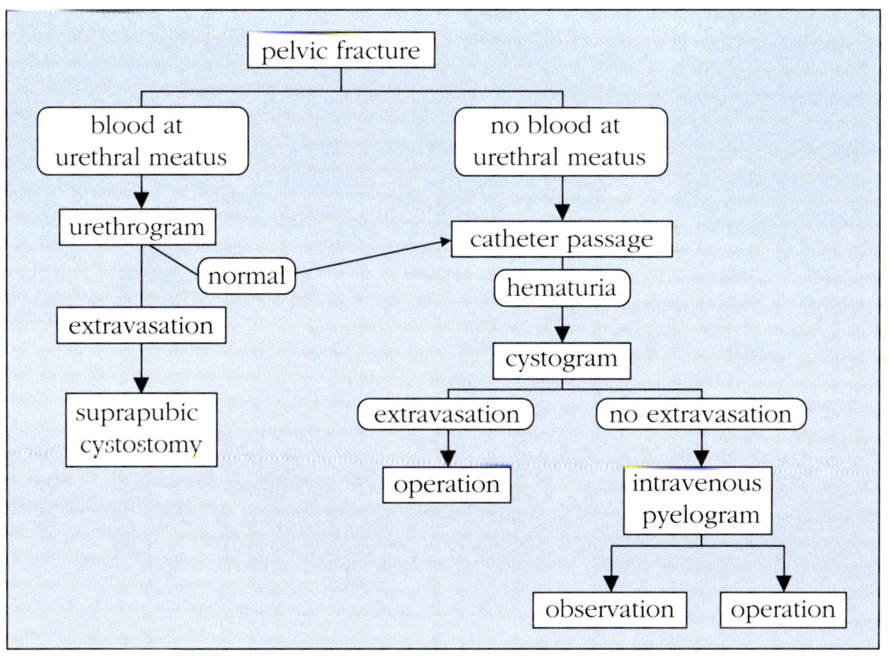

Figure 22.4 Algorithm for management of pelvic trauma.

patient without associated injuries. Its primary advantage is in possibly preventing subsequent formation of long strictures and, in certain instances, additional surgery. The disadvantage of this approach is a higher reported rate of impotence than with initial cystostomy tube drainage.[5,7]

RECONSTRUCTION

Definitive treatment of urethral strictures is usually deferred for 3 to 6 months, allowing recovery from any associated injuries and completion of collagen maturation. Not all patients will develop a clinically significant stricture after urethral trauma, and a voiding cystogram will determine the need for surgery. In most instances, however, a dense fibrotic stricture will have formed at the site of injury. The length, location, and depth of scarring can be assessed preoperatively by retrograde urethrography, magnetic resonance imaging, and sonourethrography.[8,9]

The techniques for repairing posterior urethral strictures range from endoscopic urethrotomy to perineal urethroplasty.[10,11] The preferred reconstructive approach is by combining perineal and lower abdominal incisions.[3] This is done by adhering to the following steps[12] (Fig. 22.5):

1. The patient is placed in a lithotomy position and the perineum and lower abdomen are adequately prepped and draped.
2. A vertical perineal incision is made, exposing the entire bulbar urethra.
3. The dissection is carried deep into the perineum and

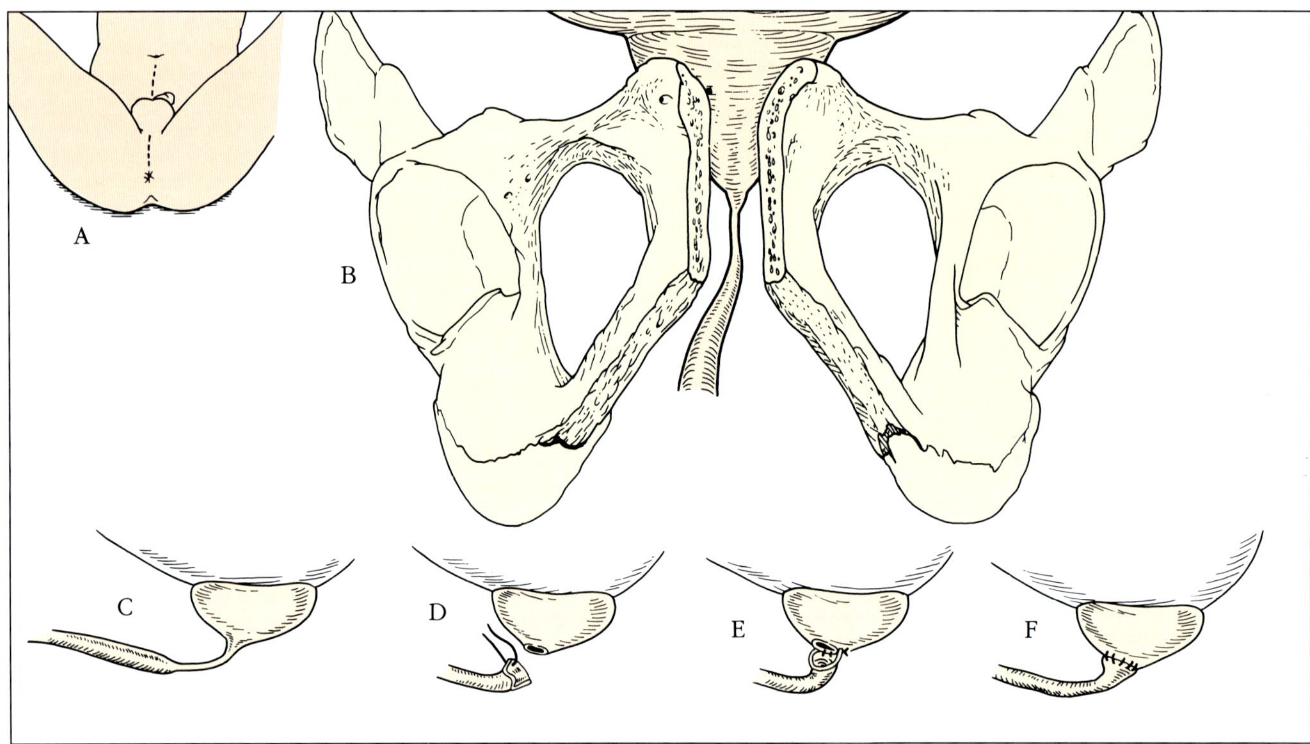

Figure 22.5 Posterior urethral reconstruction: **A** lower abdominal and perineal incisions; **B** completed pubectomy clearly exposing the entire area of stricture; **C** excised stricture; **D** urethral spatulation; **E** anastomosis begun after mobilization of the bulbar urethra; **F** completed reconstruction.

the stricture identified by antegrade and retrograde catheter instrumentation. All scar tissue is completely excised proximally and distally.

4. If visualization is poor, the pubis is removed by making a midline lower abdominal incision, extending to the penile base. The ventral surface of the pubis is exposed and the suspensory ligament of the penis is released. The dissection is extended to the posterior portion of the symphysis and a wedge of bone removed with the Gigli saw. This allows clear exposure of the entire stricture and prostatic apex without mobilizing the prostate.

5. The anterior urethra is then dissected distally, obtaining sufficient length to anastomose it directly to the prostatic apex. Interrupted 6-0 absorbable suture material is used.

6. An 18 Fr stenting urethral catheter and a suprapubic cystostomy tube are left in place.

The urethral catheter is removed in 3 weeks, and a voiding cystourethrogram obtained. The cystostomy is removed once normal voiding is documented. Postoperatively, these patients are followed at 3 and 12 months with flow rate determinations and urethrography.

Various options exist for the treatment of anterior urethral strictures. Endoscopic management includes dilation, direct-vision internal urethrotomy, and urethral stent placement.[13,14] However, most significant strictures are

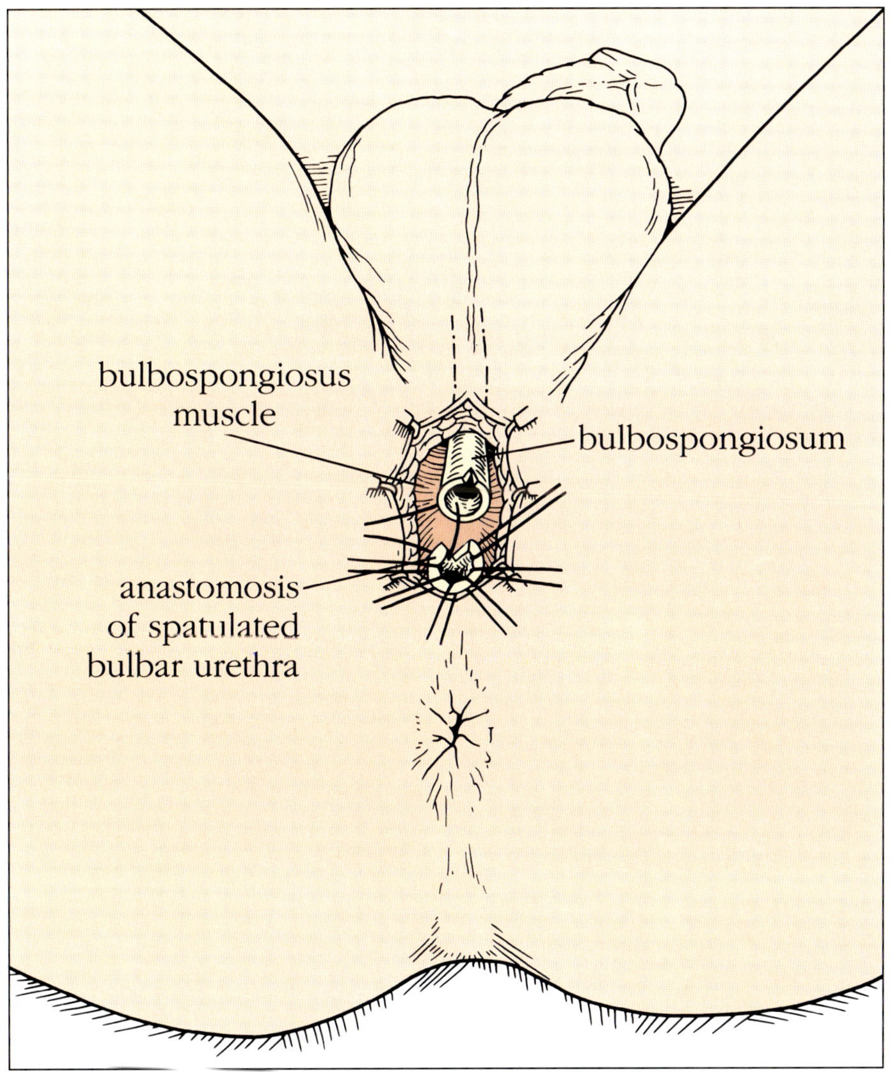

Figure 22.6 Creation of a spatulated anastomosis at the level of the bulbar urethra.

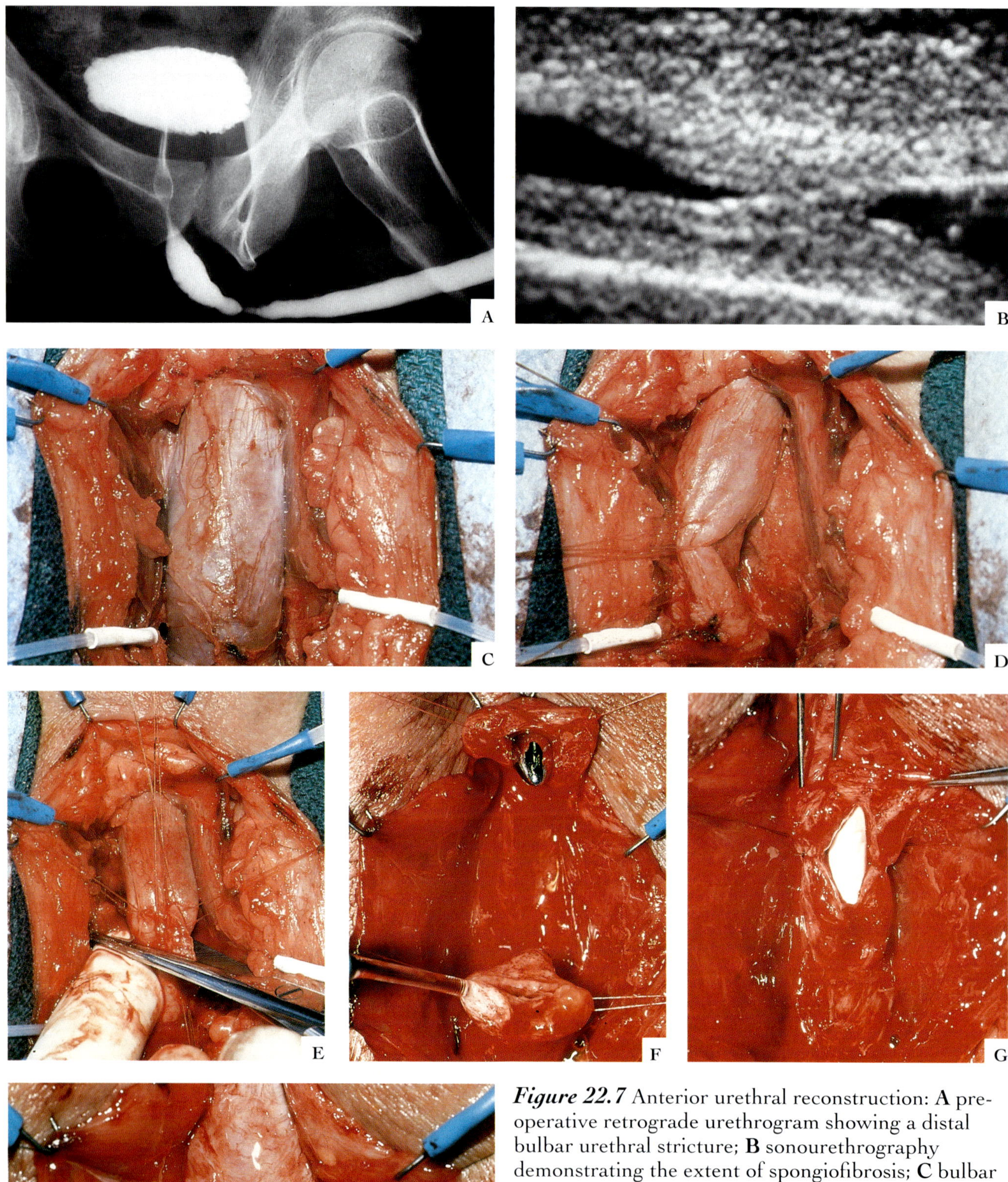

Figure 22.7 Anterior urethral reconstruction: **A** preoperative retrograde urethrogram showing a distal bulbar urethral stricture; **B** sonourethrography demonstrating the extent of spongiofibrosis; **C** bulbar urethral dissection through a midline perineal incision; **D** mobilization of the bulbar urethra; **E** urethral transection at the level of the stricture; **F** mobilized urethral ends; **G** posterior anastomosis completed over a silicone catheter; **H** completed reconstruction.

best managed with open repair. Excision with primary anastomosis is the preferred treatment of strictures up to 2 cm in length (Figs. 22.6, 22.7).[15–17] For longer urethral defects, hairless fasciocutaneous flaps should be used. These are based on a vascular pedicle, usually developed from Buck's fascia. Once fully mobilized, they can be placed as an onlay or tubularized flap, bridging up to 15 cm of stricture. Full-thickness skin grafts are limited only to reconstruction of the more vascular bulbar urethra.

Outcome

Urethral trauma can result in devastating long-term consequences. To a young person, the complications of impotence, stricture, and incontinence often create life-long morbidity. Initial cystostomy drainage with delayed repair is associated with a lower rate of impotence (10% to 20%) than immediate reconstruction (50%).[3–5] Often potency returns slowly, taking up to 1 or 2 years. Strictures recur in less than 10% of patients. Most of these can be treated by direct vision urethrotomy. Incontinence, previously reported in up to one third of patients undergoing initial primary repair, decreases to less than 5% with the delayed reconstruction described above.[3,6] With anterior urethral injury, stricture formation is the most common complication; impotence and incontinence are very rare.

Although urethral injuries often present complex problems, a favorable outcome can be achieved with careful evaluation and appropriate management. This requires a thorough knowledge of the various reconstructive techniques. In this way, normal voiding and potency can be restored.

Reference

1. Pokorny M, Pontes JE, Pierce JM Jr. Urological injuries associated with pelvic trauma. *J Urol.* 1979;121:455.
2. Pontes JE, Pierce JM Jr. Anterior urethral injuries: four years of experience at the Detroit General Hospital. *J Urol.* 1978;120:563.
3. McAninch JW. Traumatic injuries to the urethra. *J Trauma.* 1981;21:291.
4. Devine PC, Devine CJ. Posterior urethral injuries associated with pelvic fractures. *Urology.* 1982;20:467.
5. Morehouse DD, MacKinnon KJ. Management of prostato–membranous urethral disruption: 13-year experience. *J Urol.* 1980;123:173.
6. Deweerd JH. Immediate realignment of posterior urethral injury. *Urol Clin North Am.* 1977;4:75.
7. Gibson GR. Impotence following fractured pelvis and ruptured urethra. *Br J Urol.* 1970;42:86.
8. Dixon CM, Hricak H, McAninch JW. Magnetic resonance imaging of traumatic posterior urethral defects and pelvic crush injuries. *J Urol.* 1992;148:1162.
9. McAninch JW, Laing FC, Jeffrey RB Jr. Sonourethrography in the evaluation of urethral strictures: a preliminary report. *J Urol.* 1988;139:294.
10. Waterhouse K, Laungani G, Patil U. The surgical repair of membranous urethral strictures: experience with 105 consecutive cases. *J Urol.* 1980;123:500.
11. Webster GD, Ramon J. Repair of pelvic fracture posterior urethral defects using an elaborated perineal approach: experience with 74 cases. *J Urol.* 1991;145:744.
12. McAninch JW. Pubectomy in repair of membranous urethral stricture. *Urol Clin North Am.* 1989;16:297.
13. Sandozi S, Ghazali S. Sachse optical urethrotomy, a modified technique: 6 years of experience. *J Urol.* 1988;140:968.
14. Milroy EJG, Chapple C, Eldin A, Wallsten H. A new treatment for urethral strictures: a permanently implanted urethral stent. *J Urol.* 1989;141:1120.
15. Quartey JKM. One-stage penile/preputial cutaneous island flap urethroplasty for urethral stricture: a preliminary report. *J Urol.* 1983;129:284.
16. de la Rosette JJMCH, deVries JDM, Lock MTWT, Debruyne FMJ. Urethroplasty using the pedicled island flap technique in complicated urethral strictures. *J Urol.* 1991;146:40.
17. Devine PC, Sakati IA, Poutasse EF, Devine CJ Jr. One stage urethroplasty: repair of urethral strictures with a free full thickness patch of skin. *J Urol.* 1968;99:191.

CHAPTER 23

Genital Trauma

Noel A. Armenakas
Peter R. Carroll
Jack W. McAninch

Genital injuries occur rarely, constituting 7% of all genitourinary trauma.[1] Anatomically they can be divided into testicular, penile, and scrotal injuries.

Testicular Trauma

PATHOPHYSIOLOGY

Most testicular injuries result from blunt trauma and they are usually unilateral. The testicle's mobility and the strength of the tunica albuginea serve as protective mechanisms. A direct blow that forces the testicle against the pubic symphysis, however, can result in partial or complete rupture. Penetrating testicular injuries from gunshot and stab wounds are less common.

DIAGNOSIS

It is often difficult to assess the extent of testicular injury accurately by clinical means alone, as scrotal and testicular trauma are associated with significant swelling and hematoma formation. The diagnosis can be made more easily by scrotal ultrasonography. Multiple hypoechoic patterns within the testicular parenchyma are a highly sensitive but nonspecific finding.[2,3] In patients with testicular trauma who do not have a large scrotal hematoma, the sonogram may demonstrate architectural changes consistent with rupture, including parenchymal irregularity, extruded testicular tissue, or disruption of the tunica albuginea.

MANAGEMENT

All penetrating testicular injuries and any blunt testicular injury suggestive of a rupture are best managed with immediate exploration. This is done through a hemiscrotal incision during which all blood clots are evacuated. Any extruded parenchyma is debrided and the tunica albuginea is reapproximated with 2-0 or 3-0 running absorbable suture material (Fig. 23.1). Drains are seldom used. Testicular reconstruction is successful in most cases,

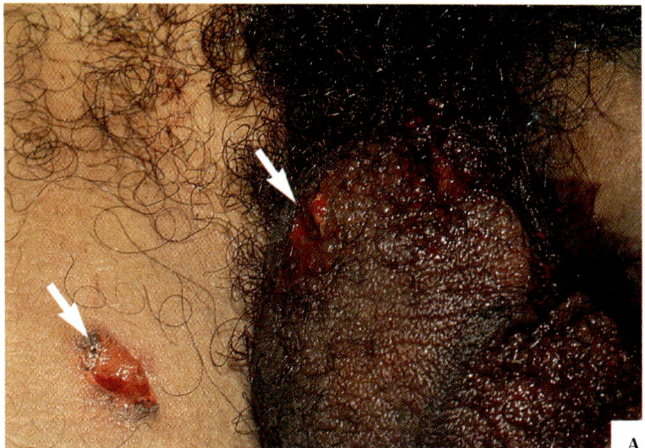

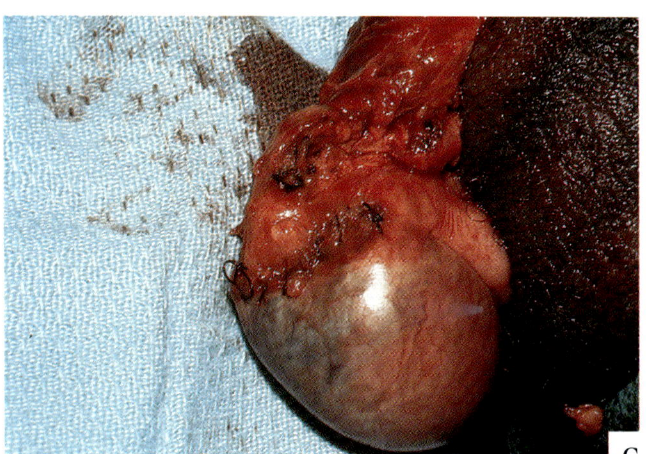

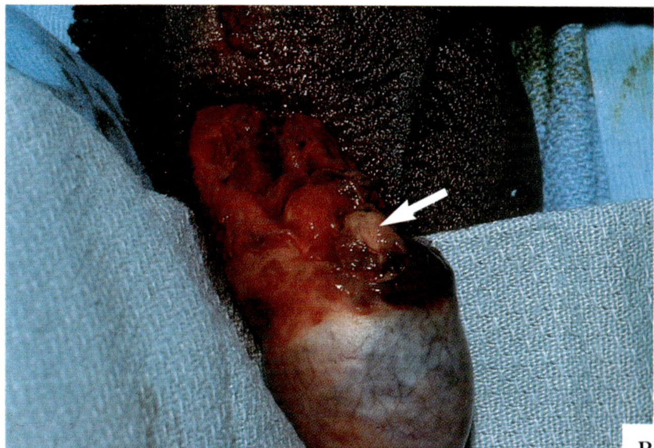

Figure 23.1 Penetrating testicular injury: **A** gunshot wound to right hemiscrotum and anterior thigh; **B** extruded seminiferous tubules; **C** debridement and closure of tunica albuginea.

although orchiectomy may be necessary for management of extensive injuries.

OUTCOME

Immediate exploration with testicular reconstruction is associated with a shorter hospital stay, better pain control, and a quicker convalescence. Moreover, the likelihood of infection is minimized and testicular function is preserved.[4]

Penile Trauma

PATHOPHYSIOLOGY

Penile injuries, although rare, have diverse mechanisms, including ruptures, amputations, strangulations, gunshot wounds, and avulsions. Ruptures, most of which occur during sexual intercourse, result from the sudden application of force to the erect penis, rupturing the tunica albuginea (Fig. 23.2). In 20% of cases, the urethra is simultane-

ously disrupted.[5] Amputations are usually self-inflicted, representing an attempt at self-emasculation. Strangulations in adults usually result from constricting penile rings used to prolong erection and increase sexual gratification (Fig. 23.3); in children, they are associated with experimentation and are commonly caused by hair, string, or rubber bands.[6,7] The penis becomes edematous and its blood flow is compromised, resulting in glanular or penile skin necrosis. Gunshot wounds usually cause little tissue destruction apart from the entrance and exit wounds (Fig. 23.4); 50% involve the urethra.[8] Avulsions result from entrapment of clothes by farm machinery or from deceleration injuries when the genitalia are caught on a stationary object.[9] They often result in extensive skin loss.

DIAGNOSIS

The diagnosis of penile injuries is usually established from the history and clinical findings. Patients with penile ruptures typically report a cracking sound during inter-

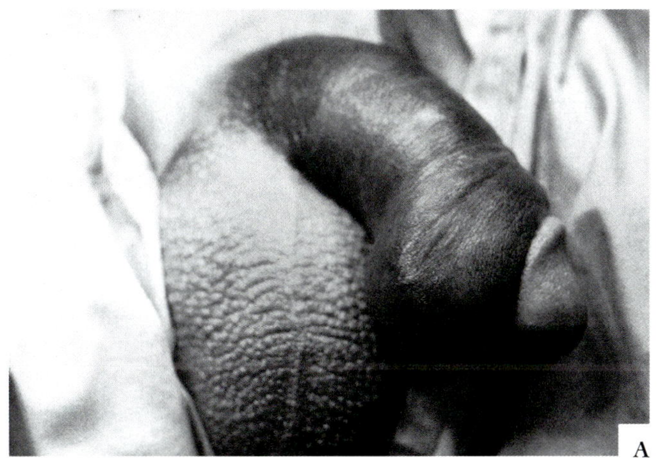

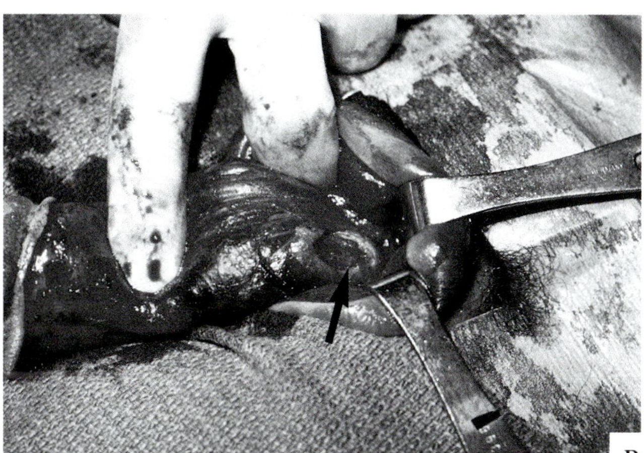

Figure 23.2 Penile rupture: **A** typical shaft ecchymosis; **B** demonstration of a tear involving the corpus cavernosum.

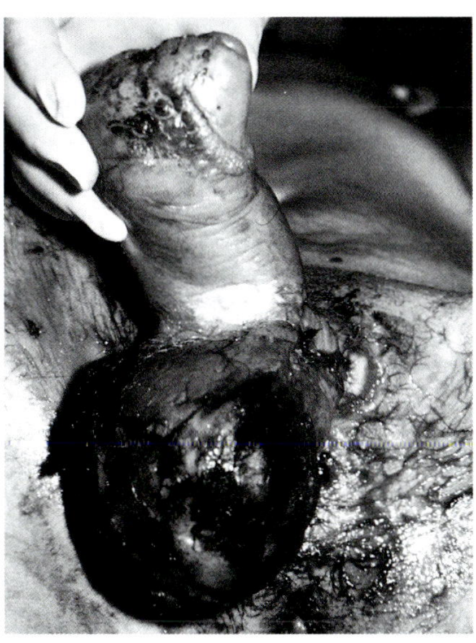

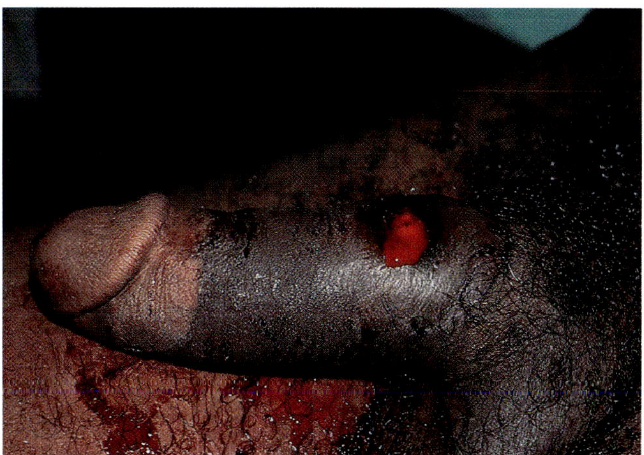

Figure 23.3 Strangulation injury to penis from a constricting ring.

Figure 23.4 Gunshot (entrance) wound to the penile shaft.

course, followed by immediate pain and detumescence. The accompanying penile hematoma and edema may compress the urethra and obstruct voiding. On physical exam, the rupture defect in the corpora cavernosa may be palpated. Other penile injuries can also be identified this way and the extent of injury established. Retrograde urethrography may be used in selected cases to define urethral involvement better.

MANAGEMENT

Penile ruptures should be explored through a circumferential subcoronal incision. The corpora are exposed and the laceration identified. The involved area is debrided and the cavernosal margins approximated with a running 2-0 absorbable suture. A coexisting urethral injury should be simultaneously repaired with 5-0 or 6-0 interrupted suture material.

Treatment of traumatic penile amputations depends on the availability and condition of the severed penile segment, as well as on the interval between injury and surgery. Ideally, reconstruction should be attempted within 6 hours.[10] Primary microvascular reimplantation yields the best results (Fig. 23.5). This can be performed by adhering to the following steps[11]:

1. Proximal vascular control is achieved by placing a Penrose drain around the penile base.
2. The penile stump and amputated segment are thoroughly irrigated with antibiotic solution.

3. The tunica albuginea is closed with 2-0 interrupted absorbable sutures and the urethra is anastomosed over a catheter with fine absorbable suture material.
4. Reanastomosis of the deep dorsal vein, at least one dorsal artery, and the dorsal nerve is completed with a microvascular technique.
5. The fascial layers are approximated to help secure a tension-free repair. Proximal urinary diversion is recommended.
6. Postoperatively, the penis is elevated and loosely wrapped to facilitate venous and lymphatic drainage.

In strangulation injuries to the penis, the constricting agent must be promptly removed. This may require the use of metal-cutting devices, including a heavy scissors, saw, or drill. Irrigation of the corpora cavernosa with heparinized saline may facilitate removal of the constricting device, as the distal corpora are engorged in such cases.[1]

Penile gunshot wounds mandate exploration and reconstruction. Because of the excellent blood supply to the penis, debridement should be minimized in an effort to preserve as much tissue as possible. Both corpora and fascia can be reapproximated precisely. The skin is closed loosely to decrease the likelihood of postoperative infection.

Avulsion injuries should be carefully cleansed and all necrotic tissue debrided. If primary closure is not feasible, skin grafts from the lower abdomen or thigh can be used to cover the defect (Figs. 23.6, 23.7). Thick (0.018 inch)

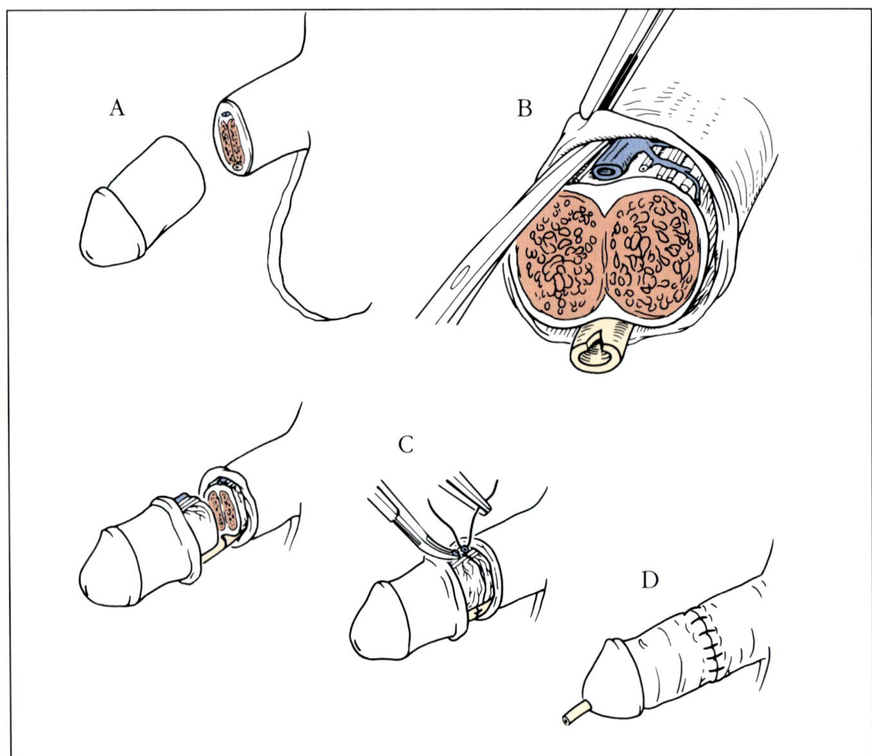

Figure 23.5 Technique of microvascular penile reimplantation: **A** complete penile amputation; **B** minimal debridement, preserving the dorsal neurovascular bundle; **C** corporal reapproximation preceding vascular reanastomosis and urethral reconstruction; **D** completed reimplantation.

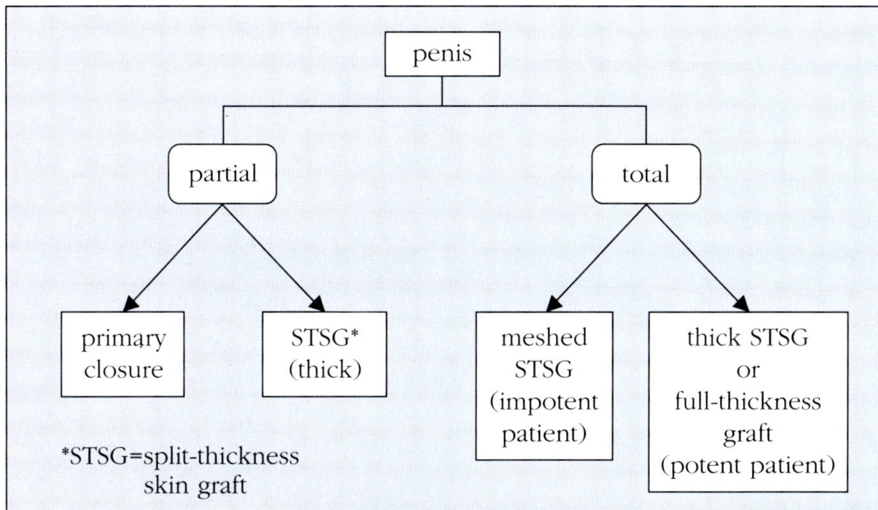

Figure 23.6 Algorithm for management of penile avulsion injuries.

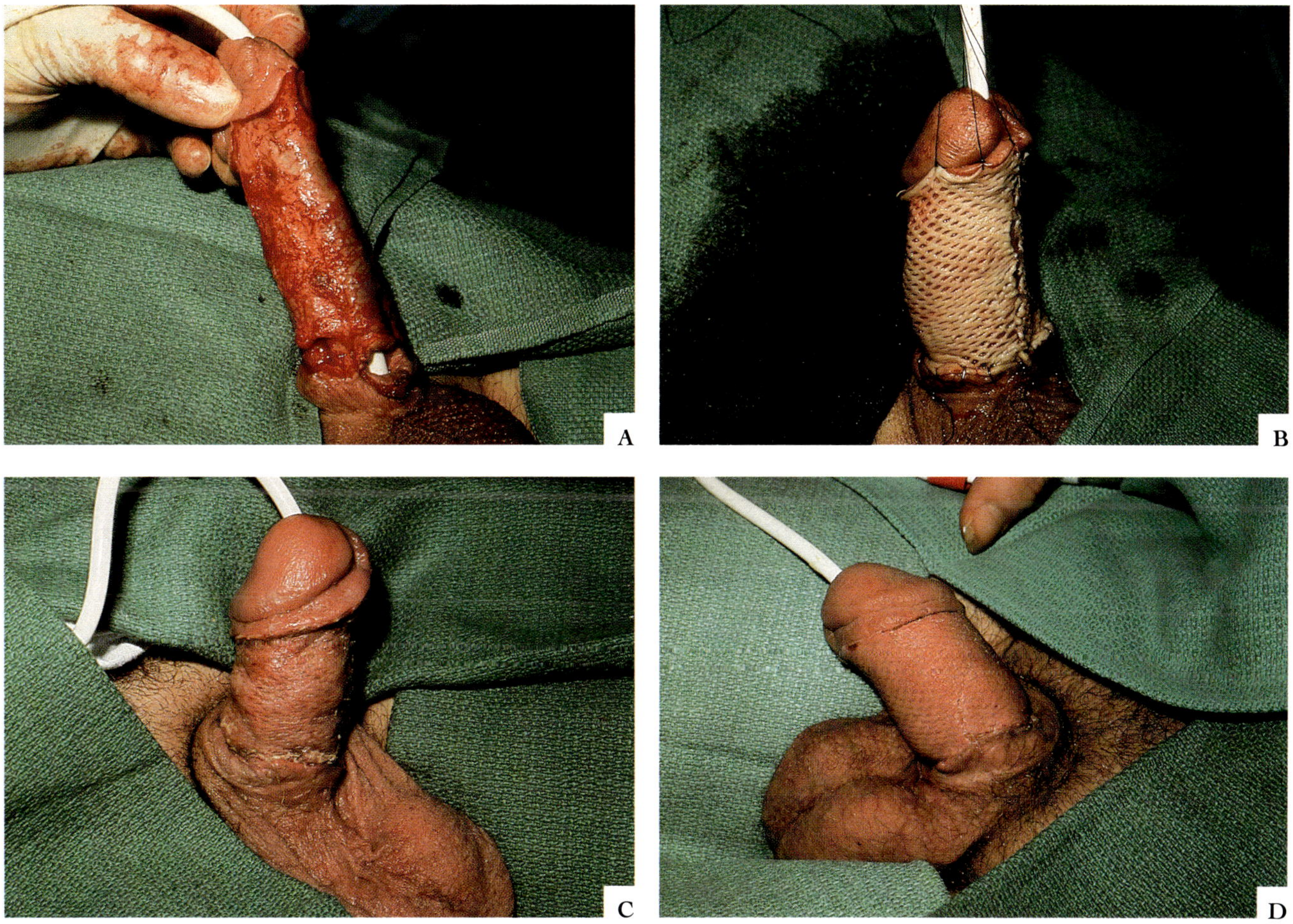

Figure 23.7 Intraoperative photographs of a penile reconstruction: **A** extensive penile skin loss from an avulsion injury; **B** meshed split-thickness skin graft; **C** 1 week postoperatively; **D** 2 weeks postoperatively, an excellent cosmetic result.

split-thickness skin grafts cause only minimal contracture and are consequently most appropriate for potent patients in whom retention of erectile function is a consideration. Meshed split-thickness grafts give excellent coverage but will result in more contracture and thus should be reserved for impotent patients.[9] Immobilization of the graft is of utmost importance in ensuring a successful take. Perioperative antibiotics are given. Postoperatively, the penile dressing is first removed after 5 days, at which time the graft is relatively fixed. Graft-take should exceed 90%.

OUTCOME

Treatment of penile injuries requires a thorough knowledge of regional anatomy and reconstructive techniques. Excellent functional and cosmetic results can be obtained. Complications such as skin necrosis, strictures, fistulas, and impotence can be minimized.

Scrotal Trauma

PATHOPHYSIOLOGY

Scrotal injuries are usually caused by either necrotizing infections or avulsion injuries. Infections are most commonly seen in older patients. In the majority of cases, a focus of infection can be identified.[12] Abscesses arising perirectally or periurethrally can penetrate Colles' or Buck's fascia, respectively, allowing rapid spread. Avulsion injuries to the scrotum are similar to those involving the penis (see above). Penetrating scrotal injuries from gunshot or stab wounds are infrequent.

DIAGNOSIS

Necrotizing scrotal infections initially manifest with pain, swelling, crepitus, and fever. Their clinical course is rapidly progressive, with skin necrosis and even septic shock. Both aerobic and anaerobic pathogens are responsible, with *Streptococcus, Bacteroides,* and *Escherichia coli* usually cultured.[12] Contributing conditions include alcohol abuse, diabetes mellitus, and prolonged bed rest in debilitated patients.

MANAGEMENT

Management of these infections is often complex (Fig. 23.8). All patients should be placed on broad-spectrum antibiotics. However, immediate surgical debridement is the mainstay of treatment, with extensive removal of all nonviable tissue. Further debridement is usually necessary within 24 hours, and it should be repeated as often as necessary to ensure removal of all infected tissue. A cystostomy is required in 83% (a diverting colostomy in 31% of these).[13] Reconstruction is performed only after the infection has been adequately controlled. Split-thickness skin grafts, rotational thigh flaps, or tissue expanders can be used to close the defect. If reconstruction is delayed, the testes can be protected by burying them in thigh pouches.

Penetrating scrotal injuries should be promptly explored. Principles of management include lavage, debridement, hemostasis, and reconstruction. Scrotal entrance or exit wounds can be safely sutured. Conservative treatment is reserved for selected cases in which clinical and sonographic findings exclude injury to the underlying structures.

OUTCOME

Aggressive wound care with control of infection and careful reconstruction are necessary in the successful management of scrotal injuries. In this way, mortality, which occurs in 20% of such patients, can be minimized.[12]

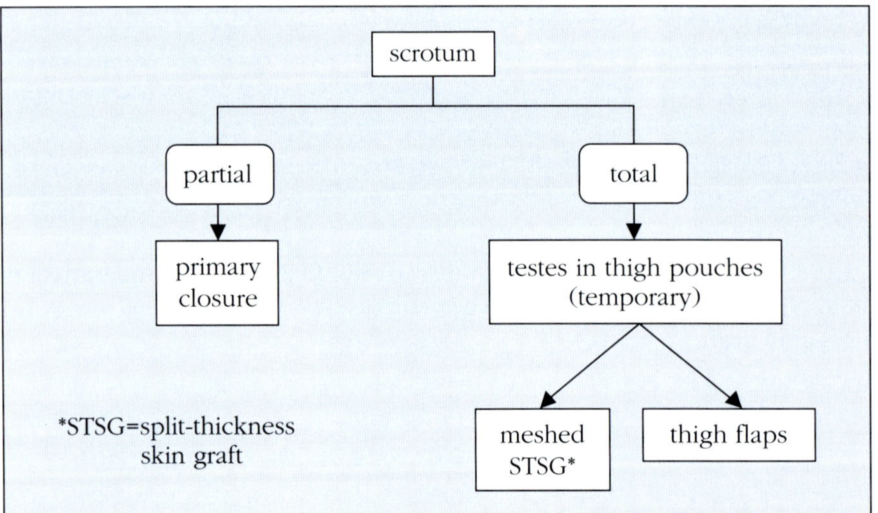

Figure 23.8 Algorithm for management of scrotal skin loss.

References

1. Cass AS. Male genital injury from external trauma. In: Cass AS, ed. Genitourinary Trauma. Boston, Mass: Blackwell Scientific Publications; 1988;257: Ch 15.
2. McAninch JW, Kahn RI, Jeffrey RB, Laing FC, Krieger MJ. Major traumatic and septic genital injuries. J Trauma. 1984;24:291.
3. Willscher MK, Conway W Jr, Daly J, DiGiacino M, Patten D. Scrotal ultrasonography. J Urol. 1983;130:931.
4. Cass AS. Testicular trauma. J Urol. 1983;129:299.
5. Nicolaisen GS, Melamud A, Williams RD, McAninch JW. Rupture of the corpus cavernosum: surgical management. J Urol. 1983;130:917.
6. Merrill DC, Palmer JM. Male genital trauma. In: Blaisdell FW, Trunkey DD, McAninch JW, eds. Trauma Management, II: Urogenital Trauma. New York, NY: Thieme-Stratton, 1985:97.
7. Singh B, Kim H, Wax SH. Strangulation of glans penis by hair. Urology. 1978;11:170.
8. Miles BJ, Poffenberger RJ, Farah RN, Moore S. Management of penile gunshot wounds. Urology. 1990;36:318.
9. McAninch JW. Management of genital skin loss. Urol Clin North Am. 1989;16:387.
10. Engelman ER, Polito G, Perley J, Bruffy J, Martin DC. Traumatic amputation of the penis. J Urol. 1974;112:774.
11. Carroll PR, Lue TF, Schmidt RA, Trengrove-Jones G, McAninch JW. Penile replantation: current concepts. J Urol. 1985;133:281.
12. Carroll PR, Cattolica EV, Turzan CT, McAninch JW. Necrotizing soft-tissue infections of the perineum and genitalia: etiology and early reconstruction. West J Med. 1986;144:174.
13. Baskin LS, Carroll PR, Cattolica EV, McAninch JW. Necrotising soft-tissue infections of the perineum and genitalia: bacteriology, treatment and risk assessment. Br J Urol. 1990;65:524.

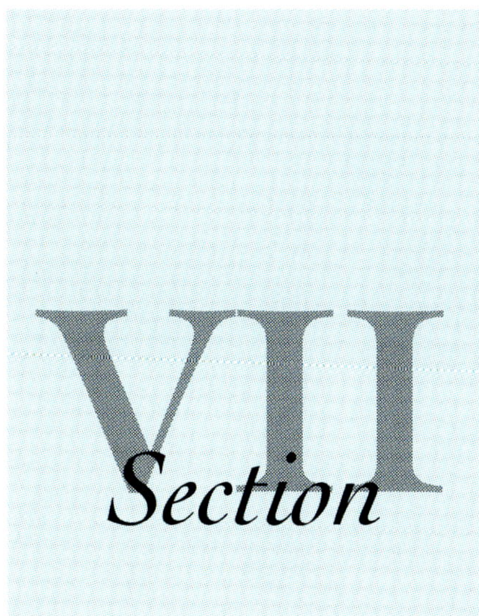

Section **VII**

Infertility

Jonathan P. Jarow, editor

CHAPTER 24

Evaluation of the Infertile Male

Michael Coburn

The evaluation of the male partner of an infertile marriage begins with a complete history and physical examination. Male sexual and reproductive function is directly dependent on an intact hypothalamic–pituitary–gonadal axis and is affected by a variety of systemic disorders. It is essential for the examining physician to have a basic understanding of male reproductive physiology to expedite the assessment of these patients. This section provides a general overview of the history and physical examination and more specific information regarding the diagnosis of varicocele, use of transrectal ultrasonography, and testis biopsy.

History

The evaluation of patients with male infertility requires a thorough general medical history with emphasis on specific factors that may affect male reproductive function by influencing the quality of sperm production, the process of ejaculation, and potency. The important aspects of the infertility history are listed in Figure 24.1.

The physiology of spermatogenesis must be kept in mind when the medical history of an infertility patient is investigated. The complete process of spermatogenesis requires 74 days for development of a mature sperm from precursor elements, and passage of sperm through the reproductive tract requires an additional 10 to 14 days. The sperm sample produced at the time of the patient's presentation may therefore have been affected by events that occurred weeks or months earlier. A history of drug use, fever, or systemic illness during the preceding months in patients with abnormal semen analysis should prompt a repeat analysis after an additional 3 months have passed before firm conclusions are reached regarding potential semen quality. It is important to inquire whether either partner in an infertile couple has exhibited fertility at an earlier time. Any previous infertility evaluation or therapy should be fully documented. Details of the couple's sexual history may reveal the use of lubricants that may have spermicidal effects, a pattern of too frequent or infrequent ejaculation, or a lack of awareness by the couple of the correct timing of ovulation. Present knowledge supports encouraging a couple to have intercourse every other day during the middle of the wife's ovulatory cycle. Ovulation monitoring by the couple should be noted.

Developmental history should include specific questions about undescended testicles, precocious or delayed puberty, and other congenital disorders. It has been well demonstrated that semen quality may be impaired even with unilateral cryptorchidism. Precocious or delayed sexual maturation at puberty can reflect an underlying endocrine disorder that may be associated with decreased fertility. Prior genital or pelvic trauma should be noted.

Systemic illness can be a contributing cause of infertility. Peripheral neuropathy secondary to diabetes mellitus may cause retrograde ejaculation or lack of emission. Spinal cord injury and multiple sclerosis can also have an adverse effect on ejaculation. Bilateral vasal agenesis is present in almost all patients with cystic fibrosis. Galactorrhea, loss of libido, or visual field impairment is suggestive of a prolactin-secreting pituitary tumor. The association of sinopulmonary infections with infertility is characteristic of several disorders. Ultrastructural defects are found in the tails of sperm in patients with Kartagener's syndrome, whereas sperm from patients with Young's syndrome have normal flagella but epididymal obstruction secondary to inspissated secretions is present.

Prior pelvic or retroperitoneal surgery, such as retroperitoneal lymphadenectomy for testicular cancer, can adversely affect seminal emission. Bladder neck surgery may be followed by retrograde ejaculation. Scrotal, inguinal, pelvic, and transurethral surgery may lead to an iatrogenically induced ductal obstruction.

As previously noted, any febrile or viral illness may cause transient impairment of testicular function, and additional follow-up data should be obtained when such effects are suspected. Other infectious conditions can have a major impact on fertility. Postpubertal mumps causes unilateral orchitis in 15% to 30% of men, resulting in severe testicular damage and subsequent atrophy. Gonorrhea or epididymitis of other etiologies can lead to vasal or epididymal scarring and reproductive tract obstruction. In addition, clinical or potentially subclinical infection with *Chlamydia, Mycoplasma,* and other agents may produce pyospermia, which can adversely affect sperm motility and function. Episodes of prostatitis can cause calcification and scarring of the ejaculatory ducts with subsequent obstruction at that level.

Germ cells are quite vulnerable to damage by drugs and environmental toxins. Certain pesticides, chemotherapeutic agents, androgenic steroids, and the chronic use of alcohol or marijuana can have deleterious effects on the germinal epithelium. Environmental exposure to heat on a chronic basis, such as use of hot tubs, can also temporarily reduce sperm count.

Physical Examination

A thorough physical examination with emphasis on the genitalia is an essential part of the infertility evaluation (Fig. 24.2). General physical characteristics that might reflect an underlying endocrine disorder should also be noted, including body habitus, gynecomastia, and distribution of body hair. The genital examination should ascertain the presence of the vas deferens bilaterally and should include careful palpation of the testis and epididymis for any mass, induration, or tenderness. The size

FIGURE 24.1 *Infertility History*

HISTORY OF INFERTILITY
Duration
Prior pregnancies
  Present wife
  Another partner
Previous evaluations
Previous treatments

SEXUAL HISTORY
Potency
Lubricants
Timing of intercourse
Frequency of intercourse

CHILDHOOD AND DEVELOPMENT
Undescended testicles; orchiopexy
Herniorrhaphy
Y-V plasty of bladder
Testicular torsion
Testicular trauma
Onset of puberty

MEDICAL HISTORY
Systemic illness
Previous/current therapy

SURGICAL HISTORY
Retroperitoneal surgery
Pelvic injury
Pelvic, inguinal, or scrotal surgery
Herniorrhaphy
Y-V plasty; TURP

INFECTIONS
Viral; febrile
Mumps orchitis
Venereal
Tuberculosis; smallpox (rare)

GONADOTOXINS
Chemicals
Drugs (chemotherapeutic; cimetidine; sulfasalazine;
  nitrofurantoin; alcohol; marijuana; androgenic
  steroids)
Thermal exposure
Radiation

FAMILY HISTORY
Cystic fibrosis
Androgen receptor deficiency

REVIEW OF SYSTEMS
Respiratory infections
Anosmia
Galactorrhea
Impaired visual fields

FIGURE 24.2 *Physical Examination*

GENERAL CHARACTERISTICS
Secondary sex characteristics
Body habitus
Gynecomastia
Body hair
Enlargement of liver
Neurologic examination

GENITAL EXAMINATION
Urethral meatus
Bilateral palpation of vas deferens
Measurement/palpation of testis and epididymis
Varicocele evaluation
Rectal examination
Prostate
Seminal vesicles

of the testes should be measured with a rule or an orchidometer. The normal size for Europeans is greater than 4×3 cm or 20 mL. Abnormal softness of the testicle may be indicative of atrophy. The inguinal and scrotal area should be inspected for old surgical scars.

The penis should be examined for plaques indicative of Peyronie's disease that may affect erectile function. The position and adequacy of caliber of the urethral meatus should also be noted. Hypospadias can adversely affect fertility by preventing normal deposition of sperm at the cervical os.

Diagnosis of Varicocele

Varicocele is an abnormal dilation of the veins of the pampiniform plexus which can be observed while the patient is standing, with or without a Valsalva maneuver. Varicocele is found in 30% to 40% of infertile patients. The standard method of diagnosing a varicocele is by physical examination. The patient is best examined in a warm room in the standing position. Having the patient stand for several minutes may enhance the examiner's ability to detect the dilated veins of the pampiniform plexus by palpation. The structures of the spermatic cord are gently palpated in the upper scrotum, and the branches of the internal spermatic vein are ballotted between the thumb and forefinger. An increase in the fullness of these venous channels during a Valsalva maneuver is diagnostic of a varicocele. A large varicocele can be detected by inspection alone; the "bag of worms" appearance is noted when multiple pampiniform plexus branches are markedly dilated. Other important physical findings to note in the course of searching for a varicocele include the firmness and relative size of the testicles, as softening and atrophy may be signs of testicular damage by the varicocele. A simple grading system for varicocele that is commonly used is listed in Figure 24.3. Although the size of a varicocele does not appear to correlate with its effect on fertility, such a descriptive system is useful for clinical and research purposes.

In addition to the physical diagnosis of varicocele, other studies can be performed to confirm the presence of a varicocele perceived on physical examination or to verify the finding of an equivocal physical examination. Varicocele diagnosed by any of these studies in patients in whom a varicocele is undetectable on physical exam is called a subclinical varicocele. The clinical significance and appropriate management of subclinical varicocele is controversial. Various noninvasive imaging modalities have been used to diagnose varicocele, including Doppler stethoscope, scrotal thermography, radioisotope angiography, and scrotal ultrasonography. The accuracy, sensitivity, and specificity of these imaging studies have not been well examined. At present, scrotal ultrasonography is the most popular noninvasive imaging study for diagnosing subclinical varicocele. Demonstration of gonadal vein diameter greater than 3 mm after a Valsalva maneuver is considered positive for a varicocele.

Venography is the current standard for testing in the diagnosis of varicocele. This test is invasive and carries the risk of contrast allergy and hemorrhage. In addition to its use in diagnosis, a percutaneous venographic approach can also be used for varicocele repair. The accuracy of venographic diagnosis has not been determined. False-positive results may occur if the intravenous catheter is pushed through a competent valve, and false-negative results may occur when the varicocele is produced by veins with aberrant anatomy. The best candidates for venography and percutaneous ablation appear to be patients with apparent or questionable persistent varicocele after previous treatment.

Transrectal Ultrasonography

Transrectal ultrasonography (TRUS) has been popularized for the diagnosis and staging of prostate carcinoma. In the evaluation of the infertility patient, it provides a highly accurate and informative means of evaluating the prostate, seminal vesicles, and ejaculatory ducts in a noninvasive manner. Such findings on initial evaluation as nonpalpable vasa deferentia, low semen volume, azoospermia, or a history of inflammatory disease involving the prostate or seminal vesicles are indications for TRUS. Both acquired and congenital defects of the male accessory sex organs can be identified by TRUS.

Patients with abnormally low semen volume (1 mL) who also have azoospermia and/or oligospermia should be evaluated for the possibility of retrograde ejaculation by examination of a postejaculatory urine sample. A nonpalpable vas deferens on physical examination suggests embryologic malformation of the mesonephric duct system, and TRUS may reveal absence or hypoplasia of the seminal vesicles, since these structures share a mesonephric duct origin. Dilation of the seminal vesicles is indicative of ejaculatory duct obstruction which can be

---

FIGURE 24.3 *Grading of Varicocele*

Small/Grade I	Palpable on Valsalva maneuver only
Moderate/Grade II	Palpable without Valsalva maneuver
Large/Grade III	Visible before palpation

either congenital or acquired as a result of prostate inflammatory disease. Calcification within the prostate overlying the course of the ejaculatory ducts may be seen on ultrasound. Müllerian duct cysts in the midline may obstruct the ejaculatory ducts by extrinsic compression. Appropriate use of TRUS in patients in whom such defects are suspected is essential, as such lesions may be readily amenable to treatment by transurethral unroofing of a cystic lesion or incision of the ejaculatory duct. TRUS is a new and vital diagnostic modality for evaluation of the infertile patient and replaces the more invasive procedure of vasography.

Testis Biopsy

Testis biopsy is most useful in providing pivotal information in the evaluation of the azoospermic patient, as it enables the urologist to distinguish between potentially correctable ductal obstruction and usually uncorrectable ablative testicular pathology. In the severely oligospermic patient, biopsy is occasionally useful in providing prognostic information to guide future medical therapy, and may be relevant when partial duct obstruction is suspected as the underlying cause of impaired semen quality.

Testicular biopsy plays a vital role in the algorithm of managing the azoospermic patient. Patients with obvious testicular failure, as identified by a markedly elevated serum FSH or bilateral testicular atrophy, do not require a testicular biopsy. Likewise, patients with obvious obstructive causes of azoospermia such as bilateral vasal agenesis also do not require a biopsy for diagnosis. In patients with at least one normal-sized testis and a vas deferens, either obstruction or testicular failure may be the cause of azoospermia, and the final diagnosis can be established only by performing testicular biopsy.

Testis biopsy can be performed under local, regional, or general anesthesia. If local anesthesia is utilized, the scrotal wall is infiltrated with lidocaine and additional lidocaine is dripped onto the testicular surface. The biopsy can be performed using a "window technique," through a small scrotal incision, or through a more generous incision through which the testis can be introduced into the operating field for direct examination of the adnexal structures. The latter technique is used only when microsurgical reconstruction is to be performed at the same time. The "window technique" is preferred when biopsy alone is to be performed, as fewer adhesions result after such limited mobilization and future scrotal exploration will be less difficult. Vasography should always be delayed until reconstructive surgery is performed. Several descriptions of needle biopsy techniques have appeared in recent years, and such techniques may be applicable in selected patients.

Unilateral biopsies may be performed but bilateral biopsy is more appropriate when the history or the physical findings suggest the presence of an asymmetric lesion, such as unilateral ductal obstruction with contralateral testicular failure.

Open surgical biopsy involves exposure of the testicular surface through a scrotal incision, after which an incision 1 cm in length is made in the tunica albuginea. With slight pressure on the testis, a small amount of testicular parenchyma can be extruded and excised sharply with fine scissors. The specimen should be carefully placed in appropriate fixative, such as Bouin's solution, glutaraldehyde, or Zinker's solution. Formalin should not be used. We perform a "touch imprint" before placement of the specimen in fixative by gently touching the exposed tubules several times to a sterile microscope slide and rapidly spraying the slide with cytofixative. This provides a cytologic preparation of testicular contents; quick staining with hematoxylin and eosin or with Papanicolaou stain allows rapid examination and documentation of the presence or absence of mature sperm, which may be important for intraoperative decision making. The testicular incision is closed with a fine running absorbable suture after careful use of cautery, and the scrotal wall is closed in a routine fashion.

Interpretation of the findings of testicular biopsy has been the subject of several major reviews. Common classification systems describe pathologic entities as displaying abnormalities of cellularity and/or maturation of the spermatogenic elements, or of the interstitial compartment. Several systems have been developed to quantify the quality of spermatogenesis, of which the Johnsen score count is the most popular system. However, most pathologists continue to use a descriptive method of classification (Fig. 24.4).

FIGURE 24.4 *Descriptive Classification of Abnormalities of Testicular Biopsy for Infertility*

Normal	(Consistent with ductal obstruction)
Germ cell aplasia	Complete absence of germ cells; "Sertoli cell only syndrome"
Hypospermatogenesis	Reduced number of germ cells although proportions and maturational pattern intact
Maturation arrest	Maturation ceases at a particular cell stage
Combined defect	Features of more than one category observed

Fine-needle aspiration and core-needle biopsy of the testis have been recommended by some authors as providing accurate diagnostic information without the need for an anesthetic and with less operative discomfort. The Tru-Cut needle, biopsy gun, and others have been described for this purpose. Specimens can be processed and examined histologically with standard techniques, although only a small number of seminiferous tubule cross-sections will be available for examination as compared with the amount of tissue obtained by an open biopsy technique. Fine-needle aspiration has been successfully combined with standard cytology or DNA flow cytometry to determine whether intact spermatogenesis is present. However, these techniques require specialized equipment and a pathologist experienced in the interpretation of the results, and have therefore not become very popular.

Vasography

Vasography can be performed at the time of testicular biopsy if spermatogenesis is demonstrated by the observation of mature sperm on frozen section or cytologic analysis of a touch imprint. Alternatively, it can be performed at the time of a subsequent surgical procedure when separate reconstruction for duct obstruction is planned. The purpose of vasography is to document the patency of the vas deferens from the site of the vasotomy to the ejaculatory duct. A partial-thickness transverse incision is made in the scrotal portion of the vas deferens. This incision is completed when an epididymovasostomy is to be performed or is closed when obstruction is found elsewhere. Proximal patency of the epididymis and vas

deferens is confirmed by finding sperm within the intravasal fluid. Distal patency can be confirmed through the infusion of saline, colored dye, or X-ray contrast into the distal vas. The advantage of X-ray contrast is that the presence and the site of obstruction are identified simultaneously. The advantage of colored dye is that resection can be performed until dye is seen in the case of ejaculatory duct obstruction. The choice of fluid or combination of fluids used should be based on clinical suspicion as to the presence and site of obstruction.

Either the vasotomy site should be repaired or the transection completed if an epididymovasotomy is to be performed. Repair using microsurgical technique is recommended in an effort to avoid leakage of vasal fluid, which could promote local inflammation and stricture formation. Fine microsurgical nylon (9-0 to 10-0) is useful for this closure. Three full-thickness sutures are usually placed, followed by several serosal–muscular sutures.

Summary

The diagnostic steps outlined provide a guide to the evaluation of the infertile male. A thorough understanding of male reproductive physiology, a detailed history and physical examination, correctly performed and interpreted semen analyses, and basic endocrinologic tests form the basis of the clinical assessment. Further studies such as scrotal ultrasonography, TRUS, and testis biopsy can then be obtained as the individual patient's needs dictate, leading to more effective and rational treatment options. As the pathophysiology of testicular dysfunction is better understood, the treatment of the infertile male will become progressively more successful.

References

1. Dubin L, Amelar RD. Etiologic factors in 1294 consecutive cases of male infertility. *Fertil Steril.* 1974;22:469.
2. Greenberg SH, Lipshultz LI, Wein AJ. Experience with 425 subfertile male patients. *J Urol.* 1978;119:507.
3. World Health Organization: Comparison among different methods for the diagnosis of varicocele. *Fertil Steril.* 1985;43:575.
4. Jarow JP, Espeland MA, Lipshultz LI. Evaluation of the azoospermic patient. *J Urol.* 1989;142:62.
5. Coburn M, Wheeler T, Lipshultz LI. Testicular biopsy: its use and limitations. *Urol Clin North Am.* 1987;14:551.
6. Carter SC, Shinohara K, Lipshultz LI. Transrectal ultrasonography in disorders of the seminal vesicles and ejaculatory ducts. *Urol Clin North Am.* 1989;16:773.
7. Johnsen SG, Agger P. Quantitative evaluation of testicular biopsies before and after operation for varicocele. *Fertil Steril.* 1978;29:58.

CHAPTER 25

Laboratory Testing

Mark Sigman

Appropriate and specific testing is an integral component of the evaluation of the infertile man. Although during the last decade many assays have been developed for evaluation of the various aspects of male infertility, it is important to stress that laboratory studies are only one component of the complete evaluation. Therefore, laboratory testing should be instituted after a complete history and physical examination of the patient. Subsequent testing should be specific for the individual couple. It is important for the physician to understand what information can be obtained from the test. Tests can be useful to diagnose specific abnormalities or to follow or alter treatment. Testing that does not fulfill any of these criteria wastes medical resources and unnecessarily increases the cost of the evaluation. Finally, it is important to realize the limitations of the various assays and to understand what they can and what they cannot tell us about a couple's infertility. When the available testing procedures are reviewed, it is apparent that there is no single test of male infertility. However, through the use of appropriate laboratory tests the physician can develop a diagnostic and therapeutic plan for the couple.

Semen Analysis

A properly performed semen analysis forms the basis of the laboratory testing of the infertile male. Although this is a commonly performed assay, it is often performed inaccurately because of lack of attention to detail. It is important to instruct the patient in the method and parameters of collection. A clean, wide-mouthed container should be supplied. Since abstinence can affect semen parameters, a specified period of abstinence should be employed, commonly 2 to 3 days. After collection, the specimen should be kept between room temperature and body temperature. Although masturbation is the preferred method of collection, some patients are unable to produce specimens by masturbation and should be supplied with seminal collection condoms. Routine contraceptive condoms often contain spermicidal lubricants and should be avoided.

Semen parameters often vary from one specimen to the next. Therefore, it is important to obtain two or three properly collected specimens. Although it would be ideal to collect these over more than one spermatogenic cycle (2 to 3 months) this is not practical, and specimens may be obtained within several weeks of the initial office visit. If there is reason to suspect a temporary insult to spermatogenesis (such as an episode of high fever), the specimens can be collected over a longer time period.

A properly performed semen analysis measures several parameters (Fig. 25.1). The viscosity of the specimen should be determined. Semen is initially produced as a coagulum, then liquefies over a 5 to 20 minute period. In patients with obstruction, dysfunction, or hypoplasia of the seminal vesicles, small-volume, noncoagulating ejaculates are produced. Hyperviscosity is often noted in semen specimens. In most instances this represents incomplete liquification and may occur because the specimen was collected in a cool container such that the prostatic enzymes responsible for liquification could not function properly. If the man's semen is hyperviscous but the postcoital test is normal, the hyperviscosity is probably not of clinical importance. Small ejaculate volumes may be a

FIGURE 25.1 *Minimal Levels of Adequacy of Semen Parameters*

Volume	1.5–5.0 mL
Sperm density	$\geq 20 \times 10^6$ sperm/mL
Motility	$\geq 60\%$
Forward progression (scale 1–4)	>2.0
Morphology	$\geq 60\%$ normal forms
Minimal agglutination	No hyperviscosity
No significant pyospermia	

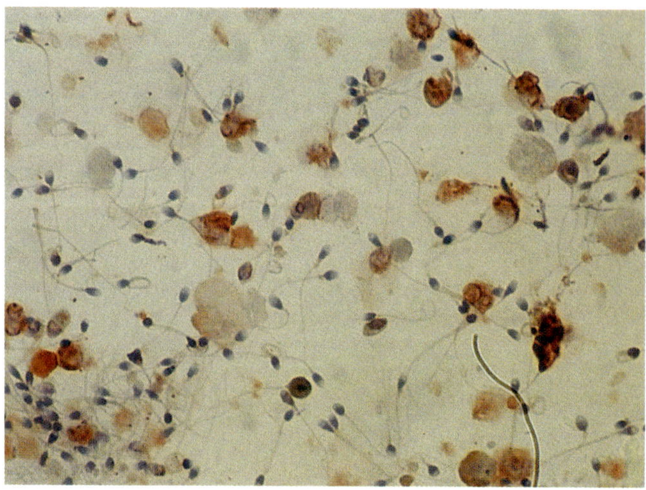

Figure 25.2 Immunohistochemical staining of white blood cells and semen. White blood cells are rust colored and immature germ cells are blue.

result of retrograde ejaculation. This possibility should be evaluated by examination of a postejaculate urine sample. Finally, high seminal volume, although anecdotally reported to be associated with male infertility, is usually not a contributory factor. Occasionally patients have very high seminal volumes that dilute the sperm density to a point of oligospermia. These couples can be treated by semen processing and intrauterine insemination.

It is important for the physician to understand the difference between average semen parameters and the minimal levels necessary for conception. Studies of sperm concentration in populations of normal fertile men have revealed average sperm counts of 70 to 80 million sperm per mL. However, it is not until the sperm density becomes less than 20 million per mL that pregnancy rates start to decrease. It is also important to realize that there is no clear cutoff between fertility and infertility, but rather a gradation from fertility through subfertility to sterility. The physician should be cautious in telling the patient that he is sterile unless there are no motile sperm in the semen specimen. Specimens in which no sperm are identified should be centrifuged and the pellet examined, since the presence of even one sperm rules out the possibility of complete bilateral duct obstruction.

Sperm motility should be measured as the percent of sperm that demonstrate movement as well as by measuring the quality of the forward progression of the sperm. These parameters are very observer-dependent, and it is important that a qualified physician or technician perform the assay. Well documented causes of retarded sperm movement include varicoceles, genital tract infection, and ultrastructural abnormalities of the spermatozoa. Other less well documented causes include the presence of antisperm antibodies and the occasional patient with a partial duct obstruction. Sperm agglutination, if excessive, should be noted, as this is often associated with the presence of antisperm antibodies.

The traditional assessment of sperm morphology uses a stained seminal smear. A normal sample has been considered one in which at least 60% of sperm demonstrate normal morphology. Although the Papanicolaou stain yields smears of excellent quality, it is a time-consuming procedure. Other, less involved procedures include DiffQuik and the use of Blutstan (prestained microscopic slides). Although spermatozoa have been classified in anywhere from six to 70 categories, these classifications have been of limited clinical value. Very few morphologic patterns are pathognomonic for specific abnormalities. Thus, although varicocele is often associated with a predominance of tapered cells and immature germ cells, varicoceles are not the only agents that cause this pattern. Recently, strict criteria have been developed to define what a normal spermatozoon should look like.[1] Sperm morphology was examined in a select group of couples undergoing in vitro fertilization. Normal in vitro fertilization rates were obtained as long as more than 14% of sperm demonstrated normal morphology by rigid criteria. Lower fertilization rates were found in samples with between 4% and 14% normal forms, whereas extremely low fertilization rates and no pregnancies were obtained from samples with less than 4% normal forms. This technique holds much promise for improving the prognostic value of sperm morphologic determinations.

Other components of semen have been measured in clinical labs. The seminal pH should be between 7.3 and 7.8 and tends to be below this in patients with obstruction or dysfunction of the seminal vesicles. Other parameters such as zinc, citric acid, acid phosphatase, aminotransferase, and magnesium levels are of no clinical value.

Pyospermia is often an overdiagnosed condition. In a normal semen specimen very few nonsperm cells should be identified; however, in about 10% of specimens excess nonsperm cells are reported (>10 cells per high-power field). Although these are often reported as being white blood cells, this is most often not the case. White blood cells (true pyospermia) and immature germ cells appear as round cells in wet-mount semen specimens. It is impossible to tell these two cell types apart without further staining procedures. These two cell types have traditionally been differentiated by use of techniques such as the Papanicolaou stain. However, these techniques require a trained observer. Recently, labeled monoclonal antibodies have been used to stain white blood cells specifically. This procedure allows easy differentiation between immature germ cells and white blood cells (Fig. 25.2).[2] The majority of samples with increased numbers of round cells contain primarily immature germ cells and are not truly pyospermic (>1 million white blood cells per mL). Patients with true pyospermia should be evaluated for genital tract infection. This evaluation should include a urine analysis and *Chlamydia* culture or smear. Performance of *Mycoplasma* cultures is often unavailable and remains controversial, since fertile males have been found to harbor this organism. Routine semen cultures for bacteria are often unproductive, exhibiting a mixture of cutaneous flora. Certainly, patients with signs or symptoms of a genital tract infection should be evaluated. When an infecting organism is identified, the patient should be treated with an appropriate antibiotic.

Computer-Assisted Semen Analysis (CASA)

The manual semen analysis has been criticized for being a subjective, time-consuming assay that requires a trained observer. Computerized systems have been developed that digitize a microscopic picture of a semen specimen and analyze sequential digitized images to determine sperm concentration and motility (Fig. 25.3). These systems are proposed as offering rapid, objective results and as reporting measurements not easily determined by manual methods. The systems often have not performed as hoped, particularly with samples that require an accurate analysis: azoospermic specimens were reported as being oligospermic, and motility measurements have often been overestimated.[3] Additional measurements such as curvilinear velocity, linear velocity, linearity, lateral head displacement, flagellar beat frequency, and circular movement analysis remain of unproven clinical value. Therefore, although these systems continue to improve, they remain primarily research tools. Recently, sperm morphology has been incorporated into the algorithms of these systems, but this will also require further clinical experience to determine its accuracy and value.

Endocrine Testing

Although the proper hormonal milieu is essential for normal spermatogenesis, hormonal abnormalities account for less than 3% of male infertility. This has resulted in controversy over what constitutes a minimum endocrine evaluation. An endocrine etiology for male infertility is rare in patients with sperm concentrations of more than 5 million sperm per mL. On the basis of these data, some investigators suggest that an endocrine evaluation is not necessary in men with sperm densities grater than 5 million per mL.

FSH is an indicator of the state of spermatogenesis and is often elevated in the presence of testicular damage.

Therefore, some investigators feel that all patients should be screened with a serum FSH measurement, and only if this is abnormal should other hormonal studies be performed. In the presence of a normal FSH level, the addition of testosterone, LH, and prolactin determinations will not add significant clinical information. Other investigators believe that a complete endocrine evaluation should be performed in most patients. It must be understood that if this approach is taken, the additional information will rarely be of clinical significance.

Prolactin elevations will be found in approximately 5% of infertile patients. In the vast majority of cases, the elevations are mild and have no identifiable etiology (idiopathic hyperprolactinemia). Normal gonadotropin and testosterone levels are present in these otherwise asymptomatic patients. Any patient with symptoms of a central nervous system tumor, such as impaired visual fields or severe headaches, should have his prolactin levels measured. In the otherwise asymptomatic patient, an isolated mild hyperprolactinemia should be confirmed with a repeat determination. If persistent mild hyperprolactinemia is identified, I recommend an endocrinologic evaluation, including a CT or MRI scan, to rule out a pituitary tumor. Since there is no convincing evidence that mild isolated prolactin elevation in the presence of normal gonadotropin and testosterone levels is responsible for male infertility, I do not recommend treating the hyperprolactinemia in these instances. In azoospermic or

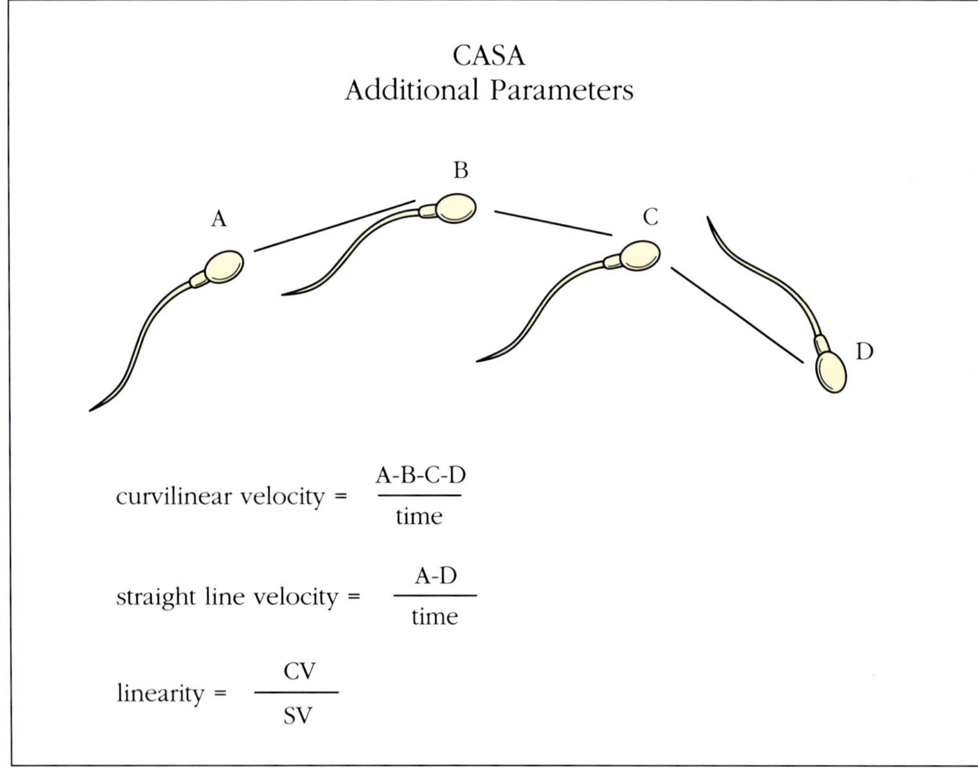

$$\text{curvilinear velocity} = \frac{A\text{-}B\text{-}C\text{-}D}{time}$$

$$\text{straight line velocity} = \frac{A\text{-}D}{time}$$

$$\text{linearity} = \frac{CV}{SV}$$

Figure 25.3 Additional semen parameters obtained through computer-assisted semen analysis techniques.

severely oligospermic patients, hormone studies may help to classify the patient's infertility as pretesticular, testicular, or posttesticular (Fig. 25.4). Although gonadotropins are secreted episodically and testosterone is secreted diurnally, with afternoon levels often higher than morning levels, this is rarely of clinical significance. I draw one serum sample for all hormone determinations at the time of the patient's office visit. If the results of these are inconsistent with the patient's history and clinical findings, repeat studies can be done using pooled samples in which a sample is drawn every 15 to 20 minutes for a total of three samples, which are then pooled. Estradiol should be measured in patients with gynecomastia. The routine determination of other hormones, such as ACTH, growth hormone, and thyroid-stimulating hormone, should not be performed unless specifically indicated by findings on the history or physical exam.

Sperm–Mucus Interaction

For a pregnancy to occur after intercourse, sperm must traverse the cervical mucus. A postcoital test examines this interaction. The examination is performed just before ovulation, at which time the cervical mucus becomes watery and clear. Most commonly the couple is instructed to have intercourse in the morning, and several hours later a specimen of cervical mucus is examined by light microscopy. There is no agreement as to what constitutes a normal postcoital test. However, the presence of 10 to 20 spermatozoa per high-power field, the majority of which demonstrate progressive motility, is usually considered normal. A normal postcoital test suggests that a cervical factor is not involved in the couple's infertility. Abnormal postcoital tests have many possible causes, the most common being inappropriate timing relative to ovulation. Anatomic abnormalities, inappropriately performed intercourse, the presence of antisperm antibodies in the semen or cervical mucus, and an abnormal semen specimen may also cause an abnormal postcoital test. The postcoital test should be performed in patients with reasonably good semen parameters, especially sperm motility, since severe defects in

these characteristics usually impair the ability of the sperm to traverse the cervical mucus, and this test will therefore add no new clinical information. The test is also indicated in patients with hyperviscous semen, abnormal penile anatomy (such as hypospadias), decreased seminal volume with good sperm density, and in couples with unexplained infertility.

To remove some of the variability from the assay, in vitro cervical mucus interaction tests have been developed. These tests involve placing cervical mucus under a cover slip or in a capillary tube adjacent to a drop of semen. The distance of sperm migration into the cervical mucus is recorded. To remove the woman as a factor from the evaluation, bovine cervical mucus has been used, because the migration of human sperm into human and bovine mucus is similar. It should be noted that sperm-bound antisperm antibodies will inhibit the ability of sperm to traverse human mucus, but their ability to traverse bovine mucus may not be impaired.

The cross-mucus test is an in vitro assay for sperm–mucus interaction which employs several controls. The patient's sperm are mixed separately with spouse and donor mucus while the spouse's mucus is mixed separately with spouse and donor sperm. In this way, the test can determine whether an abnormal postcoital test was due to male or female factors. The postcoital test should remain the initial screening test for sperm–cervical mucus interaction. If interaction is abnormal, one of the in vitro cervical mucus interaction tests can be employed to determine the cause of an abnormal postcoital test.

Antisperm Antibodies

The presence of antisperm antibodies in the male has been associated with lower pregnancy rates. A wide variety of assays have been developed to measure the presence of antisperm antibodies. Considerable controversy remains as to which assay is most appropriate, which body fluid should be assayed, and even what levels of antisperm antibodies are clinically significant (Fig. 25.5). Traditional antisperm antibody determinations required

---

FIGURE 25.4 Hormonal Studies

DIAGNOSIS	FSH	LH	T
Normal male	normal	normal	normal
Germinal cell aplasia	↑	normal	normal
Primary testicular failure	↑	↑	normal or ↓
Hypogonadotropic hypogonadism	↓	↓	↓

FIGURE 25.5 Antisperm Antibody Assays

Sperm immobilizing assay
Sperm agglutination assay
Indirect immunofluorescence assay
Radiolabeled antiglobulin assay
Enzyme-linked immunosorbent assay
Mixed agglutination reaction
Sperm panning
Immunobead binding assay

the antibodies to cause either agglutination or immobilization of the sperm. In addition, the antibodies were often measured in the serum. Over the last decade it has become clear that clinically significant antibodies can be present on the sperm surface without causing agglutination or immobilization. Therefore, most laboratories have turned to direct assays using immunologic probes that bind to human antibodies. These assays can detect the presence of surface-bound antibodies and do not require the antibodies to perform a function. The Immunobead assay has gained widespread use in the last several years (Fig. 25.6). This assay uses micron-sized polyacrylamide beads to which rabbit antihuman antibodies have been linked. When mixed with washed spermatozoa, these beads bind to the portion of the sperm containing the antisperm antibodies. Scoring is based on the percent of motile sperm with bead binding. In addition, the location of the bead binding and the class of the antisperm anti-body can be determined.[5] When more than 20% to 50% of sperm demonstrate immunobead binding, the antisperm antibodies are thought to be clinically significant.

Sperm Penetration Assay

For pregnancy to occur through normal intercourse, sperm must traverse the cervical mucus, travel through the uterus into the fallopian tube, undergo capacitation and the acrosome reaction, bind and penetrate the zona pellucida, fuse with the oolemma, and penetrate the ooplasm. The sperm penetration assay measures the ability of human sperm to penetrate hamster ova (Fig. 25.7). Since the zona pellucida prevents interspecies penetration, this assay uses zona-free hamster ova. Normal penetration requires sperm to undergo capacitation and the acrosome reaction. Therefore, this assay measures several steps required for fertilization. In the assay, zona-free

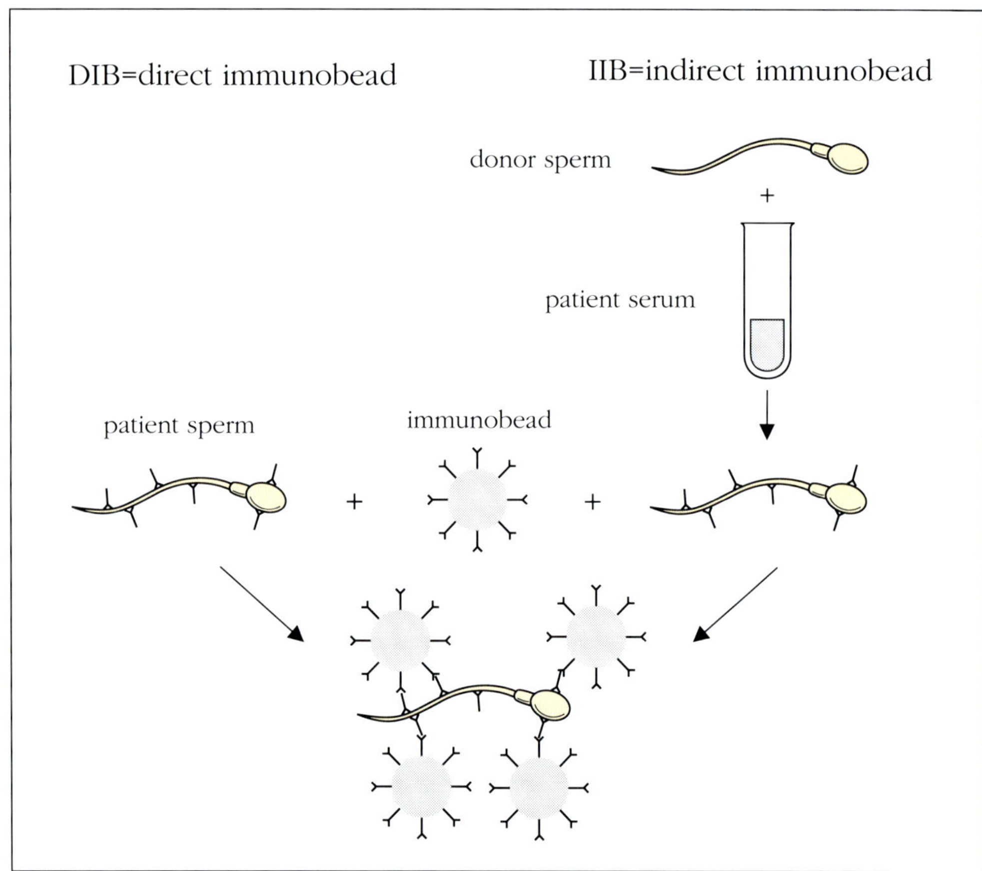

Figure 25.6 Antisperm antibody assay through the use of immunobeads.

hamster ova are inseminated with processed sperm from the patient. Scoring is then performed by determining the percent of ova with penetration and the number of penetrations per ovum. Although there are significant methodological differences between laboratories, many laboratories consider the assay normal if 10% to 30% or more of ova are penetrated. Patients with abnormal semen specimens may penetrate 100% of the ova if processing techniques are altered to enhance sperm capacitation. Thus, some laboratories find that the sperm capacitation index (the number of penetrations per ovum) is a more sensitive indicator of fertilizing capacity. Since there is no standardization among laboratories, there remains considerable controversy as to the clinical value of this assay. However, when properly performed, it can provide significant information. Pregnancy rates in couples with a normal SPA are higher whether the pregnancies are achieved through intercourse, IUI, or in vitro fertilization.

In general, 95% of men with a normal SPA will fertilize human ova in vitro. However, only 50% of men with an abnormal SPA will fertilize human ova in vitro. Finally, men whose sperm cannot penetrate any hamster ova are rarely able to fertilize any human ova in vitro. It is important to recognize that the SPA cannot detect isolated abnormalities of zona binding or zona penetration, since the assay uses zona-free hamster eggs.

The sperm penetration assay is often used in couples who are considering assisted reproductive techniques. Male-factor couples with a normal SPA can proceed with intrauterine insemination, whereas couples with an abnormal SPA may be best served by proceeding with in vitro fertilization, where an exact determination of the ability of the sperm to penetrate human ova can be made. This assay is also useful in couples with unexplained infertility (a normal male evaluation and normal semen analysis, as well as a normal female evaluation). It

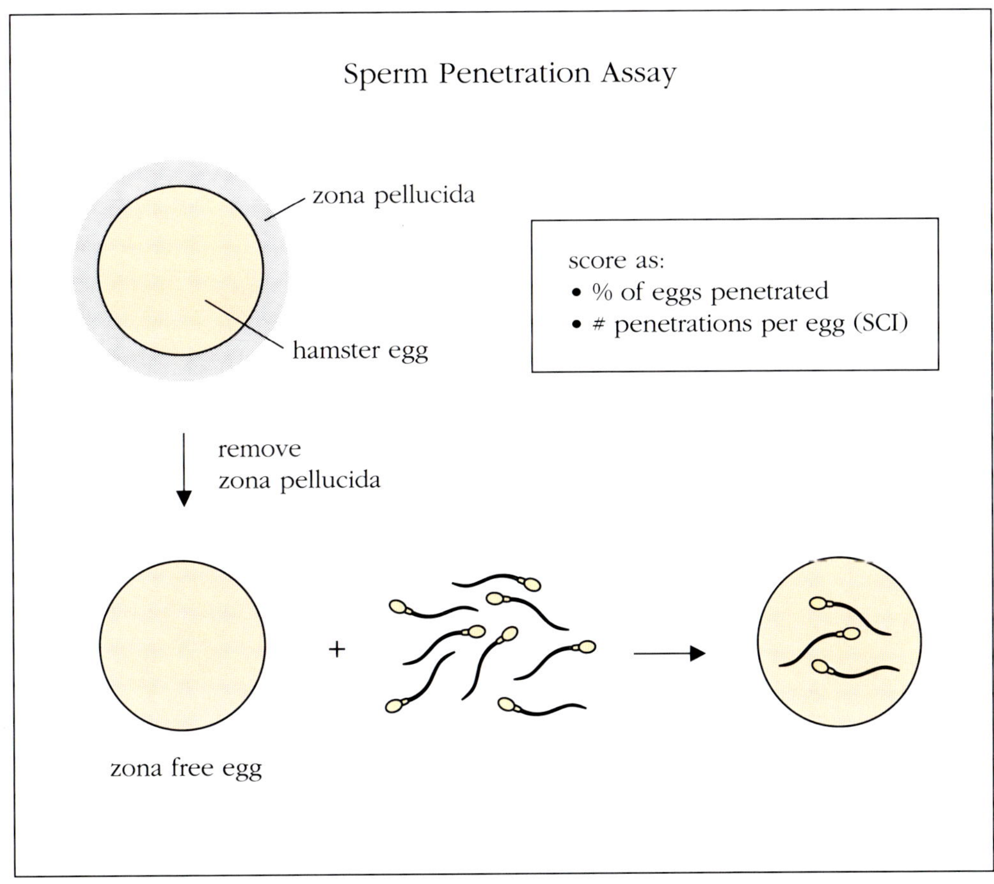

Figure 25.7 Sperm penetration assay.

should be emphasized that physicians who use the SPA should be familiar with the laboratory's method of performing the assay, as well as the false positivity and negativity of that particular assay.

Hemizona Assay

The hemizona assay determines the ability of sperm to bind to the zona pellucida (Fig. 25.8). In this assay, a human zona pellucida is microsurgically divided in half. One half is then incubated with the patient's sperm and the other half with donor sperm. By counting the number of sperm bound to each zona half and dividing the number of sperm bound from the patient by the number of sperm bound from the donor, the hemizona index is calculated. Patients with a hemizona index greater than 36% demonstrate fertilization of human ova in vitro.[4] Patients with lower hemizona assays demonstrate lower fertilization rates. This assay is labor-intensive, requires microsurgical capabilities, and has not yet gained widespread use (see Fig. 25.1).

The Future of Male Fertility Testing

With the development of bioassays to test spermatozoa function, we now have the capacity to test sequentially

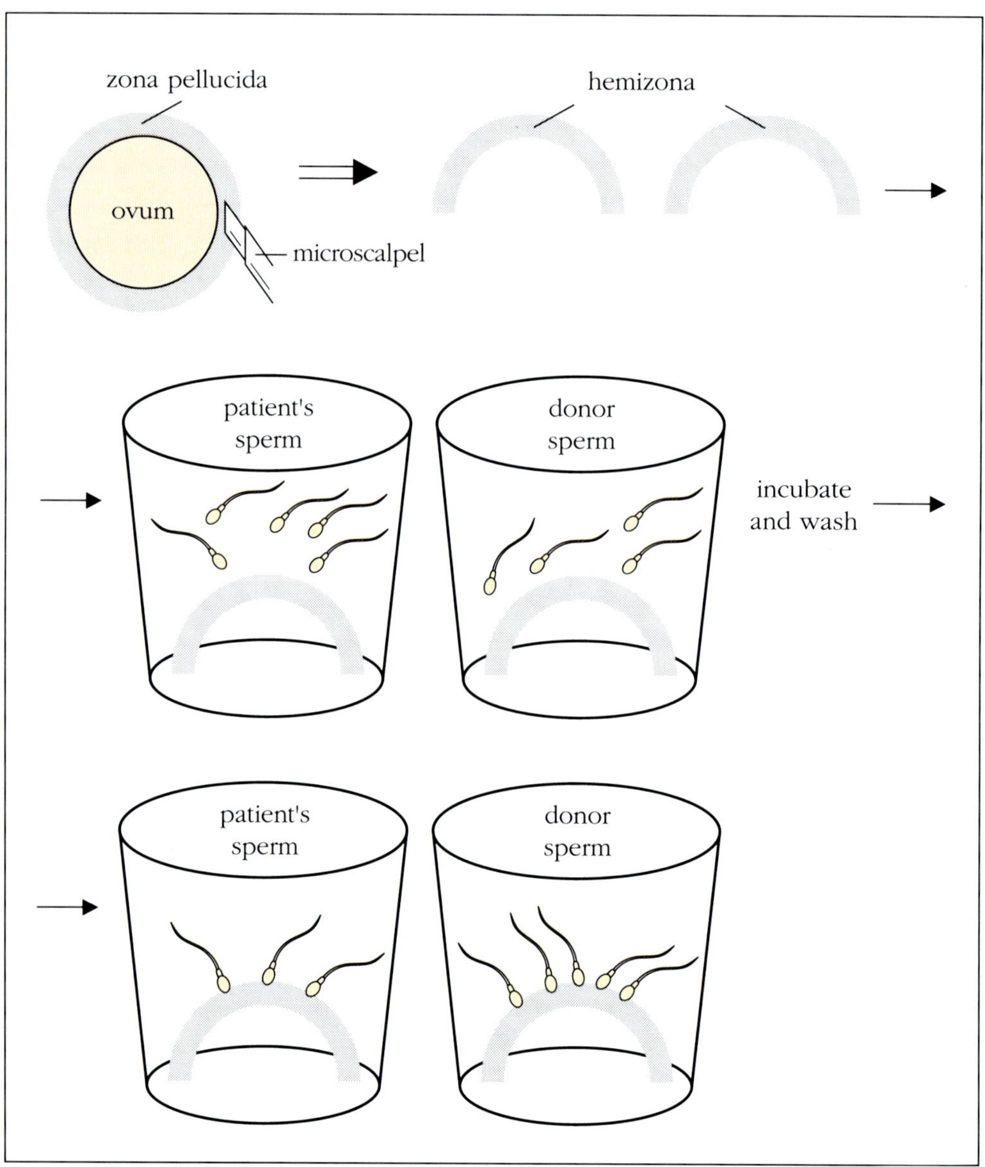

Figure 25.8 Hemizona assay.

for specific defects (Fig. 25.9). Although major defects in sperm are usually associated with abnormal results in many of the various fertility tests, specific assays are able to localize the defects. Thus, a semen analysis determines whether adequate numbers of motile sperm are available. Sperm–cervical mucus interaction testing assesses the ability of the sperm to traverse the cervical mucus and enter the female upper reproductive tract. The hemizona assay assesses the ability of the sperm to bind to the zona pellucida. The sperm penetration assay assesses the ability of the sperm to undergo capacitation, the acrosome reaction, fusion with the oolemma, and penetration into the ooplasm. In the future, we may see the use of a panel of tests to identify specific abnormalities. The results can then be used to design treatment plans to overcome these individual defects.

FIGURE 25.9 *Testing for Specific Defects*

Semen analysis	Determines numbers of motile, morphologically normal sperm
Sperm–cervical mucus interaction	Determines ability of sperm to reach female upper reproductive tract
Hemizona assay	Determines ability of sperm to bind to zona pellucida
Sperm penetration assay	Determines ability of sperm to undergo capacitation, the acrosome reaction, fusion with oolemma, and penetration of the ova

References

1. Kruger TF, Mankveld R, Stander SH, et al. Sperm morphologic features as a prognostic for in vitro fertilization. *Fertil Steril.* 1986;46:1118–1123.
2. Wolff H, Anderson DJ. Amino histologic characterization and quantification of leucocyte subpopulations in human semen. *Fertil Steril.* 1988;49:497–504.
3. Vantman D, Koukoulis G, Dennison L, Zimmerman M, Sherins RJ. Computer assisted semen analysis: evaluation of method and assessment of the influence of sperm concentrations on linear velocity determinations. *Fertil Steril.* 1988;49:510–515.
4. Franken D, Oehninger S, Burkman CJ, et al. The hemizona assay (HZA): a predictor of human sperm fertilizing potential in in vitro fertilization (IVF) treatment. *J In Vitro Fertil.* 1989;6:44–50.
5. Ayvaliotis B, Bronson R, Rosenfeld D, Cooper G. Conception rates in couples where autoimmunity to sperm is detected. *Fertil Steril.* 1985;43:739–742.

CHAPTER 26

Medical Therapy for Infertility

Jonathan P. Jarow

The primary goal in management of the infertile couple is to identify specific treatable disorders and implement therapy in a cost-effective manner. Medical therapy is used for patients with specific disorders amenable to this type of treatment, including those with ejaculatory dysfunction, hormonal abnormalities, infection, and immunologic infertility. However, many patients with male-factor infertility do not have an identifiable etiology or their disorder is irreversible, such as those with prior gonadotoxin exposure or cryptorchidism. In these patients nonspecific or empiric medical therapy can be employed. In addition, patients who do not have a satisfactory response after completion of specific therapy can be treated with empiric medical therapy.

Specific Medical Therapy

EJACULATORY DYSFUNCTION

Ejaculation is a neuromuscular process that combines autonomic and somatic nervous system functions. The process of ejaculation is divided into two phases: emission and ejaculation proper. Emission is under sympathetic autonomic control and consists of the delivery of sperm and seminal fluid to the posterior urethra with simultaneous closure of the bladder neck. Ejaculation proper results in the delivery of seminal fluid to the urethral meatus by rhythmic contraction of the pelvic floor skeletal musculature.[1] Ejaculatory dysfunction may take the form of failure of emission and/or retrograde ejaculation. The diagnosis is suspected in patients with absent ejaculate (aspermia) or low ejaculate volume (less than 1.5 mL). Retrograde ejaculation is diagnosed by the presence of many sperm in the postejaculate urine. Ejaculatory dysfunction can be caused by surgery, medical illnesses, or prescribed medications (Fig. 26.1). However, many patients have an idiopathic etiology.

Medical therapy for ejaculatory dysfunction begins with administration of α-sympathomimetic medications.[2,3] Pseudoephedrine at a dose of 60 mg q.i.d. is the usual initial therapy. Imipramine hydrochloride (25 mg b.i.d.) may be more effective in some patients, particularly diabetics. Other medications used include phenylpropanolamine (75 mg b.i.d.) and ephedrine sulfate (50 mg q.i.d.). In addition, ejaculation with a full bladder is sometimes an effective treatment for retrograde ejaculation.[4]

These drugs are typically administered in a cyclical fashion timed to the woman's ovulatory cycle. However, the treating physician should be aware of two phenomena that may occur during therapy. First, patients may require several days of therapy before an adequate response is seen. Second, the efficacy of the drugs may decline with long-term therapy (tachyphylaxis).[5–7] Therefore, therapy is usually tailored to the individual patient.

Sperm can be harvested from the bladders of patients with persistent retrograde ejaculation after α-sympathomimetic therapy by use of a bladder wash technique (Fig. 26.2). The pH and osmolality of typical urine are toxic to sperm. Therefore, the patient must be prepared with alkalinization of the urine and hydration overnight. Alkalinization can be accomplished with sodium bicarbonate at a dose of 625 mg t.i.d. starting the day before the procedure. Therefore, the hydration and alkalinization must be tailored to the individual patient; this can usually be accomplished in one or two trial procedures. An additional safeguard to preserve sperm is to wash the bladder with a physiologic buffer and leave 30 mL indwelling before the patient produces a specimen. The patient then voids the buffer, which now contains sperm, or is catheterized if he has a neurogenic bladder. Patients with neurogenic bladders should be cleared of infection or bacterial colonization before the procedure. The specimen obtained is spun down, washed, and

FIGURE 26.1 *Causes of Ejaculatory Dysfunction*

NEUROPATHIC
Spinal cord injury
Diabetes mellitus
Retroperitoneal surgery
Multiple sclerosis
Medications
Idiopathic

ANATOMIC
Bladder neck surgery
Prostatectomy
Congenital abnormality

PSYCHOGENIC

brought to a volume of 1 mL by addition of an appropriate buffer. The bladder wash is performed near the time of ovulation and the specimen obtained is used for insemination or other assisted reproductive techniques. This procedure is highly successful when it is performed carefully and when the time of ovulation has been clearly established.

Failure of emission is less amenable to therapy with medication alone. There have been several reports that failure of emission in patients after retroperitoneal lymph node dissection has been treated successfully with α-sympathomimetic medications.[1] However, spinal-cord-injured patients rarely respond to these drugs. These patients should be treated with vibratory stimulation[8] or electroejaculation,[9] which is described in depth in Chapter 27.

ENDOCRINOPATHY

Sperm production, sperm maturation, and sex accessory gland function are dependent on an intact hypothalamic–pituitary–gonadal axis (Fig. 26.3A). Sperm production is dependent on normal levels of testosterone and follicle-stimulating hormone (FSH).[10] The other functions listed above appear to be dependent on testosterone alone. The results of endocrine evaluation typically seen in infertile patients include normal endocrine function, low testosterone levels (hypogonadism), or normal testosterone with elevated serum FSH (Fig. 26.4). The endocrinopathies amenable to therapy are those resulting from inadequate gonadotropin stimulation of testicular function, hypogonadotropic hypogonadism (Fig. 26.3B), and hyperprolactinemia (Fig. 26.3C).

Hypogonadotropic hypogonadism is diagnosed by the association of a low testosterone level with low serum luteinizing hormone (LH) and FSH levels. This may be idiopathic, due to trauma, or due to a pituitary tumor. Radiologic evaluation of the pituitary gland by CT scan or MRI should be performed to rule out a tumor. In addition, a prolactin level should be obtained to rule out a prolactin-secreting pituitary adenoma.

The testis can be stimulated by administration of exogenous hormones, using two different protocols. The first protocol described stimulates testicular production of testosterone and sperm by administration of exogenous gonadotropins, human chorionic gonadotropin (HCG) and human menopausal gonadotropin (HMG).[11] Therapy is begun with HCG at a dose of 2000 units three times weekly. Testicular size, testosterone levels, and sperm counts are followed monthly. The dose of HCG should be adjusted to keep serum testosterone levels in the normal range. Many patients with postpubertally acquired hypogonadotropic hypogonadism respond to HCG alone. However, if testis size and sperm counts do not improve significantly within 6 months of normalization of serum testosterone, HMG should be started at a dose of 75 units three times weekly. The patient should be followed on this regimen for at least 1 year, since the initiation of complete spermatogenesis may take up to 20 months to appear.

An alternative protocol is the stimulation of endogenous production and secretion of pituitary gonadotropins by exogenous administration of gonadotropin-releasing hormone (Gn-RH) analogues.[12] However, this type of therapy cannot be used if the pituitary gland has been damaged by previous tumor, surgery, radiation, or trauma. Therefore, the main experience with this form of therapy has been in the subset of patients with idiopathic hypogonadotropic hypogonadism. The most efficacious form of Gn-RH administration is in a pulsatile fashion of 4 to 15 μg subcutaneously every 2 hours. This is a cumbersome form of therapy, requiring the use of a subcutaneous pulsatile pump with frequent needle changes and refilling of the pump by the patient. Patients are followed in a similar fashion as in gonadotropin therapy. It is not clear whether

FIGURE 26.2 *Bladder Wash Procedure for Retrograde Ejaculation*

Alkalinize urine
Hydrate urine

Catheterize bladder
Wash bladder with buffer

Void specimen (or catheterize)
Centrifuge specimen
Bring up to 1 mL

Inseminate

one therapy is superior to the other. Because of the difficulties associated with Gn-RH therapy, most centers use gonadotropin administration as a first line of treatment.[13]

. The success rates of both forms of therapy are high. Sperm production can be stimulated in up to 90% of patients treated. Fertility has been reported in up to 80% of patients. Patients with larger baseline testicular size, no history of cryptorchidism, and a postpubertally acquired lesion have a better prognosis.[11] The quality of sperm produced by these patients is frequently excellent despite lack of quantity. Pregnancies have been reported in couples even when the man's sperm counts are close to only 1 million/mL.

Hyperprolactinemia frequently presents with decreased libido, impotence, headache, visual changes, and galactorrhea in the male patient.[14] Fertility is adversely affected by the negative feedback of prolactin on hypothalamic secretion of Gn-RH, the destructive effect of a prolactinoma on the normal pituitary gland, and a possible direct deleterious effect of prolactin on the testis. At normal levels, prolactin is thought to have a beneficial synergistic effect with testosterone upon the reproductive organs.[15,16] However, elevated levels of prolactin appear to have an inhibitory effect. Almost all patients with significant elevations of serum prolactin (greater than 50 ng/mL) have an abnormally low serum testosterone level.[13]

Patients with significantly elevated serum prolactin levels frequently have a pituitary tumor visible on MRI. Minor elevations of serum prolactin are usually due to medication, stress, or medical illness. Treatment options for pituitary tumors include medication (bromocriptine mesylate), surgery, and radiation therapy. Historically, larger tumors were treated with radiation therapy or surgical excision. However, these treatments frequently result in panhypopituitarism and do not always normalize serum prolactin levels.[14] Management of these tumors now starts with medical therapy. Patients are followed with periodic prolactin measurements and radiologic imaging. Adverse reactions include hypotension and gastrointestinal upset. Therefore, treatment should begin at a dosage of 2.5 mg q.d. with meals and should slowly advance to a therapeutic dose while prolactin levels are monitored. The usual optimal dose falls in the range of 20 to 30 mg/d. Surgical

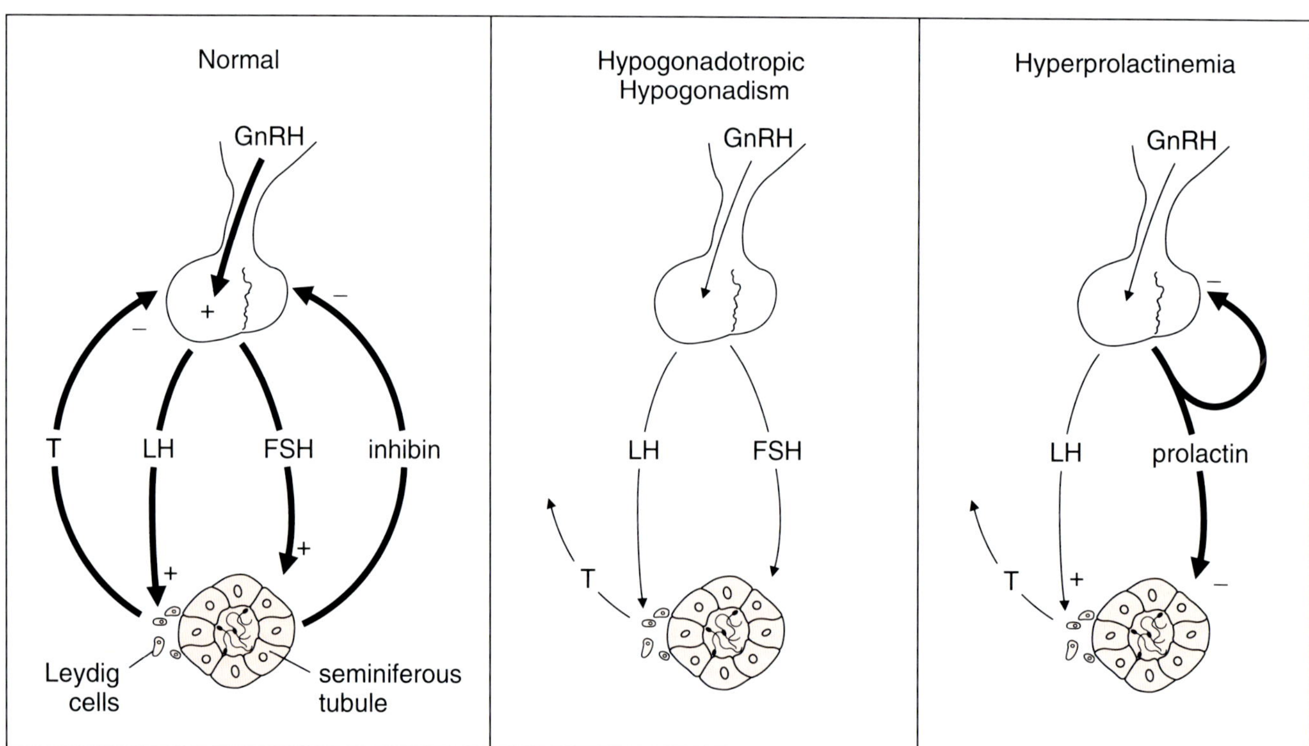

Figure 26.3 Hypothalamic–pituitary–gonadal axis. Sperm production and maturation depend on normal functioning **A**. Pathologic processes that affect fertility include hypogonadotropic hypogonadism **B** and hyperprolactinemia **C**.

therapy is indicated in the rare patient who is not adequately treated by bromocriptine or cannot tolerate its side effects. Although medical and surgical therapy are highly successful in treating prolactin-secreting pituitary tumors, the results in fertility are not as good. Unfortunately, many patients with abnormal seminal parameters at the time of diagnosis continue to have abnormal parameters after normalization of serum prolactin.[17]

INFECTION

Infections can adversely affect male fertility in two distinct ways. Prior genitourinary tuberculosis or venereal disease may produce scarring with consequent obstructive azoospermia. This entity is treated with surgical therapy and is discussed in Chapter 27. Alternatively, current infection may have a deleterious effect on sperm function. In vitro studies have demonstrated several potential pathogenic mechanisms by which this may occur in vivo. *Escherichia coli* has been shown to produce a soluble toxic factor that can reversibly immobilize sperm and over time can be spermicidal.[18] Infectious processes may also have an indirect adverse effect on sperm. White blood cells have been shown to interfere with sperm–egg interaction in vitro.[19] In fact, incubation of sperm with white blood cell cultured media inhibits penetration rates in vitro. However, other potential pathogens, *Ureaplasma* and *Mycoplasma*, have not been shown to have a significant adverse effect.[20]

The vast majority of infertile men do not present with an overt clinical infection. Chronic or acute bacterial infections of the epididymis and prostate are rarely seen in men of reproductive age.[21] However, subclinical infection or inflammation of the lower genitourinary tract is more common in infertile men.[22] Common pathogens implicated as the cause of subclinical infections include *Chlamydia*, *Ureaplasma*, and *Mycoplasma*. These organisms are difficult to grow in culture and for that reason the reported prevalence of these subclinical infections has varied greatly in the literature. However, recent studies suggest that their presence does not significantly affect sperm function.[20] Moreover, white blood cells present within the semen appear to be the major factor affecting sperm function in these patients.[23] With this in mind, it is difficult to justify the time and expense of isolating these organisms as a routine part of an infertility evaluation unless significant pyospermia is present.[24]

The best treatment for this subgroup of patients has not yet been defined. A reasonable course of action is to administer a prolonged course of antibiotics, 4 to 6 weeks, in any patient with significant pyospermia. However, one should be certain that the identified white blood cells are not actually immature germ cells, since they can easily be confused. An appropriate antibiotic would be one of the tetracyclines because of their spectrum of activity, low cost, and minimal side effects. If the pyospermia does not resolve with antibiotic therapy, a trial with nonsteroidal antiinflammatory agents is indicated. Failure to respond to either treatment is an indication for cultures and further investigation into the underlying source of inflammation.

ANTISPERM ANTIBODIES

The treatment for antisperm antibodies remains highly controversial. Autoimmunity to sperm was first described at the turn of the century. Approximately 50 years later the clinical sequela of autoimmunity to sperm was discovered.[25] During the last 30 years we have observed an evolution in the laboratory methods for antisperm antibody testing and methods for treatment.

As described in the previous chapter, only antibodies against surface-bound antigens are thought to be clinically significant. Most of the literature regarding therapy is based on outdated assays which have significant false-positive and false-negative rates.[26] The first therapy developed to treat male-factor infertility due to antisperm anti-

FIGURE 26.4 *Results of Endocrine Evaluation Typically Obtained in an Infertile Male Patient*

	T	FSH	LH	PROLACTIN
Eugonadal	Normal	Normal	Normal	Normal
Testicular failure	Normal	↑	Normal	Normal
Hypogonadotropic hypogonadism	↓	↓	↓	Normal
Hyperprolactinemia	Normal /↓	Normal	Normal	↑

bodies was steroid therapy.[27] Glucocorticoids have been shown to have significant antiinflammatory effects in vitro and in vivo. The majority of this effect is brought about by inhibition of cellular immunity. Unfortunately, steroids have only a minimal effect on antibody production within tissues. Many uncontrolled studies have demonstrated significant improvement in pregnancy rates after steroid therapy for antisperm antibodies. Almost all controlled studies of steroid therapy have been negative. However, Hendry and associates[28] recently demonstrated a significantly higher pregnancy rate, 31% versus 10%, by men taking 40 mg of prednisone per day versus placebo. None of the published controlled studies reveal a significant reduction of surface-bound antisperm antibody activity after steroid therapy. However, the efficacy of steroid therapy may be due to inhibition of cellular immunity within the seminal plasma rather than reduction of antisperm antibody production. Concern over the potentially significant side effects of high-dose steroid therapy, including aseptic hip necrosis, has encouraged development of alternative forms of therapy.

Antisperm antibodies are thought to reduce fertility by interfering with sperm transport through the female reproductive tract. The cervix normally entraps and filters sperm ejaculated into the vagina. Postcoital examination of cervical mucus usually reveals altered sperm motility. In addition, antibody-bound sperm may be more susceptible to degradation by the female immune system in the uterus and fallopian tubes. Intrauterine insemination has been used to bypass the cervical barrier. However, the pregnancy rate for intrauterine insemination in couples with male-factor antisperm antibodies has been disappointingly low.[29]

In vitro fertilization effectively eliminates female-derived immune factors, which may adversely affect sperm numbers and function even when intrauterine insemination is employed, from interfering with fertilization. The concentration of sperm incubated with the ova can be increased to compensate for functional defects in the sperm of men with male-factor infertility. Pregnancy rates as high as 33% have been reported for IVF therapy of antisperm antibodies.[30,31] Micromanipulation of the sperm and oocyte in vitro may be effective for patients with antisperm antibodies if routine in vitro fertilization fails.

Various techniques have been employed to remove antibodies from sperm after ejaculation. Ejaculation into a large volume of buffer and immediate processing have been performed in an attempt to obtain antibody-free sperm.[32] However, antibody binding appears to occur before ejaculation. Attempts at mechanically stripping antibodies from sperm have also been unsuccessful. Limited success has been obtained with enzyme digestion of sperm-associated IgA antibodies.[33] However, this technique is not yet ready for clinical application.

Nonspecific Medical Therapy

Nonspecific medical therapy for male-factor infertility, otherwise known as empiric medical therapy, consists of treatments used to correct or compensate for semen abnormalities without a specific rational basis. In other words, these therapies are instituted without clear evidence of a specific relationship to the underlying problem. Frequently, these treatments are based on the unsubstantiated but logical assumptions that increasing factors necessary for fertility or placing sperm in closer proximity to ova will improve fertility potential. These assumptions are the basis for most of the medications and reproduction-assisting techniques, such as intrauterine insemination and in vitro fertilization, presently used in the treatment of male-factor infertility. This section focuses on medications; the nonspecific use of reproduction-assisting techniques is discussed in Chapter 28.

Despite many advances in our understanding and treatment of infertility, the underlying cause of infertility remains unknown in at least 25% of men evaluated.[34] Unfortunately, empiric therapy is the only option for men without an identifiable cause of infertility. Likewise, empiric therapy is the only option for patients with a known but irreversible cause of infertility, such as cryptorchidism or gonadotoxin exposure. Finally, patients who have not been helped by specific medical or surgical therapy are candidates for nonspecific medical therapy. An important caveat is that all infertile patients should be evaluated for specific abnormalities before a nonspecific form of therapy is initiated.

ANTIESTROGENS

Follicle-stimulating hormone has been shown to be necessary for initiation and quantitative maintainance of spermatogenesis (Fig. 26.5).[35] The exact action of FSH on the germinal epithelium is still not fully understood. However, FSH receptors are located on the Sertoli cell membrane, and the Sertoli cell appears to act as the mediator of pituitary stimulation of sperm production. FSH production and secretion by the anterior pituitary are stimulated by Gn-RH secreted by the hypothalamus. Sex steroids secreted by Leydig cells and inhibin secreted by Sertoli cells exert a negative feedback inhibition on FSH release. Although the process is still incompletely understood, it appears that testosterone is aromatized to estradiol within the hypothalamus and pituitary gland, so it is primarily estradiol that exerts this negative feedback effect.[36] Therefore, administration of an antiestrogen would block this normal feedback inhibition of the pituitary gland and result in excessive production and release of both FSH and LH.[36]

The most commonly used empiric medical therapy is clomiphene citrate. Clomiphene citrate is an analogue of the nonsteroidal estrogen chlorotrianisene, which is primarily an antiestrogen but also has weak estrogenic effects. Administration of this drug results in an increase in both serum gonadotropins and testosterone. Therapy is usually begun at a dosage of 25 mg/d, although an every other day dosing has been reported to be just as effective.[37] The most common side effects reported are fluid retention, hypertension, visual distubances, and gynecomastia. Patients should be monitored with serum endocrine studies to make certain that the initial dosage is producing the desired effect, elevated serum FSH levels. In addition, seminal parameters should be checked on a monthly basis, since some patients demonstrate deterioration of sperm counts during therapy. Treatment should be continued for a minimum of 4 to 6 months. However, some patients who do not respond during this initial time period may respond by 1 year. Most placebo-controlled studies examining this therapy have not shown significant benefit. However, a study by Wang and associates[38] observed a 36% pregnancy rate in couples in whom the male partner was treated with clomiphene citrate (25 mg/d for 6 to 9 months) as compared with no pregnancies in placebo controls. Clearly, some patients do benefit from this drug. However, this probably represents only a minority, and parameters to predict a positive response have not yet been identified. The one predictor of a negative response is an elevated baseline serum FSH. Therefore, patients with an elevated baseline serum FSH should not be given clomiphene citrate.

Tamoxifen citrate is another antiestrogen that is believed to have less estrogenic effect. The recommended dose is 10 mg/d. As with clomiphene citrate, patients with normal baseline serum FSH are more likely to have a positive response and patients with azoospermia rarely respond. None of the controlled studies examining this drug have shown any efficacy over placebo.[39] Testolactone is a drug that inhibits the enzyme aromatase, which converts androgens to estrogens, with two potential beneficial effects. Inhibition of Leydig cell production of estradiol may have a direct beneficial effect on the testis. Inhibition of the conversion of androgens to estrogens partially blocks the normal negative feedback of androgens on the anterior pituitary gland and results in an increase in both serum FSH and LH. Initial reports of this drug were promising, but the only controlled trial reported was negative.[40] This drug may be potentially useful in infertile patients with altered testosterone: estradiol ratios, such as men with obesity.

GONADOTROPINS

Administration of the exogenous gonadotropins HCG and HMG to men who lack endogenous gonadotropins has been remarkably successful in restoring fertility. Gonadotropins directly stimulate all testicular functions (Fig. 26.6). Therefore, it has been an attractive hypothesis to use these drugs in infertile men to stimulate sperm production despite normal to high baseline serum gonadotropin levels. Again, the theory is that if some gonadotropins are good for spermatogenesis, more must be better. Likewise, patients with elevated levels of endogenous gonadotropins measured by radioimmunoassay may not be receiving the full biologic effect of these hormones. Many studies have demonstrated that the biologic activity

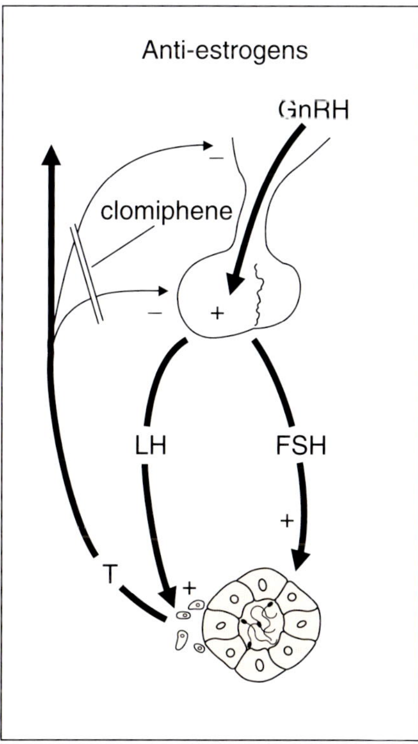

Figure 26.5 The effect of FSH on the male hypo-thalamic–pituitary–gonadal axis.

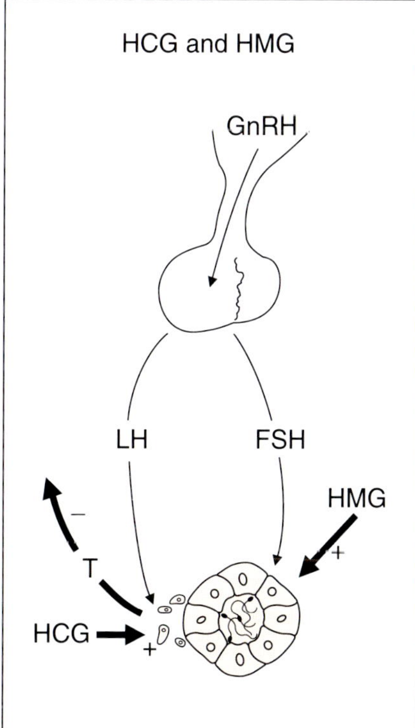

Figure 26.6 The effect of HCG and HMG on the male hypothalamic–pituitary–gonadal axis.

of gonadotropins does not always correspond to their immunologic activity.[41,42] This is particularly true in individuals with elevated levels of these protein hormones.

Both HCG and HMG must be administered parenterally. The dosage regimen is similar to that used for hypogonadotropic hypogonadism, 2500 units HCG and 150 units HMG three times weekly. Uncontrolled studies of these drugs have revealed conflicting results. However, the only controlled study performed was negative.[43] Adjunctive therapy with HCG in men with sperm counts of less than 10 million/mL who undergo varicocelectomy has shown significant benefit.[44] However, these results have not been substantiated by controlled studies.

Various regimens have been employed using HCG and HMG singly or in combination and at different dosages. A typical regimen for HCG alone is 5000 to 10,000 IU weekly divided into two or three doses. The recommended dosage of HMG is 150 IU three times weekly. However, with the possible exception of their use as adjunctive therapy in men who undergo varicocelectomy, the cost and inconvenience of these drugs prohibit their routine use in the typical infertile patient.

An alternative method to raise serum gonadotropin levels is to stimulate endogenous secretion by administration of exogenous Gn-RH (Fig. 26.7). Synthetic analogues to Gn-RH are now available. However, these drugs have a short half-life and therefore require frequent administration. Overdosing of these synthetic agents results in pituitary inhibition. The drugs can be administered via subcutaneous injection, with a portable pump, or intranasally. Early reports on the use of these drugs have not been promising and the only controlled study performed was negative.[45] However, the best dosage and method of administration have not yet been determined for this class of drugs. Until there is further information available, this drug should only be used in clinical trials.

ANDROGENS

Various preparations of androgens are available for the treatment of infertility. Similar logic is employed to justify the use of this class of drug as for drugs that increase gonadotropin levels. Clearly, testosterone is vital to maintain normal spermatogenesis and normal sex accessory gland function, and an increase may have a beneficial effect. However, most methods of delivering exogenous androgens cause a reduction of endogenous androgens. Naturally occurring testosterone cannot be administered orally. Synthetic androgens have been developed that can be absorbed through the gastrointestinal tract. However, the first-pass effect through the liver results in erratic changes in peripheral levels, and hepatic toxicity has been reported with the use of these drugs. Therefore, oral preparations of androgens should never be used in the treatment of male-factor infertility. Depot injections of testosterone esters (enanthate and cypionate) can reliably raise serum androgen levels without any significant toxicity. The usual replacement dose is 200 mg every 2 weeks.

In a normal individual there is a significant concentration gradient between testicular and peripheral levels of testosterone, due to local production. Although peripheral administration of testosterone can restore peripheral serum levels to normal, the testicular concentration of testosterone would be far below normal in this setting. Administration of testosterone in infertile patients with

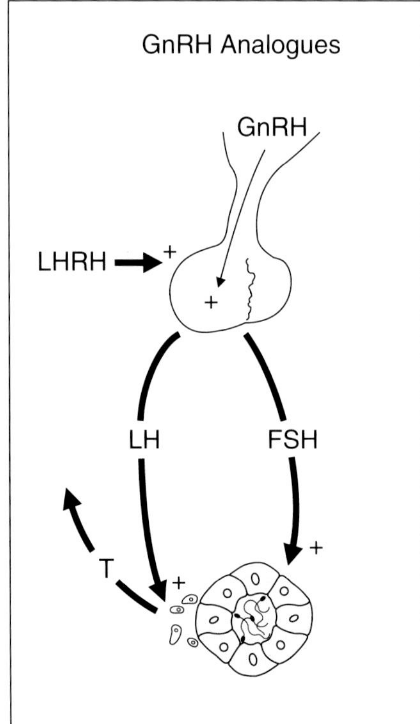

Figure 26.7 The effect of fertility drugs on the male hypothalamic–pituitary–gonadal axis.

normal androgen levels increases feedback inhibition of the anterior pituitary gland and decreases testicular production of testosterone. In fact, androgen therapy has been studied as a method for contraception in fertile men. All controlled studies of androgen therapy have been negative,[38] and this should no longer be considered part of the armamentarium of empiric medical therapy.

MISCELLANEOUS

A variety of other drugs have been employed on an empiric basis for the treatment of idiopathic male-factor infertility. Vitamins, heavy metals, thyroid hormones, and bromocriptine have all been shown to have no efficacy when employed on an empiric basis without any evidence of a specific deficiency. Several drugs have been reported to be of benefit but have received little attention. These include kallikrein, ketoprofen, and indomethacin. All of these drugs have been shown to be beneficial in at least one controlled study.

Kallikrein is a polypeptide enzyme which is active in the bradykinin pathway. Administration of 600 kU of pancreatic kallikrein produced beneficial effects in one controlled study.[46] Kallikrein may exacerbate inflammatory processes and is contraindicated in patients with either epididymitis or prostatitis.

Prostaglandin inhibitory effects of ketoprofen and indomethacin are thought to improve fertility, since early studies have shown that prostaglandins have an adverse effect on sperm motility. With a dose of 75 mg/d of indomethacin or 150 mg/d of ketoprofen, pregnancy rates were significantly better than with placebo in one controlled study.[47] Both of these drugs have the advantage of low cost and lack of serious side effects. However, a recent controlled study did not demonstrate any significant effect of these drugs on sperm motility despite significant reduction of seminal prostaglandin levels.[48] Further work is needed to determine which patients are the best candidates for these drugs.

Conclusion

The generally disappointing results obtained with non-specific medical therapy point out the importance of a thorough evaluation of the infertile patient to identify specific treatable abnormalities. It is important to limit costs and risk for the patient because infertility is not a life-threatening disorder. Likewise, each couple deserves a realistic appraisal of their potential fertility outcome and counseling on the alternatives of donor insemination and adoption. In addition to compassion and understanding, a thorough knowledge of the basic physiology of male reproduction is vital in managing the infertile couple.

References

1. Lipshultz LI, McConnell JA, Benson GS. Current concepts of the mechanisms of ejaculation: normal and abnormal states. *J Reprod Med.* 1981;26:499.
2. Proctor KG, Howards SS. The effect of sympathomimetic drugs on post lymphadenectomy aspermia. *J Urol.* 1983;129:837–838.
3. Nijman JM, Jagers S, Boer PW, Kremer J, Oldhoff J, Schraffordt Koops H. The treatment of ejaculation disorders after retroperitoneal lymph node dissection. *Cancer.* 1982;50:2967–2971.
4. Crich JP, Jequier AM. Infertility in men with retrograde ejaculation: the action of urine on sperm motility and a simple method for achieving antegrade ejaculation. *Fertil Steril.* 1978;30:572–576.
5. Innes IR, Nickerson M. Norepinephrine, epinephrine and the sympathomimetic amines. In: Goodman LS, Gilman A, eds. *The Pharmacologic Basis of Therapeutics.* New York, NY: Macmillan Press; 1975:477.
6. Urry RL, Middleton RG, McGavin S. A simple and effective treatment for increasing pregnancy rates in couples with retrograde ejaculation. *Fertil Steril.* 1986;46:1124–1127.
7. Kelly ME, Needle MA. Imipramine for aspermia after lymphadenectomy. *Urology.* 1979;13:414–415.
8. Beretta G, Chelo E, Zanollo A. Reproductive aspects in spinal cord injured males. *Paraplegia.* 1989;27:113–118.
9. Halstead LS, VerVoort S, Seager SWJ. Rectal probe electrostimulation in the treatment of ejaculatory spinal cord injured men. *Paraplegia.* 1987;25:120–129.
10. Matsumoto AM, Karpas AE, Bremner WJ. Chronic human chorionic gonadotropin administration in normal men: evidence that follicle-stimulating hormone is necessary for the maintenance of quantitatively normal spermatogenesis in man. *J Clin Endocrinol Metab.* 1986;62:1184–1192.
11. Burger HG, Baker HWG. Therapeutic considerations and results of gonadotropin treatment in male hypogonadotropic hypogonadism. *Ann NY Acad Sci.* 1984;438:447–453.
12. Schopohl J, Mehltretter G, von Zumbusch R, Eversmann T, von Weder K. Comparison of gonadotropin-releasing hormone and gonadotropin therapy in male patients with idiopathic hypothalamic hypogonadism. *Fertil Steril.* 1991;56:1143–1150.
13. Liu L, Banks SM, Barnes KM, Sherins RJ. Two-year comparison of testicular responses to pulsatile gonadotropin-releasing hormone and exogenous gonadotropins from the inception of therapy in men with isolated hypogonadotropic hypogonadism. *J Clin Endocrinol Metab.* 1988;67:1140–1145.
14. Carter JN, Tyson JE, Tolis G, Van Vliet S, Faiman C, Friesen HG. Prolactin-secreting tumors and hypogonadism in 22 men. *N Engl J Med.* 1978;299:847–852.
15. Danutra V, Harper ME, Boyns AK, Cole EN, Brownsey BG, Griffith K. The effect of certain stilbesterol analogues on plasma prolactins and testosterone in the rat. *J Endocrinol.* 1973;57:207–215.
16. Micic S, Dotlic R, Ilic V, Genbacerv O. Hormone profile in hyperprolactinemic infertile men. *Arch Androl.* 1985, 15:123–128.
17. Murray FT, Cameron DF, Ketchum C. Return of gonadal function in men with prolactin-secreting pituitary tumors. *J Clin Endocrinol Metab.* 1984;59:79–85.
18. Paulson JD, Polakoski KL. Isolation of a spermatozoal immobilization factor from *Escherichia coli* filtrates. *Fertil Steril.* 1977;28:182–185.

19. Maruyama DK, Hale RW, Rogers BJ. Effects of white blood cells on the in vitro penetration of zona-free hamster eggs by human spermatozoa. *J Androl.* 1985;6:127–135.

20. Talkington DF, Davis JK, Canupp KC, et al. The effects of three serotypes of *Ureaplasma urealyticum* on spermatozoal motility and penetration in vitro. *Fertil Steril.* 1991;55: 170–176.

21. Melekos MD, Asbach HW. Epididymitis: aspects concerning etiology and treatment. *J Urol.* 1987;138:83–86.

22. Auroux MR, DeMouy DM, Acar JF. Male fertility and positive chlamydial serology. *J Androl.* 1987;8:197–200.

23. Berger RE, Karp LE, Williamson RA, Koehler J, Moore DE, Holmes KK. The relationship of pyospermia and seminal fluid bacteriology to sperm function as reflected in the sperm penetration assay. *Fertil Steril.* 1982;37:557–564.

24. Hellstrom WJG, Schachter J, Sweet RL, McClure RD. Is there a role for *Chlamydia trachomatis* and genital mycoplasma in male infertility? *Fertil Steril.* 1987;48:337–339.

25. Rumke P, Hellinger G. Autoantibodies against spermatozoa in sterile men. *Am J Clin Pathol.* 1959;32:357–363.

26. Carson SA, Reiher J, Scommegna A, Prins GS. Antibody binding patterns in infertile males and females as detected by immunobead test, gel-agglutination test and sperm immobilization test. *Fertil Steril.* 1988;49:487–492.

27. Shulman S. Treatment of immune male infertility with methylprednisolone. *Lancet.* 1976;2:1243.

28. Hendry WF, Hughes L, Scammell G, Pryor JP, Hargreave TB. Comparison of prednisolone and placebo in subfertile men with antibodies to spermatozoa. *Lancet.* 1990;335:85–88.

29. Smarr SC, Wing R, Hammond MG. Effect of therapy on infertile couples with antisperm antibodies. *Am J Obstet Gynecol.* 1988;158:969.

30. Haas GG Jr. Immunologic infertility. *Obstet Gynecol Clin North Am.* 1987;14:1609–1085.

31. Cohen J, Edwards R, Fehilly C, et al. In vitro fertilization: a treatment for male infertility. *Fertil Steril.* 1985;43:422–432.

32. Adeghe A. Effect of washing on sperm surface autoantibodies. *Br J Urol.* 1987;60:360–363.

33. Bronson RA, Cooper GW, Rosenfeld DL, Gilbert JV, Plaut AG. The effect of an IgA$_1$ protease on immunoglobulins bound to the sperm surface and sperm cervical mucus penetrating ability. *Fertil Steril.* 1987;47:985–991.

34. Greenberg SH, Lipshultz LI, Wein AJ. Experience with 425 subfertile male patients. *J Urol.* 1978;119:507–510.

35. Sherins RJ, Loriaux DL. Studies on the role of sex steroids in the feedback control of FSH concentrations in men. *J Clin Endocrinol Metab.* 1973;36:886–893.

36. Bardin CW, Ross GT, Lipsett MB. Site of action of clomiphene citrate in men: a study of the pituitary–Leydig cell axis. *J Clin Endocrinol.* 1967;27:1558–1164.

37. Homonnai ZT, Yauetz H, Yogeu L, Rotem R, Paz GF. Clomiphene citrate treatment in oligozoospermia: comparison between two regimens of low-dose treatment. *Fertil Steril.* 1988;50:801–804.

38. Wang C, Chan CW, Wong KK, Yeung KK. Comparison of the effectiveness of placebo, clomiphene citrate, mesterolone, pentoxifylline, and testosterone rebound therapy for the treatment of idiopathic oligospermia. *Fertil Steril.* 1983; 40:358–365.

39. Ain Melk Y, Belisle S, Carmel M, Jean-Pierre T. Tamoxifen citrate therapy in male infertility. *Fertil Steril.* 1987;48: 113–117.

40. Clark RV, Sherins RJ. Treatment of men with idiopathic oligozoospermic infertility using the aromatase inhibitor, testolactone: results of a double-blinded, randomized placebo-controlled trial with crossover. *J Androl.* 1989;10:240–247.

41. Beiting IZ, Axelrod L, Ostrea T, Little R, Badger TM. Hypogonadism in a male with an immunologically active, biologically inactive luteinizing hormone: characterization of the abnormal hormone. *J Clin Endocrinol Metab.* 1981; 52:1143–1149.

42. Buch JP, Lipshultz LI, Smith RG. Evidence for altered receptor-binding activity of serum follicle-stimulating hormone in male infertility. *Fertil Steril.* 1991;55:358–362.

43. Knuth UA, Honigl W, Bals-Pratsch M, Schleicher G, Nieschlag E. Treatment of severe oligospermia with human chorionic gonadotropin/human menopausal gonadotropin: a placebo controlled double blind trial. *J Clin Endocrinol Metab.* 1987;65:1081–1087.

44. Dubin L, Amelar RD. Varicocelectomy as therapy in male infertility: a study of 504 cases. *Fertil Steril.* 1975;26:217–220.

45. Badenoch DF, Waxman J, Boorman L, et al. Administration of a gonadotropin releasing hormone analogue in oligozoospermic infertile males. *Acta Endocrinol.* 1988;117:265–267.

46. Schill WB. Treatment of idiopathic oligozoospermia by kallikrein: results of a double-blind study. *Arch Androl.* 1979;2:163–170.

47. Barkay J, Harpaz-Kerpel S, Ben-Ezra S, Gordon S, Zuckerman H. The prostaglandin inhibitor effect of anti-inflammatory drugs in the therapy of male infertility. *Fertil Steril.* 1984; 42:406–411.

48. Knuth UA, Kuhine J, Crosby J, Bals-Pratsch M, Kelly RW, Nieschlag E. Indomethacin and oxaprozin lower seminal prostaglandin levels but do not influence sperm motion characteristics and serum hormones of young healthy men in a placebo-controlled double-blind trial. *J Androl.* 1989; 10:108–119.

Surgical Therapy for Infertility

Jeffrey P. Buch

Surgical treatment for male infertility began with the first recorded varicocele repair resulting in improved semen quality, reported by Bennett in 1889.[1] The development of surgical techniques for bypassing sperm duct obstruction began in the early 1900s. Subsequently, Macomber and Sanders in 1929[2] reported the case of an oligospermic patient who underwent varicocele repair with subsequent correction of his semen quality and ultimately restoration of fertility. However, the modern era of surgical treatment for male infertility did not truly begin until the widely publicized report by Tulloch in 1952.[3] Repair of bilateral varicoceles in a man who was azoospermic before surgery ultimately returned sperm to his ejaculate and resulted in conception. More widespread acceptance of the role for varicocele repair was heralded by the work of Dubin and Amelar, reported in 1970.[4] In the 1940s, Charny[5] promoted the use of testicular biopsy in prescribing treatment for male infertility. In the 1970s, Owen[6] and Silber[7] promoted the use of the microscope for repair of vas deferens and epididymis obstructions. The most recent surgical advance is the use of laparoscopic surgery in the repair of varicoceles, with initial reports in 1992 by Donovan and Winfield[8] and Hagood et al.[9]

Varicocele Repair

Varicoceles are dilated scrotal veins that are secondary to an absence or incompetence of the venous valves within the spermatic veins. Varicoceles, present in approximately 15% of all men and in up to 40%[10] of infertile men, are the most common treatable cause of male factor infertility. The exact pathophysiology of varicoceles is still not completely understood. In fact, it appears that many men with varicoceles are fertile. However, review of the literature reveals that seminal parameters improve in approximately 66% of men who undergo varicocele repair and that pregnancy rates of approximately 50% are achieved. The most popular theory of how a varicocele causes impaired fertility is based on animal studies using surgically created varicoceles. In this model, testicular temperature is elevated by an increase in testicular blood flow.[11] Other theories include impairment of steroidogenesis, testicular hypoxia, and reflux of toxic metabolites from the kidney and/or adrenal gland.

Treatment options for varicocele repair include open surgery, percutaneous venographic approach, and laparoscopy. Each treatment modality has its own advantages and risks that may make it the most appropriate choice for select patients, depending on the availability of specialized equipment and expertise. In general, it appears that the success rates for these techniques are the same once the varicocele has been repaired.

Potential complications from varicocelectomy include hydrocele, testicular hypersensitivity, migration of embolization balloons, testicular atrophy from arterial ligation, and persistent or recurrent varicocele. The frequency of these complications varies with the different techniques

available. In addition, exposure to general anesthesia and time lost from work may influence the choice of method by which the varicocele is repaired.

OPEN SURGICAL LIGATION

Four open surgical approaches to the spermatic veins have been employed: retroperitoneal ligation superior to the internal inguinal ring, midinguinal approach, infrainguinal approach (just inferior to the external ring), and transscrotal approach (Fig. 27.1A). The transscrotal approach has been abandoned because of the difficulty in ligating the many veins present at this level and the higher complication rates.

The high retroperitoneal ligation was originally popularized by Palomo in 1949, who included ligation and transection of the internal spermatic artery with the veins at this level (Fig. 27.1B).[12] This repair is performed in the supine position with a transverse skin incision extending medially at the level of the anterior superior iliac spine. The external oblique fascia is sharply incised and a muscle-splitting technique is then used to gain entry to the retroperitoneum. It is helpful to tilt the table to the opposite side to displace the intraabdominal contents. The spermatic vessels will be found adherent to the underside of the peritoneum. The veins are individually dissected and doubly ligated with 3-0 silk suture before transection. A fine dissecting right-angle clamp is often quite helpful in these procedures. An effort should be made to identify and preserve the spermatic artery.

Advantages cited for this approach are the rapid exposure of the spermatic vessels and the fact that ligation of the spermatic artery at this level rarely has any deleterious effect on the testis, because collateral blood flow is provided by the cremasteric and deferential arteries. Disadvantages of this approach include a more difficult dissection in obese patients and a higher risk of persistence or recurrence of a varicocele from external spermatic vein collaterals. This procedure requires a major anesthetic, and approximately 2 weeks must elapse before the patient can return to full physical activity. This open approach is recommended only when the patient has had prior inguinal surgery.

The midinguinal approach through a transverse groin incision is another commonly employed approach (Fig. 27.1C). This procedure is modeled after the technique reported by the Russian surgeon Ivanissevich.[13] The incision is carried down through Scarpa's fascia onto the fascia of the external oblique, which is then incised in the direction of its fibers, allowing delivery of the spermatic cord. The veins are then individually ligated as previously noted. An intraoperative Doppler and application of topical vasodilators (i.e., lidocaine and/or papaverine) are helpful for identifying the arteries within the cord. In addition, loupe or microscopic magnification facilitates identification of small veins, lymphatics, and the spermatic artery. The advantages of the midinguinal approach include its ease and the speed with which the procedure

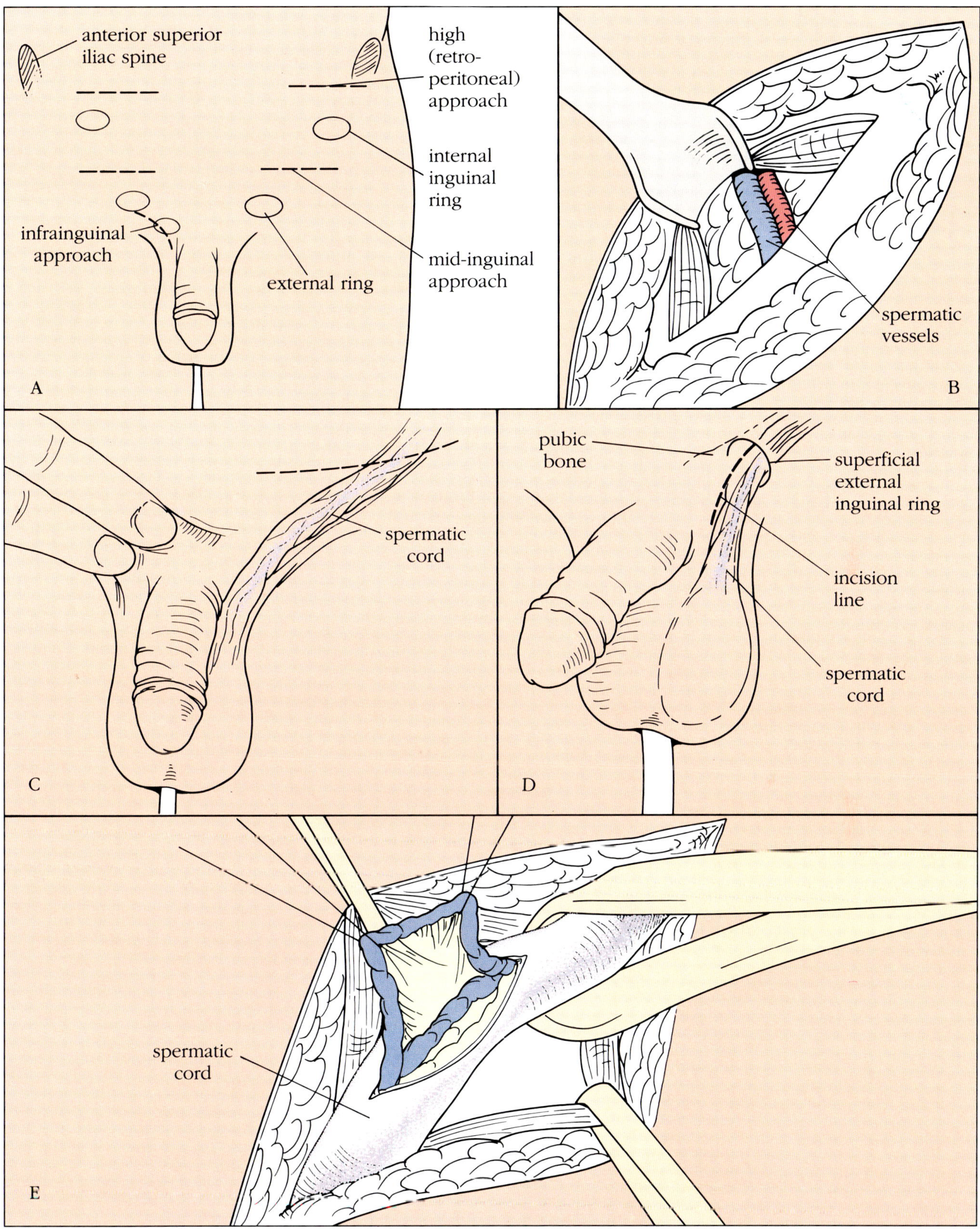

Figure 27.1 Open surgical treatment of varicocele. **A** Anatomy of surgical approaches. **B** High (retroperitoneal) approach to internal spermatic vein through a muscle-splitting incision. **C** Inguinal approach to the spermatic cord and internal spermatic veins with incision through external oblique aponeurosis with a transverse or diagonal skin incision. **D** Infrainguinal approach to spermatic cord with a transverse or diagonal skin incision. **E** Spermatic cord dissection with double ligation of internal spermatic veins from either an inguinal or an infrainguinal approach.

can be performed, a relatively low recurrence/persistence rate of only 5%, and the possibility of performing this procedure under local anesthesia with intravenous sedation. The only relative disadvantage of this approach is that it takes approximately 2 weeks until the patient is able to return to full physical activity. However, patients are usually able to return to light activity after 5 days.

The infrainguinal approach with microdissection has been popularized by Marmar et al. (Fig. 27.1D).[14] A small transverse or longitudinal incision is made inferior to the external inguinal ring over the pubic tubercle and spermatic cord. The diagonal incision extends 4 to 5 cm over the top of the spermatic cord from a point just lateral and superior to the base of the penis. This procedure is very amenable to local anesthesia with intravenous sedation, employing an inguinal cord block in addition to direct infiltration of the incision site. It is advantageous to include the scrotum in the prepped operative field, since traction on the testicle may be necessary to identify the spermatic cord. Once the spermatic cord has been isolated and the peripubic region has been examined for ligation of anomalous venous collaterals, the cord dissection is carried out as in the previously described procedures (Fig. 27.1E). Some surgeons recommend mobilization of the testis into the wound to identify and ligate gubernacular venous collaterals.

Advantages of this procedure include amenability to local anesthesia, its relative ease and rapidity, a time of approximately 1 week before return to full activity, and the lowest reported recurrence/persistence rate (only 1% to 2.5%). The disadvantage of this procedure is that it typically involves ligation of the greatest number of veins and can be tedious.

LAPAROSCOPIC VARICOCELE REPAIR

This technique, originally reported in the medical literature by Donovan and Winfield[8] and others,[9] is anatomically equivalent to the high retroperitoneal ligation. However, since it employs the laparoscope it is a transabdominal retroperitoneal ligation. This approach employs standard laparoscopic technique and equipment. The procedure requires three puncture wounds in the abdomen for trocar placement. The principal advantage of this technique is the reduction in postoperative pain and rapid return to full activity as compared with standard open procedures. This is most pronounced in the patient with bilateral varicoceles.

The procedure is performed under general anesthesia with placement of a nasogastric tube and Foley catheter. Three or four puncture sites are used. A 10 mm trocar is placed in the base of the umbilicus after insufflation of the peritoneal cavity with carbon dioxide through a Verres needle. Two accessory 10 mm trocars are placed laterally

(Fig. 27.2A). The retroperitoneum is opened 2 to 3 cm cranial to the internal ring and lateral to the spermatic vessels. The spermatic vessels are bluntly dissected in order to identify the artery before ligating the veins. An intraoperative laparoscopic Doppler and application of vasodilators may facilitate identification of the artery (Fig. 27.2B). The veins are then doubly ligated with hemoclips and divided. Smaller veins adherent to the artery can be cauterized (Fig. 27.2C). On completion of the procedure the pneumoperitoneum is evacuated and the fascia is closed at the trocar sites.

Patients can return to full activity within 48 hours. The disadvantages of this technique include the requirement for general anesthesia, subjecting the patient to the risk of bowel or major vascular injury, and the higher persistence/recurrence rate associated with the retroperitoneal approach. However, the laparoscopic technique may be advantageous in select patients who require bilateral varicocele repair.

PERCUTANEOUS ANGIOGRAPHIC OCCLUSION

The percutaneous approach has the advantage of being both diagnostic and therapeutic. Clinical reports from centers with a large experience reveal pregnancy rates comparable to those after surgical repair when the varicocele was successfully occluded. However, the occlusion rates range from only 80% to 90% and may be significantly lower at centers without much experience. These procedures use the standard Seldinger techniques employed in vascular radiology, with access to the spermatic vessels either through the groin or through the neck (Fig. 27.3). Venography is routinely performed under local anesthesia with intravenous sedation. Coils, balloons, and/or sclerosing agents can be used to occlude the veins. Advantages cited for this technique are the lack of general anesthesia, a short recuperation time (48 hours), its diagnostic potential, and the avoidance of "surgery." The main disadvantage is the lower success rate for repair and the slightly higher recurrence rate. This is the preferred technique for patients with suspected varicocele after previous surgical repair.

Electroejaculation

The need for electroejaculation has been stimulated by advances in the general rehabilitation of spinal-cord-injured men to the point that they often lead normal and productive lives. With this in mind, there have been increasing social and medical demands to enhance the fertility capabilities of this population. It is estimated that up to 90% of all spinal-cord-injured (SCI) men (complete and incomplete lesions) have failure to ejaculate. In fact, natural fertility without medical intervention is present in only 5% of spinal cord-injured men.[15] The use of electric current to achieve ejaculation in anejaculatory SCI men was first reported in 1948 by Horne et al.[16] However, it took 35 more years for a resurgence to occur in the clinical use of electric current to procure semen from neurologically anejaculatory men.[17–19] At present there are several highly successful programs around the world that employ transrectal electric stimulation of ejaculation. This technique has also been used in individuals with failure of emission due to diabetes, multiple sclerosis, retroperitoneal lymphadenectomy, and psychogenic causes who have not been helped by medical therapy. Advances in

technique and equipment offer a high degree of reliability in semen procurement (up to 90%) and minimal risk of injury. Vibratory stimulation of the frenulum of the penis has also been successfully employed to obtain sperm from SCI patients. This technique should be attempted before electroejaculation in all patients, since the risks and expense of vibratory stimulation are significantly lower than those of electroejaculation.

The application of transrectal electrical current is believed to cause ejaculation by regional stimulation of the pelvic nerves responsible for erection and ejaculation

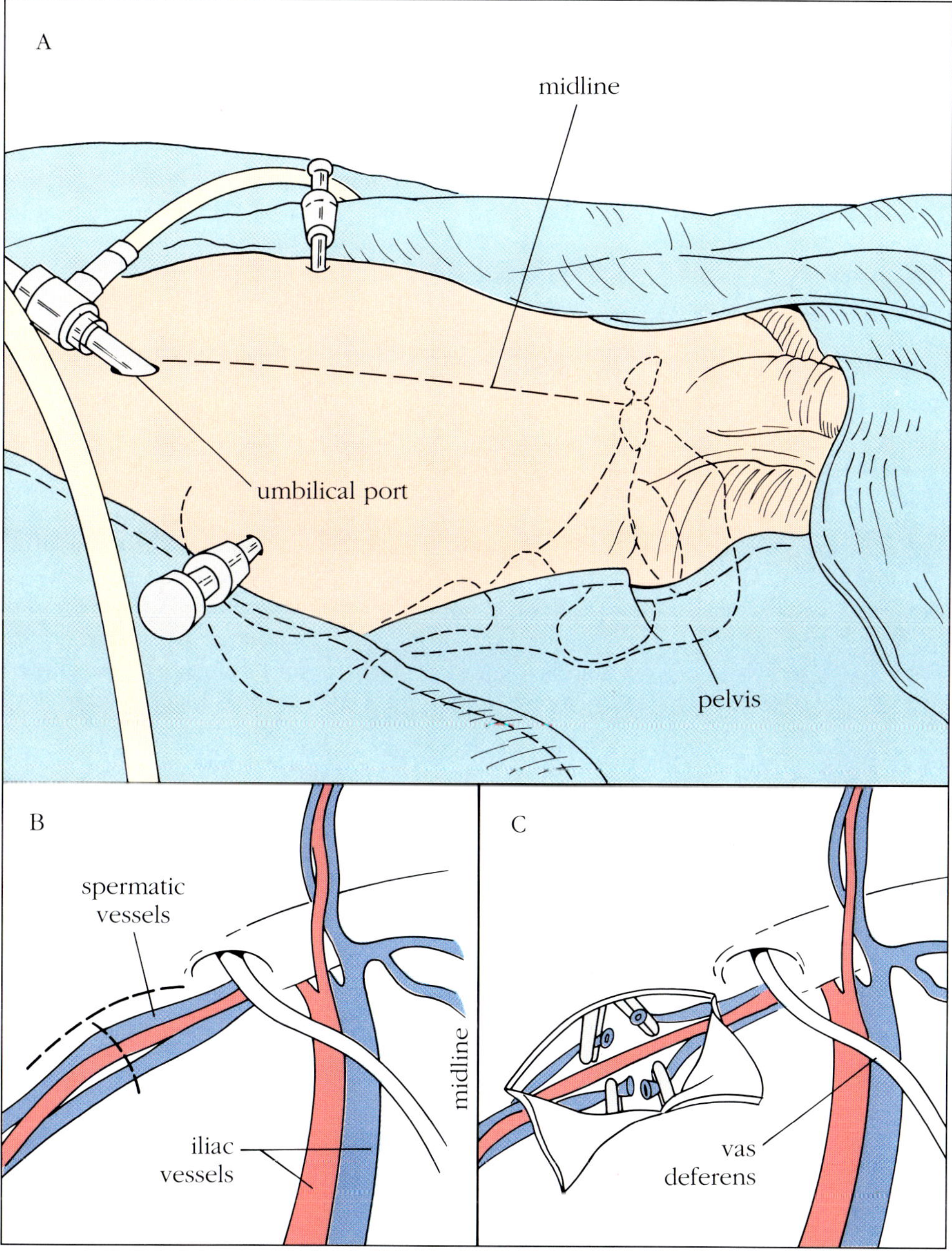

Figure 27.2
Laparoscopic treatment of varicocele. **A** Access port placement with 10 mm trocars at umbilicus (scope port) and lateral regions (clip applicators/dissecting port). **B** Intraabdominal anatomic landmarks for varicocele repair. **C** Appearance of ligated veins and preserved artery through window in peritoneum.

as they travel along the posterolateral surface of the prostate gland (Fig. 27.4). The antegrade and retrograde specimens produced can then be processed in the laboratory so that the motile sperm are isolated from dead sperm and detrimental cell contaminants, for subsequent insemination into the woman's reproductive tract at the time of ovulation. Sperm can be obtained in almost 90% of patients and many pregnancies have been reported as a result of insemination of sperm obtained with rectal probe electroejaculation (RPE).

TECHNIQUE AND EQUIPMENT

The equipment (G&S Instruments) and the basic technique were developed through application of veterinary techniques by Seager and co-workers.[20] The equipment includes a voltage generator, a temperature monitor, and multidiameter rectal probes, which contain three longitudinally oriented electrodes. In preparation, the patient is instructed to take oral antibiotics for 7 days preceding the procedure and for another day or two after the procedure. Beginning 36 hours before the procedure, he should take a minimum of 650 mg sodium bicarbonate q.i.d. to alkalinize his urine. The bowel regimen is done either the evening before or early in the morning of the procedure. The patient is instructed to minimize fluid intake so as to minimize urine production during the procedure. Patients with cardiac pacemakers or other electronic implanted devices must not be treated with RPE.

The procedure begins with sterile catheterization of the bladder in the supine position. Once the bladder has been emptied it is irrigated once with 50 mL of physiologic buffer, and 30 mL of fresh buffer is left in the bladder. The catheter is removed and the patient is placed in the lateral decubitus position. Patients at risk for autonomic dysreflexia are given sublingual nifedipine (20 mg). Blood pressure is monitored during the entire procedure. Proctoscopy is performed before and after completion of electroejaculation to assess the rectal mucosa. The most commonly used probe has a 1.25 inch diameter. The probe is introduced into the rectum with the electrodes placed anteriorly against the prostate and seminal vesicles. The electrical current is delivered in pulses lasting several seconds, with gradually increasing voltage on each pulse. The patient usually achieves an erection before ejaculation. The electrical current does not stimulate active expulsion of the semen. Therefore, the specimen must be milked out of the urethra and the bladder catheterized for the retrograde specimen.

The quality of the semen produced by this technique is usually poor. This is thought to be due to the underlying disease process, rather than to the technique itself. Sperm counts tend to be normal to high, but motility is

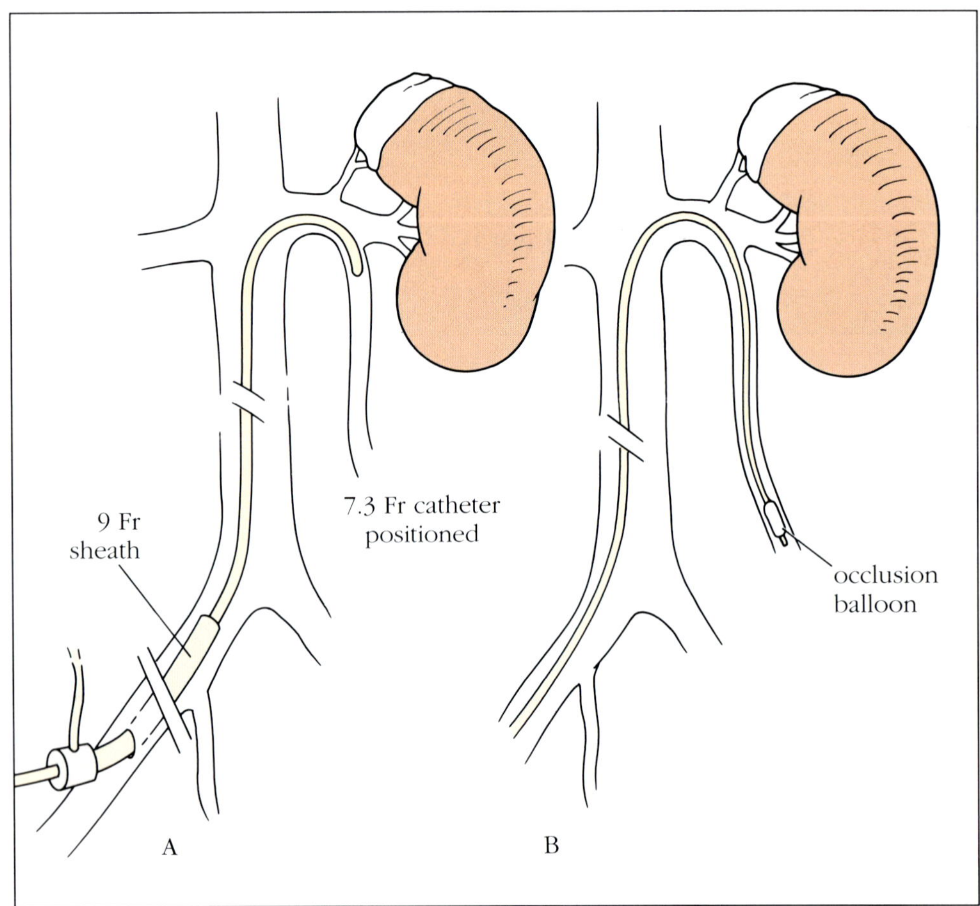

Figure 27.3
Percutaneous angiographic occlusion of left varicocele via femoral approach. **A** Position of catheter just inside origin of left internal spermatic vein. **B** Placement of occlusion balloon within spermatic vein at a level appropriate for preventing recurrence through collateral veins.

low. Almost all of the specimens require extensive processing in the laboratory to remove dead sperm cells and other cellular elements. The processed specimen is then used for insemination or other assisted reproductive techniques. It is extremely important to time these procedures well, since these sperm do not appear to survive as long in vitro or in vivo as sperm obtained from fertile men.

The exact role for assisted reproductive techniques beyond natural cycle intrauterine insemination for these couples remains to be determined. However, the majority of pregnancies currently reported in the literature from these couples have employed fertility drugs and refined ovulation monitoring of the women to enhance insemination timing and per-cycle fecundity rates. Higher per-cycle fecundity rates are especially imperative for those men with incomplete lesions who require general anesthesia in the operating room for this procedure. Early optimistic reports indicate that with assisted reproductive techniques we may be able to achieve conception in up to 50% of couples involving spinal cord-injured men.

Vasovasostomy

More than 300,000 vasectomies are performed in the United States each year. Increased rates of divorce and remarriage in the past three decades have created an increasing demand for vasectomy reversal. Initial reports of vasectomy reversal employed simple techniques using absorbable catgut sutures as stents and placement of relatively large (4-0) sutures without magnification. Despite the use of these limited techniques, the early success rate was reasonable. The microscopic techniques popularized by Owen[6] and Silber[7] in the mid 1970s dramatically improved the technical success rate of vasectomy reversal. Vasovasostomy can also be performed to bypass vasal obstruction of infectious, congenital, or iatrogenic origin.

Vasovasostomy requires identification of the site of obstruction and isolation of the patent distal and proximal ends of the vas deferens. Proximal patency can be confirmed by the identification of sperm within the intravasal fluid. Distal patency can be confirmed with vasography or injection of colored dye. The performance of vasovasostomy requires some type of magnification. Review of the literature does not reveal a significant advantage of the microscope over loupe magnification in the hands of experienced surgeons. However, an unsuspected epididymal obstruction may be present in many patients and repair of this lesion requires microsurgical techniques. Therefore, it is highly preferable to have microsurgical equipment and expertise available for all of these cases.

Vasovasostomy can be performed under local anesthesia with intravenous sedation or under general anes-

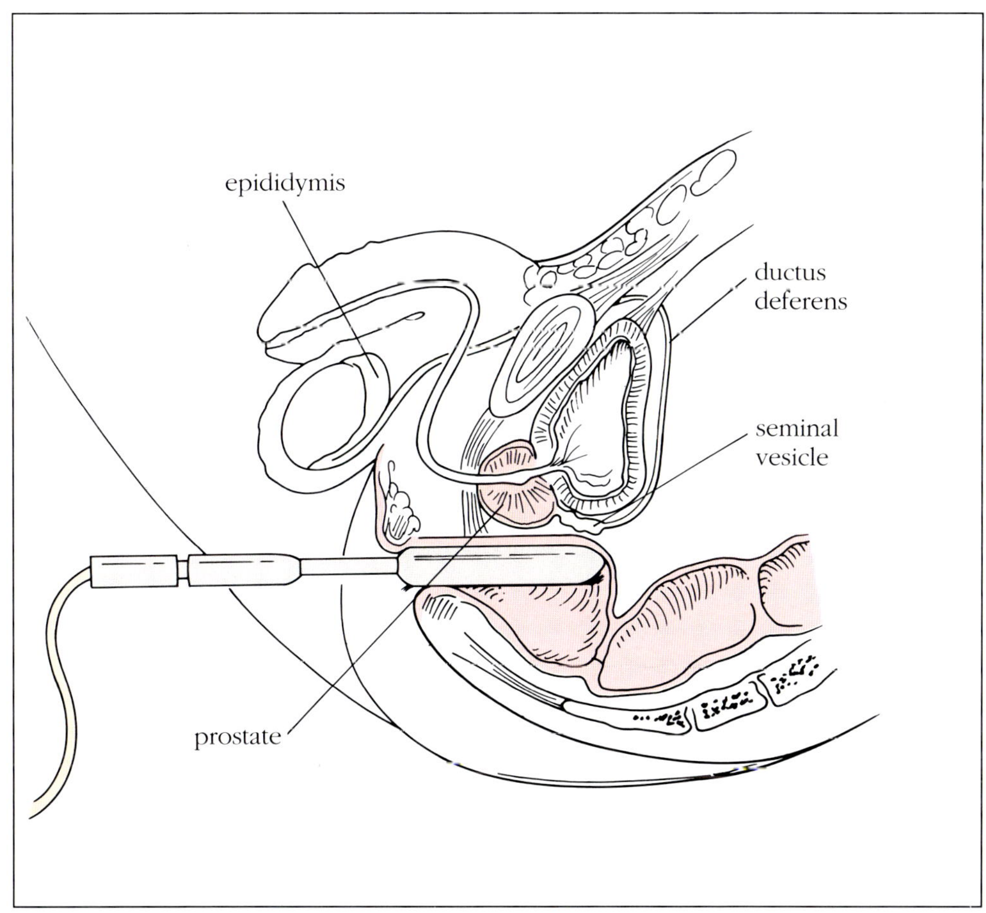

Figure 27.4 Position of probe within rectum during procedure. Electrodes are oriented longitudinally along the anterior surface of the probe.

thesia. Depending on the site of obstruction, a scrotal or an inguinal incision can be employed. The free ends of the vas should be inspected carefully to ensure adequate vascularity. The ends are then approximated using a two-layer, modified two-layer, or single-layer technique (Fig. 27.5). The main advantage of the two-layer technique is that it compensates for a disparity of lumen sizes. In the two-layer technique, six luminal sutures are placed in the mucosa and a partial thickness of muscularis, using interrupted 10-0 nylon suture. In the modified two-layer technique, four full-thickness sutures are placed using 9-0 or 10-0 nylon sutures. The outer layer is then completed with 9-0 nylon suture. A macroscopic technique with loupe magnification has been described using multiple full-thickness absorbable or nonabsorbable sutures of approximately 8-0 size.

Success is predicted by the status of the intraoperative vasal fluid, the technique used, and most of all by the experience of the surgeon. The Vasovasostomy Study Group has demonstrated that there is a difference in success rates between microscopic and macroscopic techniques.[21] However, surgical experience rather than type of technique was the better predictor of success. Patients with a duration of obstruction greater than 10 years frequently have intravasal azoospermia and require epididymovasostomy.

Epididymovasostomy (Vasoepididymostomy)

The most common situation requiring vasoepididymostomy is a case of vasectomy reversal in which a secondary "epididymal blowout" and obstruction has occurred. However, epididymal obstructions can also be secondary to inflammatory, iatrogenic, or congenital causes. Regardless of the etiology, the microscopic details for dissection and repair remain the same. However, patients with a history suggesting an inflammatory etiology should receive perioperative antibiotics and nonsteroidal antiinflammatory agents to reduce inflammation and enhance the success rate.

As with vasovasostomy, the initial reports involved the use of macroscopic repairs in which the epididymal tunic, epididymal tubules, and vas deferens were "fileted open" to make the potentially most simple and widely patent anastomosis (Fig. 27.6A). Understandably, these procedures resulted in minimal success. Not until the late 1970s did Silber and others report their initial experience with end-to-end anastomosis of the vas deferens to the specific epididymal tubule that leaked sperm when the epididymis was fully transected (Fig. 27.6B). More recently, Thomas and Howards[22] have popularized the advantages and enhanced success rates of anastomosing the side of a transected epididymal tubule to the end of the vas deferens in the so-called microscopic end-to-side vasoepididymostomy (Fig. 27.6C).

The end-to-side microscopic epididymovasostomy requires experience in determining which dilated epididymal tubules would be most likely to contain sperm in their fluid. A small portion of the epididymal tunic should be excised over the most distal portion of the epididymis at which distended tubules are visualized. Meticulous hemostasis must be maintained. Extreme caution should be exercised in using the bipolar current, since it may damage the tubules.

Once the epididymal tunic has been removed a single bulging tubule is identified, often with the assistance of staining the epididymis with indigo carmine. By use of jeweler's forceps and fine microscissors, a small piece of the side of the tubule is removed (see Fig. 27.6C). If copious amounts of sperm-containing fluid are noted, the anastomosis can be performed at this level. If there is no fluid and/or sperm within the tubule, then one should proceed proximally towards the testis until a sperm-containing epididymal tubule is isolated. Once such a tubule is identified, a marking suture is placed at the 6 o'clock position through the epididymal lumen with either 10-0 or 11-0 nylon double-armed suture. At this juncture the free cut end of the vas deferens on the abdominal side is brought into alignment with the epididymal tubule by placement of two or three 9-0 nylon sutures through the seromuscularis of the vas and the epididymal tunic between the 5 o'clock and 7 o'clock positions. These are crucial sutures for alignment— if they are properly placed the remainder of the anastomosis is not too difficult. The marking suture at 6 o'clock is placed through the lumen of the vas and tied into place. Depending on circumstance, three to five additional mucosal sutures are placed before they are all tied. The epididymal tunic is then reapproximated to the seromuscularis of the vas with several more 9-0 nylon sutures. The success rate for epididymovasostomy is a 60% patency rate and pregnancy rates approaching 30%.

Transurethral Resection of the Ejaculatory Duct

Ejaculatory duct obstruction (EDO) is primarily diagnosed on the basis of azoospermia in conjunction with low seminal volume (≤1 mL) and normal spermatogenesis on testicular biopsy. It has historically been confirmed with vasography and may be the result of congenital malformations of the Müllerian and Wolffian duct systems. EDO can be acquired as a result of genital tract infection or inflammation (e.g., from long-term indwelling catheters), and it may be partial in nature rather than a complete obstruction.[23] Transrectal ultrasonography can noninvasively diagnose EDO by the presence of markedly dilated seminal vesicles.

This procedure is performed with the patient in the lithotomy position (Fig.27.7). Transurethral resection (TUR) of the verumontanum on a pure cutting current is

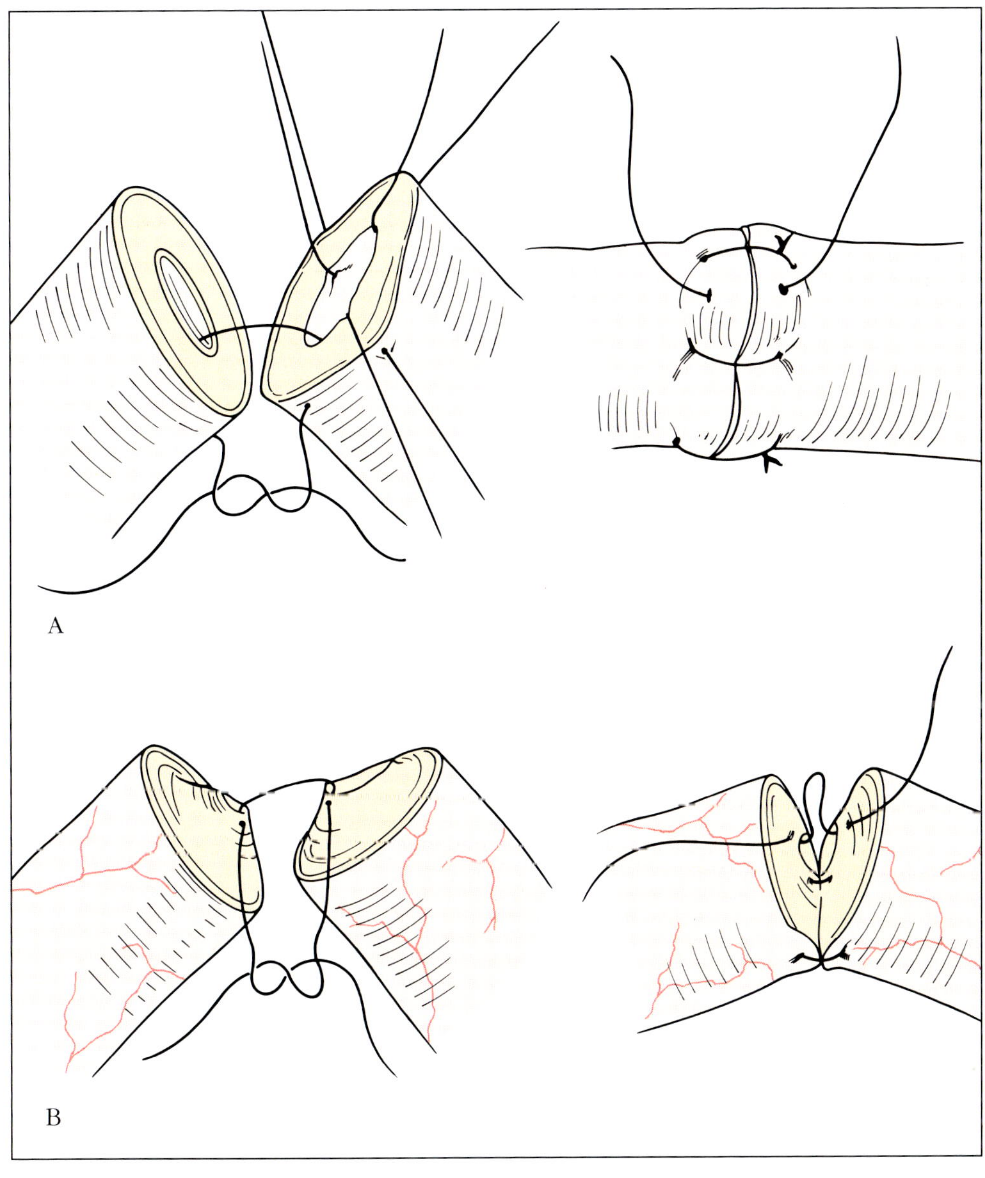

Figure 27.5 Vaso-vasostomy. **A** Placement of four-quadrant transmural sutures and reinforcing serosa–muscularis sutures once the vas deferens is positioned in a hinged vas approximator clamp (this is the same for macroscopic or modified two-layer microscopic anastomoses). **B** Suture placement for strict two-layer microsurgical anastomosis.

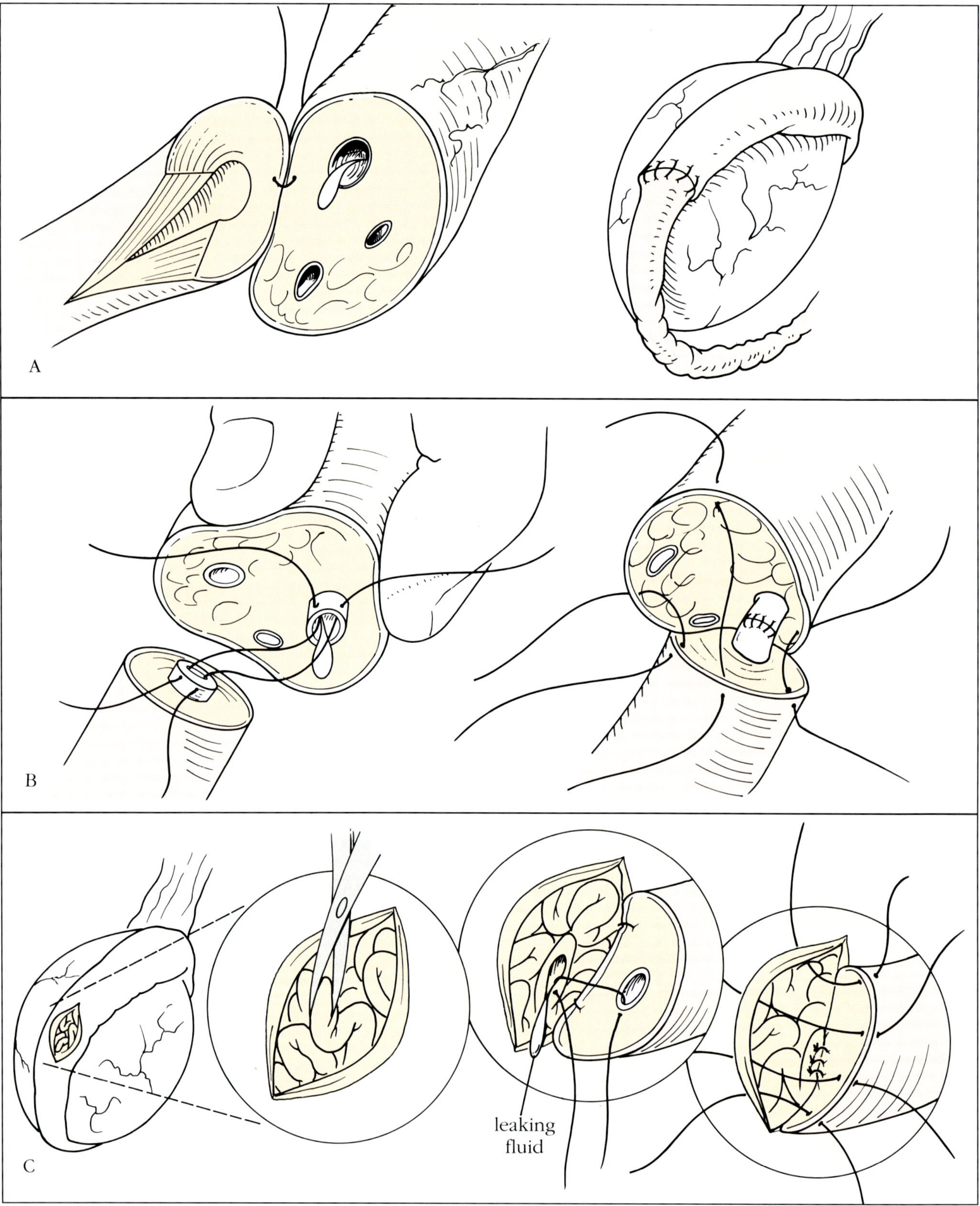

Figure 27.6 Vasoepididymostomy (epididymovasostomy). **A** Macroscopic (one-layer) anastomosis of "fish-mouthed" vas deferens to transversely cut end of epididymis (no tubule-to-tubule approximation). **B** Microscopic specific tubule end-to-end vasoepididymostomy. **C** Microscopic specific tubule end-to-side vasoepididymostomy.

performed using a 24 Fr resectoscope and a loop. An O'Conor drape is used so that the seminal vesicle can be massaged to ascertain completeness of the resection. If vasography is performed at the time of the procedure, colored dye can be mixed with the contrast to help identify the proper depth of resection. A 20 Fr three-way Foley catheter is placed in the bladder after the resection for continuous irrigation and is removed after 24 hours, just before the patient is discharged. Follow-up semen analysis may reveal normalization of seminal volume but persistent azoospermia. Epididymal obstruction should be suspected in these patients and scrotal exploration with possible epididymovasostomy should be performed.

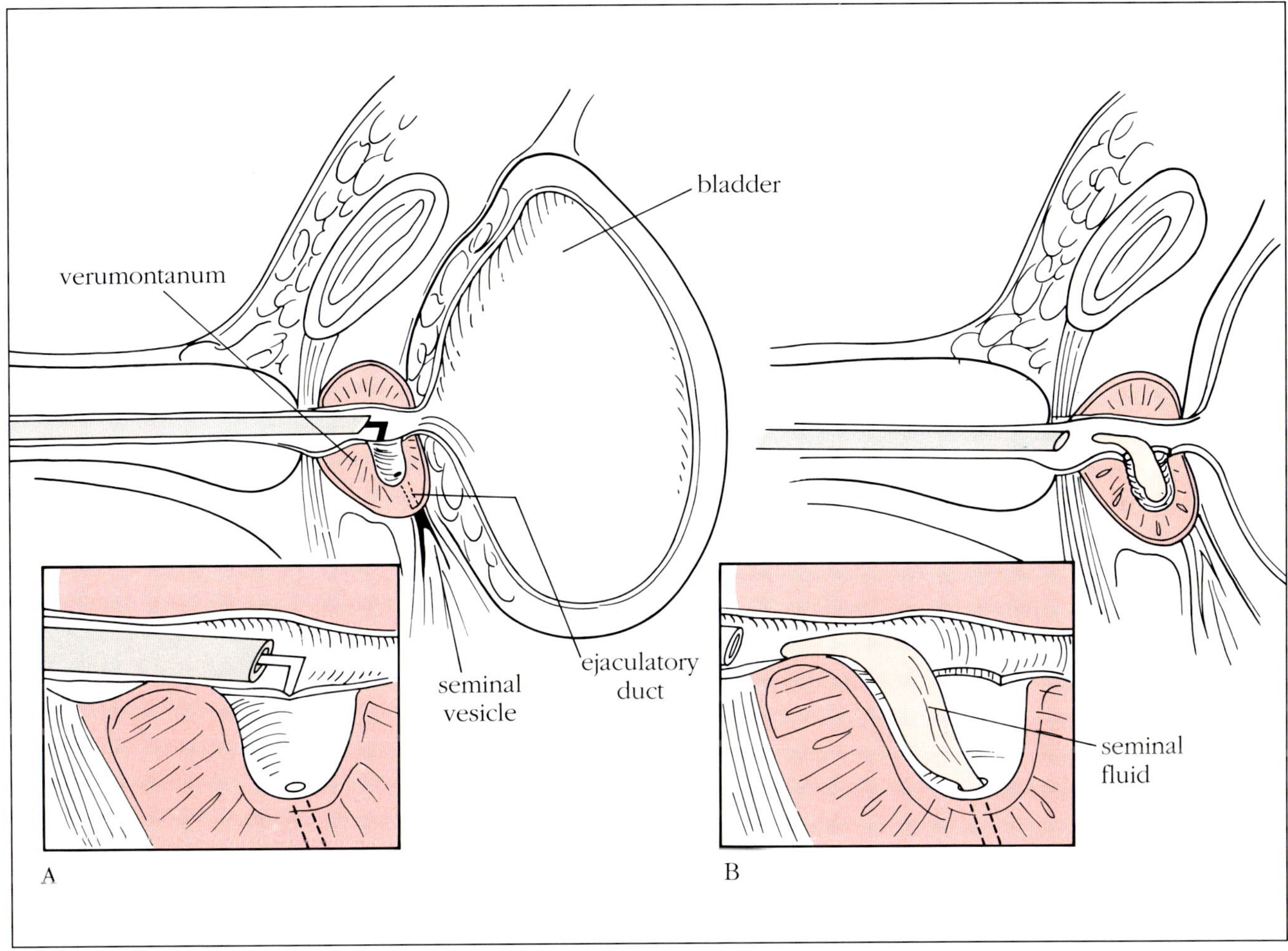

Figure 27.7 Transurethral resection (TUR) of ejaculatory duct obstruction in the case of congenital midline cyst. **A** Resection is begun distal to the bladder neck in the midline floor, often requiring resection of the verumontanum. **B** Flow of seminal fluid and/or vasography mixture is noted once the "roof" of the obstruction is resected.

References

1. Bennett WH. Varicocele, particularly with reference to its radical cure. *Lancet.* 1889;1:261–265.
2. Macomber D, Sanders MB. The spermatozoa count: its value in the diagnosis, prognosis and treatment of sterility. *N Engl J Med.* 1929;200:981–984.
3. Tulloch WS. A consideration of sterility factors in the light of subsequent pregnancies: subfertility in the male. *Trans Edinburgh Obstet Soc.* 1952;59:29–34.
4. Dubin L, Amelar RD. Varicocele size and results of varicocelectomy in selected subfertile men with varicocele. *Fertil Steril.* 1970;21:606–609.
5. Charny CW. Testicular biopsy: its value in male sterility. *JAMA..* 1940;115:1429–1433.
6. Owen ER. Microsurgical vasovasostomy: a reliable vasectomy reversal. *Aust NZ J Surg.* 1977;47:305–309.
7. Silber SJ. Microscopic vasectomy reversal. *Fertil Steril.* 1977;28:1191–1202.
8. Donovan JF, Winfield HN. Laparoscopic varix ligation. *J Urol.* 1992;147:77–81.
9. Hagood PC, Mehan DJ, Worischeck JH, et al. Laparoscopic varicocelectomy: preliminary report of a new technique. *J Urol.* 1992;147:73–76.
10. Lipshultz LI, Howards SS, Buch JP. Male infertility. In: Gillenwater JY, Grayhack JT, Howards SS, Duckett JW, eds. *Adult and Pediatric Urology.* 2nd ed. St. Louis, Mo: Mosby Year Book; 1991:1425–1477.
11. Saypol DC, Howards SS, Turner TT, Miller E. Influence of surgically induced varicocele on testicular blood flow, temperature and histology in adult rats and dogs. *J Clin Invest.* 1981;68:39–45
12. Palomo A. Radical cure of varicocele by a new technique. *J Urol.* 1949;61:604–607.
13. Ivanissevich O. Left varicocele due to reflux, experience with 4470 operative cases in 42 years. *J Int Coll Surg.* 1960;24:742.
14. Marmar JC, DeBenedictus TJ, Praiss D. The management of varicoceles by microdissection of the spermatic cord of the external ring. *Fertil Steril.* 1985;43:583–588.
15. Bors E, Comarr AE. Neurological disturbances of sexual function with special reference to 529 patients with spinal cord injury. *Urol Surv.* 1960;10:191.
16. Horne HW, Paull DP, Munro D. Fertility studies in the human male with traumatic injuries of the spinal cord and cauda equina. *N Engl J Med.* 1948;239:959–961.
17. Brindley GS. Electroejaculation: its technique, neurological implications and uses. *J Neurol Neurosurg Psychiatry.* 1981;44:9–18.
18. Perkash I, Martin DE, Warner H, et al. Reproductive biology of paraplegics: results of semen collection, testicular biopsy, and serum hormone evaluation. *J Urol.* 1985;134:284–288.
19. Bennett CJ, Seager SW, Vasher EA, et al. Sexual dysfunction and electroejaculation in men with spinal cord injury: review. *J Urol.* 1988;139:453–457.
20. Seager SW, Savastano JA, Streett JW, et al. Electroejaculation, semen quality and penile erections in normal and chronic spinal non-human primates. *J Urol.* 1984;131:234A.
21. Belker AM, Thomas AJ Jr, Fuchs EF, et al. Results of 1469 microsurgical vasectomy reversals by the vasovasostomy study group. *J Urol.* 1991;145:505–511.
22. Thomas AJ Jr, Howards SS. Microsurgical treatment of male infertility. In: Lipshultz LI, Howards SS, eds. *Infertility in the Male.* 2nd ed. St. Louis, Mo: Mosby Year Book; 1991:357–369.
23. Pryor JP, Hendry WF. Ejaculatory duct obstruction in subfertile males: analysis of 87 patients. *Fertil Steril.* 1991;56:725–730.

CHAPTER 28

Techniques of Assisted Reproduction

Peter N. Schlegel

Assisted reproduction is indicated for the treatment of infertile men when all correctable fertility factors have been addressed but pregnancy has not yet been achieved, or when semen parameters suggest that the likelihood of pregnancy with natural intercourse is very low. These techniques improve the likelihood of fertilization and pregnancy by facilitating sperm–egg interaction. This may be performed mechanically by placing sperm within the uterus, known as intrauterine insemination (IUI), or by mixing sperm and oocytes (eggs) together outside the body with in vitro fertilization (IVF), and returning any fertilized eggs to the uterus using a procedure referred to as embryo transfer (ET). Other techniques include placing retrieved oocytes and sperm together in the fallopian tube (GIFT), or returning the early fertilized oocyte (zygote) to the fallopian tube (ZIFT). Sperm–egg interaction can also be facilitated during IVF by micromanipulation of the oocyte. The most commonly used techniques include surgically opening the covering of the oocyte (zona drilling or partial zona dissection [PZD]) or injecting sperm under the zona pellucida covering the oocyte, using a technique referred to as subzonal insertion (SZI). In cases where continuity of the male reproductive tract cannot be surgically reconstructed, simultaneous surgical retrieval of sperm from the epididymis in conjunction with IVF has been performed with successful fertilizations and live births.

The techniques of assisted reproduction can be considered to be a series of progressively more invasive and expensive interventions that may increase the chance of fertilization occurring for couples with male-factor infertility. Each step in the series of assisted reproductive techniques (from natural intercourse to IUI, from IUI to IVF, and from IVF to IVF with micromanipulation) should be entertained only when specifically indicated.

A brief overview of the indications for each technique of assisted reproduction will be presented and the technique for epididymal sperm retrieval discussed in detail. Since the outcome of each treatment is affected by the technique used and patient population studied, a range of indications and expected results are presented. Figure 28.1 contains a general summary of the results of each assisted reproduction treatment. Each intervention is listed in increasing order of complexity or degree of invasiveness. Interpretation of these results requires the reader to consider that most couples do not proceed to more invasive techniques of assisted reproduction, including IUI, IVF or micromanipulation, until they have been unable to achieve pregnancy with natural intercourse or with another less invasive technique. Therefore, the "success rates" of each technique are usually not directly comparable, since they are not usually applied to the same patient populations. Rather, these numbers usually reflect success rates for couples who have failed with a less invasive approach. In addition, the results of some assisted reproductive techniques are greatly affected by initial sperm quantity and quality.

FIGURE 28.1 *Results of Natural Intercourse and Various Methods of Assisted Reproduction*

INTERVENTION	PREGNANCY RATE/CYCLE	PREGNANCY/ 3 CYCLES	EFFECT OF SEMEN PARAMETER ABNORMALITIES ON RESULTS
Natural intercourse**	<5%	10%–30%†	Marked
Intrauterine insemination (IUI)	0%–5%	5%–20%	Marked
IUI with ovarian stimulation	10%–20%	10%–40%	Marked
In vitro fertilization	11%–30%	20%–70%††	Moderate
Micromanipulation (SZI, PZD)	22%	25%–70%††	None

*Generally, these results have not been applied to similar groups of patients, and may actually represent treatment of pregnancy "failures" by less invasive treatments (or no treatment at all).

**Estimated based on published pregnancy rates for men with sperm concentration <10 million/mL, motility <40%, and normal morphology (WHO criteria) <60%, compiled from multiple sources.

†For 1 year of natural intercourse.

††Extrapolated from pregnancy rates per cycle.

Intrauterine Insemination

Intrauterine insemination (IUI) consists of placing a semen specimen, usually processed, into the uterine cavity. IUI is most effective for the treatment of couples with reproductive problems at the level of the cervix.[1] Cervical factor infertility is diagnosed by a persistently poor postcoital test in the presence of normal semen analysis and an otherwise normal female partner. IUI may also be of value, when used in conjunction with ovarian stimulation to increase oocyte production, for male-factor infertility.[2]

The reported pregnancy rates of IUI performed for male-factor infertility are highly variable, which may be due to differences in patient selection and variations in technique.[3] IUI alone has not been found to be of significant value for male-factor infertility. However, initial studies suggest that ovarian stimulation (to increase egg production) in conjunction with IUI does improve the success rate of IUI over natural intercourse alone when a male factor is present. Ovarian stimulation may be effective for some couples in whom the wife has unrecognized ovulatory dysfunction or may simply improve pregnancy rates by increasing sperm–egg interactions through the production of multiple oocytes. A risk of multiple births is present with any procedure that uses an ovarian stimulation protocol.

A couple can be considered candidates for IUI when all male factors have been corrected to the best extent possible and fertility has not been achieved. As mentioned in an earlier chapter, it is rare for men with idiopathic infertility to have a significant response to empiric medical therapy. Therefore, IUI is an alternative to nonspecific therapy with medications such as clomiphene citrate. However, it is of utmost importance to be certain that all identifiable causes of male- and female-factor infertility have been addressed before proceeding with nonspecific therapies, including IUI, because the success of IUI treatment depends on sperm quality and number.

Recent studies have indicated that the greater the number of abnormalities in semen analysis (count, motility, morphology), the smaller the chance of success with IUI.[4,5] With three abnormalities (oligoasthenoteratozoospermia) men have essentially no chance of contributing to a pregnancy via IUI with their partner. In addition, the presence of poor sperm motility alone appears to indicate a worse prognosis for IUI. This is reflected by the finding that most IUI pregnancies occur with semen specimens that have greater than 10 million motile sperm in the specimen. This information is of prognostic value for the couple, and can also suggest when other interventions should be considered.

The zona-free hamster egg penetration test may provide prognostic information helpful in counseling a couple with male factor infertility about IUI.[6] Although the predictive value of this test is not ideal, our experience is that men with a hamster egg penetration score of 0% do not achieve a pregnancy with IUI. Therefore, a couple in whom the male partner has a penetration score of 0% is counseled to proceed directly with IVF. No absolute statements can otherwise be made based on the hamster egg penetration assay, although a general correlation between pregnancy rates and hamster egg penetration scores has been reported.

Intrauterine insemination is timed to the wife's ovulation. Sperm is collected by masturbation into a sterile container and must be washed free of seminal fluid. This important step concentrates the sperm and removes reactive components in the seminal fluids that can cause vigorous and painful uterine muscle activity if placed directly in the uterine cavity. Concentrating the sperm within the seminal specimen is also important because a total volume of only 1 mL can be placed in the uterine cavity.

The seminal specimen is then introduced into the uterine cavity via the cervical canal under direct vision using a fine "Tomcat" catheter. Optimization of ovulation induction, careful sperm processing, and proper intrauterine transfer of the specimen are critical to achieving successful results with this technique.

The chances of achieving pregnancy with IUI and ovarian stimulation for male-factor infertility are approximately 10% to 40% over three cycles, although pregnancy rates as high as 50% to 70% have been reported in some series (see Fig. 28.1). Since virtually all of the pregnancies achieved occur within three cycles of IUI, no more than three or four cycles are recommended.[7] However, these results are only slightly better than the chances of male-factor couples achieving pregnancy with natural intercourse, which range from 5% to 30%.

Intrauterine insemination, in conjunction with ovarian stimulation, is a nonspecific intervention that can be of value for the treatment of male-factor infertility. It should be recommended for couples after all identifiable male factors have been corrected. Patients with extremely poor sperm motility or 0% hamster egg penetration scores should be primarily referred for IVF or IVF with micromanipulation.

In Vitro Fertilization

Male-factor infertility was initially considered a contraindication for IVF. Subsequent experience indicated that fertilization and live births were possible in couples with impaired sperm quality. However, equal numbers of sperm obtained from men with oligospermia do not fertilize at the same rate as sperm obtained from normal men, indicating that these sperm function abnormally. The usual number of sperm used to fertilize in vitro are 50 to 100×10^3 sperm/oocyte. Increasing the concentration of sperm used in male-factor couples has improved fertilization rates but not necessarily pregnancy rates.[8] Initial concerns that assisted fertilization with apparently defective sperm may lead to the development of abnormal embryos and an increase in the number of birth defects have not been confirmed.

Male-factor couples should be considered for IVF if they are unable to achieve a pregnancy with IUI or if sperm quality is too poor to make IUI a viable alternative. In general, the sperm of male-factor couples should be tested for fertility before IVF is undertaken. An alternative to the sperm penetration assay is sperm morphology using strict (Kruger's) criteria.[9] This evaluation considers sperm to be abnormal unless they have absolutely no tail, midpiece, or neck defects, an acrosome covering only 40% to 70% of the head region, and a smooth, oval sperm head between 2.5 and 3.5 μm wide and 5 to 6 μm long. Like the sperm penetration assay,[10] these criteria seem to provide a much better evaluation of the likelihood of fertilization occurring for sperm specimens than count or motility alone. Normal fertilization rates occur when more than 8% to 14% of sperm have normal morphology by these strict criteria. A set of criteria for men with semen specimens generally considered unacceptable for standard IVF is presented in Figure 28.2. At our institution, micromanipulation of oocytes to promote sperm–egg interaction is considered a standard procedure for male-factor infertility and is available for couples who do not fertilize during the first day of standard sperm–egg insemination. For the semen specimens that do not meet the criteria specified in Figure 28.2, micromanipulation should be used during IVF.

The technique of IVF has become fairly well standardized and is straightforward.[11] Ovarian hyperstimulation is achieved with a combination of FSH-stimulating agents (GnRH agonists, hMG, purified FSH, and/or clomiphene citrate) to recruit an increased number of follicles each cycle. Follicle development is evaluated directly with ultrasound and indirectly by measurement of serum estrogens and progesterone. A dose of hCG is given when optimal follicular development is obtained to stimulate final oocyte maturation, and retrieval of the oocytes is performed by transvaginal follicular aspiration with ultrasound guidance under intravenous sedation.

A semen specimen is produced and allowed to liquefy. The specimen is then processed to remove dead or dysfunctional sperm and to remove seminal fluid, which may adversely affect the fertilization process. Processing is performed using either swim-up, gravity sedimentation, Percoll gradient sedimentation, or simple washing. The sperm can be pretreated with a function-enhancing agent, such as pentoxifylline or 2-deoxyadenosine,[12] or simply inseminated with the oocytes. Pentoxifylline appears to improve sperm function by decreasing reactive oxygen-species generation from dead and dying sperm. Not only do poor semen specimens contain relatively few normally functioning sperm, but the many dead or dysfunctional sperm in a semen specimen may adversely affect the potentially normal sperm.

Swim-up is a separation technique that depends on the ability of motile sperm to swim away from dysfunctional sperm as well as from other cell components and debris in seminal fluid.[13] Sedimentation is a separation technique that relies on the propensity of debris and dysfunctional sperm to settle with gravity to the bottom of a semen specimen.[11] Thus, each technique improves the overall quality of a specimen by selecting for a fraction of motile sperm.

Percoll gradient sedimentation involves placing the semen specimen on top of a previously prepared microfuge tube containing different concentrations of Percoll.[14] Percoll is an inert component that can be prepared in predictable densities according to the concentration of Percoll used. Frequently, 50% and 95% concentrations of Percoll are used. Centrifugation of the specimen is performed for 30 to 45 minutes. These discontinuous layers of Percoll allow separation of semen specimens into white blood cell, immotile sperm, and motile sperm fractions. The separations are not perfectly pure; however, the results are equal to or better than the other techniques described.

It should be remembered that none of the separation techniques described above directly enhance sperm function, with the possible exception of Percoll gradient. These procedures are designed to subselect better-quality populations of sperm. This separation may indirectly improve sperm function by removing contaminants that can adversely affect the fertilizing ability of sperm. However, the improved quality of the resultant specimen is obtained at the expense of a significant loss of sperm quantity. Sperm fertilizing ability can be enhanced by the use of some agents that prevent sperm-related damage,

FIGURE 28.2 *Semen Parameters Considered Unacceptable for Regular IVF*

Concentration	$<2 \times 10^6$ sperm/mL
Motility	<5%
Morphology (strict criteria)	≤4% normal

such as pentoxyfilline, although the evidence supporting this finding is limited at present.

The fertilized oocytes are then incubated with sperm in vitro for 2 or 3 days. The resultant embryo is then transferred to either the uterus or the fallopian tube. Up to four embryos can be transferred to the uterus, and excess embryos can be frozen. Careful attention to detail during the embryo transfer process may prevent trauma to the uterus and improve IVF success rates. The implantation rate per embryo ranges from 20% to 30% in most IVF programs. Clinical pregnancy is defined as the presence of a functioning fetal heart, as visualized on ultrasound. Clinical pregnancies occur after 20% to 50% of all transfers. Although pregnancy rates are high, up to one third may miscarry, so that typical live birth rates are 15% to 20% per cycle.[15] Once fertilization has been achieved the results of IVF for male-factor couples are as good as those for the general IVF population.[16]

GIFT/ZIFT

Gamete intrafallopian transfer (GIFT) involves the return of retrieved oocytes and processed sperm to the fallopian tube.[17] Usually, the transfer of gametes to the fallopian tube is performed with the aid of laparoscopy, although some centers routinely cannulate the fallopian tube with a transcervical approach. Interest in GIFT arose from the realization that optimal gamete interaction appears to occur naturally in the fallopian tube. Control of sperm–egg interaction is not as great as with IVF, and multiple births as well as ectopic pregnancies are not uncommon.

Transfer of zygotes (fertilized oocytes before multiple cell divisions have occured) to the fallopian tube (ZIFT) has also been used as an assisted technique in place of standard IVF/ET. The concept behind ZIFT is that optimal early embryo development occurs within the fallopian tube. The return of the fertilized egg to the tube at its earliest possible stage may enhance embryo development and subsequent implantation. ZIFT has the advantage of more control over the potential for multiple births than GIFT.

The role of GIFT versus IVF/ET is highly controversial. The overall results with GIFT and ZIFT has been similar to that of IVF/ET performed at the best programs.[18] Therefore, GIFT and ZIFT appear to have little or no advantage over properly performed IVF/ET but have the disadvantage of requiring general anesthesia and laparoscopy at most centers.[18]

MICROMANIPULATION-ASSISTED FERTILIZATION

In men with critically poor sperm quality, conventional IVF may be inadequate to allow fertilization. For these patients, oocyte micromanipulation techniques can sometimes provide fertilizations and pregnancies. Over 200 pregnancies have now been produced after the application of microsurgical fertilization techniques in couples in whom the male partners had severely abnormal semen and who would have had little chance of producing offspring with conventional IVF. However, these techniques are still in the developmental phase at most institutions.

The development of gamete micromanipulation technology has enabled the reproductive biologist to circumvent or facilitate certain steps in the fertilization process that might prevent sperm–egg fusion in the patient with impaired sperm function. To date, three categories of assisted fertilization by gamete micromanipulation have been explored in several species (Fig. 28.3). The first involves the creation of an opening in the zona pellucida, which is an acellular protective layer surrounding the egg and a major barrier to sperm penetration. Subsequently, the micromanipulated oocyte is inseminated according to standard IVF guidelines. These procedures have been broadly termed "zona drilling." One variant of zona drilling involves mechanical piercing of the zona pellucida with a micropipet, known as partial zona dissection (PZD) (see Fig. 28.3). A second micromanipulation technique directed at facilitating sperm–egg interaction is the subzonal insertion (SZI) of sperm. Subzonal sperm insertion completely bypasses the zona pellucida and involves direct placement of sperm into the space between the zona pellucida and the oocyte (see Fig. 28.3). The application of both of these techniques has resulted in human pregnancies and live births. Finally, the third and most invasive form of microsurgical fertilization is the microinjection of single sperm into the cytoplasm of the oocyte. This method has only recently been proven to be successful in humans and holds great potential for the future.

Patients traditionally selected for micromanipulation are those who have failed to fertilize oocytes in a previous IVF cycle.[19] However, patients with extremely abnormal semen parameters are also selected for micromanipulation. For example, patients who do not fulfill the standard criteria for IVF (see Fig. 28.2) would be candidates. This would include complete absence of motility, severe oligospermia ($<1 \times 10^6$/mL), or less than 4% normal morphology by the strict Kruger criteria.

Partial zona dissection and subzonal sperm insertion have been applied by Cohen and co-workers in 250 IVF cycles for patients with consistently abnormal semen analyses.[20] Although it has been generally the aim to perform the three insemination techniques (IVF, PZD, and SZI) in parallel using sibling oocytes, this strategy was frequently hindered by the limited number of oocytes or spermatozoa available. It was found, with few exceptions, that microsurgical fertilization yielded higher rates of monospermic fertilization than routine IVF insemination. In addition, the different micromanipulation techniques were found to be complementary to each other (Fig. 28.4).

The results of micromanipulation procedures in the first 250 cycles were evaluated using a variety of analyses. Semen parameters did not appear to affect fertilization rates with these techniques. The overall incidence of embryo replacement (the frequency of having at least one embryo for transfer) was 66% (159/250) for all micro-surgical cycles combined. Sixty-one couples (61/250; 24%) had a clinical pregnancy and six of these miscarried. Of the remaining 55 couples, 15 patients have delivered 23 healthy babies, and the remaining 40 pregnancies are still ongoing.

In conclusion, techniques such as partial zona dissection and subzonal sperm insertion are advantageous in cases of extreme male-factor infertility. They can be used either simultaneously on sibling oocytes or, if indicated, individually. A substantial number of viable pregnancies have been established using semen specimens that are well below the normal cutoff values used for regular IVF procedures. Fertilization and pregnancy occurred after the use of spermatozoa without progressive motility and without normal morphology. These results provide evidence that spermatozoa from extremely oligoasthenoteratozoospermic men

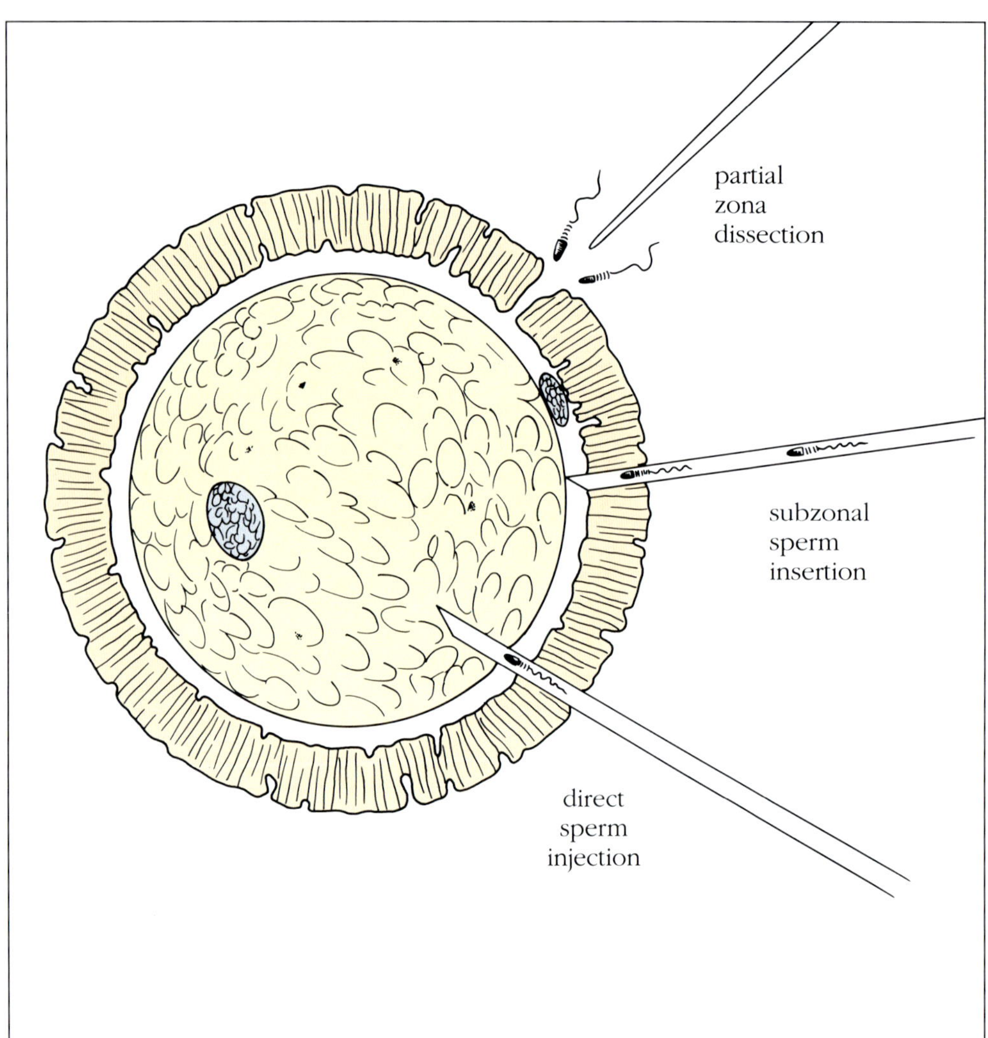

Figure 28.3 The three methods of micromanipulation-assisted fertilization. *Zona drilling.* An opening is introduced in the zona pellucida, thereby allowing sperm direct access to the oolemma. After micromanipulation, the oocyte is inseminated with spermatozoa. *Subzonal insertion.* Spermatozoa are aspirated into a hollow microneedle and are deposited directly into the perivitelline space of the oocyte. *Direct sperm microinjection.* Sperm contained within a microneedle are microinjected into cytoplasm of the oocyte.

FIGURE 28.4 *Micromanipulation Techniques for Fertilization*

Partial zona dissection (PZD) only	20/77 (26%)
Subzonal insertion (SZI) only	12/77 (16%)
PZD and SZI	17/77 (22%)
Fertilization (total)	49/77 (64%)
No fertilization	28/77 (36%)

Simultaneous use of partial zona dissection (PZD) and subzonal insertion (SZI) on sibling oocytes in 77 patients who had sufficient spermatozoa available for both procedures (Cohen J, et al).

can produce normal offspring after the application of micromanipulation techniques, even in couples with failed fertilization using standard IVF technique. Present results have not allowed identification, on the basis of conventional semen evaluations, of patient subgroups with abnormal semen parameters that would not benefit from these microsurgical techniques.

MICROPUNCTURE RETRIEVAL OF EPIDIDYMAL SPERM

Aspiration of sperm from the epididymis for in vitro fertilization of eggs was first described in a man with a surgically reconstructible obstructed reproductive tract.[21] Subsequent use of this technique has been applied to men with congenital absence of the vas deferens (CAV) or multiple previous unsuccessful attempts at vasoepididymostomy. Concerns about antisperm antibodies and

disruption of spermatogenesis from prolonged obstruction have proven to be unfounded. Most men with CAV do not have antisperm antibodies[22] and spermatogenesis is intact in the vast majority.[23]

The original technique described by Silber involved isolation and opening of a specific epididymal tubule and aspiration of sperm.[24] However, with this technique the specimen is frequently contaminated with blood. The sample was then processed using a mini-Percoll technique to eradicate contaminants. An alternative procedure is to use a micropuncture technique to obtain a relatively clean specimen initially (Figs. 28.5, 28.6).

We prepare large bore (250 to 350 µm) micropuncture pipets as described by Howards and co-workers.[25] The pipets are briefly washed in soap and then rinsed with distilled water, dried in acetone, and hand-pulled to 250 to 350 µm tip widths. The pipets are then polished

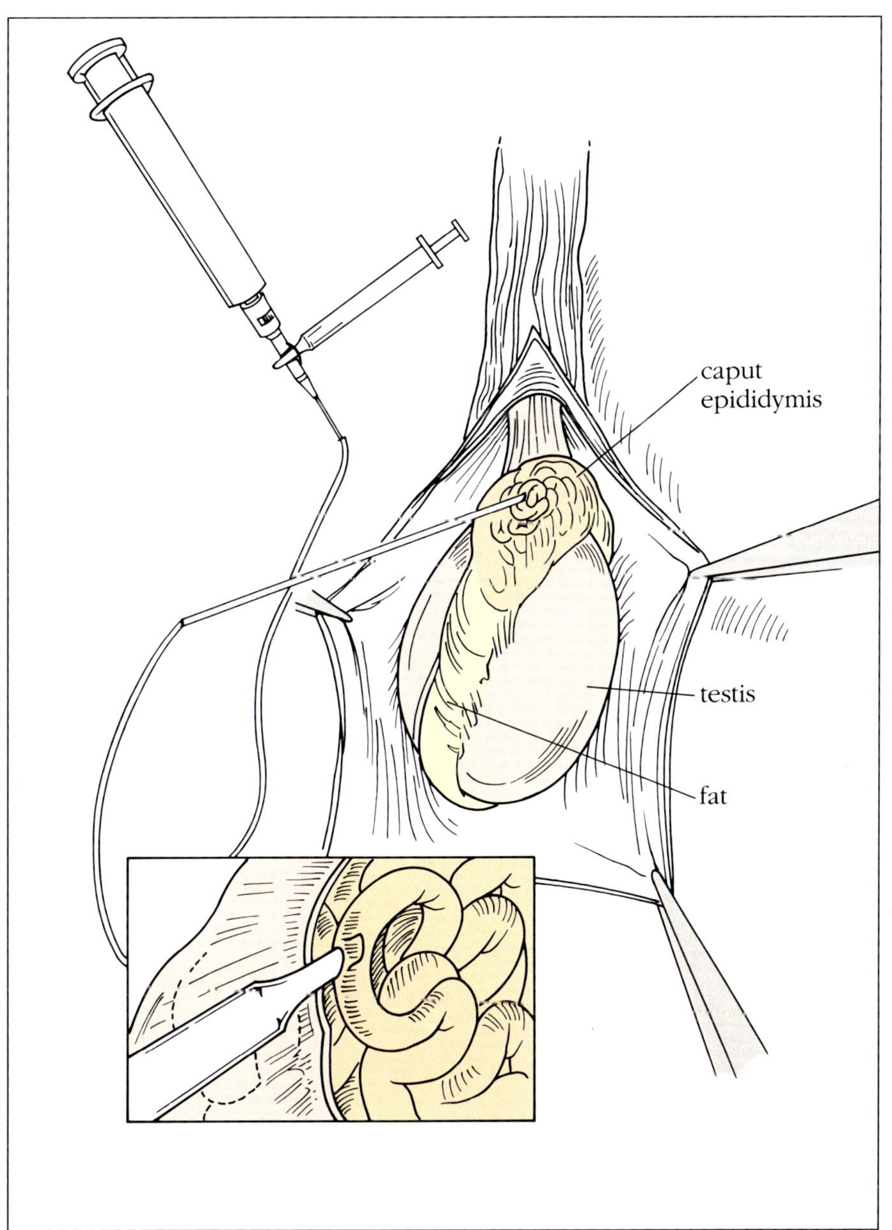

Figure 28.5 Technique for micropuncture of the human epididymis for retrieval of sperm from men with surgically unreconstructable vasal defects, including congenital absence of the vas deferens.

on a fine grinding wheel, sharpened to assist puncture of the epididymal tunics, washed again, coated with silicone, and allowed to dry completely. The pipets are autoclaved just before use. The pipets are attached via short lengths of medical grade silastic tubing to a 20-gauge needle, a three-way plastic stopcock, a 1-mL plastic tuberculin syringe, and a 10-mL glass syringe. The glass syringe allows immediate reestablishment of atmospheric pressure after aspiration of fluid from the epididymal tubule, so that no excess fluid is aspirated into the syringe during pipet removal from the lumen of the epididymal tubule, potentially contaminating the sperm specimen. It is important to avoid contact of sperm with untreated glass, since sperm will avidly adhere to glass and may clog the collection apparatus. A plastic tuberculin syringe is ideal for the collection of small volumes of fluid.

The testis and epididymis are exposed through a standard scrotal incision. In the normal unobstructed epididymis, the quality of sperm improves as it moves more distally. However, the better-quality sperm are obtained more proximally in the chronically obstructed epididymis. The distal epididymal remnant in men with CAV is filled with macrophages and degenerating sperm, which can be recognized by the yellow color of these tubules. Based on the findings by Silber and ourselves, we recommended performing micropuncture of the tubules just proximal to the region of the yellow tubules, initially. If motile sperm are not obtained in this region, proceed more proximally. Silber et al.[24] report obtaining motile sperm from as far proximal as the rete testis.

Sperm are then processed to remove any contaminants as well as dead or dying sperm. A combination of mini-Percoll gradient centrifugation, sedimentation, and swim-up has been used. These sperm are then incubated with oocytes obtained from the spouse by standard IVF technique. However, depending on the quality and quantity of sperm retrieved, micromanipulation may be necessary. In a series reported by Silber et al.[26] the pregnancy rate was 24% without micromanipulation or micropuncture retrieval. Our experience with the micropuncture technique in 42 cycles of sperm and oocyte retrieval has yielded a 29% clinical pregnancy rate, with rising β-hCG levels and fetal heartbeat on ultrasound. Seven of our twelve retrieval pregnancies occurred only with micromanipulation, demonstrating the importance of gamete laboratory manipulation techniques for men in whom the aspirated epididymal sperm quality is poor.

In summary, sperm can be obtained from the epididymis of men with CAV or unreconstructable obstruction using advanced technology. Micropuncture technique facilitates obtaining a clean specimen from these patients. The availability of micromanipulation techniques may offer the possibility of pregnancy to individuals with epididymal aspiration samples unsatisfactory for routine IVF. Optimal pregnancy rates require the use of oocyte micromanipulation.

Conclusion

Recent trends in the management of the infertile couple are towards the increased use of assisted reproduction techniques. The enhancement of sperm–egg interaction through the placement of gametes in closer proximity does appear to increase fertilization rates and subsequent pregnancy rates. However, the live birth rate for most of these techniques is below 20%.[15] With the exception of men with congenital absence of the vas deferens, these remain nonspecific therapies. In addition, there is signifi-

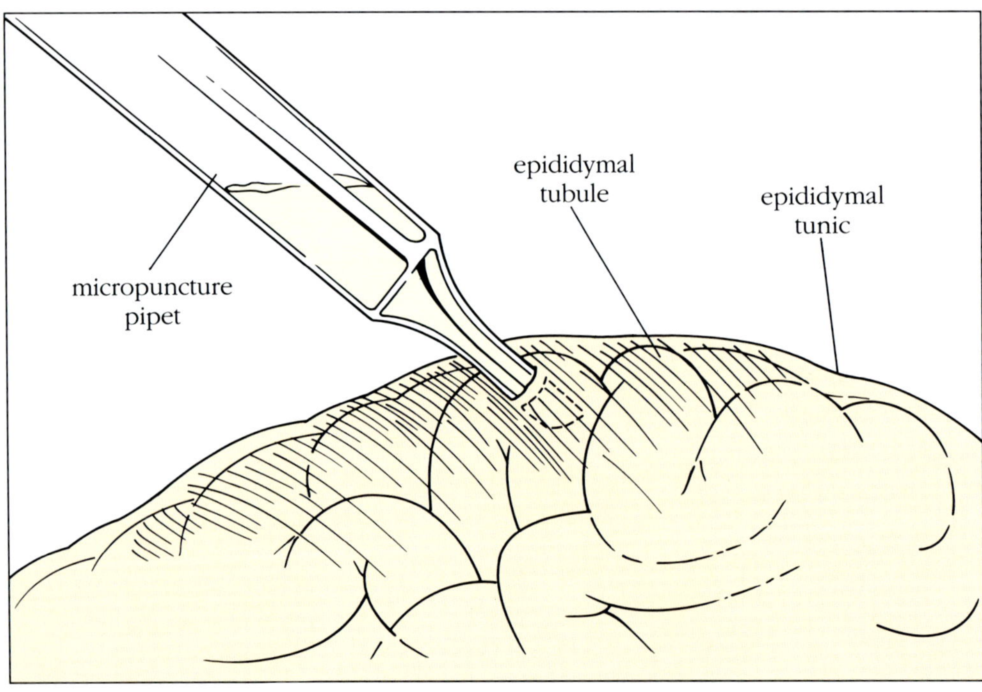

Figure 28.6 A sharpened micropipet puncturing an epididymal tubule.

cant cost and risk involved with some of these treatments. Therefore, specific therapies should always be instituted before assisted reproductive techniques are considered in the male-factor infertility couple.

The author is grateful to Jacque Cohen, Mina Alikani, Adrienne Reing, Alex Adler, Michael Suzman, Tony Ferraro, Henry Malter, Helena Kissin, Beth Talansky, Bruce Gilbert, Jamie Grifo, Owen Davis, Margaret Graf, Alan Berkeley, Zev Rosenwaks, and Marc Goldstein, as well as to the entire staff of the Cornell Center for Reproductive Medicine and Infertility, for their contributions to these studies and for providing insight into these areas of reproductive medicine.

References

1. Quagliarello J, Arny M. Intracervical versus intrauterine insemination: correlation of outcome with antecedent postcoital testing. *Fertil Steril.* 1986;46:870–875.

2. Dodson WC, Haney AF. Controlled ovarian hyperstimulation and intrauterine insemination for treatment of infertility. *Fertil Steril.* 1991;55:457–467.

3. Allen NC, Herbert CM, Masson WS, Rogers BJ, Diamond MP, Wentz AC. Intrauterine insemination: a critical review. *Fertil Steril.* 1985;44:569–580.

4. Horvath PM, Bohrer M, Shelden RM, Kemmann E. The relationship of sperm parameters to cycle fecundity in superovulated women undergoing intrauterine insemination. *Fertil Steril.* 1989;52:288–294.

5. Francavilla F, Romano R, Santucci R, Poccia G. Effect of sperm morphology and motile sperm count on outcome of intrauterine insemination in oligozoospermia and/or asthenospermia. *Fertil Steril.* 1990;53:892–897.

6. Johnson A, Smith RG, Bassham B, Lipshultz LI, Lamb DJ. The microsperm penetration assay: development of a sperm penetration assay suitable for oligospermic males. *Fertil Steril.* 1991;56:528–534.

7. Kirby CA, Flaherty SP, Godfrey BM, Warnes GM, Mathews CD. A prospective trial of intrauterine insemination of motile spermatozoa versus timed intercourse. *Fertil Steril.* 1991;56:102–107.

8. Oehninger S, Acosta AA, Morshedi M, et al. Corrective measures and pregnancy outcome in in vitro fertilization in patients with severe sperm morphology abnormalities. *Fertil Steril.* 1988;50:283–287.

9. Kruger TF, Menhueld R, Stander FSH, et al. Sperm morphologic features as a prognostic factor in in vitro fertilization. *Fertil Steril.* 1986;46:1118–1123.

10. Hirsch I, Gibbons WE, Lipshultz LI, et al. In vitro fertilization in couples with male-factor infertility. *Fertil Steril.* 1986;45:659–664.

11. Cohen J, Edwards R, Fehilly C, et al. In vitro fertilization: a treatment for male infertility. *Fertil Steril.* 1985;43:422–433.

12. Yovich JM, Edirisinghe WR, Commins JM, Yovich JL. Influence of pentoxifylline in severe male-factor infertility. *Fertil Steril.* 1990;53:715–722.

13. Oehninger S, Acosta R, Morshedi M, et al. Relationship between morphology and motion characteristics of human spermatozoa in semen and in the swimup sperm fractions. *J Androl.* 1990;11:446–452.

14. McClure RD, Nunes L, Tom R. Semen manipulation, improved sperm recovery and function with a two-layer Percoll gradient. *Fertil Steril.* 1989;51:874–877.

15. Medical Research International, Society of Assisted Reproductive Technology (SART). In vitro fertilization embryo transfer (IVF-ET) in the United States: 1990 results from the IVF-ET Registry. *Fertil Steril.* 1992;57:15–24.

16. Von Vem JFHM, Acosta AA, Swanson RJ, et al. Male factor evaluation in in vitro fertilization: Norfolk experience. *Fertil Steril.* 1985;44:375–383.

17. Asch RH, Balmaceda JP, Ellsworth LR, Wong PC. Preliminary experiences with gamete intrafallopian transfer (GIFT). *Fertil Steril.* 1986;45:366–371.

18. Leeton J, Rogers P, Caro C, Healy D, Yates C. A controlled study between the use of gamete intrafallopian transfer (GIFT) and in vitro fertilization and embryo transfer in the management of idiopathic and male infertility. *Fertil Steril.* 1987;48:605–607.

19. Ng SC, Bongso A, Sathananthan H, Ratnam SS. Micromanipulation: its relevance to human in vitro fertilization. *Fertil Steril.* 1990;53:203–219.

20. Cohen J. A review of clinical microsurgical fertilization. In: Cohen J, Malter HE, Grifo J, Talansky BE, eds. *Micromanipulation of Human Oocytes and Embryos.* New York, NY: Raven Press; 1991.

21. Temple–Smith PD, Southwick GJ, Yates CA, Trounson AO, de Kretser DM. Human pregnancy by in vitro fertilization (IVF) using sperm aspirated from the epididymis. *J IVF/ET.* 1985;2:119–122.

22. Patrizio P, Moretti–Rojas I, Ord T, Balmaceda J, Silber S, Asch RH. Low incidence of sperm antibodies in men with congenital absence of the vas deferens. *Fertil Steril.* 1989;52:1018–1021.

23. Hirsch IH, Choi H. Quantitative testicular biopsy in congenital and acquired genital obstruction. *J Urol.* 1990;143:311–312.

24. Silber SJ, Ord T, Balmaceda J, Patrizio P, Asch RH. Congenital absence of the vas deferens: the fertilizing capacity of human epididymal sperm. *N Engl J Med.* 1990;323:1788–1792.

25. Howards SS, Johnson A, Jessee S. Micropuncture and microanalytic studies of the rat testis and epididymis. *Fertil Steril.* 1975;26:13–19.

26. Asch RH, Silber SJ. Microsurgical epididymal sperm aspiration and assisted reproductive techniques. *Ann NY Acad Sci.* 1991;626:101–110.

Numbers in bold refer to figures

R

Vim-Silverman needle, **5.6**
Vinblastine, 3.16, **3.17**
    mechanism of action, **6.9**
    toxicity, 6.9
Voiding. *See* Micturition
Voiding dysfunction, management, 9.8
VP-16. *See* Etoposide

W

Whitaker test, 8.9
Whitmore-Jewett staging system, 5.3
Wilms' tumor, 3.20–3.21, **3.21**

Y

YM 617, 2.11

Z

ZIFT. *See* Zygote intrafallopian transfer
Zygote intrafallopian transfer, 28.5–28.8